HANDBOOK OF
Correctional Mental Health

Second Edition

Editorial Review Board

HANDBOOK OF
Correctional
Mental Health

Second Edition

Edited by

Charles L. Scott, M.D.

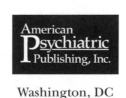

American
Psychiatric
Publishing, Inc.

Washington, DC
London, England

Copyright © 2010 American Psychiatric Publishing, Inc.
ALL RIGHTS RESERVED

Manufactured in the United States of America on acid-free paper
13 12 11 10 09   5 4 3 2 1
Second Edition

Typeset in Adobe's New Baskerville and Delta

American Psychiatric Publishing, Inc.
1000 Wilson Boulevard
Arlington, VA 22209-3901
www.appi.org

Library of Congress Cataloging-in-Publication Data
Handbook of correctional mental health / edited by Charles L. Scott. — 2nd ed.
    p. ; cm.
    Includes bibliographical references and index.
    ISBN 978-1-58562-389-1 (alk. paper)
    1. Prisoners—Mental health services—United States—Handbooks, manuals, etc. I. Scott, Charles L., 1960–
    [DNLM: 1. Mental Health Services. 2. Prisoners–psychology. 3. Prisons. WA 305.1 H236 2010]
    RC451.4.P68H356 2010
    365'.66–dc22

                                                                2009028304

British Library Cataloguing in Publication Data
A CIP record is available from the British Library.

Contents

Part I

Overview of Correctional Settings and Provision of Care

Part II
Clinical Evaluation and Care

Part III
Special Inmate Populations

Contributors

Sandra K. Antoniak, M.F.S., M.D.
Psychiatry Resident, Department of Psychiatry, University of Iowa Carver College of Medicine, Iowa City, Iowa

Kenneth L. Appelbaum, M.D.
Professor of Clinical Psychiatry; Director, Correctional Mental Health Policy and Research; Center for Health Policy and Research, Commonwealth Medicine, University of Massachusetts Medical School, Worcester, Massachusetts

Gary E. Beven, M.D.
Adult Forensic Services, Harris County Jail, Mental Health and Mental Retardation Authority of Harris County, Houston, Texas

Kathryn A. Burns, M.D., M.P.H.
Assistant Clinical Professor of Psychiatry, Case Western Reserve University School of Medicine, Cleveland, Ohio

Shama B. Chaiken, Ph.D.
Chief Psychologist, Policy and Program Development, California Department of Corrections and Rehabilitation, Sacramento, California

The Honorable Charlotte Cooksey
Judge, District Court of Maryland, Baltimore, Maryland

Henry A. Dlugacz, M.S.W., J.D.
Clinical Assistant Professor of Psychiatry and Behavioral Sciences, New York Medical College; Adjunct Professor of Law, New York Law School and St. John's University School of Law; Formerly, Director of Mental Health Services, St. Vincent's Hospital Prison Health Service; Co-Founder and Former Co-Chair, New York State Bar Association Committee on Mental Health Issues, Albany, New York

Tracy D. Gunter, M.D.
Associate Professor of Psychiatry, Department of Neurology and Psychiatry, Division of Forensic Psychiatry, St. Louis University School of Medicine, St. Louis, Missouri

Lindsay M. Hayes
Project Director, National Center on Institutions and Alternatives, Mansfield, Massachusetts

Steven J. Helfand, Psy.D.
Statewide Director of Mental Health Services, Correctional Managed Health Care, University of Connecticut Health Center, Farmington, Connecticut

James L. Knoll IV, M.D.
Director, Forensic Psychiatry and Associate Professor of Psychiatry, SUNY Upstate Medical University, Syracuse, New York; Director, Forensic Psychiatry Fellowship, Central New York Psychiatric Center, Marcy, New York

Catherine F. Lewis, M.D.
Associate Professor of Psychiatry, University of Connecticut Health Center, Farmington, Connecticut

Sharon Lipford, LCSW-C
Executive Director, Office on Mental Health, Harford County, Bel Air, Maryland

Barbara E. McDermott, Ph.D.
Professor of Clinical Psychiatry, University of California, Davis School of Medicine, Division of Psychiatry and the Law, Department of Psychiatry and Behavioral Sciences, Sacramento, California; Research Director, Forensic Psychiatry Research Division, Napa State Hospital, Napa, California

Jeffrey L. Metzner, M.D.
Clinical Professor of Psychiatry, University of Colorado School of Medicine, Denver, Colorado

Catherine Prudhomme, Ph.D.
Senior Psychologist, Policy and Program Development, California Department of Corrections and Rehabilitation, Sacramento, California

Richard Rogers, Ph.D., ABPP
Professor of Psychology, University of North Texas, Denton, Texas

Jason G. Roof, M.D.
Assistant Clinical Professor of Psychiatry, University of California, Davis School of Medicine, Division of Psychiatry and the Law, Department of Psychiatry and Behavioral Sciences, Sacramento, California

Erik Roskes, M.D.
Director, Forensic Treatment, Springfield Hospital Center, Sykesville, Maryland; Clinical Assistant Professor, Department of Psychiatry, University of Maryland School of Medicine, Baltimore, Maryland

Amanda Ruiz, M.D.
Assistant Clinical Professor, Department of Psychiatry, University of California, San Diego, California

Susan Sampl, Ph.D.
Supervising Psychologist, Correctional Managed Health Care, University of Connecticut Health Center, Farmington, Connecticut

Charles L. Scott, M.D.
Chief, Division of Psychiatry and the Law; Director, Forensic Psychiatry Fellowship; Professor of Clinical Psychiatry, University of California Davis Medical Center, Sacramento, California

Jing Shi, M.S.
Research Analyst, Center for Behavioral Health Services and Criminal Justice Research, Rutgers, The State University of New Jersey, New Brunswick, New Jersey

Humberto Temporini, M.D.
Assistant Clinical Professor of Psychiatry, Division of Psychiatry and the Law, Department of Psychiatry and Behavioral Sciences, University of California Davis Medical Center, Sacramento, California

Christopher Thompson, M.D.
Assistant Clinical Professor of Psychiatry, Child and Adolescent Division, Department of Psychiatry, David Geffen School of Medicine at UCLA, Los Angeles, California

Robert L. Trestman, Ph.D., M.D.
Executive Director, Correctional Managed Health Care; Interim Chief, Division of Public Health and Population Sciences; Interim Director, UCHC Signature Program of Public Health; Interim Co-Director, UConn Center for Public Health and Health Policy; Professor of Medicine and Psychiatry, University of Connecticut Health Center, Farmington, Connecticut

Michael J. Vitacco, Ph.D.
Associate Director of Research, Mendota Mental Health Institute, Madison, Wisconsin

Nancy L. Wolff, Ph.D.
Professor and Director, Program in Public Policy; Director, Center for Behavioral Health Services and Criminal Justice Research, Rutgers, The State University of New Jersey, New Brunswick, New Jersey

Stephen Wu, M.D.
Child and Adolescent Psychiatrist, Juvenile Justice Mental Health Program, Los Angeles County Department of Mental Health, Los Angeles, California

The following contributors to this book have indicated a financial interest in or other affiliation with a commercial supporter, a manufacturer of a commercial product, a provider of a commercial service, a nongovernmental organization, and/or a government agency, as listed below:

Shama B. Chaiken, Ph.D.—The author is employed by the California Department of Corrections and Rehabilitation.

The following contributors to this book have no competing interests or conflicts to declare:

Sandra K. Antoniak, M.F.S., M.D.
Kenneth L. Appelbaum, M.D.
Gary E. Beven, M.D.
Kathryn A. Burns, M.D., M.P.H.
Henry A. Dlugacz, M.S.W., J.D.
Tracy D. Gunter, M.D.
Catherine F. Lewis, M.D.
Sharon Lipford, LCSW-C
Barbara E. McDermott, Ph.D.
Jeffrey L. Metzner, M.D.
Catherine Prudhomme, Ph.D.
Richard Rogers, Ph.D., ABPP
Jason G. Roof, M.D.
Erik Roskes, M.D.
Amanda Ruiz, M.D.
Susan Sampl, Ph.D.
Charles L. Scott, M.D.
Jing Shi, M.S.
Humberto Temporini, M.D.
Christopher Thompson, M.D.
Robert L. Trestman, Ph.D., M.D.
Michael J. Vitacco, Ph.D.
Nancy L. Wolff, Ph.D.
Stephen Wu, M.D.

Preface

At midyear 2006, more than 2.24 million individuals were incarcerated in the United States, and 1 in every 133 U.S. residents lived in a jail or prison (Sabol et al. 2007). Correctional facilities have become the new mental health treatment centers for individuals with mental disorders. The single largest psychiatric inpatient facility in the United States is the Los Angeles County Jail (Torrey 1999). As increasing numbers of individuals with mental disorders are living behind bars, many mental health professionals are discovering that their new workplace is located inside a jail or prison.

Despite the obvious need for mental health professionals trained to provide care to those who are incarcerated, very few general psychiatry, psychology, or social work training programs provide specialized education in correctional mental health. The correctional system is a unique world, with its own terminology, laws, rules, procedures, environments, and administrative management. To provide effective care to inmates, mental health care providers must understand this world.

The first edition of this book was written to provide a practical clinical guidebook for mental health professionals working with individuals who are incarcerated or who have been involved with the criminal justice system at some point in their lives. This second edition incorporates recent and important policy trends and directions that further define the parameters of correctional mental health care. This new edition has nearly doubled the range of topics that were covered in the first edition, to keep correctional providers informed and current. Each chapter has been designed to assist the correctional practitioner with a more in-depth understanding of relevant treatment and legal issues when providing care to this population.

This handbook is divided into three basic sections. Part I contains three chapters that provide the reader with an introduction to core concepts regarding correctional systems and legal issues involved in the provision of care. Chapters 1 ("Overview of the Criminal Justice System") and 2 ("Criminal Justice System and Offenders Placed in an Outpatient Setting") specifically discuss the interrelationship of the criminal justice system and offenders in both incarcerated and outpatient settings. Chapter 3 ("Legal Issues Regarding the Provision of Care in a Correctional Setting") gives a practical translation of legal issues that govern why and how mental health professionals must provide care to those incarcerated.

Part II includes 12 chapters that focus on the evaluation and care of inmates. The wide-ranging topics are all extremely important. Chapter 4 ("The Mental Health Professional in a Correctional Culture") describes how practicing mental health care in a correctional culture differs from treatment in the outside world to include system challenges that are unique to this setting. Chapter 5 ("Conducting Mental Health Assessments in Correctional Settings") highlights fundamentals of mental health assessment. Chapter 6 ("Continuous Quality Improvement and Documentation"), which is new to this edition, provides practical guidelines on the role of continuous quality improvement and documentation principles for correctional providers. Chapters 7–11 provide thorough reviews of the most common diagnostic and behavioral presentations of inmates. Many of these chapters are new in this edition, and the topics include evaluating and treating substance use disorders, managing disruptive and aggressive inmates, suicide prevention, the assessment of malingering, and the impact of trauma on incarcerated persons. Chapters 12 ("Pharmacotherapy in Correctional Settings") and 13 ("Creating Wellness Through Collaborative Mental Health Interventions") focus on psychopharmacological and mental health interventions. Both chapters highlight considerations that must be taken into account when organizing a mental health treatment plan in a jail or prison. Chapter 14 ("Monitoring a Correctional Mental Health System") discusses how to provide care in a correctional system monitored under a consent decree. The last chapter in Part II is also new to this book and focuses on the increasingly growing emphasis on clinically oriented reentry planning for inmates being released from jail or prison.

Part III covers an expanded range of special populations and includes chapters focusing on offenders housed on supermaximum security (supermax) units and death row, female offenders, offenders with developmental disabilities, juvenile offenders, and geriatric offenders.

To create a meaningful, state-of-the-art text, I invited contributors who are recognized as national experts in their topics. A distinguished editorial review board was created to review and comment on each chapter prior to its submission for publication. Members of the editorial board were Joel A. Dvoskin, Ph.D.; Jeffrey L. Metzner, M.D.; Phillip J. Resnick, M.D.; and Nancy L. Wolff, Ph.D.

The chapters in this second edition were chosen to address common issues faced by mental health professionals and to focus on relevant clinical and legal issues. Each chapter provides a combination of basic background information for professionals new to the world of corrections and more advanced material for seasoned correctional caregivers. Key issues are emphasized in tables throughout the chapters and in summary points at the end of each chapter. Hypothetical clinical case examples are provided to emphasize important aspects of evaluating and treating offenders with mental illness. An important strength of this book is the incorporation of varying viewpoints on potentially controversial treatment topics, such as the prescription of benzodiazepines to incarcerated inmates. Extensive legal and clinical references are provided that reflect current trends in correctional psychiatry.

This text is intended for a wide-ranging audience, to include psychiatrists, psychologists, social workers, nurses, correctional officers and administrators, attorneys, and judges interested in mental health issues facing inmates. The focus of this text is on synthesizing the vast literature on the treatment of offenders with mental illness into a useful practical handbook for providers. Individuals preparing for forensic psychiatry or psychology boards may also find this text helpful, because it summarizes the most important forensic clinical issues and relevant legal cases.

REFERENCES

Sabol WJ, Minton TD, Harrison PM: Prison and jail inmates at midyear 2006. Bureau of Justice Statistics Bulletin, June 2007 (NCJ 217675). Available at: http://www.ojp.usdoj.gov/bjs/pub/pdf/pjim06.pdf. Accessed March 13, 2009.

Torrey EF: Reinventing mental health care. City Journal, Autumn 1999. Available at: http://www.city-journal.org/html/9_4_a5.html. Accessed March 13, 2009.

Acknowledgments

Once again I am extremely grateful to Robert E. Hales, M.D., M.B.A., editor-in-chief of American Psychiatric Publishing, Inc., for his continued wisdom in understanding the importance of a clinical textbook that focuses on correctional mental health. His appreciation of this topic translates into a handbook that can assist those providers who work in this environment to provide the best mental health care possible. I am honored to have worked with such a distinguished editorial review board; the members provided insightful and valuable input for every chapter. I also wish to thank the many wonderful chapter authors who met the various deadlines and my seemingly endless revision requests with great professionalism.

As with many projects in which I am involved, the administrative foundation that supports the hard work of so many people rests squarely on the very capable shoulders of editorial assistant and forensic coordinator David Spagnolo. All who have worked with him are fortunate to experience an individual who remains calm throughout all storms, keeps in good humor despite rocky waves, and never loses focus on the horizon ahead.

Although this second edition is greatly expanded and nearly double the length of the first edition, this time a seemingly impossible obstacle had faded away. Finally, I wish to thank with all my heart my All Wise support system, which gave me the motivation to bring this project forward and a desire to never give up.

PART I

Overview of Correctional Settings and Provision of Care

CHAPTER 1

Overview of the Criminal Justice System

Charles L. Scott, M.D.

To work with offenders involved in the criminal justice system, mental health care providers not only must assess them as individuals but also must understand the context in which they live. Joel Dvoskin (personal communication, January 2005) described this unique context when he noted,

> In many ways, the criminal justice system creates "communities." In some ways, these communities are similar to neighborhoods in the free world, but in other ways they are very, very different. For a person with post-traumatic stress disorder, the first day in jail can create terror that is almost beyond description. For first time offenders, confusion about rights and expectations can dramatically increase anxiety, to pathological levels. For these reasons, it is important for mental health providers serving criminal justice clients to understand the criminal justice system itself.

The need for mental health professionals who understand the challenging world of individuals who have been arrested, charged, or sentenced for a criminal act cannot be understated. Consider that in 1955, state mental hospitals in the United States institutionalized 559,000 persons out of a U.S. population of 165 million. During the next 45 years, these numbers dropped dramatically. For example, in December 2000, only

55,000 persons with mental illness were in a state hospital, although the U.S. general population had expanded to greater than 275 million (Lamb et al. 2004).

In what setting do these individuals now find their treatment? The evidence increasingly suggests that many are housed in the nation's jails and prisons. During the period that state psychiatric inpatient beds were dramatically declining in the United States, the number of jail and prison beds was on the rise. In 1985, the total number of inmates in custody was 744,208 (Gilliard and Beck 1997). At the end of 2007, U.S. prisons and jails incarcerated over 2.4 million persons, a significant number of whom had a mental disorder (West and Sabol 2008). According to Torrey (1999), the Los Angeles County Jail houses 3,400 inmates with mental illness, making it the largest psychiatric inpatient facility in the United States.

The increased prevalence of individuals with mental illness entering the criminal justice system has been referred to as the criminalization of the mentally ill. Reasons cited for the increasing numbers of individuals with mental illness in the criminal justice system include 1) the deinstitutionalization movement beginning in the 1960s that resulted in a massive discharge of psychiatric patients from state hospitals to the community; 2) more restrictive civil commitment criteria that make it more difficult to involuntarily hospitalize persons with mental illness *and* that result in briefer hospital stays; 3) a lack of adequate community support systems; and 4) an increased role of police officers in determining whether an arrested individual is transported to a jail or to a hospital (Lamb et al. 2004).

To provide effective mental health care in the correctional setting, the provider needs to understand this unique environment in which many patients now live. This chapter begins this education process by providing a definition of *corrections*, explaining theories of punishment, describing types of correctional settings, reviewing stages of the criminal justice system, explaining inmate classification schemes, and outlining the process governing the return of inmates to society.

DEFINITION OF *CORRECTIONS*

What does the term *corrections* actually mean? *Corrections* refers to those agencies and programs at the local, state, and federal levels that interface with individuals who have been either accused of crimes (detention) or convicted of them (correction). The correctional process is integrally related to three other areas of the criminal justice system: police, prosecutors, and courts. Each of these three components plays a significant role in determining whether an individual enters the legal system at all and/ or is subject to imposed controls from a correctional agency (Silverman 2001).

Correctional settings are wide-ranging and include lockups, jails, and prisons. Other programs that may interface with the criminal justice system include mandated community alcohol and drug treatment programs and community mental health supervision and treatment. *Correctional mental health* refers to the provision of mental health assessment and clinical treatment in a correctional setting. The term *penology* predates the concept of corrections and originates from the Latin word *poena*, which means "penalty." Whereas *penology* represents the study of punishment, the term *corrections* encompasses a much broader area that includes both the management and treatment of offenders, and implies an effort to "correct" the person and his or her misbehavior, presumably through some sort of rehabilitation.

The criminal justice system was created to address those actions committed by individuals that violate laws against society. These violations of laws are generally referred to as *crimes*. All states and the federal government have criminal codes that define specific crimes and associated sentences. In general, charges are likely to be filed in *federal* court when either 1) the alleged violation broke federal as opposed to state law or 2) the alleged crime took place on federal property. The most common crimes referred to federal court include controlled substance violations, immigration law violations, mail or wire fraud, gun law violations, postal offenses, child pornography, counterfeiting, and crimes that occur on federal property or in federal buildings (Federal Crime Cases 2009). Charges are filed in *state* court when an individual has violated a specific state statute and the alleged crime is not covered under federal jurisdiction.

How commonly are U.S. citizens victimized by crime? According to the 2005 National Crime Victimization Survey, 14% of U.S. households had experienced at least one violent or property crime. This victimization rate represents a substantial drop from 1994, when 25% of U.S. households had experienced a violent or property crime (Klaus 2007). Proposed theories to explain this drop include changing demographics, with fewer Americans in the younger age group traditionally associated with most crime; a decline in drug trafficking; an increased police presence in the community; and longer periods of incarceration for offenders in a correctional environment.

THEORIES OF PUNISHMENT

Why punish an individual? The most common answer is because someone has done something wrong. Although this response may seem sufficient at face value, theories underlying the purposes of punishment are
much more complex. In *Regina v. Dudley and Stephens* (1884), an English
court grappled with the meaning and purpose of punishment in an interesting case. Two Englishmen, Thomas Dudley and Edwin Stephens,
were indicted for the murder of a 17-year-old boy named Richard Parker.
All three were sailing on an English yacht when they encountered a severe storm on the high seas 1,600 miles from the Cape of Good Hope. As
a result of the storm, they were lost and stranded. There was no supply of
water on the boat and only two 1-pound tins of turnips. After 21 days of
virtually no food or water, the men realized that they all would die without some type of sustenance. The 17-year-old boy was the weakest of the
three and was lying at the bottom of the boat, extremely malnourished
by famine. Dudley and Stephens agreed that if they were not rescued by
the following day, the boy would have to be killed so they could potentially survive. On the day of the murder, the two men told the fragile boy
that his time had come, put a knife to his throat, and killed him. For 4 days,
the two men fed on the body and blood of the boy, and on the fourth day
they were rescued by a passing vessel. Both men were subsequently
charged with the murder of Richard Parker, whom they had eaten. At
their trial, testimony was presented that the boy would probably have
died from severe famine during the 4 days prior to the rescue and therefore he would not have lived anyway. Further testimony was provided that
had the two men not eaten the boy, they likely would have died from starvation. Should these men be punished considering these circumstances?
If so, what purpose would punishing them serve? Four general principles
of punishment help answer these difficult questions. These classic theories of punishment include retribution, deterrence, rehabilitation, and
incapacitation (see Table 1–1).

TABLE 1–1. Theories of punishment

Retribution	Person deserves punishment for breaking the law
Deterrence	Person receives punishment to help prevent future law-violating behaviors
Rehabilitation	Person utilizes punishment as a growth and learning opportunity
Incapacitation	Person is housed to stop him or her from offending

Retribution

The concept of retribution can be traced to the Latin word *retribuo*, which means "I pay back." The theory of retribution involves the use of punishment in response to a law-violating act simply because the offender deserves it. This philosophy can be summarized by the belief that an individual causing harm should be harmed. Historically, early legal systems almost exclusively used retribution as the guiding principle to punish. This approach was referred to as *lex talionis*, or "the law (*lex*) of retaliation." Under the law of *lex talionis*, equal and exact retribution was exacted as demonstrated in the words of the Hebrew scripture: "An eye for an eye, a tooth for a tooth, an arm for an arm, a life for a life" (Hooker 2004).

The concept known as "just deserts" is the modern equivalent of *lex talionis*. Although the individual is punished because his or her act deserves punishment, the "just deserts" approach allows consideration of punishment proportional to the severity of the crime, whereas this is not typically considered under strict retribution theory. Notably, the retribution principle is nearly entirely retrospective. Under the retribution theory, what purpose would punishing the two seamen discussed above serve?

Deterrence

Under the theory of deterrence, punishment is imposed to deter or prevent the commission of future criminal acts. The concept of deterrence involves both specific and general deterrence. The theory of *specific deterrence* holds that punished individuals are less likely to reoffend if imposed sanctions exist on their law-violating behavior. The theory of *general deterrence* proposes that by an individual's being held accountable for his or her illegal actions, other members of the general public will be less likely to offend, due to their fear of legal consequences. In the example of the lost and hungry seamen, specific deterrence theorists would argue that punishment will help deter these men from eating other people in the future in the unlikely event that they run out of food. Under the general deterrence principle, citizens, upon learning that punishment was imposed on these men, would theoretically be deterred from cannibalism, even if near starvation.

Does the theory of deterrence work in reality? An argument that specific deterrence is not achieved through punishment is supported by the high rearrest rate of U.S. prisoners after they are released from incarceration. In a study of 300,000 prisoners released in 15 states in 1994, nearly 68% were rearrested within 3 years (Langan and Levin 2002). At the same time, nearly one-third of all offenders did not reoffend, suggesting that a significant minority of them seem to have been deterred from future criminal acts. Other studies indicate that in some situations, punished individuals are specifically deterred from future offenses. For example, arrested drunk drivers (Shapiro and Votey 1984), first-time offenders (Smith and Gartin 1989), and spouse abusers (Sherman and Berk 1984) who received severe punishment were less likely to violate the law upon release than were those who received more lenient sentences. Three factors that are believed to affect the success or failure of criminal sanctions are the severity, the certainty, and the swiftness of punishment (Silverman 2001).

Rehabilitation

According to the rehabilitative theory of punishment, individuals are incarcerated so they have an opportunity to learn alternative behaviors to curb their deviant lifestyles. Corrections, therefore, is a system designed to correct those traits that result in criminal behavior. The rehabilitative model argues that the purpose of incarceration is to reform inmates through educational, training, and counseling programs. Under a rehabilitative model, would the English seamen require punishment? Considering the unusual circumstances of their having been lost at sea, a training program most likely would not be necessary to prevent them from eating others in the future. Therefore, if rehabilitation were the sole theory of punishment applied in this case, incarceration would not be justified.

The rehabilitative approach to managing criminal offenders was prominent following World War II up until the 1960s (Silverman 2001). As recidivism of released prisoners continued, Americans became increasingly skeptical of the rehabilitative approach. A published review of rehabilitation programs for inmates by New York sociologist Robert Martinson and colleagues contributed to the belief that rehabilitation programs for offenders had minimal benefit. This research reviewed 231 studies of offender rehabilitation programs conducted between 1945 and 1967 (Lipton et al. 1975). In his famous 1974 article titled "What Works? Questions and Answers About Prison Reform," Martinson interpreted the results from this research. In this article, he concluded, "With few and isolated exceptions, the rehabilitative efforts that have been reported so far have had no appreciable effect on recidivism." He emphasized that "our present strategies...cannot overcome, or even appreciably reduce, the powerful tendencies of offenders to continue in criminal behavior" (Martinson 1974, p. 49).

Martinson's (1974) article was widely read and his published findings on rehabilitation were quickly renamed "Nothing works!" His persuasive arguments had far-reaching effects and played a significant role in the U.S. penal system's moving away from the rehabilitative approach for offenders. Subsequent reviews of rehabilitation programs did not replicate Martinson's findings but used statistical analyses of treatment outcome not available to Martinson. In their survey of 200 studies on rehabilitation conducted from 1981 to 1987, Gendreau and Ross (1987) concluded that successful rehabilitation of offenders was possible and that an up to 80% reduction in recidivism had been noted in research studies examining effective programs. Despite these more encouraging results, the pendulum had already moved away from rehabilitation as a purpose of punishment. As a result, a harsher theory of punishment, known as incapacitation, became increasingly popular throughout the United States.

Incapacitation

Under the incapacitation principle, individuals are prevented from committing future criminal acts against free citizens through detention in a secure environment. A sentence of life without the possibility of parole is an extreme form of incapacitation. The ultimate form of incapacitation is the imposition of the death penalty. Applying the incapacitation theory to the hungry yachtsmen described above would result in their detention for the primary purpose of preventing them from ever repeating a criminal act. In reality, how likely are they to repeat this type of behavior? If their risk of eating another person in the future is actually very low, then lengthy incarceration under the incapacitation theory would not be justified.

With public concern increasing alongside the rising crime rate during the late 1980s and 1990s, many state legislatures passed laws that resulted in longer sentences—that is, increased incapacitation. Not all incapacitation, however, is the same. In general, three forms of incapacitation exist. Under a schema known as *collective incapacitation*, all offenders convicted of the same crime receive exactly the same sentence. The anticipated effect of collective incapacitation is a substantial increase in the prison population because no attempt is made to distinguish between high-risk and low-risk offenders (Cohen 1983; Silverman 2001). In contrast, *selective incapacitation* results in the incarceration of only those offenders who are predicted to be at higher risk for reoffending. Legislative efforts to increase the length of incapacitation for higher-risk offenders have resulted in significant sentencing reform over the last three decades. These reforms include "truth in sentencing" schemes and the passage of "three strikes you're out" statutes. Truth-in-sentencing laws require offenders to serve a substantial portion of their prison sentence with restrictions on both parole eligibility and good-time credits (Ditton and Wilson 1999). Under "three strikes you're out" statutes, felons found guilty of a third serious crime would be incarcerated for 25 years to life, even if the felonies were relatively minor. A third incapacitation approach is called *criminal career incapacitation.* Under this scheme, classes of criminals (rather than all criminals) with known high rates of crime receive longer sentences (Silverman 2001).

The increasing use of incapacitation as punishment is reflected in the growing prison population. For example, from 2000 through 2007, the general population increased by 6.4%, whereas the number of sentenced prisoners increased by 15%. At the end of 2007, a total of 2,293,157 persons were incarcerated in U.S. jails and prisons. To put these numbers into perspective, 1 in every 132 U.S. residents was in prison or jail at year-end 2007 (West and Sabol 2008).

And what punishment was given to the two English seamen who were both charged with and stood trial for the murder of young Richard Parker? The English legal system struggled with what sentence might fairly fulfill any of the four theories of punishment outlined above. Eventually a compromise solution was reached. The men were found guilty of murder and sentenced to death with a subsequent commutation of their sentence to 6 months in prison. The ultimate outcome balanced the importance of finding the lost seamen responsible for their acts while also considering the circumstances that led to their offense.

TYPES OF CORRECTIONAL FACILITIES

The U.S. correctional system is complex and includes a federal system, 50 separate state systems, and thousands of local systems. Because each state determines its own criminal justice and correctional system, states differ in how crimes are defined, who is arrested, and what consequences are imposed for law-violating behavior (Silverman 2001). Correctional housing facilities vary and are broadly classified into three types of facilities: lockups, jails, and prisons.

Lockups and Local Jails

Lockups are local temporary holding facilities that constitute the initial phase of the criminal justice system in a significant number of jurisdictions. The lockup is the most common type of correctional facility, with an average stay usually lasting less than 48 hours. Lockups are often located in the local police station, where only temporary detainment (e.g., with arrestees charged with drunk driving) is required. Approximately 30% of local police departments operate at least one lockup facility for adults separate from a jail. In jurisdictions with 500,000 or more residents, local lockups can detain up to 70 individuals, whereas lockups in jurisdictions with fewer than 10,000 residents typically house about three persons (Reaves and Goldberg 2000). In jurisdictions that do not have a local lockup, arrested individuals are usually detained in the local jail.

Jails

Jails are locally operated correctional facilities that confine persons before or after adjudication. Individuals who are convicted of a misdemeanor (minor crime) may receive a sentence of a year or less and complete their sentence in a jail, not a prison. Jails serve a variety of functions, including holding persons awaiting trial; punishing persons convicted of a misdemeanor; detaining violators of probation, parole, or bail; temporarily detaining juveniles pending transfer to juvenile authorities; holding mentally ill persons pending movement to appropriate health facilities; holding inmates before transfer to federal, state, or other authorities; holding individuals for the military, protective custody, or contempt; holding witnesses for the courts; and sometimes serving as community-based programs as alternatives to incarceration.

In some circumstances, individuals facing federal charges may be detained in a local jail. For example, the U.S. Citizenship and Immigration Services has the authority to detain certain categories of noncitizens. The U.S. Marshals Service assumes custody of persons arrested by all federal agencies. The Marshals Service houses over 58,000 federal unsentenced detainees in federal, state, and local jails. In jurisdictions where detention space is limited, the Marshals Service utilizes Cooperative Agreement Program funds to improve local jail conditions in exchange for guaranteed space for federal prisoners (U.S. Marshals Service 2009).

Of the total incarcerated population in the United States, approximately one-third are held in local jails (Harrison and Karberg 2004). At midyear 2007, approximately 780,700 persons were being held in local U.S. jails (Sabol et al. 2007). Of individuals detained in jail, approximately 62% are awaiting some type of court action on their current charge, while the remainder are serving time for their conviction (Sabol et al. 2007). The following findings characterize the U.S. jail inmate population: nearly half (46%) are on probation or parole at the time of their arrest; half have been using drugs or alcohol at the time of their offense; half are being held for a violent or drug offense; over half grew up in a single-parent household; and nearly half (46%) had a family member who had been incarcerated (James 2004). Of jail inmates identified as mentally ill, over 30% were homeless in the year prior to the arrest, compared with 17.3% of jail inmates without an identified mental disorder (Ditton 1999).

Female jail inmates are more likely than male inmates to be drug offenders (29% of females vs. 24% of males). Furthermore, female drug
offenses more commonly involve drug possession, whereas male drug offenses more commonly involve drug trafficking. Female jail inmates are
more likely to report a past history of physical or sexual abuse than are
male jail inmates. In 2002, among jail inmates, 55% of women reported
a history of abuse, compared with 13% of men (James 2004).

Prisons

Prisons are confinement facilities that maintain custodial authority over
individuals who have been convicted of felonies. A felony is considered a
more serious crime than a misdemeanor. The imposed sentence for a felony is greater than 1 year at a minimum. Prisons are operated by both
state and federal governments and are typically large facilities, often with
over 500 beds. Approximately two-thirds of inmates serve their time in
prison (Harrison and Beck 2004).

The Federal Bureau of Prisons was established in 1930. The federal
prison system includes a nationwide system of prisons and detention facilities for the incarceration of inmates who are awaiting trial or sentencing in federal court or who have been sentenced to a federal facility after
conviction for a federal crime (Federal Bureau of Prisons 2009a).

As of 2009, the Federal Bureau of Prisons had 114 facilities housing
over 201,000 inmates throughout the country. As of February 21, 2009,
the percentage breakdown of offenses committed by federal inmates
was as follows: drug offenses (52.4%); crimes involving weapons, explo-
sives, or arson (15.1%); robbery (4.7%); homicide, aggravated assault,
and kidnapping offenses (2.9%); and sex offenses (3.5%). Drug offenders represented the majority of federal inmates in 2009, whereas they
represented only 16% of offenders in 1970 (Federal Bureau of Prisons
2009b).

Thirty states and the federal system contract with private agencies to
hold prisoners in privately operated facilities. An increase in private con-
tracting of correctional beds has arisen to alleviate overcrowding in the
state and federal systems and to quickly obtain beds as the incarcerated
population increases (McDonald et al. 1998). In 2006, a total of 111,975
inmates were housed in private facilities, a number that represents 7.2%
of all prisoners under state or federal jurisdiction, up from 6.5% in 2003
(Sabol et al. 2007).

Prison demographic data demonstrate inequalities based on ethnicity, age, and gender. For decades, minority males have been overrepresented among prison inmates, although black imprisonment rates in
2007 had decreased since 2000. At year-end 2007, 18.2% of the sentenced

males were Hispanic, 30.8% were white, and 36.3% were black (down from 40% in 2000) (West and Sabol 2008). Men continue to dominate the prison population and are nearly 14 times more likely than women to be incarcerated in a state or federal prison. However, the face of the typical prison inmate as one of a young male is slowly changing. In particular, the rate of female incarceration has been increasing faster than the rate for males. Since 1995, the total number of male prisoners has increased 29%, whereas the number of female prisoners has increased 48% (Harrison and Beck 2004).

Prison inmates are also getting older. In their review of prison inmates, Harrison and Beck (2004) found that inmates ages 55 and older represent the age group with the largest percentage increase. Since 1995, this particular sector of the prison population has increased 85%. The increasing length of sentences under mandatory sentencing schemes has contributed to the aging of the correctional population. Because inmates have a constitutional right to medical care, states and counties will likely face substantial financial burdens as offenders age and require costly medical interventions.

Table 1–2 provides definitions of important aspects of the correctional system.

OVERVIEW OF THE CRIMINAL JUSTICE PROCESS

Throughout their incarceration, detainees face numerous court procedures and hearings that are stressful and can significantly impact the detainees' emotional state. An understanding of the sequence of events facing an individual journeying through the criminal justice system is important for clinicians working with this population.

Although the U.S. system of justice originates from English common law, no uniform criminal justice system exists in the United States. Often criminal actions are not discovered or reported to law enforcement agencies (Bureau of Justice Statistics 2005). The majority of crimes are not solved. Under the Uniform Crime Report Program, once a crime is reported to law enforcement, it is designated as "cleared" if at least one person is arrested, charged with the commission of the offense, and turned over to the court for prosecution. In 2007, law enforcement agencies cleared 44.5% of violent crimes (murder, forcible rape, robbery, and aggravated assault), 16.5% of property crimes (burglary, larceny-theft, and motor vehicle theft), and 18% of arson offenses (Federal Bureau of Investigation 2008).

Despite some variation in the handling of criminal cases across various jurisdictions, the most common sequence of steps in response to

TABLE 1–2.	Important definitions
Lockup	A temporary holding facility with an average stay of less than 48 hours
Jail	A locally operated correctional facility that confines persons before or after their adjudication
Prison	Confinement facility that houses individuals convicted of felonies
Misdemeanor	A crime with a sentence of 1 year or less
Felony	A crime with a sentence of greater than 1 year

known criminal behavior is as follows. An individual becomes a suspect in a crime following reports from victims or other witnesses, discovery by a police officer, or investigative work. For most crimes, especially minor crimes, police officers serve as gatekeepers in determining which persons will formally enter into the justice system. This discretionary arrest authority provides officers options other than taking the person into custody. For example, officers can warn offenders and release them or divert an offender to a mental health treatment program. In dealing with juveniles, the officer can bring the youth home and meet with the family (Finn and Sullivan 1988).

An arrest involves the taking of an individual into custody under the legal authority granted by the government. Law enforcement practices regarding who is arrested and why vary according to the jurisdiction. In 2007, law enforcement made approximately 14.2 million arrests in the United States. Drug abuse violations represented the most common offense type for which individuals were arrested. Young adults are overrepresented among those arrested. For example, nearly 40% of individuals arrested in 2007 in a metropolitan area were younger than age 25, and persons under age 21 accounted for nearly half (49.4%) of all robbery arrests (Federal Bureau of Investigation 2008).

Individuals who are arrested or charged with an offense are usually required to appear at the police station or local jail for booking. The booking process has many administrative steps following the arrest of a person. This process includes taking the individual's mug shot, recording personal information, fingerprinting, assigning identifying case numbers, conducting medical and psychiatric screening, and beginning a new file for first-time arrestees. Nearly half of arrested individuals leave the jail within 24–48 hours after they are booked. Inmates who are not released are thoroughly searched, their property is removed, and they are issued standard jail clothing (Silverman 2001). The booking process, particularly for first-time offenders, is often frightening for the arrestee. As discussed in Chapter 9, "Suicide Prevention in Correctional Facilities," the risk of suicide during the first 24–48 hours after a person is detained in a lockup or jail is exceptionally high due to the high stress level and overwhelming emotions.

Following an individual's arrest and subsequent booking, law enforcement agencies provide information regarding the accused to the prosecutor. Prosecutors have broad discretionary authority. They play a significant role in determining whether to initiate prosecution and what specific charges are filed with the court. If no charges are filed, the accused must be released. At this stage, there are several alternatives to a formal filing of charges. First, the prosecutor may request that the judge enter a *nolle prosequi*. In this case, the prosecuting officer in a criminal action declares that he or she will "not further prosecute" the case against some or all of the defendants. This is commonly referred to as "nol pros" (Silverman 2001; Bureau of Justice Statistics 2005). Second, for individuals already involved in the criminal justice system, the prosecutor may decide to revoke probation or parole rather than initiate new charges. Third, the suspect may be civilly committed to a mental health treatment facility. Fourth, a decision to invoke civil sanctions, such a revocation of a person's license, may substitute for processing the arrestee through the criminal justice system. Charges may also be reduced or dismissed when the victim is unwilling to cooperate with the prosecution or when a suspect agrees to testify for the prosecution or to act as an informer (Silverman 2001).

If a suspect is charged with a crime, he or she is taken before a judge or magistrate. At this initial appearance, the judge must inform the accused of the charges and decide whether probable cause exists to detain the individual. Probable cause exists when there is a reasonable belief that a crime has or is being committed, and such cause is the basis for all lawful searches, seizures, and arrests. For nonserious offenses, the judge or magistrate may determine guilt and assess a penalty at this stage. Defense counsel may also be assigned at this initial appearance. As stated in the Sixth Amendment of the U.S. Constitution, all suspects charged with serious crimes have a right to be represented by an attorney (Bureau of Justice Statistics 2005). The court assigns an attorney for indigent suspects who cannot afford their own counsel (Bureau of Justice Statistics 2005).

Following the assignment of a defense attorney, the accused has an initial court appearance, where the court may decide to release the accused prior to trial. For individuals released prior to trial, the court may set bail (Bureau of Justice Statistics 2005). *Bail* is money that a defendant must provide up front (often through a contract with a bail bondsman) and that must be forfeited if the accused fails to appear in court for trial. The amount of bail set is governed by multiple factors, including the seriousness of the charges, the risk of the defendant's flight from the governing jurisdiction, the defendant's past legal history, and the defendant's financial status.

Depending on the locality, a preliminary hearing may follow the initial appearance of the defendant in court. The primary purpose of this hearing is for the court to determine if there is sufficient evidence of probable cause that the accused committed a crime. In situations where the judge does not find probable cause, he or she must dismiss the case. If probable cause is found or if the accused waives his or her right to a preliminary hearing, then the case may be forwarded to a grand jury (Bureau of Justice Statistics 2005).

During the hearing before the grand jury, the prosecutor presents the evidence against the accused, and the grand jury decides whether the evidence warrants bringing the accused to trial. If the grand jury determines that sufficient evidence exists, it submits an indictment to the court. An indictment is a written summary of the facts of the offenses charged against the accused. In some jurisdictions, both misdemeanor and felony cases move forward after a document known as the "issuance of information" is provided. The issuance of information is a formal written accusation that the prosecutor submits to the court. The accused may choose to waive a grand jury indictment and accept the issuance of information (Bureau of Justice Statistics 2005).

Following an indictment or filing of an issuance of information with the court, the accused is scheduled for an arraignment. An arraignment is a hearing where the accused is informed of the charges, advised of his or her rights, and requested to enter a plea. In some situations, the defendant may choose to enter either a guilty plea or a plea of *nolo contendere.* A plea of *nolo contendere* indicates that the defendant accepts the penalty without admitting guilt. If the judge accepts a guilty or *nolo contendere* plea, a trial is not held and the case proceeds to the sentencing phase (Bureau of Justice Statistics 2005).

If the defendant pleads not guilty or not guilty by reason of insanity, a trial date is scheduled. In serious crimes, the defendant is guaranteed a right to trial by jury but may choose to have a "bench trial," in which the judge rather than a jury hears the case and determines guilt. At the trial, the defense and prosecution both present evidence, and the judge decides on issues of law. At the conclusion of the trial, a finding of guilty or not guilty is made. Next, the defendant is scheduled for a sentencing hearing where both mitigating and aggravating factors are presented.

In deciding the appropriate sentence for the convicted offender, courts often review presentence investigations, completed by probation agencies, along with victim impact statements. Mental health professionals are frequently asked to present information regarding the defendant's psychiatric history as part of the sentencing process. Following the trial, the defendant may appeal his or her conviction or sentence. In all states with a capital punishment provision, appeals are automatic for defendants who receive the death penalty (Bureau of Justice Statistics 2005).

Sentencing options include incarceration in a prison, jail, or other confinement facility, or release into the community on probationary status. Probation allows those convicted to remain in the community under specified restrictions, such as drug testing or required treatment programs. At year-end 2007, approximately 4,293,200 men and women were on probation in the United States (Glaze and Bonczar 2008). The court may also require the convicted offender to pay a fine or make restitution through financial compensation to a victim. Certain jurisdictions provide other alternatives to incarceration that are more intense than regular probation requirements but do not require actual incarceration. Such programs include boot camps, house arrest with electronic monitoring, intense supervision with mandated drug and/or psychiatric treatment, and community service. Jurisdictions vary significantly in how time periods of incarceration are determined. In general, convicted offenders who receive a sentence of less than 1 year are sent to a jail, whereas those who are sentenced to more than 1 year serve their time in prison (Bureau of Justice Statistics 2005).

INMATE CLASSIFICATION

At some point after an individual is placed into a correctional facility, a process known as classification occurs. Classification attempts to match inmates with the appropriate level of security, custody supervision, and services necessary to meet their needs. Appropriate classification is important for the following five reasons: protection of inmates; protection of the public; maximizing efficient use of resources; controlling inmate behavior; and providing planning information for budgets, staffing, and program development (Silverman 2001).

For individuals who are serving time in jail, the classification procedure typically occurs in the jail in which they are housed. As a result of this process, the inmate may be placed in a particular housing unit within the jail based on either security, medical, and/or mental health needs. For those individuals sentenced to prison, the location of the classification process depends largely on the inmate's jurisdiction. In some areas, an inmate is sent to a central reception and diagnostic center after being sentenced. Following an evaluation of the level of security and special services required, the inmate is transferred to the most appropriate facility. In other jurisdictions, an inmate undergoes the classification process in a prison reception unit, where he or she is kept until this process is completed. The inmate is then placed in general population or transferred to another facility if needed.

Classification involves determination of both the security and the custody level appropriate for the inmate. *Facility security level* describes the type of physical barriers designed to prevent escape and control inmate behavior (Henderson et al. 1997). Jurisdictions vary regarding how they define security levels for their correctional institutions. For example, the Federal Bureau of Prisons devised a security classification scheme that includes four recommended security levels. Level I prisons are referred to as minimum security facilities or federal prison camps. These facilities have dormitory housing, no surrounding fence, and a relatively low inmate:staff ratio. Level II facilities are termed low-security institutions and are typically surrounded by double-fenced perimeters. These facilities have strong work and program components and a higher inmate:staff ratio than do minimum security facilities. Level III facilities—that is, medium-security institutions—have more secure perimeters with electronic detection systems, cell-type housing, and greater inmate:staff ratios than do lower-level facilities. Level IV facilities are considered high-security institutions. Their perimeters are often significantly reinforced and may consist of walls with towers at each corner that are manned by armed correctional officers. Patients in a level IV facility are housed primarily in single- or multiple-occupant cells, with close staff supervision and movement control (Silverman 2001).

Whereas *security level* refers to the number of environmental barriers to prevent escape or manage behavior, an inmate's custody level is determined by the degree of staff supervision necessary to provide adequate control of the inmate (National Institute of Corrections 1987). Under the Federal Bureau of Prisons' classification scheme, inmates noted as "out custody" have a relatively greater degree of movement of freedom compared with higher-level custody inmates. For example, such inmates may be assigned to less secure housing because they are eligible for work detail outside the secure perimeter of the institution, with decreased levels of staff supervision. Inmates classified as "in custody" are typically assigned to regular quarters, may have work assignments under normal levels of supervision, and are not allowed to participate in work programs outside the confines of the institution. "Maximum custody" is the highest custody level assigned, and inmates with this classification require intense control and supervision. This classification is generally given to those inmates who demonstrated violence or disruptive behavior, or who pose a serious escape risk (Silverman 2001).

Prison environments vary regarding the type of inmate received, as well as the level of security and staffing. Traditionally, inmates who have received the death penalty have been segregated into separate housing areas known as death row. Because persons who receive the death penalty are viewed as dangerous or as an increased escape risk, separate secure housing pods with increased supervision and correctional officer staffing are often deemed necessary. However, with the increasing financial burdens associated with longer periods on death row, some states have developed opportunities for inmates who have received the death penalty to be mainstreamed into the general inmate population and/or to participate in work programs while on death row. Benefits of these policy changes for correctional administration have included cost savings, reduction in legal expenses regarding defense of standard of care law suits, and greater flexibility with the use of bed space; advantages for death row inmates include increased access to legal resources, recreation time, commissary use, visitation, medical care, and work programs (Lombardi et al. 1997; Silverman 2001).

No longer do inmates have to be convicted of a capital crime to be housed on a special security unit. During the last few decades, several jurisdictions have built or modified existing prison facilities to create highly isolated environments for those inmates considered too dangerous to be maintained in a general prison population. These facilities are known by various names, including extended control facilities, supermax units, maxi-max units, and security housing units. Often labeled a prison within a prison, these tightly managed facilities provide control of inmates who have exhibited violent or seriously disruptive behaviors while incarcerated and, as a result, cannot be maintained in a less restrictive environment. In 1963, the U.S. Penitentiary at Marion, located in southern Illinois, was opened to replace Alcatraz and was the highest maximum security prison in the United States. Inmates in these types of facilities are often kept in their cell for up to 23 hours a day and have minimal, if any, interaction with other inmates. The authors of Chapter 16, "Supermax Units and Death Row," describe in greater detail this type of prison environment and relevant mental health issues.

RELEASE FROM PRISON

The amount of time an offender serves in prison depends on the type of sentencing scheme outlined in the reviewing jurisdiction. Each state's penal code provides sentencing guidelines, which are minimum and maximum time frames to be imposed for each offense. An indeterminate sentencing scheme provides a minimum time period the inmate must serve and a maximum time period after which the inmate must be released (Silverman 2001). Under an indeterminate sentencing scheme, a parole board (or other reviewing agency) periodically considers whether an individual can be released and placed into the community.

As a result of increasing public skepticism regarding the rehabilitative potential of inmates and the appropriateness of early release, indeterminate schemes have lost their popularity over the last several decades. More jurisdictions are now adopting determinate sentencing schemes. A determinate sentencing scheme specifies the number of years that the individual must serve based on the offense. Under a determinate sentencing scheme, the time sentenced cannot be increased or decreased. Although determinate sentences are fixed, an inmate may be granted an earlier release date through the accumulation of "good time." Depending on each jurisdiction's statutory provision, this good time can be earned through either automatic or earned credits. Credits can be earned through participation in work or treatment programs (Silverman 2001).

Under both determinate and indeterminate sentencing schemes, a prisoner may be released prior to completing his or her sentence through the process known as parole. Parole represents the conditional release of the offender into the community. Under an indeterminate sentencing scheme, a parole board (or similarly designated authority) decides whether the inmate should be granted an early release. If the inmate is released, a separate process known as parole supervision begins, which provides support, monitoring and supervision, and services to the newly released offender. Two important components often considered when deciding the appropriateness of parole include the severity of the offense and the inmate's risk of reoffending.

Inmates who have been sentenced under a determinate sentencing scheme are required to serve out their full sentence less any good-time credits for participation in programs. Those convicted offenders who are released into the community under parole remain under the supervision of the parole officer. They must adhere to specified conditions of parole for the remainder of their unexpired sentence. Failure to adhere to the conditions of parole can cause the offender to be returned to prison to complete his or her sentence.

As of year-end 2007, the U.S. parole population was 824,364, a 3.2% increase from the prior year. During this same time period, Rhode Island, Indiana, and West Virginia experienced more than a 20% increase in their parole populations. In line with the increasing rates of incarceration among women, the female parole population is also increasing. In 2007, female parolees represented 12% of all parolees, compared with 10% in 1995. Unfortunately, less than half of all parolees successfully meet the conditions of their supervision, and 38% of parolees in 2007 were returned to prison or jail (Glaze and Bonczar 2008).

CONCLUSION

Correctional environments are multifaceted organizations. Societies have utilized various theories of punishment to justify the incarceration of offenders, some with the hopeful goal of decreasing future crime. Mental health practitioners play a variety of vitally important roles in the assessment, treatment, and management of offenders at virtually every point along their journey through this complex and sometimes frightening world. Among the many reasons to provide mental health treatment in a correctional environment are easing the inmate's suffering, lessening the offender's disability so that he or she can participate in jail and prison programs, increasing safety within the institution, and providing care for serious medical needs as constitutionally required. Understanding this special environment improves providers' ability to assist inmates as they travel through the criminal justice system.

SUMMARY POINTS

- The four theories of punishment are retribution, deterrence, rehabilitation, and incapacitation.
- The criminal justice system is complex and includes multiple entry and exit points.
- Classification attempts to match inmates with the appropriate level of security, custody supervision required, and services necessary to meet their needs.

REFERENCES

Bureau of Justice Statistics: The justice system. 2005. Available at: http://www.ojp.usdoj.gov/bjs/justsys.htm. Accessed March 14, 2009.

Cohen J: Incapacitating criminals: recent research findings. National Institute of Justice, Research in Brief. Washington, DC, U.S. Department of Justice, December 1983

Ditton PM: Mental health treatment of inmates and probationers (NCJ 174463). Washington, DC, U.S. Department of Justice, Office of Justice Programs, Bureau of Justice Statistics, 1999

Ditton PM, Wilson DJ: Truth in sentencing in state prisons (NCJ 170032). Washington, DC, U.S. Department of Justice, Office of Justice Programs, Bureau of Justice Statistics, 1999

Federal Bureau of Investigation: Crime in the United States, 2007. September 2008. Available at: http://www.fbi.gov/ucr/cius2007/index.html. Accessed March 14, 2009.

Federal Bureau of Prisons: About the Bureau of Prisons. 2009a. Available at: http://www.bop.gov/about/index.jsp. Accessed March 14, 2009.

Federal Bureau of Prisons: Quick facts about the Bureau of Prisons. February 2009b. Available at: http://www.bop.gov/about/facts.jsp. Accessed March 14, 2009.

Federal Crime Cases. Available at: http://www.gottrouble.com/legal/criminal/federal/federalcases.html. Accessed March 14, 2009.

Finn PE, Sullivan M: Police respond to special populations: handling the mentally ill, public inebriate, and the homeless. National Institute of Justice Reports 209:2–8, 1988

Gendreau P, Ross RR: Revivification of rehabilitation: evidence from the 1980s. Justice Quarterly 4:349–407, 1987

Gilliard DK, Beck AJ: Prison and jail inmates at midyear 1996 (NCJ 162843). Washington, DC, U.S. Department of Justice, Office of Justice Programs, Bureau of Justice Statistics, January 1997

Glaze LE, Bonczar TP: Probation and parole in the United States, 2007 (NCJ 224707). Washington, DC, U.S. Department of Justice, Office of Justice Programs, Bureau of Justice Statistics, December 2008

Harrison PM, Beck AJ: Prisoners in 2003 (NCJ 203947). Washington, DC, U.S. Department of Justice, Office of Justice Programs, Bureau of Justice Statistics, November 2004

Harrison PM, Karberg JC: Prison and jail inmates at midyear 2003 (NCJ 203947). Washington, DC, U.S. Department of Justice, Office of Justice Programs, Bureau of Justice Statistics, May 2004

Henderson JD, Rauch WD, Phillips RL: Guidelines for the Development of a Security Program, 2nd Edition. Lanham, MD, American Correctional Association, 1997

Hooker R: Lex talionis, in World Cultures, General Glossary. 2004. Available at: http://www.wsu.edu:8080/~dee/GLOSSARY/LEXTAL.HTM. Accessed March 14, 2009.

James DJ: Profile of jail inmates, 2002 (NCJ 201932). Washington, DC, U.S. Department of Justice, Office of Justice Programs, Bureau of Justice Statistics, July 2004

Klaus PA: Crime and the nation's households, 2005 (NCJ 217198). Washington, DC, U.S. Department of Justice, Office of Justice Programs, Bureau of Justice Statistics, April 2007

Lamb HR, Weinberger LE, Gross BH: Mentally ill persons in the criminal justice system: some perspectives. Psychiatr Q 75:107–126, 2004

Langan PA, Levin DJ: Recidivism of prisoners released in 1994 (NCJ 193427). Washington, DC, U.S. Department of Justice, Office of Justice Programs, Bureau of Justice Statistics, June 2002

Lipton DS, Martinson R, Wilks J: The Effectiveness of Correctional Treatment: A Survey of Treatment Validation Studies. New York, Praeger, 1975

Lombardi G, Sluder RD, Wallace D: Mainstreaming death-sentenced inmates: the Missouri experience and its legal significance. Fed Probat 61:3–10, 1997

Martinson R: What works? Questions and answers about prison reform. Public Interest 35:22–54, 1974

McDonald D, Fournier E, Russell-Einhourn M, et al: Private prisons in the United States: executive summary. July 16, 1998. Available at: http://www.abtassoc.com/reports/ES-priv-report.pdf. Accessed March 14, 2009.

National Institute of Corrections: Guidelines for the development of a security program. Washington, DC, Department of Justice, National Institute of Corrections, July 1987

Reaves BA, Goldberg AL: Local police departments 1997 (NCJ 173429). Washington, DC, U.S. Department of Justice, Office of Justice Programs, Bureau of Justice Statistics, February 2000

Regina v Dudley and Stephens, Queen's Bench Division, 14 Q.B.D. 273 (1884)

Sabol WJ, Minton TD, Harrison PM: Prison and jail inmates at midyear 2006 (NCJ 217675). Washington, DC, U.S. Department of Justice, Office of Justice Programs, Bureau of Justice Statistics, June 2007. Available at: http://www.ojp.usdoj.gov/bjs/pub/pdf/pjim06.pdf. Accessed March 13, 2009.

Shapiro P, Votey H: Deterrence and subjective probabilities of arrest: modeling individual decisions to drink and drive in Sweden. Law Soc Rev 18:111–149, 1984

Sherman L, Berk R: The specific deterrent effects of arrest for domestic assault. Am Sociol Rev 49:261–272, 1984

Silverman IJ: The correctional process, in Corrections: A Comprehensive View, 2nd Edition. Belmont, CA, Wadsworth/Thomson Learning, 2001

Smith D, Gartin P: Specifying specific deterrence: the influence of arrest on future criminal activity. Am Sociol Rev 54:94–105, 1989

Torrey EF: Reinventing mental health care. City Journal, Autumn 1999. Available at: http://www.city-journal.org/html/9_4_a5.html. Accessed March 14, 2009.

U.S. Marshals Service: Major responsibilities of the U.S. Marshals Service. 2009. Available at: http://www.usmarshals.gov/duties/index.html. Accessed February 22, 2009.

West HC, Sabol W: Prisoners in 2007 (NCJ 224280). Washington, DC, U.S. Department of Justice, Office of Justice Programs, Bureau of Justice Statistics, December 2008

CHAPTER 2

The Criminal Justice System and Offenders Placed in an Outpatient Setting

Erik Roskes, M.D.

The Honorable Charlotte Cooksey

Sharon Lipford, LCSW-C

Henry A. Dlugacz, M.S.W., J.D.

The challenges that offenders with mental illness pose to the penal system are obvious (Human Rights Watch 2003). The penal system, designed to provide safety and security, is not well equipped to manage the needs of individuals with severe mental illness. Correctional employees are often not trained to identify or assist detainees or inmates who are experiencing psychiatric symptoms. Correctional personnel vary in their response but frequently lack the knowledge, experience, and patience to provide a therapeutic intervention. In addition, the physical plant and layout of most jails and prisons are not conducive to the provision of quality mental health care. As a result, mechanisms to encourage the release of individuals with mental illness from incarceration may practically promote more effective mental health care in the community.

Although much of the remainder of this book focuses on the delivery of mental health care within correctional settings, this chapter focuses on the management of offenders with mental illness in the community. By any accounting, far more offenders are in community settings (on parole, probation, or another form of supervised release) than in jails or prisons. For example, in the United States in 2007, approximately 2,293,000 inmates were in federal or state prisons or in local jails, whereas about 5,118,500 individuals were on probation (court-ordered terms of community supervision, with conditions, in lieu of a sentence of incarceration) or parole (proactive early release from incarceration with conditions and supervision) (Bureau of Justice Statistics 2007). Figure 2–1 demonstrates the dramatic increase seen in both incarcerated and community-based correctional populations over the past quarter century.

The incidence and prevalence of mental illness among offenders who reside in community settings are vastly understudied compared with those among incarcerated individuals. According to the Bureau of Justice Statistics, in 1998 an estimated 16% of individuals on probation, or 547,800 individuals, were mentally ill. In this study, mental illness was defined by the inmate's self-report of having a "mental or emotional condition" or as having stayed overnight in a mental hospital (Ditton 1999). Skeem and Louden (2006) concurred with this prevalence estimate. In an earlier study, Fulton (1996) found that many states did not track parolees and probationers with mental health problems and as a result were unable to determine the prevalence rate of mental illness in this population. In the 15 states that collected this type of epidemiological information, the prevalence rates for mental illness ranged from 1% to 11% (mean 5%) for parolees and from 3% to 23% (mean 6%) for probationers. Recognizing the difficulty of comparing information across jurisdictions that may use different definitions of mental illness, Fulton (1996) recommended use of the following definition for adults with mental illness, promulgated by the National Coalition for Mental Health and Substance Abuse Care in the Justice System: "adults having a disabling mental illness, which includes schizophrenia and/or an affective disorder." In addition to having mental illness, most offenders have a comorbid substance use disorder. According to the Epidemiologic Catchment Area study (Regier et al. 1990), 90% of incarcerated inmates with mental illness also met criteria for a substance use disorder at some point during their lifetime. Therefore, integrated or concurrent mental health and substance use treatment are critical interventions for the vast majority of offenders when they are released into the community.

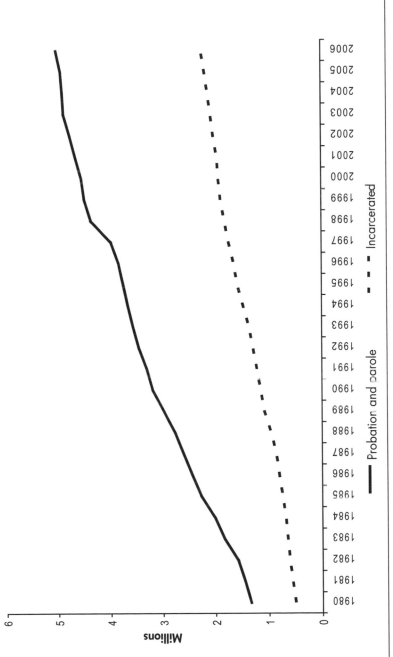

FIGURE 2–1. Correctional populations, 1980–2006.

POINTS OF CONTACT BETWEEN THE CRIMINAL JUSTICE SYSTEM AND COMMUNITY MENTAL HEALTH CARE PROVIDERS

Individuals with mental illness may be diverted from the criminal justice system at a variety of points. Broadly defined, these opportunities can be divided into prebooking and postbooking diversions. All diversions occur because some participant in the criminal justice system (not a mental health care provider) recognizes a mental health issue in a defendant or detainee. In functioning diversion programs, this recognition leads to a referral to a mental health professional for a definitive evaluation and potential diversion from the criminal justice system into the mental health treatment system. Thus, all diversion programs require some degree of partnering between agents of the criminal justice and mental health care systems. The role of the criminal justice system in deciding whether to apply legal sanctions or to divert individuals away from the system is based primarily in a balancing of the principles of *police power* (the power and responsibility to protect the safety and welfare of the public) and *parens patriae* (the responsibility to protect persons who are disabled or otherwise unable to care for themselves).

An ideal diversion model includes interventions for offenders with mental illness at all stages of the criminal justice process (Buchan 2003; Munetz and Griffin 2006). The foundation for diverting individuals from the criminal justice system begins with a system of best clinical practices, the importance of which is emphasized in the following quote: "An accessible, comprehensive, effective mental health treatment system focused on the needs of individuals with serious and persistent mental disorders is undoubtedly the most effective means of preventing the criminalization of people with mental illness" (Munetz and Griffin 2006, p. 545).

Assuming that no set of clinical services will be able to prevent all individuals with mental illness from entering the criminal justice system, diversion at any point will require a partnership and genuine collaboration among the law enforcement, mental health care, and judicial systems. In response to the increasing cycle of recidivism, these three systems are beginning to work together to find solutions to the growing crisis. Buchan (2003) described several counties in which a variety of agencies have begun collaborations to respond more effectively to individuals with mental illness. Many other programs have been described by the Council of State Governments, both in their landmark Criminal Justice/Mental Health Consensus Project (Council of State Governments 2002) and on their interactive Consensus Project Web site (http://consensusproject.org). Formal and informal mechanisms can be established to create a positive relationship between the professions. Strategic planning and partnering occur in a variety of ways, including formal agreements with memorandums of understanding, contracts, stakeholder meetings, and sharing of staff persons by two agencies. More informal agreements can include joint meetings with criminal justice and mental health staff representatives, seeking opportunities to find commonalities between criminal justice and mental health care systems, and simply having the name of a contact person from a different system to consult.

A variety of barriers complicate community-based coordinated management of offenders with mental illness. One of the most important barriers is the mutual distrust that exists between mental health care providers and community corrections officials (Roskes et al. 1999, 2005). Mental health professionals often view criminal justice and community corrections personnel as harsh and punitive, whereas criminal justice officials tend to view mental health counselors as "soft" or "bleeding hearts." At times, confidentiality issues are raised as reasons for noncooperation by both health care and criminal justice agencies involved in the care and supervision of such individuals. In addition, mental health agencies have understandable concerns regarding the cost of mental health care for court-ordered clients. Finally, mental health care providers may hesitate to serve individuals with legal problems due to liability concerns.

One suggested intervention for many of these difficulties is cross-training, whereby professionals from each side of the equation are trained together and train each other. These efforts serve to open communication and break down barriers. Another potential solution is the development of specialized or intensive caseloads, in which closer monitoring and more intensive services can be provided to offenders with mental illness. Small specialized caseloads offer community corrections officers an improved opportunity to establish more effective relationships with providers of mental health care (Council of State Governments 2002). A growing literature supports reduced caseloads of 25–35 cases for a mental health specialist officer (Slate et al. 2003, 2004).

Unfortunately, many jurisdictions have little effective diversion capacity, both because services are not ideal and because collaborations between the mental health care and criminal justice systems are difficult and slow to develop. For example, in 1998, the National Institute of Justice, in a study examining the interactions between the mental health care and law enforcement systems, found that less than half of the 176 big-city police departments had specific protocols for handling calls with persons exhibiting emotional disturbances (Psych Job 2000). More recently, Teller et al. (2006) reported that, in 2004, only 70 police departments in the United States had specialized crisis intervention programs designed to assist officers in dealing with situations involving persons with mental illness.

Similarly, many judges and court officers are unfamiliar with the issues raised by defendants with mental illness. Many professionals falsely assume that the insanity defense is a strategy to move defendants with mental illness out of the correctional system, when in fact as few as 1 in 10,000 defendants mounts a successful insanity defense (Janofsky et al. 1996). This lack of awareness, coupled with a legitimate concern for public safety, may lead to a decision that incarceration is the safest course of action. Additionally, many judges and defense attorneys may incorrectly believe that while incarcerated, detainees and inmates will receive medication and other forms of mental health treatment. Because of these basic misunderstandings, courts are likely to treat defendants with mental illness similarly to the way they treat defendants who are not mentally ill, both at trial and at sentencing. Defendants with mental illness frequently do not receive the treatment and support that might prevent recidivism, improve their mental health, and safeguard the community (Denckla and Berman 2001).

Conventional probation supervision and services are often insufficient for offenders with serious mental illness or mental retardation (Skeem and Louden 2006). Many people with mental illness who commit criminal offenses are reluctant to participate in psychiatric treatment. They often miss appointments, refuse medication, and do not fully comply with probation conditions. Moreover, because many mental health agencies are reluctant to accept individuals with criminal histories into their programs, arranging treatment in the community after their release can be difficult (Jemelka et al. 1989). The lack of discharge planning combined with the ineffectiveness of traditional probation may play a role in the quick return of offenders with mental illness to the criminal justice system. Recidivism rates are much higher than average for offenders with mental illness than for those without mental illness. In one study, researchers found that 49% of federal inmates who were mentally ill had three or more prior probations, incarcerations, or arrests, compared with 28% of those without mental illness (Ditton 1999). Of incarcerated individuals with mental illness, only 17% of prison inmates and 11% of jail inmates reported receiving any treatment while incarcerated (Ditton 1999). Furthermore, correctional facilities are often not equipped to handle people who, because of mental disabilities, cannot conform their behaviors to the rules of the institution. As a result, these inmates are more likely to incur disciplinary infractions than inmates who do not have serious mental illness. Additionally, because of their symptoms or their treatment with medications, offenders with mental illness are ineligible for many programs that would permit them to earn time off their sentence through programming or educational credits. These individuals tend to stay in jail longer than other people charged with similar offenses, and the confinement often leads to further decompensation (Bazelon Center for Mental Health Law 2003).

Because of the challenges posed by offenders with mental illness to the criminal justice system and correctional agencies, several innovative approaches are being used to divert such individuals. These approaches include prearrest diversion; postarrest and postbooking diversion; mental health services in jails; specialized mental health courts; and collaboration among probation, parole, and mental health care systems. These approaches seek to address the criminal behaviors of offenders with mental illness and to link the individuals to treatment and services. Interventions are developed to address the underlying causes of an offender's behavior in an effort to prevent recidivism.

Prebooking Diversion

Police Involvement With Individuals With Mental Illness

Law enforcement officers are routinely dispatched to respond to persons with mental illness as a peacekeeping function. In some jurisdictions, these interactions occur on a daily basis. By default, police officers are often the first responders to persons experiencing a psychiatric crisis. Ron Honberg, director of legal services for the National Alliance for the Mentally Ill (now National Alliance on Mental Illness), reportedly said, "In effect, police have become the 'front-line crisis respondents' in many jurisdictions....It's really a reflection of the lack of appropriate treatment options for people" (Psych Job 2000).

During these police encounters, as in others, societal expectations are that if a crime has been committed, an arrest of the alleged perpetrator of that crime is warranted. However, since the late 1980s, the law enforcement profession has been challenged to develop alternatives to arresting and detaining individuals whose illegal behaviors apparently stem from mental illness. This is especially true when the crime committed is a misdemeanor or nuisance crime. In the absence of *formalized* agreements or partnerships, mental health care and law enforcement systems are not likely to find mutually acceptable alternatives to arrest (Psych Job 2000).

Both mental health and law enforcement professionals have speculated that individuals with mental disorders have increasingly been shifted from the mental health care system into the criminal justice system. This phenomenon has been termed the "criminalization of mentally disordered behavior" (Teller et al. 2006; Teplin 2000) and is sometimes referred to as "transinstitutionalization." According to Teplin (2000), the probability of being arrested was 67% greater for people who exhibited signs of a mental disorder than for those without an apparent disorder. Both police and mental health professionals emphasize the role of prebooking diversion as an ideal alternative to the "criminalization" of people with mental illness.

According to the Criminal Justice/Mental Health Consensus Project (Council of State Governments 2002), written protocols should be developed to include approaches to assist officers in effectively managing situations involving individuals with mental illness. These policies should include guidelines for law enforcement to effectively assess the situation, assurance of on-scene safety, developing partnerships with the mental health care and judicial systems, implementation of appropriate responses, and comprehensive training.

Types of Police–Mental Health Collaborations

The first opportunity for prebooking diversion occurs at the scene of the disturbance. On-scene expertise in mental illness is crucial for the effective management of a person with mental illness who is suspected of committing a crime. This type of expertise can be provided by specially trained police officers or by mental health professionals (Council of State Governments 2002). Three major models of police–mental health collaboration have been developed in various jurisdictions around the United States:

1. Specialized police response teams
2. Specialized mental health response teams
3. Blended police and mental health response teams

Although pros and cons exist for each of the various models, each jurisdiction should determine what components best suit its needs. Factors involved in deciding what type of collaboration is most appropriate include geographic size, location, types of law enforcement departments, community resources, and funding. Regardless of the approach accepted, law enforcement officers are responsible for ensuring safety at the scene, recognizing the presence of mental illness, determining whether a serious crime has been committed, and formulating an appropriate disposition (Council of State Governments 2002).

Specialized police response teams. Following the tragic shooting of a person with mental illness by a police officer in Memphis, Tennessee, an innovative program for jail diversion and improvement of police response for mentally ill persons in crisis was developed (Cochran et al. 2000). Patrol officers in Memphis volunteer for and are selected to participate in a 40-hour specialized training program given by mental health care providers, family advocates, and mental health consumer groups. Having completed the training, these patrol officers become part of an elite specialized response team. Rather than having only a few officers available to respond to a crisis (as with other models), the Memphis model has multiple officers trained who are accessible for a quick response. These officers are on duty during all shifts, and they perform routine patrol duties when not involved in the specialized crisis intervention tasks for which they are trained.

Through emergency communication dispatchers, a crisis intervention team officer is deployed to each crisis call. The officer responds to the scene immediately, assesses the situation to determine the nature of the complaint and the degree of risk, ensures safety, and determines the most appropriate intervention (Cochran et al. 2000). A National Institute of Justice study examined the effectiveness of various crisis response models (Steadman et al. 2000). Although the results indicate that all three models diverted persons with mental illness from jail, the Memphis model resulted in the lowest arrest rate from calls involving a subject with mental illness. Similar models exist in other jurisdictions, including Los Angeles, California (Lamb et al. 1995, 2002).

In the Memphis model, one important systems change has been the development of the "no wrong door" or "single point of entry" approach. In researching the problems of access to mental health care for individuals in police custody, the collaborating law enforcement and mental health care systems found that a major barrier faced by police officers was that the treatment systems could easily refuse to accept individuals for clinical and fiscal reasons. For example, when an individual with a psychotic illness who is also high on cocaine is stopped by police for a nuisance crime, such as loitering or trespassing, he or she could be refused by mental health care providers because of the substance use disorder, and could also be refused by substance abuse providers because of having untreated mental illness. This issue was resolved in Memphis by the development of a "single point of entry" to the treatment system at the University of Tennessee Hospital psychiatric emergency department. This entry point permits the police officer to rapidly divert this individual, without arrest, into the treatment system.

Specialized mental health response teams.   In the second model, mental health clinicians, who are typically part of the local mental health service system, respond in pairs to persons in crisis. The mobile response teams work to develop a relationship with the police department (Cochran et al. 2000). The mobile crisis team can be dispatched through a hotline, by the local mental health authority, or by police or emergency dispatchers, or the team can be called directly by police officers. If a crime has not been committed, the mobile crisis team can provide transportation to a community crisis bed program, hospital, or other mental health care facility (Council of State Governments 2002).

Blended police and mental health response teams. A blended response model includes pairing a police officer with a civilian mental health professional. The civilian clinician rides along with officers as part of a specialized team or meets the officer on the scene once it has been deemed safe (Council of State Governments 2002). The crisis team can be dispatched through the emergency communication dispatchers, a crisis hotline, or the mental health authority.

The Baltimore County (Maryland) model. Baltimore County Crisis Response was developed through the partnership of the local mental health care authority, police department, and a community mental health care provider. Similar to the Memphis model, clinical and police members of the Baltimore County mobile crisis team participate together in a specialized 40-hour training program. In addition, team members receive joint training in police officer survival tactics. This joint training in mental health and law enforcement results in an innovative, hybrid mobile crisis team model. A first responder team composed of police officers and mental health professionals, both dressed in similar street attire, responds together in an unmarked police car. If the situation can be stabilized following an initial response by the police–mental health team, a separate mental health team (composed only of clinicians) provides follow-up services for a period of 10 days to ensure that the person in crisis is connected to mental health services.

Establishing a Police–Mental Health Collaboration Program

Jurisdictions interested in improving overall police response and increasing the likelihood of diversion of offenders with mental illness from the criminal justice system can begin by establishing cross-training programs between law enforcement and mental health professionals (Council of State Governments 2002). Police training should be provided in three forums: academy level upon admission to the police department; mandatory annual in-service; and specialized programs (elective participation in advanced training on mental illness). Training should include, at a minimum, an overview of mental illness, substance abuse, and psychotropic medications; communication/crisis de-escalation techniques; role-playing of actual responses; and an overview of treatment resources (Cochran et al. 2000). The purpose of training officers is not for them to become diagnosticians, but rather to educate them about mental illness and ways in which mental illness may contribute to criminal activity (Council of State Governments 2002). Cross-training enhances police officers' knowledge of mental illness, improves mutual understanding with the mental health system, and provides officers with an understanding of the rationale behind and the importance of implementing the least restrictive alternative possible to prevent the unnecessary incarceration of a mentally ill person in crisis. Psychiatrists and other mental health care providers are encouraged to participate in this training and can thereby contribute to improved communication between clinicians and officers. This improved communication will ultimately lead to an increase in diversion and a reduction in the criminalization of behaviors related to mental illness. Additionally, administrators of mental health and law enforcement agencies can work together to improve the systemic response as demonstrated by the Memphis "no wrong door" approach (Cochran et al. 2000).

Outcomes

Police–mental health collaborations have demonstrated improved outcomes on a variety of measures. For example, these joint efforts have reduced the arrest rates from incidents of police intervention in situations involving citizens with mental illness. A 21% arrest rate occurs with nonspecialized police interventions (Sheridan and Teplin 1981), whereas a 2%–13% arrest rate results when the police response involves a specialized, collaborative model (Lamb et al. 1995; Steadman et al. 2000). In Los Angeles in 2001, less than 2% of police–mental health evaluations resulted in an arrest (114 arrests in 6,575 interventions) (Pacific Clinics 2002).

Police time is also reduced in such models. For example, in Los Angeles, the initial responding nonspecialized officers are able to transfer control of the situation to the specialized team within 40 minutes, compared with a total time of 3.2 hours required for the average involuntary civil commitment (Pacific Clinics 2002).

Postbooking, Pretrial Diversion

Background

Diversion can be accomplished at a variety of points once a person has been arrested and processed into the criminal justice system (postbooking). The first possibility for diversion is upon the completion of the book-

ing process, when the commissioner or magistrate is setting bail or permitting release of the defendant on recognizance. During this hearing,
the commissioner can refer a defendant to a mental health professional
or team for consideration for diversion. Based on the findings of the evaluation, a commissioner has the authority to release a defendant, pending
trial, under special conditions, which may require a mental health treatment plan. To remain at liberty, the defendant must comply with these
conditions until trial. Monitoring of the treatment plan can be assigned
to a monitoring agency to ensure that the defendant is in fact following
the order for release. A consequence of noncompliance can be a revocation of the recognizance order and incarceration pending trial. Oversight
of the plan and support of the individual are often critical in helping the
defendant to remain motivated and engaged in treatment.

A second opportunity for postbooking diversion can occur at the formal bail review, at which time a judge is reconsidering the bail amount
or release with or without conditions. This process is consistent with the
pretrial process described above. Often the diversion team is consulted
by the court, defense counsel, prosecutors, or correctional staff.

A different mechanism for postbooking diversion requires the cooperation of the prosecutor's office. In this case, an accelerated hearing
date is sought for the defendant with mental illness. Bringing the defendant before the court earlier than the scheduled court date allows for
expedited release if the court is in agreement with the plan. This accelerated processing may help such a defendant remain engaged in prearrest community services and benefits that would be lost if he or she were
forced to spend more time incarcerated pending trial.

Monitoring is a key component of any successful diversion program
in that it allows the court to feel confident that the diverted defendant or
probationer is complying with conditions of release. Monitoring agencies can include a general or trained probation agent or officer and/or a
clinical team employed by the court and tasked with monitoring compliance and ensuring adequate and appropriate clinical care.

According to the National GAINS Center (2008), as of mid-2007, ap-
proximately 500 jail diversion programs were in operation in the United
States. Key elements of successful diversion programs are included in
Table 2–1.

The Forensic Alternative Services Team in Baltimore

The Forensic Alternative Services Team (FAST) is a program run under
the auspices of the Medical Service of the Circuit Court of Maryland for
Baltimore. The program is grant funded through Baltimore Mental
Health Systems, the mental health authority for the city, and has been in

---

TABLE 2–1. Key elements of successful diversion programs

The target group is defined.

Individuals are identified as early as possible in criminal justice processing.

Community-based treatment alternatives are negotiated in lieu of incarceration.

Linkages are made to comprehensive systems of care and an appropriate level of supervision consistent with the disposition of the criminal case.

Source. Adapted from National GAINS Center 2009.

---

operation since approximately 1995. Staffing includes six licensed clinicians and one administrative assistant. The program diverts defendants at the booking/bail review phase, at accelerated trial dates, and at existing trial dates. Occasionally, the team is asked to consider a sentence modification to divert previously sentenced defendants to the Division of Corrections, which could be considered postsentence diversion. Staff personnel are located in the Baltimore jails and in two of the three district courts (the lower-level trial court) in the city. FAST can also be called to the circuit court (the higher-level trial court, and the venue for all jury trials in Maryland) to divert the offender as needed. Criteria for entry into FAST are outlined in Table 2–2.

As with most diversion programs, FAST prefers the defendant's participation in the diversion agreement to be voluntary. A level of coercion on the part of the court to "convince" the defendant to accept the conditions of release may occur under certain circumstances. To determine program eligibility, the clinician conducts psychosocial evaluations, during which the clinician balances individual defendant characteristics and history, program criteria, and community safety risks. If the defendant is eligible, an individualized treatment plan is created and offered to the court at the designated hearing. With the court's approval, the defendant is released under court order to comply with the terms of the release agreement.

The clinician who presents the original treatment plan to the court becomes the monitor of the defendant's compliance with release conditions. The clinician typically meets with the defendant and receives written and telephone documentation from the community mental health care provider. The clinician also provides support to the community providers by making home visits, encouraging compliance, and helping to modify plans when needed. If the defendant does not adhere to the

TABLE 2–2.   Criteria for entry into FAST program

Offender is 18 years or older.

Offender is diagnosed with major mental illness and/or trauma-related illness.

Offense level is relatively minor.

Offender is amenable to community-based treatment.

Offender is willing to participate in community supervision by FAST staff.

Note.   FAST=Forensic Alternative Services Team (Baltimore, Maryland).

terms of his or her agreement, FAST personnel respond quickly and the presiding judge is notified. Depending on the stage at which the defendant was diverted to community treatment, the responses by FAST can include an upgrade in the level of mental health or substance abuse treatment, a request for a bail revocation, or a recommendation for probation revocation. FAST presents information to the court regarding compliance, and the court may modify the original disposition.

Clinical Case 2–1

Mr. J is a 46-year-old man who was observed demonstrating clear signs of mental illness in the hallway of the courthouse by a FAST clinician (the mental health worker in the courthouse). When approached, Mr. J stated that he thought he was supposed to be in court but was not sure where. The FAST clinician determined that Mr. J was 2 days late for a court hearing on a trespassing charge, for which the judge had issued a bench warrant. With the assistance of the public defender, the judge agreed to recall the bench warrant. A new court date was assigned.

In the interim, Mr. J was evaluated as having bipolar disorder and AIDS dementia. Given his continued behavioral disorder, he required the assistance of the FAST clinician to appear for and sit through his hearing several weeks later. At that time, the case was postponed for 90 days to give the FAST clinician time to obtain appropriate treatment. The treatment plan ultimately developed included supportive housing, psychiatric and medical care, mobile treatment, and a day program (with transportation). Mr. J responded well to these interventions, and the case was dismissed at the time of the postponed hearing.

FAST continues to face challenges, primarily regarding the inability of the program to meet the demands and difficulties of serving individuals with comorbid mental illness and substance use disorders. Finally, supervised housing with an appropriate level of program structure is extremely limited. These shortcomings present the court, and FAST by extension, with the dilemma of needing to achieve rapid case disposition but being unable to do so because of inadequate community resources.

Outcomes and Caveats

Data regarding the effectiveness of jail diversion programs are beginning to emerge. The Department of Health and Human Services, through the Substance Abuse and Mental Health Services Administration, has undertaken a multisite study of jail diversion programs across the country (Steadman et al. 1999b). Although the evaluation of the effectiveness of jail diversion is a complex task (Draine and Solomon 1999), initial results indicate that jail diversion 1) decreases jail time and 2) results in no increase in arrest rates or recidivism, but, based on available evidence, 3) does not appear to be associated with clinical or social improvements (F. Osher, personal communication, December 1, 2003; Steadman et al. 1999a). The most parsimonious explanation of these findings is that unless improvements are made in the mental health and social service system to which people are diverted and unless coordination is improved between the institutional and community care systems, jail diversion programs have only limited impact on the lives of people with mental illness. This is often termed the "Diversion to what?" question. However, the importance of these data should not be minimized, because jail time alone is traumatizing for many, and reducing it has some value. That this reduction in incarceration time occurs without an apparent decrease in public safety, even in the absence of positive clinical outcomes, is cause for optimism.

Mental Health Courts

Origin and Rationale

Over the previous few decades, a few jurisdictions have made attempts to manage defendants with mental illness in a less punitive and more therapeutic way. In the 1960s, courts in Chicago and New York practiced what was known as "therapeutic disposition" of such cases. Chicago courts could order psychiatric screening, allow psychiatrists and social workers to make sentencing suggestions, and give nonpenal sentences such as outpatient treatment or civil commitment to offenders with mental illness. Often, when the referrals resulted in these therapeutic dispositions, the criminal charges were dismissed (Mathews 1970).

In New York, offenders with mental illness were diverted to health care treatment at the time of arrest and avoided the courts entirely. Police officers had the option of taking arrestees to Bellevue or Elmhurst hospitals' prison wards, which were administered by the Department of Corrections and which linked the mental health and criminal justice systems' efforts on behalf of these individuals. The court could also refer defendants for competency to stand trial and criminal responsibility evaluations. Under these orders, the hospital treatment team prepared a report that answered the court-ordered legal question and made recommendations regarding appropriate treatment (Mathews 1970).

These early initiatives were the precursors to the modern mental health court. Like other diversion programs, mental health courts seek not only to address the criminal behaviors of the defendant with mental illness but also to link the defendant to treatment and services. These specialty courts attempt to address the underlying problems of each individual defendant in an effort to prevent recidivism and to promote ongoing connection to community mental health services.

Development of Mental Health Courts

Mental health courts are modeled after the drug courts created in southern Florida in the early 1990s (Denckla and Berman 2001). As with approaches adopted by the drug court model, the mental health court judge takes a hands-on role in managing the defendant's case and uses treatment as a public safety tool rather than relying solely on incarceration, fines, or other forms of punishment (Goldkamp and Irons-Guynn 2000). Under this new model, mental health courts attempt to attack the root of the problem by focusing on reasons that underlie why the defendant became involved in the criminal justice system (Goldkamp and Irons-Guynn 2000). The first mental health court began operation in Broward County, Florida, in 1997. Since that time, these courts have proliferated around the country in recognition of the need for this type of initiative. In 2000, the U.S. Congress passed America's Law Enforcement and Mental Health Project Act (Public Law 106-515), allowing local jurisdictions to receive federal funds to create or expand existing mental health courts (Bazelon Center for Mental Health Law 2003).

The mental health court model is based on the premise that the criminal and juvenile justice systems are ineffective providers of mental health services. The rationale behind the development of this specialized court system is twofold: 1) a mental health court can properly address the mental illness underlying a criminal defendant's actions, and 2) this specialty court can assign an appropriate treatment for that criminal defendant (Bazelon Center for Mental Health Law 2003). Rather than imprisoning or fining the defendant with mental illness, the mental health court can provide that individual with psychiatric treatment and other necessary services. With such assistance, the system aspires to address each defendant's mental illness and thereby hopes to reduce the recidivism of defendants with mental illness. Unlike the regular criminal court, the mental health court seeks to help the defendant who is mentally ill on a long-term basis. Once the defendant is in the program, the court retains jurisdiction over him or her, enabling the judge to monitor the defendant's progress until the completion of the program by the offender (Goldkamp and Irons-Guynn 2000).

Screening and Evaluation for Mental Health Court Admission

All mental health courts share common features. The identification of potential candidates for the mental health court requires screening and referrals of defendants soon after their arrests. This initial stage is vital if the offender is to be offered a timely opportunity to participate in the program. Newly incarcerated detainees must be screened for mental illness within 24–48 hours of their entry into the criminal justice system (Goldkamp and Irons-Guynn 2000). Jail staff, family members, and defense attorneys are generally responsible for identification of appropriate candidates (Denckla and Berman 2001).

After being identified as potentially eligible, these offenders must be evaluated to determine if their illness is severe enough to qualify for services and if they have a history of violence. Criteria for "serious mental illness" vary from state to state. In some jurisdictions, participants must have organic brain impairment, a developmental disability, or an Axis I diagnosis as assessed under the *Diagnostic and Statistical Manual of Mental Disorders*, 4th Edition, Text Revision (American Psychiatric Association 2000a). In other jurisdictions (e.g., King County, Washington), the defendant need only have a diagnosis of mental illness or obvious signs of serious mental illness (Goldkamp and Irons-Guynn 2000). In many mental health courts, a history of a violent offense would exclude a potential candidate for consideration for entry, although exceptions to this approach exist, most notably the Nathaniel Project in New York (Council of State Governments 2002).

The second factor considered in determining eligibility is the nature of the crime with which the defendant is charged. Most jurisdictions limit eligibility to those persons with mental illness who are charged with a nonviolent misdemeanor, although a few jurisdictions allow participation of individuals with a nonviolent felony charge. The target populations of these courts include perpetrators of minor crimes, generally misdemeanors or "quality of life" ordinance violations, such as disorderly conduct. Either the mental health court judge or the treatment team has the final decision about eligibility (Goldkamp and Irons-Guynn 2000).

Finally, all mental health courts require a defendant's voluntary assent or consent to participation. As discussed in detail below, this consent may be "coerced" or negotiated rather than truly voluntary.

Mental Health Court Program

Entry into a mental health court program varies by jurisdiction and generally occurs either prior to or after conviction. Some jurisdictions use a nonconviction approach, in which the person with mental illness is sentenced before the case is adjudicated; if the defendant completes the program, the charges may be dismissed. Other jurisdictions require the defendant to plead guilty before entering the program; however, the plea may be withdrawn or expunged upon successful completion. Another approach is to allow a deferred adjudication or deferred sentence to be entered pending completion of the program (Goldkamp and Irons-Guynn 2000).

Once the defendant is admitted into the mental health court program, a treatment team oversees the case. This treatment team may include the judge, probation officers, clinical supervisors or coordinators, case managers, defense attorneys and prosecutors, and jail liaisons, each of whom is accountable to the court. This team works together to link the participants with appropriate treatment services, often including residential or other supportive housing placements. The participation of the court ensures the presence of a central figure to coordinate these services, monitor the defendant's progress, and provide accountability for the treatment process. The judge presides formally over any legal matters at the entry and completion stages of the process. The judge also meets routinely with the participant and provides rewards or sanctions as appropriate. Sanctions may be of a punitive nature (e.g., time in jail) or of therapeutic orientation (e.g., increased intensity of treatment). Treatment providers in such settings can assist judges in determining whether therapeutic approaches or criminal justice sanctions are indicated. Most mental health court programs last from 12 to 18 months and have a subsequent probation period (Goldkamp and Irons-Guynn 2000).

Outcomes and Caveats

The development of mental health courts reflects a change in attitude in the criminal justice system toward offenders with mental illness. These mental health courts represent a fundamental philosophical shift away from the traditional adversarial "process and punish" orientation of the judiciary to a more hands-on therapeutic jurisprudence approach.

The key intervention provided by mental health courts is not identifying and processing defendants, but connecting them to treatment.

Accordingly, whichever diagnoses the court decides to include, it must consider whether the corresponding treatment is available in the community and how that treatment will be accessed and monitored (Bureau of Justice Assistance 2005). For example, the Bazelon Center for Mental Health Law, in a review of 20 mental health courts, concluded that no diversion or alternative disposition program can be effective unless it makes available the services and supports that individuals with serious mental illness need to live in the community (Selzer 2005).

Additionally, clinical outcome research and program evaluation are required to determine if mental health courts are having the desired effect or if, as has been found in some studies of intensive supervision probation (Draine and Solomon 1994; Solomon et al. 1994), the increased focus on these defendants may result in their being more likely to remain involved in the criminal justice system. Although drug courts have been operating for nearly 20 years and have been the subject of more than 100 evaluations, only recently have the research designs and methods approached scientific standards for reliability and validity (Wolff and Pogorzelski 2005). Because mental health courts are new to the problem-solving court arena, they can benefit from the evolution of the drug court evaluation methodology.

The design of mental health courts is not research based, however, so conducting objective scientific studies of their effectiveness is difficult. Only recently have courts realized that collecting and analyzing outcome data can provide empirical verification of the positive impact of the mental health court. Some studies are under way, and more are being planned, to better understand the operation and impact of mental health courts (Bureau of Justice Assistance 2005; Redlich et al. 2005). An evaluation of the Broward County mental health court measured success in terms of involvement in treatment. The study found that the portion of participants engaged in treatment increased from 36% in the 8 months prior to the first mental health court appearance to 53% during the 8 months following that appearance; individuals in a comparison group undergoing regular case processing did not show any change between equivalent periods (29% and 28%, respectively) (Boothroyd et al. 2003; O'Keefe 2006).

A study involving the mental health court in Santa Barbara, California, incorporated a prospective, randomized experimental design and evaluated for broader measures of success. In the study, 235 defendants were randomly assigned either to the mental health court or to standard case processing, and outcomes were tracked over a 2-year follow-up period. Results indicated that a majority of the defendants in both study groups spent less time in jail and showed improved psychosocial functioning from preenrollment to postenrollment periods. However, no differences were found when the two experimental groups were compared (Cosden et al. 2003). In contrast, a study in San Francisco found that mental health court involvement "was associated with longer time without any new criminal charges or charges for violent crimes" and that "successful completion of the mental health court program was associated with maintenance of reductions in recidivism and violence after graduates were no longer under supervision of the mental health court" (McNeil and Binder 2007, p. 1395). Finally, in a study in Allegheny County, Pennsylvania, findings indicated that a mental health court did not increase costs to the jurisdiction in the short term (months), and suggested that over the long term, the jurisdiction may experience a cost saving when both mental health care and criminal justice costs are considered (Ridgely et al. 2007). Taken together, these studies suggest that mental health courts may improve criminal justice outcomes and that they may do so in a cost-effective fashion. However, because every mental health court program is different, findings from one setting cannot be applied to any other.

More research is needed to determine whether mental health courts are truly succeeding in preventing recidivism or whether the treatment programs are successful in helping offenders with mental illness stabilize in the community. Such alternative methods should continue to be considered, explored, and modified. Jurisdictions considering adopting a mental health court model are encouraged to build a program that includes evaluation components, so that a true understanding of the effectiveness of the intervention can be developed.

SENTENCED INDIVIDUALS

Presentence Investigation

The sentencing of defendants varies by jurisdiction. Historically, in the 1920s and 1930s, a medical model of corrections developed in which sentencing was based on a defendant's individual characteristics rather than the crime committed. During that time, the use of a presentence investigation (PSI) report came into common use. The two basic approaches to PSI reports are offender based and offense based. An offender-based PSI report is prepared for the sentencing court to describe the offender and to offer background information to be used by the judge in making sentencing decisions. The philosophy behind this approach to the PSI report is that individualized factors in each defendant's life and background are useful in determining his or her amenability to rehabilitation and community integration. As sentencing approaches became more punitive during the 1950s and 1960s, determinate sentences with less judicial discretion were emphasized. Guideline sentencing, legislated in a more conservative social environment, encouraged more uniform punishment for offenders. In addition, the individuality of offenders was felt to be less important in sentencing than the nature of the offense and the role of the convicted offender in that offense. This philosophy gave rise to the offense-based PSI report, wherein factors related to the offense itself and the offender's involvement in it became more relevant, while factors related to the offender himself or herself became relatively less important in determining the sentence (Center on Juvenile and Criminal Justice 2002).

In jurisdictions that continue to allow for substantial judicial discretion in sentencing, or in cases in which diminished capacity may be at issue, mental health evaluations are beneficial supplements to PSI reports. Mental health evaluations are usually requested by defendants seeking to establish mental illness as a mitigating factor in the commission of an offense, to rebut expert testimony by the state, or to assist in determining postsentence treatment requirements in the community (U.S. Sentencing Commission 2007). Such evaluations may be used by judges to determine appropriateness for probation with mandated community treatment as opposed to (or in addition to) a term of incarceration. As an example, federal probation officers, in the preparation of a PSI in which mental health is to be raised as a possible mitigating factor arguing for release, base a recommendation for release on the following factors (Federal Judicial Center 2003):

1. Does the severity of the mental illness have an impact on managing risk or compliance with standard conditions of release?
2. Does a disorder create a risk issue?
3. Is an offender willing to submit voluntarily to treatment?

These reports often play a major role in the development of specialized conditions of probation or, eventually, parole.

Court-mandated supervision of an offender in a community setting has been described as "a means to engage the offender [in] improving compliance with general societal norms, including conditions of release" (Taxman 2002, p. 20). For positive outcomes, interventions and supervision strategies must address each individual's specific needs. Ideally, these individuals should be provided with a plan that integrates or coordinates a variety of services and approaches, including psychiatric treatment, psychotherapy, substance use treatment, case management, and rehabilitative (including psychosocial, vocational, and residential) services.

Types of Postconviction Release

Judges can impose a term of *probation* as an alternative to incarceration for defendants convicted of minor crimes. Probation can also be imposed before judgment, in cases where sentencing is offered before a trial to offer a defendant a chance to reform. In each of these cases, conditions are imposed on the defendant. The defendant must comply with the conditions or return to court for a violation of probation hearing. *Parole*, by contrast, is a form of early release from jail or prison, with conditions similar to those of probation imposed on the offender. Parole is affirmatively granted by an official body (often called a parole commission or parole board), and an offender must demonstrate a level of compliance with conditions of incarceration and a degree of readiness to return to the community. Finally, in many jurisdictions, incarcerated individuals can be released early based on behavioral requirements during their time in jail or prison. This form of release is often called *mandatory* or *supervised release*. This form of release is distinguished from parole in that it is a passive process. In other words, no decision is made about an individual defendant. Instead, "good time" can be earned based on behavior within the correctional setting, and additional time can be earned by participation in programs while incarcerated, based on statutorily defined calculations. Noncompliance with conditions of parole or supervised release can result in a return to incarceration and imposition of the remainder of the sentence.

In all of these forms of release, standard and special conditions may be imposed. Examples of standard and special conditions are listed in Table 2–3.

Collaborative Programs

Programs that have demonstrated success in the management of court-ordered individuals have a high degree of collaboration and cross-training (Roskes and Feldman 1999; Roskes et al. 1999; Skeem and Louden 2006; Slate et al. 2003). These programs include personnel from a variety of treatment disciplines, including psychiatrists, nurses, social workers, case managers, addiction counselors, and rehabilitation staff, as well as community corrections officials. In addition, these programs have a highly developed treatment-first orientation. A treatment-first philosophy forces providers from both mental health and criminal justice to seek a treatment intervention when a client is doing poorly rather than jumping quickly to a punitive or correctional intervention. Often, this approach

TABLE 2–3. Potential release conditions

Standard conditions	Special conditions
Living situation	Participation in mental health assessment and, if appropriate, treatment
Work obligations	
Reporting to supervising agency or officer	
	Participation in substance abuse assessment and, if appropriate, treatment
Payment of fees	
Avoidance of firearms	Provision of urine specimens
Avoidance of drugs	Compliance with prescribed medications
Obedience to the law	
	Avoidance of victim
	Registration as a sex offender
	Participation in anger management program

takes the form of a good cop/bad cop conversation with a client, in which the client is placed in a forced-choice situation. Roskes et al. (1999) described a number of successful interventions under this paradigm.

Clinical Case 2–2

Mr. A, a 45-year-old man with bipolar disorder and cocaine dependence, was on parole, having been convicted of bank robbery a number of years before. He had spent about 8 years in prison prior to his first parole. He was reincarcerated after only 8 months in the community, having had a relapse in cocaine use and discontinued his psychiatric treatment. He had two more cycles of release and reincarceration. The latest parole was by far the most successful, lasting over 2 years.

He presented one day with racing thoughts, disorganized thinking, and denial of his illness. He repeatedly denied cocaine use and insisted that he was taking his medications, lithium and olanzapine, as prescribed. He readily agreed to provide urine and blood samples to confirm his abstinence and compliance with the medication regimen. Because his psychiatrist was concerned, he contacted Mr. A's parole officer, who came to the clinic. The psychiatrist offered Mr. A a voluntary hospitalization in an attempt to intervene in an apparent manic decompensation. Mr. A refused. The parole officer indicated that given what he was seeing, he had serious concerns about Mr. A's adherence to treatment and compliance with other conditions of his release. The probation officer said to Mr. A, "If you don't go into the

hospital, I will have to give some serious thought to seeking a revocation of your parole. I don't want you to go back to prison, but..." After
some discussion, it became apparent that Mr. A was concerned about
not being home the following week when his disability check was due
to come in the mail. He stated, "Where I live, if you aren't home when
your check comes, you won't ever see that check."

Given Mr. A's reality-based concerns, the psychiatrist offered Mr. A
a course of partial hospitalization. Mr. A agreed and was accepted into
a local partial program, where his medications were readjusted. The
decompensation resolved in about 4 weeks, and Mr. A continued his
outpatient treatment. He remained in the community, fully compliant
with the conditions of his parole, for 3 more years, until he died of a
sudden heart attack.

At times, relationships between mental health care providers and community corrections can be formalized through contractual agreements.
The federal probation system has been at the forefront in the development
of the specialized probation officer. In 1978, the Administrative Office of
the U.S. Courts was authorized by federal legislation to contract for drug
treatment services. This contractual capacity was expanded to include
mental health treatment. Later, the authority to enter into such contracts
was delegated by federal district courts to each local or regional probation
office, thus permitting flexibility in meeting the needs of each office
(Hughes and Henkel 1997). Over time, the federal probation offices developed both mental health and substance abuse specialists, among others
(Freitas 1997). In some jurisdictions, informal relationships develop between parole and probation officers and mental health care providers or
agencies. These agencies work with clients and come to view the officer as
another referral source.

SPECIAL TOPICS

Medication Management of the
Court-Ordered Outpatient

Many, if not most, individuals who are court ordered to community treatment will be required by that court order to take medication as prescribed. Some court orders may be much more specific, including the
type or name of the medication and even the dosage or a dosage range.
Highly specific court orders are less preferable than court orders written
with more general requirements, because the specific court order precludes the clinician from reacting to changes in the individual patient's
clinical condition. In addition, a specific court order eliminates the col-

laborative negotiation about medication issues that must take place in community care between the doctor and the patient.

In the community care of court-ordered patients, a common strategy to ensure that these patients follow their medication regimen is the use of long-acting intramuscular antipsychotics. In addition, for appropriate patients, medications that require serum monitoring of therapeutic concentrations can be useful in that the blood level serves as a proxy for medication compliance.

Newer antipsychotics (e.g., risperidone, olanzapine, quetiapine, ziprasidone, aripiprazole) are often preferred by patients due to their improved tolerability. Although not without disadvantages, when used in appropriate cases, these medications can lead to more successful community tenure of court-ordered patients. Clozapine, in addition to successfully treating many patients with previously treatment-resistant psychosis, may have a specific neurochemical role in the treatment of aggression (Hector 1998; Spivak et al. 1997). One study identified a reduction in arrest rates of patients with psychotic disorders taking clozapine compared with those taking other antipsychotics (Frankle et al. 2001). As the authors noted, the requirement for regular blood testing for patients taking clozapine necessitates frequent contact with mental health care providers; this frequent contact may result in an improved therapeutic alliance, closer monitoring, and an improved ability to detect early decompensations that might have led to recurrent criminal behaviors if undetected.

Working With the Insanity Acquittee in the Community

Although not technically a part of the correctional system, the insanity defense system mirrors the criminal justice system in many ways. However, several key differences may be relevant to the community provider working with such patients.

The similarities begin at the onset of the legal process. An individual is charged with a crime, but rather than pleading not guilty or engaging in a plea bargaining process, the individual, his or her attorney, other legal actors including the judge or even the prosecuting attorney, or correctional staff raise concerns regarding mental health issues. This may happen at any point prior to trial and may result in a competency to stand trial assessment. Some individuals, but remarkably few, plead insanity in those states permitting such a defense. For example, Janofsky et al. (1996) found that only 190 defendants out of more than 60,000 (0.3%) indictments in Baltimore during 1991 entered a plea of insanity. Nearly all withdrew the plea prior to trial. Many fewer will be adjudicated as "not guilty by reason of insanity" (NGRI) or "not criminally responsible." These investigators also reported that only eight defendants (0.01%) were ultimately adjudicated not criminally responsible by reason of mental disease or defect.

Upon this adjudication, the defendant is transferred out of the criminal justice system and into the mental health system, often to a forensic high-security hospital that has many of the same security issues that apply to jails and prisons. Maryland's statute governing length of confinement of NGRI acquittees is characteristic of these confinement laws. According to this statute, the NGRI acquittee is hospitalized until he or she is no longer "a danger, as a result of mental disorder or mental retardation, to self or to the person or property of others if discharged" [Maryland Annotated Code, Criminal Procedure Article, § 3-114(b) 2009]. Unlike a sentence to prison, in which the term of confinement is defined, confinement to a psychiatric hospital subsequent to a successful insanity defense may be indeterminate and does not depend on the nature of the crime committed (*Jones v. United States* 1983). However, some states, such as Oregon, have restricted the maximum length of criminal hospital commitment to the maximum prison sentence a defendant could have received for the offense (Oregon Advocacy Center 2001).

States vary in their approach to conditional release of NGRI acquittees. Some states, such as Maryland, use a judicial process, in which the burden is on the detained patient to demonstrate by a preponderance of the evidence that, if released, he or she would not pose "a danger, as a result of mental disorder or mental retardation, to self or to the person or property of others" (Maryland Annotated Code 2009). Other states, such as Oregon, commit the individual determined insane under state law to the supervision of an administrative board. This board, which in Oregon is termed the Psychiatric Security Review Board, bears responsibility for all decisions as to release and rehospitalization (Oregon Advocacy Center 2001).

Upon release from a criminal hospital commitment, the individual is subject to a variety of conditions, which generally include a specified housing arrangement and required participation in mental health and substance abuse treatment, as well as many of the standard conditions of probation, described above. Clinicians working with such individuals in community settings may have a dual role as clinical providers and as agents of public safety, although in some areas, these roles are functionally separate. This situation is functionally identical to working with individuals who are court ordered to treatment by judges as a condition of probation or by parole boards as a condition of parole or supervised release (see subsection "Types of Postconviction Release" earlier in this chapter).

Managing Individuals With Complex Comorbidities

One of the issues facing all community mental health care providers is the difficulty of working with people who have mental illness as well as comorbid conditions. In forensic populations, as noted previously, a significant majority of individuals with mental illness also have substance use disorders. For example, in a study of 16 individuals under federal supervision requiring psychiatric treatment, 94% had comorbid mental illness and addiction (Roskes and Feldman 1999). These disorders must be managed in an integrated fashion in community settings to maximize the chances for the individual to succeed in his or her community placement (Minkoff 2001; Pita and Spaniol 2002). Ideally, a single program should integrate the treatment of the mental illness and substance use disorders. Random urine screens can be extremely helpful in ensuring that the patient is remaining abstinent and can also serve as a tool to maintain a connection between the patient and the clinical program.

Medical comorbidity is also very common among offenders with mental illness. Roskes and Feldman (1999) found that nearly 60% of the individuals in their study had a variety of medical problems, ranging from quiescent hepatitis C infection to recurrent metastatic lung cancer. The role of the psychiatrist and other members of the mental health team, in both assisting in the diagnosis and ensuring adequate medical care, is significant and often undervalued in community mental health settings.

Coercive Treatment in a Community Setting

Like clinicians working in correctional institutions, those working with patients under a court order may find themselves in a dual agency role when providing mandated treatment. Treatment under any kind of court order presents moral and ethical dilemmas unique to the coerced treatment paradigm (Monahan et al. 2003, 2005). When working in a court-mandated treatment setting, clinicians must recognize that the therapeutic relationship is itself influenced by the coercive nature of the court order that brings the patient into treatment. This coercion can be used to assist the patient in achieving his or her goals, such as obtaining stable housing (which is often initially court mandated) or avoiding a return to jail, prison, or the hospital. Notably, in some circumstances outside of a criminal justice setting, treatment must be, and ethically is, provided against a patient's stated desires (see, e.g., Guarda et al. 2007).

Clinicians serving court-ordered clients serve two masters: the patient and the public safety monitoring agency (Packard 1989). Such dual agency dilemmas can arise in several ways:

- A provider may find that a patient has encountered legal problems, and the court may order compliance with ongoing treatment. This provider now serves as a public safety agent in addition to having the preexisting purely clinical role.
- A forensic evaluator may recommend treatment to the court, and then the court may order the defendant to undergo that treatment with the evaluator.
- A clinician providing court-mandated treatment may be asked to answer ongoing public safety questions or to testify regarding public safety issues.

The last item above is probably the most common situation and is the only one that a clinician working with court-ordered patients should expect as a matter of course. In these treatment situations, the clinician must be responsive to questions from public safety agents regarding the patient's attendance, adherence to treatment requirements, and maintenance of sobriety. Many public safety agencies send regular questionnaires to providers treating court-ordered patients and expect feedback on these questionnaires. These providers must provide patients with ongoing information regarding communication between the provider and the public safety agency and obtain ongoing consent for that communication. Refusal to give such consent should be clarified with the patient, and the patient should be made aware that the clinician will be required to report the patient's refusal to consent to information transfer.

Clearly, treatment under these paradigms may be coercive. Many individuals come to treatment under these court orders as less than fully willing participants, and the provider faces a challenge in engaging such clients. The degree of coercion even among court-ordered patients is rather variable, however. For example, individuals found not guilty by reason of insanity and then conditionally released generally will not be released until they assent to ongoing care in the community. In contrast, people released on probation may not have undergone nearly as much institutionally based treatment. In our experience, such individuals are much more likely to test the clinician's ability to provide structure and safety because they have not received the intensive treatment and psychoeducation in the jail or while released on bail awaiting trial. Indirect support for this concept comes from the very low rate of rearrest (3.4%–7.8% per year) among conditionally released NGRI acquittees (Wiederanders et al. 1997). In comparison, during 2006, half of all parolees were rearrested or otherwise had an unsatisfactory end to their parole (Glaze and Bonczar 2008). Of note, however, is that some research is demonstrating that 1) recidivism among offenders with mental illness is lower than among offenders without mental illness and 2) the risk factors for recidivism are no different for individuals with mental illness than for those without mental illness (Bonta et al. 1997).

The Testifying Clinician

At times, clinicians caring for individuals under court order may be called to testify regarding a patient. Most of the time, the clinician is being asked to testify as a fact witness—that is, to advise the court as to details of compliance with treatment as defined by the court order requiring that treatment. On less frequent occasions, the clinician may be asked to provide opinion testimony as an expert witness. In general, clinicians working with court-ordered patients should testify only under court order and should strenuously attempt to avoid being drawn into other, nonmandatory witness roles.

Testifying as a fact witness generally raises no issues for the treating clinician, provided that the clinician has advised the patient of the need to share information with the court or the supervising agency from the outset of the court-ordered treatment and on a frequent basis during that treatment. Requests for such testimony may be built into the court order, which may require periodic reports to the court or an administrative body such as a Psychiatric Security Review Board (this may happen, e.g., in a mental health court model or in a supervised release model that requires monthly or quarterly reports). Alternatively, a clinician may be called only when things are going badly. Most patients treated under this rubric are aware of the need for such information sharing. When done well, this open sharing of information, with the consent of the patient, serves to improve the care delivered to the patient and to result in improved chances for successful community treatment (Heilbrun and Griffin 1998).

Assuming the role of an expert witness raises more difficult ethical issues, because the expert role calls for more than simple reporting of facts. The expert witness can be asked to provide opinions on a variety of questions, such as an offender's dangerousness risk and competency to proceed with trial in new cases. As in many areas of correctional psychiatric practice, this is a form of dual agency that is ethically challenging. The clinician asked to testify as an expert witness has two potentially conflicting obligations: a fiduciary responsibility toward the patient and a legal mandate to testify truthfully. Most forensic academicians strongly discourage blending the clinician and expert roles. For example, the ethics guidelines of the American Academy of Psychiatry and the Law (2005) expressly recommend "referral to another evaluator" if possible when a treating psychiatrist is asked to render a forensic opinion. Similarly, in

Psychiatric Services in Jails and Prisons, the American Psychiatric Association (2000b) explicitly endorses this separation of roles. However, at times, a clinician cannot avoid such court requests. The clinician must recognize that such expert testimony, regardless of the content, may irrevocably alter the quality of the therapeutic relationship. Therefore, the clinician should explain such risks to the court prior to testifying, in an attempt to preserve the therapeutic alliance for future treatment efforts.

A clinician who chooses to work with court-ordered patients can do several things to minimize the damage that may result from testifying about one's patient. First and foremost, clear communication with the patient that the clinician will be sharing information with a supervising agency or court must occur from the outset and throughout the course of treatment. This serves to keep the court-ordered nature of the treatment at the forefront of the patient's and clinician's minds and avoids subsequent misunderstandings. Ideally, patients who are court mandated to participate in treatment understand the need for information sharing between the clinician and the supervising agent and consent to this sharing. Should a patient refuse consent, efforts to treat the patient should be terminated and only the refusal to grant consent should be communicated to the court or supervising agency.

Although one may argue that consent for this communication is not needed in a court-mandated treatment setting, we disagree with that contention, from a clinical perspective. In a forensic evaluation, the evaluator is not the defendant's provider but instead is working on behalf of the court or counsel, whereas in a court-mandated treatment setting, the provider works for the patient and must report to an outside authority. This is akin to the dual agency related to working in a correctional setting or in the military, and in our view, with certain exceptions, consent for communication must be obtained. Although the clinician's reporting without the patient's consent may be technically legal (e.g., if the court order specifies that the provider will report), we believe that an ongoing discussion of the communication and the patient's consent for that communication will enhance the therapeutic relationship and may be inherently therapeutic for the patient.

Second, adherence to reporting schedules should be maintained. These reports should be made completely and in a timely fashion. If this approach is adopted when things are going well, the supervising agency will be able to respond quickly if and when things begin to turn sour (missed appointments, noncompliance with medications, etc.).

Finally, reporting of problems as soon as they happen is imperative. This communication permits the clinician and the supervising agency or court to work together to craft a clinical intervention under a treatment-first philosophy before legal action becomes necessary. For example, if a patient develops early signs of mania or substance use, or is suspected of failing to take prescribed medication, a conference can be held between the patient, the clinician, and the supervising agent. Various clinical options, such as increased frequency of visits to the clinician, partial or inpatient hospitalization, emergency medication levels, or random urine toxicology screens, can be presented to the patient. Only when all clinical interventions fail should legal consequences be considered. Provided that good communication exists between the clinician and the supervising agency, such interventions result in improved community tenure and minimal use of legal sanctions (Roskes et al. 1999).

Offenders Referred for Treatment Without a Court Order

The majority of individuals who are incarcerated will be released from incarceration without a mandate to participate in treatment. As a rule, this population is similar to both the court-mandated population and the more usual community mental health population. These individuals may be released without any attention to their postrelease mental health needs. In some cases, these individuals may be provided with discharge planning services (*Brad H. et al. v. City of New York et al.* 2003; Roskes et al. 2001). In such cases, community providers should collaborate with their correctional counterparts in creating appropriate transition plans that attend to clinical, rehabilitative, and supportive needs of the individual to be released. Where feasible, such collaborations should include "inreach" by community providers (Roskes et al. 2001). In communities that lack such services, community mental health care providers and administrators may wish to engage with their correctional counterparts to develop such collaborative approaches (Council of State Governments 2002).

One of the most complex groups of offenders includes those who, by virtue of mental illness, developmental disability, or character pathology, lose all of their "good time" while incarcerated and are released having "maxed out" their sentence. This small group of individuals must be released without any supervision by statute, yet they include some of the most impaired, and most dangerous, individuals in the criminal justice system. Correctional providers should prepare such individuals for release and, if possible, refer them for appropriate postrelease services. In some cases, they may be civilly committed at the end of their sentence to a psychiatric hospital. In addition, some specific training and therapeutic models have been used to ease the transition of incarcerated individuals back into their communities (Draine and Herman 2007; Rotter et al. 2005). The principles related to the preparation of noncommitted individuals for release from incarceration are discussed more fully in Chapter 15, "Clinically Oriented Reentry Planning."

CONCLUSION

In this chapter, we have described a variety of collaborative models between criminal justice and mental health professionals in the community along the entire criminal justice spectrum. Although a number of difficulties are involved in taking on this work, these difficulties can be overcome with adequate motivation, interest, and training. Some of the common denominators in successful collaborative programs include a willingness for the parties to develop an understanding of each other's system, the motivation to learn each other's language, and an ability to set aside stereotypes and take each case as it comes. Mental health care providers must have an ability to see the human being behind the rap sheet and to develop a relationship with that human being. In the end, working with such individuals has obvious public safety implications: people with mental illness and legal involvement are common in communities. Clearly, both these individuals and society are better and safer if mental health care providers assist in their return to and retention in communities.

SUMMARY POINTS

- Diversion represents an opportunity for persons with mental illness to be diverted from the criminal justice system.
- Mental health courts examine underlying mental illness that contributes to a defendant's action and assign treatment.
- Probation is an alternative to incarceration.
- Parole is a form of early release from jail or prison.

REFERENCES

American Academy of Psychiatry and the Law: Ethics guidelines for the practice of forensic psychiatry. May 2005. Available at: https://www.aapl.org/pdf/ETHICSGDLNS.pdf. Accessed March 15, 2009.
American Psychiatric Association: Diagnostic and Statistical Manual of Mental Disorders, 4th Edition, Text Revision. Washington, DC, American Psychiatric Association, 2000a

American Psychiatric Association: Psychiatric Services in Jails and Prisons: A Task
Force Report of the American Psychiatric Association, 2nd Edition. Washington, DC, American Psychiatric Association, 2000b
Bazelon Center for Mental Health Law: Criminalization of people with mental illnesses: the role of mental health courts in system reform. January 2003.
Available at: http://www.bazelon.org/issues/criminalization/publications/
mentalhealthcourts/mentalhealthcourts.pdf. Accessed March 15, 2009.
Bonta J, Law M, Hanson K: The prediction of criminal and violent recidivism
among mentally disordered offenders: a meta-analysis. Psychol Bull 123:123–142, 1997
Boothroyd R, Poythress N, McGaha A, et al: The Broward Mental Health Court:
process, outcomes, and service utilization. Int J Law Psychiatry 26:55–71, 2003
Brad H. et al. v. City of New York et al. Index No. 117882/99, Stipulation of Settlement, January 8, 2003. Available at: http://www.urbanjustice.org/pdf/litigation/BradSettlementMHP.pdf. Accessed March 16, 2009.
Buchan L: Ending the cycle of recidivism: best practices for diverting mentally ill
individuals from county jails. June 2003. Available at: http://ws1000.
psych.org/cgi-bin/patience.cgi?id=7dd05698-7545-11de-840a-9371de0de5e7.
Accessed March 15, 2009.
Bureau of Justice Assistance: A Guide to Collecting Mental Health Court Data.
New York, Council of State Governments, 2005
Bureau of Justice Statistics: Correctional Surveys 2007. Available at: http://
www.ojp.usdoj.gov/bjs/glance/tables/corr2tab.htm. Accessed June 5, 2009.
Center on Juvenile and Criminal Justice: The history of the presentence investigation report. 2002. Available at: http://www.cjcj.org/files/the_history.pdf.
Accessed March 16, 2009.
Cochran S, Deane MW, Borum R: Improving police response to mentally ill people. Psychiatr Serv 51:1315–1316, 2000
Cosden M, Ellens JK, Schnell JL, et al: Evaluation of a mental health treatment
court with assertive community treatment. Behav Sci Law 21:415–427, 2003
Council of State Governments: Criminal Justice/Mental Health Consensus
Project. June 2002. Available at: http://consensusproject.org/downloads/
Entire_report.pdf. Accessed March 15, 2009.
Denckla D, Berman G: Rethinking the revolving door: a look at mental illness in
the courts. 2001. Available at http://www.courtinnovation.org/pdf/
mental_health.pdf. Accessed March 15, 2009.
Ditton PM: Mental health and treatment of inmates and probationers (NCJ
174463). Washington, DC, U.S. Department of Justice, Office of Justice Programs, Bureau of Justice Statistics, 1999
Draine J, Herman DB: Critical time intervention for reentry from prison for persons with mental illness. Psychiatr Serv 58:1577–1581, 2007
Draine J, Solomon P: Jail recidivism and the intensity of case management services among homeless persons with mental illness leaving jail. J Psychiatry
Law 22:245–261, 1994
Draine J, Solomon P: Describing and evaluating jail diversion services for persons
with serious mental illness. Psychiatr Serv 50:56–61, 1999

Federal Judicial Center: Supervising defendants and offenders with mental disorders: participant guide (DVD #4416-V/03). Washington, DC, Federal Judicial Center, 2003

Frankle WG, Shera D, Berger-Hershkowitz H, et al: Clozapine-associated reduction in arrest rates of psychotic patients with criminal histories. Am J Psychiatry 158:270–274, 2001

Freitas SI: Mentally disordered offenders: Who are they? What are their needs? Fed Probat, March 1997, pp 33–35

Fulton B: Persons with mental illness on parole and probation: the importance of information, in Community Corrections in America: New Directions and Sounder Investments for Persons with Mental Illness and Codisorders. Edited by Lurigio A. Seattle, WA, National Coalition for Mental and Substance Abuse Health Care in the Justice System, 1996. Available at: http://www.nicic.org/pubs/1996/014000.pdf. Accessed March 15, 2009.

Glaze LE, Bonczar TP: Probation and parole in the United States, 2006. Bureau of Justice Statistics Bulletin, December 2007, NCJ 220218. Washington, DC, U.S. Department of Justice, 2008. Available at: http://www.ojp.usdoj.gov/bjs/pub/pdf/ppus06.pdf. Accessed March 15, 2009.

Goldkamp JS, Irons-Guynn C: Emerging judicial strategies for the mentally ill in the criminal caseload: mental health courts in Fort Lauderdale, Seattle, San Bernardino, and Anchorage (NCJ 182504). Washington, DC, U.S. Department of Justice, Office of Justice Programs, Bureau of Justice Assistance, April 2000. Available at: http://www.ncjrs.org/pdffiles1/bja/182504.pdf. Accessed March 15, 2009.

Guarda AS, Pinto AM, Coughlin JW, et al: Perceived coercion and change in perceived need for admission in patients hospitalized for eating disorders. Am J Psychiatry 164:108–114, 2007

Hector RI: The use of clozapine in the treatment of aggressive schizophrenia. Can J Psychiatry 43:466–472, 1998

Heilbrun K, Griffin PA: Community based forensic treatment, in Treatment of Offenders With Mental Disorders. Edited by RM Wettstein. New York, Guilford, 1998, pp 168–210

Hughes J, Henkel K: The Federal Probation and Pretrial Services System since 1975: an era of growth and change. Fed Probat, March 1997, pp 103–111

Human Rights Watch: Ill-equipped: U.S. prisons and offenders with mental illness. New York, Human Rights Watch, 2003. Available at: http://www.hrw.org/reports/2003/usa1003/usa1003.pdf. Accessed March 15, 2009.

Janofsky JS, Dunn MH, Roskes EJ, et al: Insanity defense pleas in Baltimore City: an analysis of outcome. Am J Psychiatry 153:1464–1468, 1996

Jemelka R, Trupin E, Chiles J: The mentally ill in prison: a review. Hosp Community Psychiatry 40:481–491, 1989

Jones v United States, 463 U.S. 354, 103 S.Ct. 3043 (1983)

Lamb HR, Shaner R, Elliott DM, et al: Outcome for psychiatric emergency patients seen by an outreach police–mental health team. Psychiatr Serv 46:1267–1271, 1995

Lamb HR, Weinberger LE, DeCuir WJ: The police and mental health. Psychiatr Serv 53:1266–1271, 2002

Maryland Annotated Code, Criminal Procedure, § 3-114 et seq, undated. Available at: http://law.justia.com/maryland/codes/gcp/3-114.html. Accessed March 15, 2009.

Mathews AR: Mental Disability and the Criminal Justice System. Chicago, American Bar Foundation, 1970. Cited in Goldkamp JS, Irons-Guynn C: Emerging judicial strategies for the mentally ill in the criminal caseload: mental health courts in Fort Lauderdale, Seattle, San Bernardino, and Anchorage (NCJ 182504). Washington, DC, U.S. Department of Justice, Office of Justice Programs, Bureau of Justice Assistance, April 2000. Available at http://www.ncjrs.org/pdffiles1/bja/182504.pdf. Accessed March 15, 2009.

McNeil DE, Binder RL: Effectiveness of a mental health court in reducing criminal recidivism and violence. Am J Psychiatry 164:1395–1403, 2007

Minkoff K: Developing standards of care for individuals with co-occurring psychiatric and substance use disorders. Psychiatr Serv 52:597–599, 2001

Monahan J, Swartz M, Bonnie RJ: Mandated treatment in the community for people with mental disorders. Health Aff 22:28–38, 2003

Monahan J, Redlich A, Swanson J, et al: Use of leverage to improve adherence to psychiatric treatment in the community. Psychiatr Serv 56:37–44, 2005

Munetz M, Griffin P: Use of the sequential intercept model as an approach to decriminalization of people with serious mental illness. Psychiatr Serv 57:544–549, 2006

National GAINS Center, TAPA Center for Jail Diversion: Ten Years of Learnings on Jail Diversion From the CMHS National GAINS Center. Delmar, NY, GAINS, 2008. Available at: http://www.nicic.org/Library/022928. Accessed June 5, 2009.

National GAINS Center: What is jail diversion? Available at: http://gainscenter.samhsa.gov/html/jail_diversion/what_is_jd.asp. Accessed March 16, 2009.

O'Keefe K: The Brooklyn Mental Health Court Evaluation: Planning, Implementation, Courtroom Dynamics, and Participant Outcomes. New York, Center for Court Innovation, 2006

Oregon Advocacy Center: Mental health law in Oregon: a guide for consumers and families. August 2001. Available at: http://psychrights.org/States/Oregon/MHLawGuide.htm. Accessed March 16, 2009.

Pacific Clinics: Mental Health Law Enforcement Programs, 2002. Available from the authors.

Packard WS: Forensic evaluation and treatment in the same institution: a moral dilemma, in Correctional Psychiatry. Edited by Rosner R, Harmon RB. New York, Plenum, 1989, pp 187–195

Pita DD, Spaniol L: A Comprehensive Guide for Integrated Treatment of People With Co-occurring Disorders. Boston, MA, Boston University Center for Psychiatric Rehabilitation, 2002

Psych Job: The Memphis PD's Crisis Intervention Team reinvents police response to EDPs. Law Enforcement News, John Jay College of Criminal Justice, December 15/31, 2000. Available at: http://www.lib.jjay.cuny.edu/len/2000/12.31. Accessed March 16, 2009.

Redlich AD, Steadman HJ, Monahan J, et al: The second generation of mental health courts. Psychol Public Policy Law 11:527–538, 2005

Regier DA, Farmer ME, Rae D, et al: Comorbidity of mental disorders with alcohol and other drug abuse. JAMA 246:2511–2518, 1990

Ridgely MS, Engberg J, Greenberg MD, et al: Justice, treatment, and cost: an evaluation of the fiscal impact of Allegheny County Mental Health Court. 2007. Available at: http://www.rand.org/pubs/technical_reports/2007/RAND_TR439.pdf. Accessed March 16, 2009.

Roskes E, Feldman R: A collaborative community based treatment program for offenders with mental illness. Psychiatr Serv 50:1614–1619, 1999

Roskes E, Feldman R, Arrington S, et al: A model program for the treatment of mentally ill offenders in the community. Community Ment Health J 35:461–472, 1999

Roskes E, Craig R, Strangman A: A prerelease program for mentally ill inmates. Psychiatr Serv 52:108, 2001

Roskes E, Cooksey C, Feldman R, et al: Management of offenders with mental illnesses in outpatient settings, in Handbook of Correctional Mental Health. Edited by Scott CL, Gerbasi JB. Washington, DC, American Psychiatric Publishing, 2005, pp 229–258

Rotter M, McQuistion HL, Broner N, et al: The impact of "incarceration culture" on reentry for adults with mental illness: a training and group treatment model. Psychiatr Serv 56:265–267, 2005

Selzer T: Mental health courts: a misguided attempt to address the criminal justice system's unfair treatment of people with mental illnesses. Psychol Public Policy Law 11:570–586, 2005

Sheridan EP, Teplin L: Police-referred psychiatric emergencies: advantages of community treatment. J Community Psychol 9:140–147, 1981

Skeem J, Louden JE: Toward evidence-based practice for probationers and parolees mandated to mental health treatment. Psychiatr Serv 57:333–342, 2006

Slate R, Roskes E, Feldman R, et al: Doing justice for mental illness and society: federal probation and pretrial services officers as mental health specialists. Fed Probat, December 2003, pp 13–19

Slate RN, Feldman R, Roskes E, et al: Training federal probation officers as mental health specialists. Fed Probat, December 2004, pp 9–15

Solomon P, Draine J, Meyerson A: Jail recidivism and receipt of community mental health services. Hosp Community Psychiatry 45:793–797, 1994

Spivak B, Mester R, Wittenberg N, et al: Reduction of aggressiveness and impulsiveness during clozapine treatment in chronic neuroleptic-resistant schizophrenic patients. Clin Neuropharmacol 20:442–446, 1997

Steadman HJ, Cocozza JJ, Veysey BM: Comparing outcomes for diverted and nondiverted jail detainees with mental illnesses. Law Hum Behav 23:615–627, 1999a

Steadman HJ, Deane MW, Morrissey JP, et al: A SAMHSA research initiative assessing the effectiveness of jail diversion programs for mentally ill persons. Psychiatr Serv 50:1620–1623, 1999b

Steadman HJ, Deane MW, Borum R, et al: Comparing outcomes of major models of police responses to mental health emergencies. Psychiatr Serv 51:645–649, 2000

Taxman F: Supervision: exploring the dimensions of effectiveness. Fed Probat, September 2002, pp 14–27

Teller JLS, Munetz MR, Gil KM, et al: Crisis intervention team training for police officers responding to mental disturbance calls. Psychiatr Serv 57:232–237, 2006

Teplin LA: Keeping the peace: police discretion and mentally ill persons. National Institute of Justice Journal, July 2000. Available at: http://www.ncjrs.org/pdffiles1/jr000244c.pdf. Accessed March 16, 2009.

U.S. Sentencing Commission: Determining the sentence (Chapter 5), in U.S. Sentencing Commission 2007 Federal Sentencing Guideline Manual. Washington, DC, U.S. Sentencing Commission, 2007. Available at: http://www.ussc.gov/2007guid/CHAP5.html. Accessed March 16, 2009.

Wiederanders MR, Bromley DL, Choate PA: Forensic conditional release programs and outcomes in three states. Int J Law Psychiatry 20:249–257, 1997

Wolff N, Pogorzelski W: Measuring the effectiveness of mental health courts: challenges and recommendations. Psychol Public Policy Law 11:539–569, 2005

CHAPTER 3

Legal Issues Regarding the Provision of Care in a Correctional Setting

Charles L. Scott, M.D.

For nearly two centuries in the United States, inmates' legal rights were significantly limited during their incarceration, with the government rarely interfering with a penal institution's inmate management on behalf of the inmate. This approach became known as the "hands-off approach." In 1871, a Virginia court articulated this approach in the case of *Ruffin v. Commonwealth* (1871) when writing,

> A convicted felon...punished by confinement in the penitentiary instead of with death...is in a state of penal servitude to the State. He has, as a consequence of his crime, not only forfeited his liberty, but all his personal rights except those which the law in its humanity accords to him. He is for [the] time being a slave of the state.

During the turbulent times of the 1960s, the courts moved away from this hands-off attitude. A closer scrutiny of inmates' rights emerged in a new judicial "hands-on" approach that involved more oversight by the legal system. The U.S. Supreme Court strengthened the foundation for this philosophical change in the case of *Cooper v. Pate* (1964). In *Cooper,*

63

the Court ruled for the first time that state prison inmates have standing to sue in federal court to address their grievances. The Court specified that inmates' legal rights were not left behind as they crossed the threshold from their life in the community into the world of corrections.

Mental health care providers and correctional officials should be familiar with common legal mechanisms used by inmates to address concerns regarding the care they are provided. This chapter focuses on five areas related to inmate litigation:

1. The government's legal duty to protect inmates
2. Tort claims alleging medical negligence
3. Claims alleging a violation of constitutional rights
4. Involuntary treatment and transfer of inmates
5. Prison litigation reform

Common legal terms that are often used in litigation are defined in Table 3–1.

TABLE 3–1. Correctional litigation terminology

Legal term	Definition
Pro se	Translated as "for oneself." The filing of a complaint unrepresented and unassisted by legal counsel. The majority of prisoners' complaints are pro se complaints.
In forma pauperis	Translated as "in the manner of a pauper." In pleadings, in forma pauperis grants an inmate the right to sue without assuming the costs or formalities of pleading.
Sua sponte	Translated as "of one's own will." Refers to a court's acting of its own volition, without a motion being made by either of the adverse parties.
Consent decree	A recorded agreement of parties to a lawsuit concerning the form that the judgment should take.
Magistrate judge	A judge who has jurisdiction over federal 42 U.S.C. §1983 claims with consent of both parties.[a]
Special master	A person often appointed in prison condition cases to oversee court-mandated remedial measures.

[a]See section "Inmates' Constitutional Right to Treatment" for further discussion.

LEGAL DUTY TO PROTECT INMATES

The government does not have an affirmative obligation to protect its citizens absent a "special relationship." That is, the U.S. government has no constitutional duty to provide income, food, health care, housing, or employment to its citizens, even if the government elects to do so. Taking someone into custody, however, changes this dynamic. In this situation, a special relationship is created that obligates the government to protect inmates from harm (Cohen and Gerbasi 2005).

The U.S. Supreme Court articulated this affirmative obligation in *DeShaney v. Winnebago County Department of Social Services* (1989), a case that actually involved a small child rather than an adult prisoner. Joshua DeShaney was a 3-year-old child living with his father, Randy, and stepmother. Joshua's stepmother reported that Joshua's father had hit Joshua and left marks on him. Randy denied all accusations to the investigating social workers, and Joshua was maintained in Randy's custody. A year later, Joshua was admitted to a local hospital with multiple bruises and abrasions, and the Winnebago County Department of Social Services (DSS) was notified of suspected child abuse. A child protection team recommended that Joshua be returned to his father's care. Despite repeated in-home observations by DSS of suspicious bruising and another emergency room visit for injuries believed to be a result of child abuse, Joshua was maintained under the care of his father. In March 1984, Randy DeShancy beat 4-year-old Joshua so severely that the child entered into a life-threatening coma. Although Joshua lived, he experienced permanent brain damage that resulted in his being confined to an institution for individuals with profound retardation.

Joshua and his mother brought a civil rights claim against the Winnebago County DSS. They alleged that by failing to protect Joshua from his father, DSS had deprived Joshua of his liberty without due process of law, in violation of his rights under the Fourteenth Amendment.

The U.S. Supreme Court held that a state's failure to protect an individual against private violence does not constitute a violation of the due process clause. Joshua and his mother had argued that because the state had known that Joshua had faced a special danger of abuse at his father's hand, a special relationship had existed, and therefore the state had had a duty to protect Joshua. The Court emphasized that because the state had not actually taken Joshua into protective custody, the state had no affirmative obligation to protect him. Chief Justice William Rehnquist specifically noted,

> The affirmative duty to protect arises not from the State's knowledge of the individual's predicament or from its expression of intent to help him,

but from the limitation which it has imposed on his freedom to act on his behalf.…In the substantive due process analysis, it is the State's affirmative act of restraining the individual's freedom to act on his own behalf—through incarceration, institutionalization, or other similar restraint of personal liberty—which is the "deprivation of liberty" triggering the protections of the Due Process Clause, not its failure to act to protect his liberty interest against harms inflicted by other means. (*DeShaney v. Winnebago County Department of Social Services* 1989, p. 201)

The *DeShaney* Court specifically noted that incarceration represents a form of state restraint that triggers a constitutional duty to protect inmates. This legal concept is important in how courts have subsequently analyzed harms that inmates have experienced while incarcerated.

TORT CLAIMS ALLEGING MEDICAL NEGLIGENCE

Tort law governs the legal resolution of complaints regarding medical treatment. A *tort* is a civil wrong. Tort law seeks to financially compensate individuals who have been injured or who have suffered losses due to the conduct of others. Inmates maintain the right to sue for medical negligence during their incarceration. In cases involving the death of an inmate, the plaintiff is generally a surviving spouse or family member who seeks financial compensation for the loss of his or her loved one. Torts are typically divided into one of three categories: 1) strict liability, 2) intentional torts, and 3) negligence.

Strict liability imposes liability on defendants without requiring any proof of lack of due care, and this standard is not used in malpractice litigation. The most common example of strict liability is harm caused to an individual resulting from a product proven to be unreasonably dangerous and defective (Schubert 1996).

Intentional torts involve actions in which an individual either intends harm or knows that harm may result from his or her behavior (Schubert 1996). Examples of intentional torts that involve mental health care include assault (an attempt to inflict bodily injury), battery (touching without consent), false imprisonment, and violation of a person's civil rights.

Negligent torts occur when a clinician's behavior unintentionally causes an unreasonable risk of harm to another. Medical malpractice is based on the theory of negligence. The four elements required to establish medical negligence are commonly known as the "four Ds": **D**ereliction of **D**uty that **D**irectly results in **D**amages (see Table 3–2). A *duty* is most commonly established for a clinician when the patient seeks treatment, and treatment is provided. The provision of services does not require

TABLE 3–2.   The "four D's" of negligence

Dereliction	Deviations from minimally acceptable standards of care
Duty	Established when there is a professional treatment relationship between a clinician and patient
Directly causing	Relationship between dereliction of duty and harm caused
Damages	The amount of money awarded the plaintiff to compensate for harm caused

the patient's presence and can even extend to assessment and treatment provided over the telephone.

Dereliction of duty is usually the most difficult component of negligence for the plaintiff to establish. Dereliction of duty is divided into acts of commission (providing substandard care) and acts of omission (failure to provide care). Acceptable care does not have to be perfect care but is care provided by a reasonable practitioner. This standard requires that the provider exercise, in both diagnosis and treatment, that reasonable degree of knowledge and skill that ordinarily is possessed and exercised by other members of the profession in similar circumstances (Black 1979). An important issue is whether the standard of mental health care for inmates should be lower than, the same as, or higher than that provided for individuals who are not incarcerated. In an important policy statement regarding the treatment provided to those incarcerated, a task force established by the American Psychiatric Association (2000) provided guidance on this issue when noting the following:

> The fundamental policy goal for correctional mental health is to provide the same level of mental health services to each patient in the criminal justice process that should be available in the community. This policy goal is deliberately higher than the "community standard" that is called for in various legal contexts. (p. 6)

Two aspects of causation generally cited as establishing negligence include the foreseeability of the bad outcome and the clinicians' role in *directly* causing the harm.

Damages are the amount of money the plaintiff is awarded in a lawsuit. Various types of damages may be awarded. *Special damages* are for those actually caused by the injury and include payment for lost wages and medical bills. *General damages* are more subjective in nature and provide financial compensation for the plaintiff's pain and suffering, mental anguish, loss of future income due to injury, and loss of companionship. A third category of damages includes *exemplary* or *punitive damages*. Punitive damages may be awarded when the defendant has been determined to have acted in a malicious or grossly reckless manner. Because punitive damages generally involve harm that is intentionally caused, they are rarely awarded in suicide malpractice cases.

INMATES' CONSTITUTIONAL RIGHT TO TREATMENT

Legal Overview

Inmates may also sue correctional providers claiming that the care provided, or not provided, violated their constitutional rights. Lawsuits alleging that the care provided was unconstitutional have important differences from medical malpractice lawsuits described above. The two constitutional amendments that are most commonly cited as potentially being violated in these types of claims are the Eighth Amendment and the Fourteenth Amendment.

The Eighth Amendment to the U.S. Constitution was ratified as part of the Bill of Rights in 1791. One provision of this amendment prohibits the federal government from imposing cruel and unusual punishment on those convicted of a crime. In 1878, the U.S. Supreme Court provided examples of cruel and unusual punishments, which included publicly dissecting, burning alive, or disemboweling a convicted person (*Wilkerson v. Utah* 1878).

How does the Eighth Amendment now relate to constitutional standards of medical care provided to convicted inmates? Consider the following scenario: An inmate is alone in his cell and notices the onset of a squeezing severe chest pain, accompanied by a tingling in his left arm and hand and shortness of breath. He believes he is suffering from an acute heart attack and experiences pain that becomes increasingly intolerable. He contacts the correctional officer and requests help. The correctional officer ignores his request. Because the inmate is incarcerated, he has no other capability to obtain care for the pain he is experiencing. He is "tortured" by this ripping chest pain. As a result, this lack of care by his prison providers exposes him to a cruel and unusual punishment in violation of the Eighth Amendment. Consequently, convicted prisoners are the only category of individuals in the United States who have a constitutional right to health care.

The legal mechanism that authorizes an inmate to sue a provider or correctional official for failing to provide constitutionally adequate care originates from a federal statute known as 42 U.S.C. § 1983. This statute, also known as the Ku Klux Klan Act, was passed in 1871 to help protect black individuals by providing them a civil remedy for abuses the Klan committed against them. Section 1 of this federal statute reads as follows:

> Every person who, under color of any statute, ordinance, regulation, custom, or usage, of any State or Territory or the District of Columbia, subjects, or causes to be subjected, any citizen of the United States or other person within the jurisdiction thereof to the deprivation of any rights, privileges, or immunities secured by the Constitution and laws, shall be liable to the party injured in an action at law…. (Federal Statute 42 U.S.C. § 1983 [1871])

The importance of this statute is that it established a legal mechanism to sue an individual for a violation of a constitutional right. In 1964, the U.S. Supreme Court held that state inmates could also bring forth a civil rights suit against prison officials for a violation of their constitutional rights (*Cooper v. Pate* 1964). Thus, the door was opened for prison inmates to sue for a violation of their Eighth Amendment rights if the conditions of their medical care represented cruel and unusual punishment. These particular claims are often referred to as "Section 1983" claims.

How, then, do correctional providers know when their care, or lack of care, equates with a violation of an inmate's Eighth Amendment right to such care? In the case of *Estelle v. Gamble* (1976), the U.S. Supreme Court attempted to answer this question. J.W. Gamble, an inmate in the Texas prison system, was allegedly injured when a bale of cotton fell on him while he was unloading a truck as part of his prison work. Although he continued to work for 4 hours, he later complained of back stiffness and was given a pass to go to the prison hospital for evaluation and treatment. During the ensuing 3 months, inmate Gamble was seen by medical personnel on 17 different occasions and received a variety of treatments for his back injury and other problems.

On February 11, 1974, Gamble brought a civil rights action under 42 U.S.C. § 1983 against two correctional officials and the medical director, claiming that he was subjected to cruel and unusual punishment in violation of the Eighth Amendment because of the care, or lack thereof, provided to him. In particular, Gamble complained that a failure to request an X ray of his back resulted in inadequate assessment and treatment, causing his condition to worsen and thereby subjecting him to cruel and unusual punishment.

The *Gamble* Court majority noted that although a failure to conduct an X ray or use additional diagnostic techniques may represent negligence, the presence of medical malpractice *alone* does not constitute cruel and unusual punishment. The Court specifically stated, "Medical malpractice does not become a constitutional violation merely because the victim is a prisoner" (*Estelle v. Gamble* 1976). Therefore, the standard establishing a violation of an inmate's Eighth Amendment rights in regard to the medical care provided *is higher than* what is required to establish medical negligence, which was discussed in the previous section of this chapter.

The *Gamble* Court noted that a violation of an inmate's constitutional rights was established if prison personnel demonstrated "deliberate indifference" to a prisoner's "serious illness or injury." Table 3–3 summarizes key points of the *Gamble* Court ruling, in an attempt to clarify the "deliberate indifference" standard.

The phrase "serious medical need" has been defined by at least two lower courts. The First Circuit Court of Appeals commented that a serious medical need is one that

> has been diagnosed by a physician as mandating treatment, or one that is so obvious that even a lay person would easily recognize the necessity for a doctor's attention....The "seriousness" of an inmate's needs may also be determined by reference to the effect of the delay of treatment. (*Gaudreault v. Municipality of Salem* 1990)

This definition has been criticized because a layperson may not find "so obvious" the signs and symptoms of mental illness and understand how such an illness could affect an inmate's behavior (Cohen and Dvoskin 1992).

Two years later, the Ninth Circuit provided an alternative definition to what constitutes a "serious medical need":

> A "serious" medical need exists if the failure to treat a prisoner's condition could result in further injury or the "unnecessary and wanton infliction of pain."...Either result is not the type of "routine discomfort [that] is 'part of the penalty that criminal offenders pay for their offenses against society.'"...The existence of an injury that a reasonable doctor or patient would find important and worthy of comment or treatment; the presence of a medical condition that significantly affects an individual's daily activities; or the existence of chronic and substantial pain are examples of indications that a prisoner has a "serious" need for medical treatment. (*McGuckin v. Smith* 1992)

After the enunciation of the deliberate indifference standard, some confusion arose across jurisdictions regarding how to more precisely evaluate the mind-set of prison officials accused of being deliberately indifferent to an inmate's needs. As previously emphasized, the U.S. Supreme Court in *Estelle v. Gamble* (1976) specified that the deliberate indifference

TABLE 3–3.   "Deliberate indifference" defined

Deliberate indifference to serious medical needs constitutes the unnecessary and wanton infliction of pain, and such indifference must offend evolving standards of decency.

An inadvertent failure to provide adequate medical care does not constitute deliberate indifference.

Deliberate indifference may be established by
— Prison doctors in their response to a prisoner's needs,
— Correctional officers in intentionally denying or delaying access to medical care, or
— Personnel who intentionally interfere with treatment once proscribed.

Source.   *Estelle v. Gamble* 1976.

standard was higher than the negligence standard used in medical malpractice cases. The next highest standard in evaluating someone's mindset (i.e., *mens rea*, or guilty mind) in regard to his or her actions involves analyzing whether the person had a "reckless" mind at the time of his or her acts. Two types of recklessness have been defined:

1. *Subjective recklessness:* A person knows of a particular situation or risk and disregards it
2. *Objective recklessness:* A person does not know of a particular situation or risk but, based on the circumstances, should have known

Because the *Gamble* Court did not provide specific guidance as to which recklessness standard was to be used in evaluating inmates' deliberate indifference claims, courts have varied in how they analyzed deliberate indifference claims, resulting in a confusing trail of court rulings.

Eventually, this confusion was resolved by the U.S. Supreme Court in the interesting case of *Farmer v. Brennan* (1994). Dee Farmer, a biological male, was a preoperative transsexual who received a federal sentence for credit card fraud. For years prior to Farmer's conviction and sentence, Farmer wore women's clothing, took female hormones, received silicone breast implants, and even underwent a botched black market testicle removal. After being convicted, Farmer was eventually transferred to the U.S. Penitentiary in Terre Haute, Indiana, and was placed in the general population of male inmates without voicing objection to this placement. During this time, Farmer allegedly smuggled hormone drugs into prison and wore the prison clothing off one shoulder, in a "feminine manner." Within

2 weeks of being placed in the facility, Farmer was beaten and raped by another inmate. Farmer subsequently filed a civil rights claim alleging that prison officials were deliberately indifferent to the placement of Farmer in this potentially harmful situation. In particular, Farmer asserted that because this penitentiary had a violent environment and a history of inmate assaults, correctional officials should have known that Farmer was at high risk for sexual victimization.

A critical issue in analyzing this case was what standard of recklessness would apply in determining whether prison personnel were deliberately indifferent to Dee Farmer. Was the standard *subjective recklessness*, whereby the inmate must show that the prison officials had *actual knowledge* of the risk or potential danger, or was it *objective recklessness*, indicating that the inmate must only show that the prison officials *should have known* of the risk or potential danger, even when they did not have actual knowledge?

The U.S. Supreme Court ruled that the appropriate test in evaluating an inmate's deliberate indifference claim is *subjective recklessness*. According to the *Farmer* Court,

> A prison official may be held liable under the Eighth Amendment for acting with "deliberate indifference" to inmate health or safety only if he knows that inmates face a substantial risk of danger of serious harm and disregards that risk by failing to take reasonable measures. (*Farmer v. Brennan* 1994)

The Court also commented that a fact finder could conclude that the prison officials had the necessary knowledge, despite claims to the contrary, in situations that involved obvious dangers to inmates. In other words, although the deliberate indifference standard requires knowledge of the risk, prison officials cannot escape liability by pretending that they did not know of the risk when it is actually obvious that they did know.

"Serious Medical Need" and Mental Health Needs

In the *Estelle v. Gamble* (1976) holding, the U.S. Supreme Court stated that prison officials may not be deliberately indifferent to an inmate's serious *medical* needs. Although the Court did not specifically note that mental health needs were equivalent to medical needs, lower courts have held that no distinction should be made between medical and mental health needs when considering deliberate indifference claims.

In *Bowring v. Godwin* (1976), Larry Bowring, who was serving a sentence for robbery, attempted robbery, and kidnapping, claimed that his Eighth and Fourteenth Amendment rights were violated because his denial of parole was based, in part, on a psychological evaluation that stated he would not successfully complete a parole period. Bowring asserted that the state must provide him with a psychological diagnosis and treatment so that he would qualify for parole, and a failure to do so constitutes cruel and unusual punishment. In conducting an analysis of Bowring's claim, the Fourth Circuit Court of Appeals specifically noted,

> We see no underlying distinction between the right to medical care for physical ills and its psychological or psychiatric counterpart. Modern science has rejected the notion that mental or emotional disturbances are the products of afflicted souls, hence beyond the purview of counseling, medication and therapy. (*Bowring v. Godwin* 1976)

This same court noted that a prisoner is entitled to psychological or psychiatric treatment if a physician or other health care provider concludes that

1. the prisoner's symptoms are evidence of a serious disease or injury,
2. such disease or injury is curable or may be substantially alleviated, and
3. the potential for harm to the prisoner by reason of delay or the denial of care would be substantial.

The *Bowring* court also emphasized that the right to mental heath treatment was limited to treatment that could be provided on a reasonable cost and time basis and was medically necessary rather than merely desirable.

Deliberate Indifference and Pretrial Detainees

The Eighth Amendment discussion above applies only to *convicted* prisoners. Does this mean that pretrial detainees serving their time in a jail are not afforded the same constitutional protections and right to be free from deliberate indifference that are given to convicted prisoners? Obviously, the answer is "no." In fact, the U.S. Supreme Court has noted that pretrial detainees have a right to be free from punishment altogether (*Bell v. Wolfish* 1979) because they have not been convicted of a crime. In *City of Revere v. Massachusetts General Hospital* (1983), the U.S. Supreme Court emphasized that the due process clause of the Fourteenth Amendment

> does require the responsible government or governmental agency to provide medical care to persons...who have been injured while being apprehended by the police. In fact, the due process rights of a [pretrial detainee] are at least as great as the Eighth Amendment protections available to a convicted prisoner.

Therefore, in cases involving pretrial detainees, deliberate indifference claims are analyzed under the Fourteenth Amendment's due process clause, and such reviews are conducted in a manner similar to those involving convicted prisoners.

Inmate Suicides and Deliberate Indifference

When an inmate attempts or actually commits suicide, the possibility of a civil rights action claiming deliberate indifference by correctional staff should be anticipated, in addition to claims of medical negligence. Does a risk of suicide equate with the required "serious medical need" component to establish deliberate indifference? In *Partridge v. Two Unknown Police Officers* (1986), the Fifth Circuit Court evaluated a case involving the suicide of Michael Partridge, a pretrial detainee arrested by a Houston police officer on suspicion of burglary and theft. Upon his arrest, Michael was described as hysterical. Michael's father was at the scene of the arrest and informed the arresting officer that his son had had a nervous breakdown. When placed into the police car, Michael became agitated and violent and tried to kick the windows and doors out of the car. During the drive to the jail, he intentionally struck his head against the Plexiglas divider, but he appeared composed by the time he arrived at the jail.

The transporting officers did not report Michael's behavior at the scene or during transport to anyone at the jail, and he was subsequently placed in solitary confinement. Three hours later, Michael tied a pair of socks to the upper bars of his cell and hanged himself. Clinical records within the jail documented that Michael had attempted suicide during a prior confinement. Michael's parents filed a Section 1983 claim alleging that the Houston police officers were deliberately indifferent to their son's risk of suicide.

The Fifth Circuit Court noted the following in evaluating if a suicide risk represents a serious medical need:

> A serious medical need may exist for psychological or psychiatric treatment, just as it may exist for physical ills. A psychological or psychiatric condition can be as serious as any physical pathology or injury, especially when it results in suicidal tendencies. And just as a failure to act to save a detainee from suffering from gangrene might violate the duty to provide reasonable medical care absent an intervening legitimate government objective, failure to take any steps to save a suicidal detainee from injuring himself may also constitute a due process violation under *Bell v. Wolfish*. (*Partridge v. Two Unknown Police Officers* 1986)

Section 1983 claims have also been forwarded for failure to adequately train governmental employees in the identification and appropriate interventions for potentially suicidal inmates. In the case of *Colburn v. Upper Darby Township* (1991), the Third Circuit Court of Appeals noted that to establish deliberate indifference to an inmate's constitutional rights based on failures in a training program, "the identified deficiency must be closely related to the ultimate injury." The *Colburn* court noted that in this type of Section 1983 claim, the plaintiff must 1) identify specific training not provided that could reasonably be expected to prevent the suicide that occurred and 2) demonstrate that the risk reduction associated with the proposed training is so great and so obvious that it can reasonably be attributed to deliberate indifference.

In this same case, the *Colburn* court provided their methodology regarding how to analyze Section 1983 claims that involved pretrial detainees who committed suicide. According to the standard outlined by this court, the plaintiff must prove that

1. the inmate had a particular vulnerability to suicide,
2. the custodial officers knew or should have known of this vulnerability, and
3. the officers acted with "reckless indifference" to the inmate's particular vulnerability.

The court emphasized that the vulnerability to suicide could not be a "mere possibility" but must represent a "strong likelihood." In addition, the court noted that in evaluating if the officers should have known that the inmate was vulnerable to suicide, the vulnerability had to be "so obvious that a lay person would easily recognize the necessity for preventative action" (*Colburn v. Upper Darby Township* 1991).

Common acts of omission or commission involving inmate suicide that are noted both in tort claims and in Section 1983 claims are highlighted in Table 3–4.

Deliberate Indifference and Other Clinical and Custodial Care Issues

Claims of deliberate indifference are not limited to inmate suicides or suicide attempts. Section 1983 claims alleging violation of an inmate's constitutional rights are potentially wide-ranging and may include failure to appropriately diagnose, treat, or monitor care given. In addition, courts may consider if a correctional facility was deliberately indifferent to the impact of placement in isolation or segregated units such as security housing units. For example, in the case of *Jones'El v. Berge* (2001), a federal district court noted that the confinement conditions in a Wisconsin supermax prison may be unconstitutional for inmates with serious

TABLE 3–4.   Common tort and Section 1983 claims involving inmate suicide

Failure to properly screen for suicide

Failure to adequately train custodial staff in suicide recognition and prevention

Failure to communicate information regarding suicide potential

Failure to identify risk of suicide

Failure to appropriately intervene to diminish suicide risk

Failure to adequately treat a suicidal inmate

Failure to provide a safe environment

Failure to provide an appropriate emergency intervention following a suicide attempt

Source.   Cohen 2008.

mental illness. The authors of Chapter 16, "Supermax Units and Death Row," in this handbook further discuss legal rulings related to the constitutional violations associated with the placement of inmates with mental illness in such settings.

Continued Care After Release From Incarceration

One might expect that the constitutional obligation to provide care to an inmate ceases upon his or her release from incarceration, particularly in light of the previously discussed case of *DeShaney v. Winnebago* (1989), which held that an affirmative obligation of the state was created when the person was taken into the state's *custody*. However, three more recent cases indicate that the grasp of this custody requirement may reach beyond the walls of a jail or prison. In the first case, *Wakefield v. Thompson* (1999), the Ninth Circuit Court addressed a Section 1983 claim by Timothy Wakefield that a correctional officer at San Quentin Prison was deliberately indifferent to his serious medical needs by refusing to provide him with prescription psychotropic medication upon his release from prison. According to Wakefield, his prison psychiatrist had written a 2-week prescription for thiothixene for treatment of his diagnosed organic delusional disorder. In his lawsuit, Wakefield asserted that on the day of his release, the correctional officer told him that no medication was available and refused to call the medical staff to check on his prescription. Wakefield claimed that because he was without his necessary antipsychotic medication, he had a relapse of his mental condition, which led to a violent outburst and his rearrest.

The Ninth Circuit Court concluded that Wakefield did have an adequate Section 1983 claim that the officer was deliberately indifferent to his serious medical needs by failing to provide his prescribed medications, in violation of Wakefield's Eighth and Fourteenth Amendment rights. In explaining why the state may have an obligation beyond medical care required during actual incarceration, the court noted,

> It is a matter of common sense, however, that a prisoner's ability to secure medication "on his own behalf" is not necessarily restored the instant he walks through the prison gates and into the civil world. Although many patients must take their medication one or more times a day, it may take a number of days, or possibly even weeks for a recently released prisoner to find a doctor, schedule an examination, obtain a diagnosis, and have a prescription filled. Accordingly the period of time during which prisoners are unable to secure medication "on their own behalf" may extend beyond the period of actual incarceration. Under the reasoning of Estelle and DeShaney, the state's responsibility to provide a temporary supply of medication to prisoners in such cases extends beyond that period as well. (*Wakefield v. Thompson* 1999)

The court in *Wakefield* held that the state must provide an outgoing prisoner (who needs medication) a "sufficient supply" of medications for a period of time reasonably necessary to permit the inmate to consult a doctor and obtain a new supply. This ruling neither stated exactly how many days of medication must be prescribed nor required that a doctor or doctor's appointment be provided.

In what appears to be an extension of the *Wakefield* holding, the New York case of *Brad H. v. City of New York* (2000) addressed obligations by jail personnel in regard to discharge planning for jail inmates. In 1999, a class action lawsuit was brought forward on behalf of the nearly 25,000 inmates with mental illness who are released annually from New York City jails. According to the plaintiffs, inmates with mental illness were released with minimal, if any, coordinated follow-up care. The alleged practice of jail discharge involved releasing the inmates with mental illness in the isolated Queens Plaza between 2 A.M. and 4 A.M. with $1.50 in cash and a $3 Metrocard. The complaint alleged that this practice violated inmates' rights under New York State laws and regulations that require discharge planning by providers of mental health treatment.

In January 2003, a settlement agreement was reached that provided various services to qualifying class members. Services included connection with community mental health services, assistance in obtaining medications upon discharge, a discharge summary, aftercare appointments, and assistance with public housing. For additional information regarding discharge placement obligations of correctional personnel, see Chapter 15, "Clinically Oriented Reentry Planning," in this handbook.

The third case, *Lugo v. Senkowski* (2000), represents yet another view regarding what care, if any, clinicians are obligated to provide after an inmate's discharge. Mr. Lugo was a New York prison inmate who was paroled from New York's Clinton Prison. His release occurred shortly after he underwent surgery for removal of a kidney stone. As part of his surgery, a metal stent was left in the kidney. Mr. Lugo's physician informed him that he would need subsequent surgery to remove this stent. Mr. Lugo's parole release occurred before this surgery could be arranged. Mr. Lugo subsequently sued, alleging that he was not provided any assistance in obtaining the surgery that had been recommended by his doctor. The judge interpreted the *Wakefield* (1999) ruling as requiring the state to provide care that they had initiated, and this continued obligation should remain for a "reasonable period of time."

Although this case did not involve an inmate with mental illness, it raises the question of how future courts may interpret psychiatric care that is initiated and requires ongoing monitoring for safety upon release. For example, might a mental health care provider have an obligation to arrange for white blood cell monitoring in the community for a released inmate who has recently started taking the antipsychotic clozapine? The cases outlined above suggest that a mental health practitioner should consider the following when an inmate under his or her care is going to be released:

1. Provide psychiatric medications long enough for an inmate to reasonably access a treating provider in the community.
2. Coordinate discharge planning and reentry into the community when feasible.
3. Consider what monitoring may be necessary for treatment that is begun but not yet completed, and that requires further intervention for completion of the treatment.

CONSTITUTIONAL ISSUES REGARDING SYSTEMS OF CARE

In addition to Section 1983 claims involving specific failures in individual cases, the entire mental health care system can be evaluated to determine if it meets a constitutionally acceptable standard. One of the most famous cases that provided guidelines for adequate mental health care was that of *Ruiz v. Estelle* (1980). David Ruiz was a Texas prison inmate repeatedly incarcerated for aggravated robbery. In 1972, he filed a 15-page handwritten civil rights complaint alleging numerous violations of his constitutional rights, to include the lack of medical care, unlawful placement in solitary confinement, and harassment by prison officials. His lawsuit was later combined with six other lawsuits into a class action on behalf of all Texas prisoners. After a yearlong trial, the judge ruled in favor of Ruiz and the prisoners. Texas was ordered to make massive changes in its prison system. The federal government's monitoring of the Texas prison system lasted until 2002, when the federal court turned the system back over to state control. The court outlined six requirements of a constitutionally acceptable mental health program; these are described in Table 3–5.

INVOLUNTARY TREATMENT AND TRANSFER OF INMATES

Involuntary Medication for Treatment Purposes

Inmates do not give up their right to refuse treatment as a condition of their confinement; however, involuntary treatment may be administered in a life-threatening situation if the failure to treat could result in the inmate's death or serious harm. In addition, most jurisdictions provide a review mechanism that allows the involuntary treatment of an inmate when he or she poses a threat of danger to self or others, or is gravely disabled (e.g., unable to attend to his or her basic needs of daily living). The provider should be familiar with his or her jurisdiction's legal requirements for the involuntary administration of medications in both jail and prison settings, because the mechanism for forced treatment may differ in the two environments.

In some jail settings, the involuntary administration of medication to jail inmates in nonemergency settings follows a process similar to that used for individuals being considered for involuntary psychotropic medication in the community. For example, in California, providers who recommend involuntary medicating of a jail inmate must first present their reasoning for doing so to a judge at a court hearing.

Are such judicial hearings constitutionally *required* for prison inmates before involuntary medications may be given? The U.S. Supreme Court ruled that a nonjudicial administrative review mechanism is constitutionally permissible, as outlined in the case of *Washington v. Harper* (1990). Walter Harper was a convicted robber incarcerated in the Washington State penal system who had episodes of violent behavior when he did not take his antipsychotic medication. He was transferred on two occasions to the Special Offender Center (SOC), a state institution for offenders with mental illness, where he was diagnosed with manic-depressive disorder. The SOC had an institutional review policy for evaluating when anti-

---

TABLE 3–5. Guidelines for a constitutionally acceptable mental health program

---

1. The prison must have a systematic program of screening and evaluations of prisoners to identify those who need mental health treatment.

2. Treatment for a prisoner must entail more than just segregation and close supervision.

3. The prison must employ enough mental health professionals to be able to identify and treat the mentally ill in an individualized manner.

4. The treating professionals must keep accurate, complete, and confidential records of the mental health treatment process.

5. A prisoner cannot be treated with a prescription for behavior-altering medications in dangerous amounts, by dangerous methods, or without acceptable supervision and periodic evaluations.

6. The prison must have a basic program to identify, treat, and supervise inmates with suicidal tendencies.

Source. Ruiz v. Estelle 1980.

---

psychotic drugs could be administered against an inmate's wishes. According to this policy, a special review committee examined the involuntary medication recommendations made by the treating psychiatrist. The review committee consisted of a psychiatrist, psychologist, and SOC official, none of whom could be involved in the inmate's current diagnosis or treatment. This special committee decided to approve the involuntary administration of medication only if 1) the committee psychiatrist was in the majority recommending medication and 2) the inmate had a "mental disorder" and was "gravely disabled" or posed a "likelihood of serious harm" to self or others.

This SOC policy also provided inmates with many procedural due process rights, including the following:

- Right to notice of the hearing
- Right to attend the hearing
- Right to present evidence and cross-examine witnesses
- Right to representation by a disinterested lay adviser versed in the psychological issues
- Right to appeal the decision to the SOC's superintendent
- Right to periodic review of any involuntary medication ordered

Harper filed a Section 1983 suit claiming that the SOC's failure to provide a judicial hearing before the involuntary administration of antipsychotic medication violated the due process clause of the Fourteenth Amendment. The U.S. Supreme Court held that the due process clause permits the state to treat a prison inmate who has a serious mental illness with antipsychotic drugs against his or her will, if he or she is dangerous to self or others and if the treatment is in his or her medical interest. The major point of this case is that prison officials are *not* constitutionally required to arrange a judicial hearing to obtain court approval of involuntary medication of a prisoner with mental illness.

Involuntary Medication for Competency to Stand Trial Restoration

Occasionally, jail providers may be faced with a situation in which a pretrial detainee who has been found incompetent to stand trial has a court order that authorizes the involuntary administration of psychotropic medications even when the inmate has not been found to be a danger to self or others or to be gravely disabled. This order, referred to as a *Sell* order, arises out of the case of *Sell v. United States* (2003). In this case, the U.S. Supreme Court provided guidance on when pretrial detainees may be involuntarily medicated to restore their competency to stand trial even when they are not considered a danger to themselves or others and are not gravely disabled. Charles Sell was a St. Louis dentist who had a long-standing history of delusional disorder. He was eventually charged with multiple counts of Medicaid fraud and one count of money laundering. While Sell was released on bail, his mental status reportedly deteriorated, and he was eventually charged with one count of conspiring to murder the FBI agent who had arrested him.

Sell was found incompetent to stand trial. After being ordered to a hospital for competency restoration, he refused to take the antipsychotic medication prescribed for his delusional disorder. Sell challenged any involuntary medication administration, and the case was appealed to the U.S. Supreme Court. The issue before the court was whether the U.S. Constitution permits the government to involuntarily administer antipsychotic drugs to a criminal defendant with mental illness for the purpose of rendering the individual competent to stand trial. The U.S. Supreme Court outlined conditions that must be met prior to the involuntary administration of medication, and these factors are sometimes referred to as the *Sell* criteria:

1. The court must find that an important government interest is at stake. Both person and property crimes can be viewed as serious offenses that justify the government's interest in adjudicating criminality.

2. The court must find that the medication significantly furthers the state's interests. For example, the medication should likely render the defendant competent to stand trial and not have severe side effects that would interfere with the trial competency.
3. The medication must be the most appropriate method of restoring trial competency, which cannot be achieved with less intrusive treatments.
4. The medication must be medically appropriate, based on its efficacy and side effects.

If a jail provider receives a *Sell* order from the court authorizing involuntary medication, he or she should carefully review the order to verify that it allows such administration in the jail setting as opposed to a hospital setting. Some orders specify that forced medication for trial competency may be given only in a hospital setting. In this circumstance, the provider should seek guidance from the court regarding whether or not the *Sell* order permits forced medication at the jail. Individuals found incompetent to stand trial are often sent to a state hospital for competency restoration and may be involuntarily medicated under a *Sell* order in that setting. After the hospital determines that the defendant is trial competent, the inmate is usually returned to jail to await his or her competency hearing. Such defendants sometimes refuse the medications that were forced on them at the hospital. Does the *Sell* order still apply while they await their trial in jail? In other words, does a hospital's opinion that the inmate is no longer incompetent to stand trial negate the conditions of the *Sell* order? No clear rule on this issue exists, and providers should contact the court to clarify whether or not such continued involuntary medication administration is permitted at the jail while the inmate awaits the competency hearing.

Involuntary Transfer of Prisoners to a Psychiatric Hospital

Prisoners also have constitutional rights in regard to their being transferred to a psychiatric facility against their will. In the case of *Vitek v. Jones* (1980), the U.S. Supreme Court provided criteria to be considered before a prisoner could be involuntarily sent to a psychiatric hospital. At issue was a Nebraska statute that authorized a state prisoner's transfer to a state mental hospital without the inmate's consent. Mr. Jones had been convicted of robbery and sentenced to a prison term of 3–9 years. Eight months after he began serving his sentence, he was transferred to the prison hospital, and 2 days later, he was housed in solitary confinement at the prison adjustment center. While there, he suffered serious burns after he set his mattress on fire. He was subsequently sent by ambulance to the burn unit of a private hospital, where he remained for approximately 4 months. Mr. Jones was then considered for a possible transfer from the burn unit to a nonprison psychiatric hospital.

Under the governing Nebraska statute, if a physician or psychologist finds that an inmate has a mental disease or defect and determines that the inmate cannot be given proper treatment at the prison, the director of correctional services may arrange for the inmate's transfer to a psychiatric facility. Mr. Jones was examined by a psychiatrist, who recommended that Mr. Jones be sent to a psychiatric hospital, and Mr. Jones reportedly told the psychiatrist that he agreed with this decision. A year later, he challenged his transfer under the due process clause of the Fourteenth Amendment, arguing that inadequate procedures were afforded him regarding the decision to have him serve his sentence in a psychiatric facility as opposed to a state prison.

The U.S. Supreme Court agreed with Mr. Jones that he had a protected liberty interest under the Fourteenth Amendment and noted that Nebraska's reliance on the opinion of a physician or psychologist in determining the conditions for transfer did not provide adequate due process protections. The *Vitek* Court commented,

> Involuntary commitment to a mental hospital is not within the range of conditions of confinement to which a prison sentence subjects an individual. While a conviction and sentence extinguish an individual's right to freedom from confinement for the term of his sentence, they do not authorize the State to classify him as mentally ill and to subject him to involuntary psychiatric treatment without affording him additional due process protections. Here, the stigmatizing consequences of a transfer to a mental hospital for involuntary psychiatric treatment, coupled with the subjection of the prisoner to mandatory behavior modification as a treatment for mental illness, constitute the kind of deprivations of liberty that requires procedural protections. (*Vitek v. Jones* 1980, pp. 491–494)

The *Vitek* Court upheld minimum procedures outlined by the district court that must be followed before transferring a prisoner to a mental hospital (see Table 3–6). The procedural guidelines summarized in Table 3–6 are typically provided to inmates who are being considered for transfer to a psychiatric facility. Hearings to consider this move are commonly referred to as *Vitek* hearings. *Vitek* hearings are not required for prison-to-prison transfers or in psychiatric emergencies where short-term crisis stabilization is required.

TABLE 3–6. *Vitek* procedures required for prisoner transfer to a psychiatric hospital

---

1. Written notice that a transfer to a mental hospital is being considered.

2. A hearing after the prisoner is given written notice that a transfer is being considered and sufficient time to prepare for this hearing. At the hearing, the evidence being relied upon for the transfer must be presented and the inmate must have an opportunity to be heard in person and to present documentary evidence.

3. An opportunity to present testimony of witnesses by the defense and to confront and cross-examine witnesses called by the state, unless there is a good cause finding for not permitting such presentation, confrontation, or cross-examination.

4. A right to an independent decision maker at the hearing.

5. A written statement by the fact finder as to the evidence relied on and the reasons for transferring the inmate.

6. Availability of "qualified and independent assistance" provided by the state (a licensed attorney is not required).

7. Effective and timely notice of all of the above rights.

Source.   Vitek v. Jones 1980.

PRISON LITIGATION REFORM

As noted at the beginning of this chapter, the U.S. Supreme Court held in *Cooper v. Pate* (1964) that prison inmates could sue for a violation of their constitutional rights under the Civil Rights Act of 1871. As time passed, concern arose that inmates were increasingly using this mechanism to file frivolous civil rights claims. In 1994, the U.S. Department of Justice conducted a study to evaluate Section 1983 claims made by inmates. In 96% of these lawsuits, the inmate proceeded *pro se* (without counsel). In 94% of the cases, the inmate won nothing as a result of his or her claim (Hanson and Daley 1994). Additional findings from this study are highlighted in Tables 3–7 and 3–8.

In 1995, Congress passed the Prison Litigation Reform Act (PLRA) as one mechanism to address concerns regarding the costs and time demands associated with frivolous civil rights lawsuits brought by inmates. When Senator Bob Dole introduced the PLRA as a Senate bill, he stated that the PLRA was necessary "to provide for appropriate remedies for prison condition lawsuits, to discourage frivolous and abusive prison lawsuits, and for other purposes" (Dole 1995). Senator Dole provided vari-

TABLE 3–7.   U.S. Department of Justice report on Section 1983 litigation

Inmate plaintiffs in Section 1983 lawsuits	
State prison inmates	62%
Jail inmates	36%
Parolees (released inmates)	2%
Defendants in Section 1983 lawsuits	
Correctional officers	26%
Wardens/jail administrators	22%
Medical staff (doctors and nurses)	9%
Elected officials	7%
Arresting officers	6%

Source.   Hanson and Daley 1994.

TABLE 3–8.   Top five issues in Section 1983 lawsuits

Issue	Percentage of lawsuits
Physical security	21%
Medical treatment	17%
Due process	13%
Challenges to conviction	12%
Physical conditions	9%

Source.   Hanson and Daley 1994.

ous examples of inmate lawsuit abuses: an inmate sued because he preferred creamy rather than chunky peanut butter, another sued a prison barber for a defective haircut, and yet another claimed a civil rights violation because prison officials had failed to invite him to a pizza party for a departing prison employee (Dole 1995).

The PLRA was not unanimously lauded by members of the U.S. Senate, and some senators expressed their concerns regarding the potential consequences of this legislation. For example, Senator Ted Kennedy (1996) warned that the PLRA effectively stripped federal courts of their remedial power, and he argued that the bill was "patently unconstitutional, and a dangerous legislative incursion into the work of the judicial branch."

Likewise, Senator Joe Biden (1995) cautioned that the PLRA could prevent meritorious lawsuits from being heard by courts.

In reality, the PLRA does contain several key provisions designed to discourage or prevent prisoners from bringing lawsuits into court. First, the statute requires indigent inmates to pay the filing fee (up to $150). The entire fee can be paid in installments over time. Second, the PLRA requires that before a prisoner forwards a case to court, he or she first exhaust all administrative remedies that are available. Third, this statute restricts attorneys' fees, making it potentially more difficult for inmates to find legal representation. Fourth, the PLRA contains a "three strikes" provision, which bars prisoners who have previously filed three or more frivolous complaints or appeals from filing *in forma pauperis* (Latin for "in the manner of a pauper"). Federal and state courts grant this status to individuals without funds so they can pursue litigation with a waiver of the normal costs. The PLRA restricts this ability in defined circumstances.

In regard to claims for mental or emotional injuries, the PLRA (1995) specifies the following: "No Federal civil action may be brought by a prisoner confined in a jail, prison, or other correctional facility for a mental or emotional injury suffered while in custody without a prior showing of physical injury." The PLRA does not define what constitutes a "mental or emotional injury," explain what is meant by "prior showing," or define "physical injury." One could envision a scenario in which an inmate was threatened with a shank to his throat or witnessed the brutal stabbing of his cell mate. Under the PLRA, if no physical injury resulted, the inmate might be restricted from filing a claim for a mental or emotional injury.

Has the PLRA achieved its goal of decreasing the frequency of inmate lawsuits? In a study examining data made available by the federal court system and the Bureau of Justice Statistics, Schlanger (2005) examined jail and prison inmate civil rights suits filed in federal court both before and after the passage of the PLRA. She noted a sharp decline in inmate lawsuit rates immediately following passage of the PLRA, in marked contrast to a nearly 25-year history of increasing inmate lawsuits prior to this legislation. It remains unclear whether this decline represents a decrease in only frivolous litigation or a drop in some genuine lawsuits due to the higher hurdles of the PLRA.

CONCLUSION

This chapter has highlighted important aspects involving the standard of care provided to inmates and their legal rights to care as they traverse through the criminal justice system. Because incarceration prevents inmates from independently accessing care as they might in the community, the courts have ruled that they have a constitutional right to treatment. Clearly, an inmate does not lose the right to appropriate mental health care because he or she has been charged with or found guilty of a crime. This point was clearly emphasized by the U.S. Supreme Court in the case of *Wolff v. McDonnell* (1974): "There is no iron curtain drawn between the Constitution and the prisons of this country."

SUMMARY POINTS

- Mental health care providers can be sued for negligence regarding the care they provide inmates.
- Mental health care providers can be sued for violating an inmate's constitutional rights if they are found "deliberately indifferent" to an inmate's serious medical needs.
- The standard for deliberate indifference is higher than that for medical negligence and requires an awareness and disregard of the risk or situation alleged to cause the harm.
- Inmates have a constitutional right to treatment.
- Providers should be familiar with their jurisdictional requirements for involuntary medication administration and transfer of inmates.
- The Prison Litigation Reform Act was passed to decrease frivolous inmate lawsuits, and trends do show a subsequent decrease in inmate lawsuit filings.

REFERENCES

American Psychiatric Association: Psychiatric Services in Jails and Prisons: A Task Force Report of the American Psychiatric Association, 2nd Edition. Washington, DC, American Psychiatric Association, 2000
Bell v Wolfish, 441 U.S. 520 (1979)
Biden J: Statement of Senator Joe Biden. 141 Congressional Record S14, 628 (September 29, 1995)
Black HC: Black's Law Dictionary. St. Paul, MN, West Publishing, 1979
Bowring v Godwin, 555 F.2d 44 (4th Cir. 1976)
Brad H v City of New York, 712 N.Y.S.2d 336 (Sup. Ct. 2000); 716 N.Y.S.2d 852 (N.Y. App. Div. 2000)
City of Revere v Massachusetts General Hospital, 463 U.S. 239 (1983)
Cohen F: Suicide, in The Mentally Disordered Inmate and the Law, 2nd Edition. Edited by Cohen F. Kingston, NJ, Civic Research Institute, 2008, pp 14–16
Cohen F, Dvoskin J: Inmates with mental disorders: a guide to law and practice. Ment Phys Disabil Law Rep 16:339–341, 1992

Cohen F, Gerbasi J: Legal issues, in Handbook of Correctional Mental Health. Edited by Scott CL, Gerbasi JB. Washington, DC, American Psychiatric Publishing, 2005, pp 259–283

Colburn v Upper Darby Township, 946 F.2d 1017 (3d Cir. 1991)

Cooper v Pate, 378 U.S. 546 (1964)

DeShaney v Winnebago County Department of Social Services, 489 U.S. 189 (1989)

Dole R: Statement of Senator Robert Dole. 141 Congressional Record S14, 413, Daily Edition, September 27, 1995

Estelle v Gamble, 429 U.S. 97 (1976)

Farmer v Brennan, 555 U.S. 825 (1994)

Federal statute 42 U.S.C. § 1983 (1871)

Gaudreault v Municipality of Salem, Massachusetts, 923 F.2d 203, 208 (1st Cir. 1990)

Hanson RA, Daley HWK: Challenging the conditions of prisons and jails: a report on Section 1983 litigation. Washington, DC, U.S. Department of Justice, Office of Justice Programs, Bureau of Justice Statistics, December 1994

Jones'El v Berge, 164 F.Supp.2d 1096 (W.D. Wis. 2001)

Kennedy T: Statement of Senator Ted Kennedy. 142 Congressional Record S2296, Daily Edition, March 19, 1996

Lugo v Senkowski, 114 F.Supp.2s 111 (N.D. N.Y. September 25, 2000)

McGuckin v Smith, 974 F.2d 1050 (9th Cir. 1992)

Partridge v Two Unknown Police Officers, 791 F.2d 1182, 1187 (5th Cir. 1986)

Prison Litigation Reform Act, 42 U.S.C. § 1997e(e), 1995

Ruffin v Commonwealth, 62 Va.790 (1871)

Ruiz v Estelle, 503 F.Supp. 1265 (S.D. Tex 1980)

Schlanger M: Prison conditions lawsuits: subject matter and time trends, December 15, 2005. Available at: http://law.wustl.edu/courses/Schlanger/Prisons2006/Reading/Prison_Lawsuits_trends.pdf. Accessed March 25, 2009.

Schubert FA: Grilliot's Introduction to Law and the Legal System, 6th Edition. Boston, MA, Houghton Mifflin, 1996, pp 537–541

Sell v United States, 539 U.S. 166 (2003)

Vitek v Jones, 445 U.S. 480 (1980)

Wakefield v Thompson, 177 F.3d 1160 (9th Cir. 1999)

Washington v Harper, 494 U.S. 210, 215–217 (1990)

Wilkerson v Utah, 99 U.S. 130 (1878)

Wolff v McDonnell, 418 U.S. 539 (1974)

PART II

Clinical Evaluation and Care

CHAPTER 4

The Mental Health Professional in a Correctional Culture

Kenneth L. Appelbaum, M.D.

As described in Chapter 1, "Overview of the Criminal Justice System," correctional facilities include lockups and jails for pretrial defendants, houses of correction for inmates convicted of misdemeanors, and prisons for sentenced felons. Institutions are typically segregated by gender, and the custodial levels range from prerelease centers to minimum, medium, or maximum security. The purpose of each of these types of facilities can have a significant effect on the overall environment. The pace and relatively rapid turnover of population in a jail, for example, contrasts with the stability of a prison population. The atmosphere in a female facility often differs from that in a male facility. Also, as a general rule, higher-security facilities feel more stark, bleak, and oppressive.

Despite their differences, correctional institutions have many cultural similarities. Each contains a "society of captives" (Sykes 1958), subject to varying degrees of surveillance and control depending on the setting. As with any society, jails and prisons have unique rules, routines, and hardships. The inhabitants, both correctional staff and inmates, have well-defined roles and their own jargon.

Entering the correctional subculture for the first time can be daunting for the new mental health professional. The loud, crowded, and austere environment typical of many institutions may lead to unease and apprehension. In the absence of clearly defined expectations, the newcomer can feel at a loss for how to behave. With the proper preparation and attitude, however, clinicians can find correctional work surprisingly stimulating and rewarding.

I begin this chapter by examining the correctional environment, including its mission, rules, routines, and deprivations. I then review the role of the mental health professional in the correctional culture from the perspectives of custody staff, inmates, and clinicians themselves. I also explore the recent growth and evolution of academic opportunities in correctional mental health. The emphasis throughout is on the special challenges and rewards encountered by the correctional mental health care provider. My focus in this chapter is on higher-security prisons, which tend to have the most pronounced cultural differences from noncorrectional settings.

ENVIRONMENT AND CULTURE

Containment and security are central to the mission of all correctional facilities, and the environment reflects this priority. Prisons are fortresses that carefully control who gets in and, more importantly, who gets out. Without proper clearance and identification, outsiders will not make it past the "front trap." Similar to the entryway of a castle across a moat, the front trap is the passage through the razor-wire-topped outer perimeter walls. A correctional officer in a separate control station regulates entrance to and exit from the trap through the security doors on either end of the passageway. At least one door is always closed, literally trapping, at least temporarily, all traffic as it transits through the trap. Another officer assigned to the trap may search visitors and staff as they enter or leave the facility. Additional inner traps control movement within the facility. Officers control all movement. The clinician usually does not have a key.

Although the distance between two points in a prison may be short, transit time can vary considerably. Many factors affect the ease of movement. For example, delays can occur when visitors in the trap require more extensive searching and processing. Sometimes, the control officer or the trap officer is temporarily distracted by other tasks. At other times, a freeze on all movement within the institution occurs because of a medical emergency, a fight, or another disturbance. These delays cannot be avoided, but even during normal operations, the speed of movement may be directly proportional to the quality of the relationship the mental health professional has with the officers in charge. Good rapport with officers can go a long way toward improving a clinician's efficiency, and, as described later in this chapter, rapport can be critical in the efficacy of clinical assessments and interventions.

Regardless of the ease or speed of movement within a prison, one transits through a generally stark and drab environment. Whether old and dilapidated or modern and pristine, most prisons have an oppressive austerity. The architecture and the limited furnishings are utilitarian and institutional. Although inmates may attempt, within limits, to decorate their individual cells, the hallways and common areas typically remain unadorned and bleak. With little to soften them, sounds usually echo into a background din and cacophony. Musty odors of a densely populated community and the chemical scent from large-scale use of cleansers are often the prevailing smells. The overall impression of a harsh and impersonal setting strikes at both conscious and visceral levels.

Some prisons, however, provide a more enriched experience. They take a broader view of their mission than mere incapacitation. All effective prisons seek to incapacitate inmates through containment, which prevents criminal activity in society at large, and through security, which prevents criminal activity in the prison itself. In a broader sense, however, prisons serve functions other than incapacitation. Several justifications for incarceration have waxed and waned in popularity (Packer 1968). These justifications include rehabilitation, based on the assumption that incarceration can be a reforming experience. The reference to penal institutions as correctional facilities reflects the goal of rehabilitation. Thus, more enlightened institutions offer educational and vocational programming. Such programming helps to keep inmates constructively occupied; this can minimize the time and energy inmates spend making mischief, and it also helps prepare them for reintegration into society.

The routines and rules of a prison mirror the institutional feel of the physical environment. Daily activities, such as meals, medication lines, and inmate counts, typically occur on an unchanging schedule. Controlled movement periods may limit the times when an inmate can go from one location to another. The predictable regularity of prison life adds to the dullness of incarceration.

Prison rules complement the security functions of the physical plant. Rules and guidelines typically address contraband, staff behavior, and interactions with inmates. Weapons, drugs, and handcuff keys cannot be brought into facilities, but prohibitions may also exist against bringing other, less obvious items into facilities. Cell phones, computers with modems, and other devices that might allow inmates to communicate with people outside the institution can pose security risks. Large sums of money and items that can easily be fashioned into weapons, such as binder clips, may also qualify as contraband. Personal mail, magazines, or other written materials that contain home addresses or phone numbers can compromise safety. Taking photographs of the prison or its inmates will likely require the knowledge and approval of the superintendent or warden.

Other behavioral guidelines may admonish staff to stay alert and to avoid potentially dangerous situations. Such situations can include entering areas without looking for possible setups, allowing an inmate to become positioned behind the back of a staff person, and allowing an inmate to become positioned between the staff person and the exit to an area.

Significant prohibitions generally apply to relationships with inmates, former inmates, and people outside the institution. Boundary violations can include touching or being touched by an inmate, except as part of a security or medical activity; bringing items into the facility for an inmate or transporting items, such as mail, out of the facility for an inmate; discussing a staff member's personal life with an inmate; providing an inmate with special favors or receiving such favors from an inmate; or becoming overly familiar in other ways with inmates. Prohibitions also apply to contact with former inmates, and when such contact occurs, it should be reported to supervisors. Sharing information or messages with people outside the institution or with an inmate's family or friends also can breach rules and security. For example, dangerous situations can arise if an inmate or his or her associates learn details of a pending outside medical appointment or other external trips.

The correctional culture also includes its own jargon, which the mental health professional must learn. Examples of such terminology are provided in Table 4–1.

Failure to use proper terminology can cause offense and strain relationships. Correctional officers, for example, generally bristle if referred to as guards, a term perceived as not appreciating the challenges and professionalism of their work. Sergeants, lieutenants, and captains, who are recognizable, respectively, by two chevrons, a silver bar, and two gold bars on the sleeve or collar, might take umbrage if addressed in a way that does not acknowledge their superior rank. Mastery of the language specific to the institution helps convey familiarity with and sensitivity to the culture and can lessen the perception of the mental health professional as an interloper.

New health care staff generally receive an orientation that informs them about many of the aspects of the correctional environment and culture. All new employees must receive orientation for each of the prison

TABLE 4–1. Sample correctional culture jargon

Term	Definition
Bugs	Derogatory term used for inmates with mental illness
CO	Corrections officer; COs generally should not be referred to as "guards"
Count	A regularly occurring facility-wide census that typically requires inmates to be on their housing unit while the count occurs
Freeze	A cessation of all movement within a facility, including entrance and egress from "traps" (see below), often in response to an incident such as a fight
IMU	Intensive management unit
Lockdown	A facility-wide confinement of all inmates to their cells
Lugs	An officer "lugs" (rather than takes) an inmate to segregation
Med line	The line where nurses dispense medications
PC	Protective custody
Pop	General population housing unit
Reception	The process of arrival at a facility (e.g., at the start of an incarceration, at return from a court appearance, or upon transfer from another facility)
Seg	A segregation unit that keeps some inmates isolated from the general population of the facility; usually results in an inmate's being locked down for 23 hours a day for disciplinary or administrative reasons
Shakedown	A search, such as a search of a cell to look for contraband
Shank	A homemade knife or stabbing weapon
SHU	Special housing unit
Skinners	A term used for sex offenders, who generally have a low status within the inmate subculture
SMU	Special management unit
Trap	A holding area with security doors on either end that are opened one at a time from a control booth to allow secure passage
Wrap	To complete a sentence of incarceration

accreditation standards of the National Commission on Correctional Health Care (2008; see Standard P-C-09) and the American Correctional Association (2003; see Standards 4-4082 and 4-4088). Topics covered during orientation typically include security policies and procedures, contraband regulations, emergency situations, and inmate–staff relationships.

HOW OTHERS VIEW THE MENTAL HEALTH PROFESSIONAL'S ROLE IN THE CORRECTIONAL CULTURE

Custody Staff

As noted in the preceding section, the core mission of correctional staff involves containment and security. Custody staff sometimes view clinicians as guests: welcome and appreciated when relationships are good, but rejected and resented when relationships are poor. Correctional officers have the authority to enforce rules, regimentation, and sanctions. Unlike health care providers, who typically seek negotiated compliance from their patients, correctional officers have an authoritarian basis for their relationship with inmates. These disparate ideologies sometimes lead to conflict between officers and clinicians (Cormier 1973; Culbertson 1977; Cumming and Solway 1973; Kaufman 1973; Powelson and Bendix 1951; Roth 1986). Officers may view mental health professionals in particular as naive or even indulgent with inmates, and mental health professionals may view officers as overly harsh and punitive.

The two professional groups, however, have many common interests despite their often disparate training, beliefs, methods, and purposes (Steadman et al. 1989). Neither can function effectively without the other. Correctional officers, for example, have extremely stressful jobs (Finn 2000). They identify the threat of violence by inmates as their most frequent source of stress (Finn 2000). Only police officers experience a higher rate of nonfatal workplace violence (Warchol 1998). Dysfunctional behavior and poor adaptation by inmates with mental disorders, described in the following subsection, add to officer stress. Competent mental health treatment results in fewer behavioral disturbances and more tranquil facilities. Mental health professionals, for their part, cannot readily provide their services in an unsafe environment.

Effective correctional officers, of whom there are many, perform their tasks with professionalism. They are firm but fair. They support humane health care services, and they appreciate the contribution that psychiatrists and other mental health professionals make to operational efficiency (Steadman et al. 1989).

Achieving harmonious and collaborative relationships, however, takes time and effort. A new prison mental health professional will likely face scrutiny by correctional officers, as well as by inmates (Robey 1998). Staff and inmate observers will closely note the clinician's appearance, behavior, opinions, reactions, and interpersonal style. Showing professional respect for the challenges faced by custody staff and for their knowledge and expertise can play a critical role in the ultimate acceptance of the clinician. The newcomer's attitude toward security constraints, his or her temperament, and his or her approach to advocacy, privilege requests, medication use, consultation-liaison situations, forensic questions, and confidentiality, as described later in this chapter, will all affect the quality of relations with security staff.

Inmates

The deprivations of the prison environment can take a toll on inmates. In addition to tedium and boredom, inmates must cope with separation from family and social supports, limited privacy and autonomy, and fear of assault. Rape, which can have especially devastating physical and psychological consequences, is an understudied but endemic problem in correctional settings (Dumond 2003). Overcrowding, a common occurrence in many prisons (Harrison and Beck 2003), adds to the stress. Even in the absence of other traumatic events, the inherently dehumanizing experience of incarceration itself can have intensely negative psychological effects (Haney and Zimbaro 1998).

Inmates who have mental disorders are especially vulnerable to the hardships of incarceration (Human Rights Watch 2003). They risk rape (Dumond 2003) and victimization by higher-functioning inmates. The challenges of prison life can overwhelm their already limited coping skills and lead to exacerbation of symptoms, functional deterioration, and poor adaptation (Morgan et al. 1993; Sowers et al. 1999; Toch and Adams 1987). Some inmates with mental disorders have difficulty understanding and following rules and expectations. Those with schizophrenia (Morgan et al. 1993), mental retardation (Santamour and West 1982), or mental illness in general (Ditton 1999) commit more rule infractions, spend more time in lockup, and are less likely to obtain parole.

Despite the predominantly negative effects of incarceration, some inmates obtain tangible benefits (Human Rights Watch 2003). Although conditions can vary dramatically across states, many correctional systems offer services that may exceed those received by inmates prior to incarceration. Prisons sometimes provide better access to treatment, shelter, structure, and even safety than is available to homeless or unemployed people in the general community. Many inmates with mental disorders receive their first comprehensive treatment services during their incarcerations.

Attitudes of inmates toward their health care providers depend, in part, on the quality of care in the system and on the manner in which clinicians approach their role. Similar to correctional officers, inmates usually try to appraise the attitude of a new mental health professional. In some instances, they may test the provider in one of several ways: How will a new psychiatrist respond to requests for medications or special privileges? Will a clinician inappropriately bend rules or regulations with inmates and become open to exploitation? How will a mental health professional handle questions of confidentiality? Will a clinician treat inmates in an overly punitive or an overly indulgent manner? Although only some inmates will engage in schemes or testing involving the newcomer, the mental health care provider's reputation will likely spread quickly. For the most part, however, inmates show appreciation and respect to competent, caring, and professional health care providers who offer appropriate services. A capable and considerate clinician provides welcome relief in an often harsh environment.

Relationships between inmates and health care providers, however, do not always achieve such harmony. Inmate patients can have both legitimate and frivolous grievances against their clinicians. Poor services and disrespectful or incompetent providers will likely receive a catalogue of complaints. Even appropriate care may result in grievances when inmates pursue demands for unnecessary services, medications, or privileges.

Dissatisfaction with care may lead some inmates to seek legal redress. Unlike free persons in the general community, inmates cannot choose their medical caregivers or switch providers when displeased with services. A similar lack of alternatives binds the caregiver, who cannot refuse to provide services to the inmate patient. Thus, malpractice lawsuits or complaints to state licensing boards may represent an inmate's attempt to gain leverage when seeking a denied service. Some clinicians with unblemished records and histories of good rapport with their patients may begin to accumulate legal complaints from working in prisons.

Correctional employment also exposes the mental health professional to a legal course of action rarely encountered in other practice settings. Inmates, in comparison with other patients, disproportionately file allegations of constitutional violations against their medical and mental health caretakers. The basis for these allegations generally derives from the 1976 U.S. Supreme Court decision *Estelle v. Gamble* (1976). In *Estelle*, the Supreme Court held that deliberate indifference by prison personnel to a prisoner's serious illness or injury constitutes cruel and unusual punishment that contravenes the Eighth Amendment to the U.S. Constitution. No other patient group in the United States has a constitutionally recognized right to health care. Although the Supreme Court did not explicitly include a right to treatment for mental disorders in the *Estelle* decision, which dealt with a nonpsychiatric problem, a federal court of appeals quickly found no reason to distinguish between rights to treatment for medical and psychiatric conditions (*Bowring v. Godwin* 1977). In the ensuing years, no court has found that the constitutional right to care does not extend to psychiatric cases (Cohen 1998). This constitutional right provides inmate litigants with access to federal courts. Because of the prevalence of such litigation, correctional health care providers should seek insurance that covers at least the expenses involved in defending against accusations of civil rights violations, along with standard malpractice coverage.

The neophyte correctional clinician may fear assault more than litigation. Although this fear is not entirely without basis, such concerns usually exceed the real risk. Inmates have little to gain and much to lose from harming health care providers. Security measures, including close monitoring and rapid response by officers, also help limit the risk. Correctional clinicians who have worked in other public sector mental health programs often feel much safer practicing in prisons than in other inpatient or outpatient settings.

THE MENTAL HEALTH PROFESSIONAL'S ROLE IN THE CORRECTIONAL CULTURE

Appeal of Correctional Mental Health

Although the challenges of working in a prison can seem daunting, the rewards more than compensate for many clinicians. Correctional work appeals to some individuals for a mix of altruistic, clinical, financial, and lifestyle-related reasons. Many health care providers have a commitment to public service for historically underserved populations, such as inmates. In a system with adequate resources and reasonable caseloads, the practitioner can focus his or her time and energy on delivery of good clinical care instead of having to concentrate on processing paperwork and overcoming restrictions of managed care. The predictable income of a salaried position, absence of the expenses and demands of running a practice, and limited on-call responsibilities can add to the attractiveness.

Not all prison systems, however, have the same appeal. In addition to the typically stark environment, many correctional health care programs have insufficient funding and resources, which can limit staffing and services. The consequences of inadequate staffing include high caseloads that allow for little more than cursory psychopharmacological or case management and insufficient time to treat any but the most seriously disturbed inmates. Other important psychiatric tasks, such as providing diagnostic consultations or serving as a liaison with correctional staff, cannot readily occur in understaffed facilities. Shortages of other licensed professionals that compose the multidisciplinary mental health treatment team also can significantly detract from the appeal of correctional employment. Underfunding in some systems affects not only staffing levels but the quality of services and programming. Such systems may have severely restricted formularies and limited access to hospitalization or intermediate care programs for inmates with rehabilitation needs. A paucity of educational, vocational, and other correctional programming can add to distress and dysfunction among inmates, compounding the effects of unmet treatment needs.

Temperament

Even in well-staffed and well-funded programs, however, the correctional health care provider must recognize that the prison is not primarily a medical or mental health center (Start 1998). Security constraints will almost always trump clinical agendas. For example, appointments commonly cannot be scheduled during inmate counts or other lockdown situations, and inmates sometimes fail to show for scheduled appointments because of freezes on movement within a facility or other security-related impediments. Some prisons can have surprisingly high rates of such no-show appointments, considering the captive nature of the patient population.

Just as a prison's characteristics can influence its attractiveness as a work site, a clinician's temperament can affect the success of adaptation to correctional work. Some individuals may experience the harsh environment, security constraints, and relationships with correctional staff and inmates as too overwhelming and stressful (Bell 1989). Attitudes and demeanor remain important even for those who do not feel overwhelmed by the overall climate. Expressed respect for correctional officers, a flexible style, acceptance of sometimes antiquated furnishings, and low expectations for special accommodations all increase the likelihood of positive adjustment.

A clinician's temperament will also affect the quality of relationships with inmate patients. Like any other patients, inmates usually respond positively when treated with respect by a competent and caring professional, but maintaining harmonious relationships poses challenges at times. Some inmates have committed heinous crimes that engender feelings of disgust. Even the most compassionate professional will have difficulty overcoming such feelings in some circumstances. Successful adaptation to prison work usually involves an ability to sustain a caring and professional attitude despite an inmate's reprehensible past. At the very least, the mental health care provider needs to resist any inclination to withhold appropriate professional care because of negative feelings.

Preserving professional perspective can become even more difficult when an inmate tries to exploit the treatment relationship to obtain a desired, but often unstated, goal. With limited access to the goods, services, and privileges that free persons typically take for granted, some inmates will use any available opportunity to gain sought-after commodities. Such inmates may get branded as manipulative, but this label rarely serves a useful purpose. Instead, it conveys a pejorative and adversarial attitude toward the inmate. At best, using the term *manipulative* represents a shorthand communication that the described behavior has its roots in external incentives instead of an underlying mental disorder. Thus, treatment interventions that might be appropriate for behavior associated with a serious mental disorder become inappropriate, and even contraindicated, when the behavior denotes a calculated deception. This economy of communication comes with a price. The relationship between the inmate and the mental health professional may become a contest with an inevitable winner and loser. Because few people enjoy losing, the clinician's focus may shift away from understanding the reasons for the inmate's disruptive behaviors and toward resisting exploitation.

A more clinically useful approach begins by acknowledging that all people, including inmates, have needs. In an effort to meet those needs, people often try to manage, or manipulate, the impressions they make within a relationship. Inmates, who have few luxuries and little autonomy, may have even greater motivation than most people have to seize whatever advantages possible. By interpreting an inmate's behavior as an attempt to meet identifiable needs, the mental health professional can better understand those needs while depersonalizing and disengaging from, as much as possible, the struggle for power and control.

An explicit identification of the inmate's goals provides a foundation for a behavior management approach to the situation. As described in the following subsection on advocacy, for example, a thoughtful and professional approach to privilege requests or to goal-directed self-injurious behavior is more helpful than pejorative labeling and adversarial interactions.

Advocacy

An especially critical aspect of the mental health professional's temperament involves patient advocacy. Either excessive or insufficient advocacy can cause problems. A clinician who overly champions the interests of inmates may lose credibility and persuasiveness as a clinical proponent. An effective advocate uses discretion when choosing which battles to fight. In the absence of some restraint, the clinician may squander the ability to have influence over more significant concerns.

Excessive reticence about advocacy can also create problems. Mental health professionals have special expertise and a unique perspective about quality of care and the mental health needs of inmates. In the absence of active involvement by mental health professionals in clinical policy and administration, both inmates and correctional systems lose the benefit of an important voice. Inmates may receive less than adequate care, and systems expose themselves to potential public health, safety, and legal problems because of substandard services. Distinguishing minor concerns from important matters that affect quality of care is not always easy.

In addition to advocating for adequate resources and systemic services, correctional clinicians occasionally must recommend special privileges for inmates who have mental illnesses. Inmates sometimes request adjustments in housing, work assignments, or recreational opportunities, as well as allotment of extra services or commodities. The clinician walks a fine line between supporting appropriate requests that can help inmates deal with disabling symptoms or treatment side effects and encouraging excessive demands and accommodations that can disrupt facility operations. Table 4–2 provides some recommended guidelines for responding to privilege requests (Pinta 1998).

Medication Use

An area of advocacy that falls uniquely within the competence and responsibility of psychiatrists involves access to medications. Because inmates should be able to obtain the full range of psychotropic medications available in the broader community, psychiatrists need to play a key role in helping to ensure that correctional formularies and policies do not compromise care through unreasonable restrictions. For example, clinically acceptable standards of care allow patients to receive first-line medications without first having to fail in treatment on less expensive second-line agents. At the same time, however, financial and operational concerns also warrant careful consideration.

Formulary costs have become a major fiscal challenge not only for correctional systems but also for private insurers, public mental health systems, and other community organizations. In recent years, costs have significantly increased for medications used in the treatment of mental disorders, HIV disease, hepatitis C, and other disorders. Pharmaceutical expenses, however, represent only one of many expenses associated with such

TABLE 4–2. Guidelines for responding to requests for special privileges

1. Explore alternatives to granting privileges.
2. Base privilege decisions on objective data.
3. Use privileges mostly for patients with serious mental disorders.
4. Involve custody staff in special privilege decisions.

disorders. Systems that fail to provide adequate access to medications will likely incur added expenses in other areas. For example, substandard pharmacological treatment of mental disorders, infectious diseases, and other serious conditions can result in otherwise avoidable suffering, disability, hospitalizations, staff injuries, and lost productivity. Because most inmates eventually return to the community, poor treatment in prison can jeopardize the health and safety of the general public. Psychiatrists can advocate for modern formularies by providing educational information about these broader costs and considerations.

Prescribing practices also have operational effects, especially for nursing and security staff. Controlled substances, such as benzodiazepines and stimulants, require special procedures for storage, monitoring, and administration. These procedures, along with additional precautions, such as crushing of medications, all add to the demands on often-limited nursing time. The potential for misuse and the black market sale of controlled substances also has security implications. Predatory inmates might steal controlled substances from other inmates by pressuring those inmates into hiding pills in their mouths instead of swallowing them. Some inmates also feign symptoms in attempts to get medications that they do not need. Crushing controlled substances, whenever possible, eliminates much of the potential for medication stealing and black market diversion, but it does require additional nursing time, as noted.

Despite appropriate precautions, prescribing controlled substances, such as benzodiazepines and stimulants, creates vexing problems for many correctional psychiatrists. Responding to inmate demands for controlled substances and attempting to distinguish truly symptomatic inmates from malingerers often requires considerable clinical time. Security staff, nurses, and nonmedical clinicians may view even appropriate prescribing practices with skepticism, and they might pressure psychiatrists to decrease or eliminate orders for these medications. Formal or de facto prohibitions on the use of these agents, however, would deprive inmates of access to safe and effective treatments that are available and widely used for patients in the general community (Moller 1999; Posternak and Mueller 2001). Careful selection of patients for treatment (Appelbaum 2008a) and development of treatment protocols (Appelbaum 2009) can minimize some of the problems associated with stimulant use, and similar approaches can help with the prescription of other controlled substances.

Regarding benzodiazepines, in addition to their well-established efficacy in treating generalized anxiety disorder, panic disorder, and sleep disorders, they can play a role in the treatment of many other conditions, including social phobia, mood disorders, schizophrenia, seizure disorders, and muscle spasms. Withholding treatment exposes patients to unnecessary suffering, and alternative pharmacological treatments often have less efficacy and/or lower safety than benzodiazepines. Although benzodiazepines are among the most widely prescribed medications in the United States, with millions of prescriptions per year, relatively few patients seek dosage increases or engage in drug-seeking behavior (U.S. Drug Enforcement Administration 2009; Soumerai et al. 2003). Even many former substance abusers can safely benefit from treatment with benzodiazepines (Posternak and Mueller 2001). In addition, compared with people in the general community, inmates have less opportunity to misuse benzodiazepines, or other medications, by obtaining multiple prescriptions from different physicians or by combining benzodiazepines with illicit substances. As with any other treatment modality, both the psychiatrist and the patient need to weigh the risks and benefits of benzodiazepines against the risks and benefits of alternative interventions. The acknowledged problems associated with the prescription of controlled substances in prisons, as well as in community settings, do not justify blanket restrictions on their availability.

Correctional psychiatrists can show sensitivity to many fiscal and operational concerns in several ways without compromising clinical care. For example, strategies that focus on dosage strength and frequency can lower medication costs and demands on nursing time. For many of the newer psychotropic agents, such as the atypical antipsychotic medications, the selective serotonin reuptake inhibitors, and other novel antidepressants, the cost per pill does not substantially differ based on the dosage strength. Thus, providing a medication as a once-a-day dose often costs half as much as providing the same total quantity divided into two doses. Limiting the number of doses also diminishes the time that inmates spend in medication lines and nurses spend dispensing medications. Similarly, dosages that require use of multiple-tablet strengths, such as 75 mg of a medication that comes only in 25-, 50-, and 100-mg strengths, can dramatically increase expenses. Fiscal sensitivity also includes careful attention to evidence-based practices that 1) avoid use of medications without empirical or clinical justifications or 2) substitute equally effective generic or alternative medications for expensive preparations.

Although correctional systems have an obligation to provide inmates with access to the same care and services that should be available in the community, incarceration can provide an opportunity to reassess an inmate's mental health needs and discontinue unnecessary treatment. Many inmates arrive in prison after accumulating multiple medications in the community, often within the context of active substance abuse that complicates their symptom and diagnostic presentation. Controlled medication tapering and observation in the prison represent a rare opportunity to carefully reassess inmates' clinical needs. This process can reasonably occur, however, only in systems that have adequate professional staff to ensure comprehensive evaluation and ongoing follow-up to monitor the effect of these changes.

Consultation and Liaison Roles

As noted in the previous subsection, sufficient staffing levels allow mental health professionals, including psychiatrists, to provide more comprehensive services and to play broader roles within correctional systems. In addition to prescribing and monitoring psychotropic medications and responding to psychiatric emergencies, psychiatrists can participate in policy development and assist with difficult diagnostic questions and with strategies for managing disruptive behaviors. Nonpsychiatric physicians, other mental health professionals, and correctional staff can all benefit from access to psychiatrists' training and expertise.

A particularly challenging consultative situation involves inmates who engage in disruptive behaviors (e.g., flooding cells, setting fires, smearing body wastes and fluids) or self-injurious behaviors (e.g., cutting, inserting or swallowing inappropriate objects, interfering with medical treatment). Although several psychiatric disorders can be accompanied by self-injurious behavior (Winchel and Stanley 1991), other precipitants and motivators that often occur in correctional settings include isolation, loss of a sense of control, anxiety, situational stress, and attention- or drug-seeking behavior (Fulwiler et al. 1997; Martinez 1980; Thorburn 1984). Most self-injurious behavior in prisons occurs in isolation or segregation settings (Jones 1986). An inmate's autonomy is severely limited by segregation, and incarceration in general, but controlling what an inmate does to his or her own body is difficult, if not impossible. Self-harm can return some control to the inmate, such as the chance to obtain a transfer to a medical unit. These behaviors also sometimes relieve tension and anxiety due to situational stresses, and they may occur in reaction to sexual intimidation or assaults. Some inmates enjoy the commotion caused by their behaviors or seek the attention or medications they receive after hurting themselves.

The most difficult cases of self-injurious behaviors in prisons involve power struggles between the inmate and the correctional administration. Inmates with ulterior motives have higher rates of recurrence of these behaviors than do inmates who self-injure with suicidal intent (Franklin 1988; Fulwiler et al. 1997). The presence of ulterior motives, however, does not necessarily indicate an absence of suicidal intent or a low risk of lethality (Dear et al. 2000; Haycock 1989; Karp et al. 1991). Some inmates miscalculate the risks of their behaviors, and others are willing to risk death in an attempt to get what they want. Regardless of the underlying intent, however, serious episodes of self-harm generally require a freeze in movement and suspension of normal operations during the response to the incident. Staff and other inmates risk exposure to potentially infectious blood and body fluids, and the need to transfer the inmate to a health services unit, emergency room, or hospital can drain staff time and financial resources.

The challenge of dealing with self-injurious inmates or with inmates who engage in other disruptive behaviors can be a source of ongoing conflict between mental health care and custody staff or an opportunity for communication and collaboration. Polarized and dichotomous disputes about whether the behavior represents a mental health or security problem serve little purpose except to create splitting and divisiveness. Interventions with self-injurious inmates must involve shared responsibility among medical, mental health, and custody personnel, or they will have little chance of effectiveness. The role of the mental health professional can include diagnostic assessment to rule out an underlying mental disorder as a cause of the behavior, elucidating the environmental contingencies that reinforce the behavior, and helping to develop intervention plans that reshape those contingencies.

Forensic Roles

Unlike consultations that focus on management of disruptive behaviors, dual-agency consultations create fundamental conflicts for correctional clinicians (Belitsky 2002; Dvoskin et al. 1995; Krelstein 2002; Metzner 2002). A mental health professional who treats inmates cannot appropriately conduct, with the same inmates, forensic evaluations, such as parole assessments or formal determinations of competence or responsibility in disciplinary proceedings. Clinical, ethical, professional, and programmatic contraindications preclude such formal assessments or opinions. The therapeutic alliance with inmate–patients would likely weaken if treatment providers assumed forensic responsibilities. Clinical care can suffer if inmates become less trusting and less willing to share information. In part because of the adverse effect that a forensic evaluation can have on the therapeutic relationship, ethical guidelines assert that treating psychiatrists should generally avoid performing evaluations of their patients for forensic purposes (American Academy of Psychiatry and the Law 2005). In addition, forensic evaluations usually require third-party interviews that are not commonly a part of a therapeutic relationship and specialized knowledge, training, skills, and experience that general clinicians do not necessarily possess. Examiners who lack the requisite background often reach conclusions based on an unsophisticated understanding of the forensic issues. Conducting formal forensic assessments can also foster tensions between custody and mental health staff and drain programmatic resources away from the primary mission of providing treatment services.

Role boundaries do not necessarily restrict appropriate informal sharing of clinical information. For example, limited sharing of information may help disciplinary hearing officers to appreciate an association between an inmate's symptoms and behavior that might otherwise result in a disciplinary sanction such as placement in segregation. Even when symptoms do not have a direct relationship to the proscribed behavior, they may impair the ability of an inmate to tolerate segregation or other sanctions. Mental health professionals have an obligation to inform correctional staff of these mitigating and dispositional factors, without undertaking formal forensic roles or offering formal forensic opinions.

These informal, but potentially valuable, consultations with disciplinary officers and correctional administrators can involve general education about mental health matters, as well as information about the functioning of a specific inmate in active mental health treatment. For example, inmates may receive disciplinary sanctions for failing to comply with instructions and regulations, such as providing urine samples for drug screening. Some inmates, however, may claim that for psychological reasons they cannot produce a urine specimen while observed, a frequently occurring condition known as paruresis (Bohn and Sternbach 1997; Labbate 1996–1997; Zgourides 1987). Difficulty with public urination is one of several common social fears and phobias (Kessler et al. 1998), and it can occur with a wide range of severity among individuals or within the same person in different circumstances and times. No definitive or objective test is available to confirm or refute the presence of paruresis. The absence of prior treatment or the ability to void in some social situations but not in others does not rule it out. Although modalities associated with the treatment of social phobias help some individuals, no universally effective medication or other treatment exists. Coercive interventions, such as forcing fluids while observing a person with paruresis, are ineffective and can cause serious medical complications. Alternatives to observed urine specimen collection for individuals who self-report paruresis include unobserved collections in a dry room, testing of hair specimens, saliva testing, sweat testing with a patch, and blood testing ("Tests for Drugs of Abuse" 2002). These alternatives preclude the need for futile attempts to differentiate inmates with true paruresis from those who fabricate complaints. Mental health professionals provide a valuable service to the disciplinary process and to inmates when they provide information about such conditions and helpful suggestions about their management.

Confidentiality

Limitations on confidentiality exist in prisons, just as they do in other settings. In addition to universally recognized exceptions to confidentiality, such as the duty to protect, some exceptions arise uniquely in correctional facilities. For example, mental health professionals may need to report to authorities serious inmate rule violations and plans for escapes or disturbances.

Some information is hard to keep confidential in a prison. Because of medication lines and scheduled clinic visits, correctional officers and other inmates have little difficulty determining which inmates take medications or have appointments with mental health care providers. Inmates at maximum security facilities may require special transport and monitoring by officers during mental health appointments. The medical record itself is often accessible to security staff. In Massachusetts, for example, the medical record, including the mental health notes, belongs to the Department of Correction. Health care personnel have access to the record as needed for the performance of their duties. Designated correctional administrators have unrestricted access to the record, and other custody personnel can receive authorization to review the record for reasons that include preserving the health or enhancing the care of the patient, protecting the health of others, and exercising a duty to warn (Commonwealth of Massachusetts Regulations, 103 DOC 607.05, Inmate Medical Records).

In addition, correctional officers cannot adequately fulfill their important role in observing and intervening with inmates who have mental disorders unless mental health professionals share some clinical information with them (Appelbaum et al. 2001). Compared with clinicians, who have relatively brief contact with inmates, correctional officers typically spend many hours a day in close proximity to inmates. They may have the first opportunity to observe significant changes in an inmate's behavior or mental status. Their observations can aid in diagnostic assessments and alert clinical staff to potential crisis situations. Officers can also assist inmates with functional impairments and encourage treatment compliance if they know about inmates' mental health needs. For officers to fulfill these roles effectively, clinicians must sometimes share confidential information to apprise them of concerns about an inmate. If appropriate communication between clinical and security staff does not occur, the treatment of inmates suffers and their safety can be compromised (Geller et al. 1997). Successful collaboration requires clinical staff to exercise discretion about the type and amount of information to share, and requires security staff to handle the clinical information that they receive with the same degree of care and confidentiality that applies to clinicians. Under Massachusetts law, for example, Department of Correction employees must keep "strictly confidential" any information that they learn regarding an inmate's medical condition (Commonwealth of Massachusetts Regulations, 103 DOC 607.05; General Laws of Massachusetts, Chapter 111, section 70E: Patients' and Residents' Rights).

THE MENTAL HEALTH PROFESSIONAL'S EVOLVING ROLE AS STUDENT, TEACHER, AND RESEARCHER

As with correctional medicine in general, correctional mental health has struggled to establish its academic base. Scholars and researchers have contributed to the field with varying degrees of recognition and success. Although many competent and dedicated professionals have chosen penal settings for their clinical and academic work, they have had to contend with a historically poor, and often undeserved, image (Roth 1986; Yarvis 1996–1997). Recent developments, however, bode well for enhancing the academic foundations of correctional mental health and the stature of its practitioners. Progress continues to occur in areas that include standards and certifications, involvement by medical schools, training opportunities, and research. Each of these areas provides correctional clinicians with opportunities to learn and to advance the field.

Standards and Certifications

Several national organizations, including the American Public Health Association (2003) and the American Correctional Association (2003), have promulgated standards for correctional health services. Especially noteworthy contributions have come from the American Psychiatric Association (APA) and the National Commission on Correctional Health Care (NCCHC).

The APA guidelines, which were first published in 1989, are now in their second edition (American Psychiatric Association 2000). Components of the APA have also begun to address challenging aspects of correctional psychiatry, such as the use of seclusion and restraint for mental health reasons (Metzner et al. 2007), which has led to commentary and debate in the professional literature (Appelbaum 2007; Champion 2007; O'Grady 2007; Vlach and Daniel 2007).

NCCHC, which was first incorporated in 1983, arose out of a project by the American Medical Association in the 1970s. Thirty-eight national organizations from the fields of health, law, and corrections appoint representatives to NCCHC's board of directors. In addition to a certification process for correctional health professionals and publications that include national standards and guidelines and a peer-reviewed journal, services offered by NCCHC include a voluntary accreditation program for correctional institutions, conferences and educational programs, and consultations and technical assistance.

Involvement by Medical Schools

Some correctional systems have increased the desirability of employment for health care providers by partnering with medical schools (Appelbaum et al. 2002). Recruiting and retaining adequate numbers of qualified providers for jails and prisons have often been challenging (King 1998; Moore 1998; Roth 1986). Involvement by a medical school, however, can enhance the prestige of correctional work and help to attract practitioners with an interest in learning, teaching, and research. Medical school affiliations can assist with continuing education programming and ensure up-to-date practices. The presence of students and trainees also provides a stimulus for professional staff to maintain their knowledge and skills. Thus, correctional health care providers in these systems have encouragement to continue their development both as students and as teachers.

Medical schools also have the ability to provide unique training activities that attest to the growing recognition of correctional health care as an area of special skill and expertise. In 1997, for example, the Accreditation Council for Graduate Medical Education (ACGME) began formal accreditation of fellowship programs in forensic psychiatry. These programs must provide trainees with experience treating individuals involved in the criminal justice system, and many programs provide this experience through rotations based in penal institutions. In conjunction with ACGME recognition of forensic psychiatry training programs, the American Board of Psychiatry and Neurology began certifying psychiatrists with added qualifications in forensic psychiatry in 1994. Graduates of accredited fellowship programs may take the certification examination, which includes correctional psychiatry as one of the tested content areas. Although advanced training and certification in forensic psychiatry are not prerequisites for practice in penal settings, the number of correctional psychiatrists who have this training will likely increase over time, and the establishment of a recognized subspecialty curriculum can have broader benefits.

Other Training Opportunities

In addition to training programs run by medical schools and other professional health care schools, practitioners have growing opportunities for ongoing training and continuing education. As already noted, NCCHC runs conferences and educational programs, and other national organizations, such as the American Academy of Psychiatry and the Law, include correctional mental health among the topic areas covered at national and regional conferences. In addition, medical schools have not limited their activities to formal training programs for students and residents. The University of Massachusetts Medical School, for example, has taken a leading role in organizing an ongoing series of annual national conferences on academic correctional health (Appelbaum 2008b). These meetings have attracted academicians, clinicians, researchers, and correctional personnel from all over the United States and increasingly from abroad.

Research

The expanding involvement by medical schools and the growing focus on correctional health in national conferences also provide opportunities to advance research in medical and mental health care. Significant gaps exist in knowledge of critical areas such as epidemiology, research methodology, assessment of functional impairments in penal settings, efficacy of treatment interventions, and factors related to safety and risk reduction (Appelbaum 2008b). Despite the broad need, many barriers stand in the way of ongoing research. Funding difficulties, resistance from stakeholders, restricted access to subjects, limited information technology, ethical concerns, and institutional review board requirements can all impede studies with correctional populations. Historical exploitation of vulnerable inmates (Hornblum 1997; Kalmbach and Lyons 2003), for example, understandably led to protective federal regulations (U.S. Department of Health and Human Services 2005). The Institute of Medicine (Gostin et al. 2006) has come out with recommended revisions to the 30-year-old conclusions of the National Commission for the Protection of Human Subjects of Biomedical and Behavioral Research (1976) regarding research with prisoners, but these recommendations may do little to ease the hurdles in the way of correctional research. Although substantial barriers to research remain, hopefully correctional mental health professionals may have increasing opportunities to do clinically relevant and ethically sound research that will close some of the gaps in current knowledge.

FACTORS FOR A MENTAL HEALTH PROFESSIONAL TO CONSIDER BEFORE SEEKING EMPLOYMENT IN CORRECTIONS

This chapter has included an exploration of some of the challenges and rewards for mental health professionals who choose to work in correctional settings. Clinicians who contemplate such employment would be well served by giving careful thought to these factors. Not everyone is well suited for work in a jail or prison. A careful and honest self-assessment may help clarify whether this is the right place for one to work. For example, will an austere environment, patient scheduling disruptions, or a lack of uppermost status be sources of irritation or taken in stride? Is one prepared to generally accept the sometimes harsh and detrimental realities that inmates can experience and advocate selectively on their behalf, in a constructive way, and only on significant clinical issues? Table 4–3 lists both positive and negative aspects of correctional employment that warrant consideration by mental health professionals.

CONCLUSION

Mental health professionals venture into a different world when they enter a prison. Within the often stark, regimented, and utilitarian environment exists a culture with its own rules, customs, jargon, roles, and relationships. Medical services have historically occupied a peripheral place in the overall mission and organization of a prison, unlike in the health care facilities with which clinicians typically have the greatest familiarity. Nevertheless, psychiatrists and other mental health care providers play an increasingly recognized and central role in correctional institutions. They can make valuable contributions to the health and well-being of inmates and to the safety and efficiency of the institution. Although not every clinician has the temperament or desire to pursue a successful career in corrections, those who possess these characteristics may find rewarding opportunities in correctional work. Openness and sensitivity to the cultural differences and constraints increase the likelihood of harmonious relationships. The topics covered in this chapter provide an overview to some of the areas that make this work both challenging and interesting.

TABLE 4–3.   Pros and cons of working in a correctional setting

Pros	Cons
Public service for a historically underserved population	Safety concerns (often exaggerated)
Ability to focus primarily on clinical care	Inadequate clinical staffing in some correctional systems
Often less nonclinical paperwork and fewer managed care restrictions compared to general community settings	Sometimes limited resources, including information technologies
Working with complex clinical and behavioral situations	Coping with potentially negative feelings about inmate behaviors
Inmate appreciation for receipt of good professional care	Increased likelihood of board complaints and litigation, including allegations of civil rights violations
Interesting systems and subculture challenges	Practicing in frequently drab settings that are not devoted primarily to health care, and dealing with security-related disruptions to clinical schedules
Working with a team of other health care and custody professionals	Potential for interdisciplinary conflicts
Predictable income of a salaried position and usually limited on-call responsibilities	Limitations on autonomy, including ability to select patients
Increasing involvement of medical schools and expanding opportunities for teaching, research, and continuing education	Paucity of research-based knowledge and impediments to conducting research
Growing prestige and recognition of correctional health care as an important subspecialty area	Historically poor, even if undeserved, reputation of correctional health care providers

SUMMARY POINTS

An effective correctional mental health professional

- Understands the correctional culture.
- Complies with institutional rules and regulations.
- Maintains appropriate boundaries.
- Uses correctional jargon appropriately.
- Treats inmates, security staff, and other health care professionals with respect.
- Collaborates with security staff.
- Approaches patients in a professional, nonadversarial way.
- Adapts with flexibility to the prison environment.
- Advocates selectively.
- Practices with sensitivity to fiscal and operational concerns.
- Provides consultation and liaison services.
- Balances confidentiality with sharing of necessary information.
- Contributes to compliance with evolving standards of care.
- Participates in continuing education activities.

REFERENCES

American Academy of Psychiatry and the Law: Ethics Guidelines for the Practice of Forensic Psychiatry. Bloomfield, CT, American Academy of Psychiatry and the Law, 2005

American Correctional Association: Standards for Adult Correctional Institutions, 4th Edition. Lanham, MD, American Correctional Association, 2003

American Psychiatric Association: Psychiatric Services in Jails and Prisons: A Task Force Report of the American Psychiatric Association, 2nd Edition. Washington, DC, American Psychiatric Association, 2000

American Public Health Association: Standards for Health Services in Correctional Institutions, 3rd Edition. Washington, DC, American Public Health Association, 2003

Appelbaum KL: Commentary: the use of restraint and seclusion in correctional mental health. J Am Acad Psychiatry Law 35:431–435, 2007

Appelbaum KL: Assessment and treatment of correctional inmates with ADHD. Am J Psychiatry 165:1520–1524, 2008a

Appelbaum KL: Correctional mental health research: opportunities and barriers. Journal of Correctional Health Care 14:269–277, 2008b

Appelbaum KL: ADHD in prison: a treatment protocol. J Am Acad Psychiatry Law 37:45–49, 2009

Appelbaum KL, Hickey JM, Packer I: The role of correctional officers in multidisciplinary mental health care in prisons. Psychiatr Serv 52:1343–1347, 2001

Appelbaum KL, Manning TD, Noonan JD: A university-state-corporation partnership for providing correctional mental health services. Psychiatr Serv 53:185–189, 2002

Belitsky R: Commentary: mental health in the inmate disciplinary process. J Am Acad Psychiatry Law 30:500–501, 2002

Bell MH: Stress as a factor for mental health professionals in correctional facilities, in Correctional Psychiatry. Edited by Rosner R, Harmon RB. New York, Plenum, 1989, pp 145–154

Bohn P, Sternbach H: Current knowledge and research directions in the treatment of paruresis. Depress Anxiety 5:41–42, 1997

Bowring v Godwin, 551 F.2d 44 (4th Cir. 1977)

Champion MK: Commentary: seclusion and restraint in corrections—a time for change. J Am Acad Psychiatry Law 35:426–430, 2007

Cohen F: The Mentally Disordered Inmate and the Law. Kingston, NJ, Civic Research Institute, 1998

Cormier B: The practice of psychiatry in the prison society. Bull Am Acad Psychiatry Law 1:156–183, 1973

Culbertson R: Personnel conflicts in jail management. Am J Correct 39:28–39, 1977

Cumming R, Solway H: The incarcerated psychiatrist. Hosp Community Psychiatry 24:631–632, 1973

Dear GE, Thomson DM, Hills AM: Self-harm in prison: manipulators can also be suicide attempters. Crim Justice Behav 27:160–175, 2000

Ditton PM: Mental Health and Treatment of Inmates and Probationers (BJS Special Report, NCJ 174463). Washington, DC, U.S. Department of Justice, Office of Justice Programs, Bureau of Justice Statistics, July 1999

Dumond RW: Confronting America's most ignored crime problem: the Prison Rape Elimination Act of 2003. J Am Acad Psychiatry Law 31:354–360, 2003

Dvoskin JA, Petrila J, Stark-Riemer S: Case note: Powell v Coughlin and the application of the professional judgment rule to prison mental health. Ment Phys Disabil Law Rep 19:108–114, 1995

Estelle v Gamble, 429 U.S. 97 (1976)

Finn P: Addressing correctional officer stress: programs and strategies (NJC 183474). December 2000. Available at: http://www.ncjrs.org/pdffiles1/nij/183474.pdf. Accessed March 17, 2009.

Franklin RK: Deliberate self-harm: self-injurious behavior within a correctional mental health population. Crim Justice Behav 15:210–218, 1988

Fulwiler C, Forbes C, Santangelo SL, et al: Self-mutilation and suicide attempt: distinguishing features in prisoners. J Am Acad Psychiatry Law 25:69–77, 1997

Geller J, Appelbaum K, Dvoskin J, et al: Report on the Psychiatric Management of John Salvi in Massachusetts Department of Correction Facilities 1995–1996. Submitted to the Massachusetts Department of Correction by the University of Massachusetts Medical Center, January 31, 1997.

Gostin LO, Vanchieri C, Pope A (eds): Ethical Considerations for Research Involving Prisoners. Washington, DC, Institute of Medicine, National Academies Press, 2006

Haney C, Zimbaro P: The past and future of U.S. prison policy: twenty-five years after the Stanford Prison Experiment. Am Psychol 53:709–727, 1998

Harrison PM, Beck AJ: Prisoners in 2002 (NCJ 200248). Washington, DC, U.S. Department of Justice, Office of Justice Programs, Bureau of Justice Statistics, July 2003, p 7

Haycock J: Manipulation and suicide attempts in jails and prisons. Psychiatr Q 60:85–98, 1989

Hornblum AM: They were cheap and available: prisoners as research subjects in twentieth century America. BMJ 315:1437–1441, 1997

Human Rights Watch: Ill-equipped: U.S. prisons and offenders with mental illness. October 21, 2003. Available at: http://www.hrw.org/en/reports/2003/10/21/ill-equipped. Accessed March 17, 2009.

Jones A: Self-mutilation in prison: a comparison of mutilators and nonmutilators. Crim Justice Behav 13:286–296, 1986

Kalmbach KC, Lyons PM: Ethical and legal standards for research in prisons. Behav Sci Law 21:671–686, 2003

Karp JG, Whitman L, Convit A: Intentional ingestion of foreign objects by male prison inmates. Hosp Community Psychiatry 42:533–535, 1991

Kaufman E: Can comprehensive mental health care be provided in an overcrowded prison system? J Psychiatry Law 1:243–262, 1973

Kessler RC, Stein MB, Berglund P: Social phobia subtypes in the National Comorbidity Survey. Am J Psychiatry 155:613–619, 1998

King LN: Doctors, patients, and the history of correctional medicine, in Clinical Practice in Correctional Medicine. Edited by Puisis M. St Louis, MO, Mosby, 1998, pp 3–11

Krelstein MS: The role of mental health in the inmate disciplinary process: a national survey. J Am Acad Psychiatry Law 30:488–496, 2002

Labbate LA: Paruresis and urine drug testing. Depress Anxiety 4:249–252, 1996–1997

Martinez ME: Manipulative self-injurious behavior in correctional settings: an environmental treatment approach. Journal of Offender Counseling, Services and Rehabilitation 4:275–283, 1980

Metzner JL: Commentary: the role of mental health in the inmate disciplinary process. J Am Acad Psychiatry Law 30:497–499, 2002

Metzner JL, Tardiff K, Lion J, et al: Resource document on the use of restraint and seclusion in correctional mental health care. J Am Acad Psychiatry Law 35:417–425, 2007

Moller H-J: Effectiveness and safety of benzodiazepines. J Clin Psychopharmacol 19 (suppl 2):2S–11S, 1999

Moore J: Considering the private sector, in Health Care Management Issues in Corrections. Edited by Faiver KL. Lanham, MD, American Correctional Association, 1998, pp 41–67

Morgan DW, Edwards AC, Faulkner LR: The adaptation to prison by individuals with schizophrenia. Bull Am Acad Psychiatry Law 21:427–433, 1993

National Commission for the Protection of Human Subjects of Biomedical and Behavioral Research: Report and Recommendations: Research Involving Prisoners. Washington, DC, National Commission for the Protection of Human Subjects of Biomedical and Behavioral Research, 1976

National Commission on Correctional Health Care: Standards for Health Services in Prisons. Chicago, National Commission on Correctional Health Care, 2008

O'Grady JC: Commentary: a British perspective on the use of restraint and seclusion in correctional mental health care. J Am Acad Psychiatry Law 35:439–443, 2007

Packer HL: Justifications for criminal punishment, in The Limits of the Criminal Sanction. Stanford, CA, Stanford University Press, 1968, pp 35–61

Pinta ER: Evaluating privilege requests from mentally ill prisoners. J Am Acad Psychiatry Law 26:259–265, 1998

Posternak MA, Mueller TI: Assessing the risks and benefits of benzodiazepines for anxiety disorders in patients with a history of substance abuse or dependence. Am J Addict 10:48–68, 2001

Powelson H, Bendix R: Psychiatry in prison. Psychiatry 14:73–86, 1951

Robey A: Stone walls do not a prison psychiatrist make. J Am Acad Psychiatry Law 26:101–105, 1998

Roth L: Correctional psychiatry, in Forensic Psychiatry and Psychology: Perspectives and Standards for Interdisciplinary Practice. Edited by Curran WJ, McGarry AL, Shah SA. Philadelphia, PA, FA Davis, 1986, pp 429–468

Santamour MB, West B: The mentally retarded offender: presentation of the facts and a discussion of issues, in The Retarded Offender. Edited by Santamour MB, Watson PS. New York, Praeger, 1982

Soumerai SB, Simoni-Wastila L, Singer C, et al: Lack of relationship between long-term use of benzodiazepines and escalation to high dosages. Psychiatr Serv 54:1006–1011, 2003

Sowers W, Thompson K, Mullins S: Mental Health in Corrections: An Overview for Correctional Staff. Lanham, MD, American Correctional Association, 1999

Start A: Interaction between correctional staff and health care providers in the delivery of medical care, in Clinical Practice in Correctional Medicine. Edited by Puisis M. St Louis, MO, Mosby, 1998, pp 26–31

Steadman HJ, McCarty DW, Morrissey JP: Scope and frequency of conflict between mental health and correctional staffs, in The Mentally Ill in Jail: Planning for Essential Services. New York, Guilford, 1989, pp 90–104

Sykes GM: The Society of Captives: A Study of a Maximum Security Prison. Princeton, NJ, Princeton University Press, 1958

Tests for drugs of abuse. Med Lett Drugs Ther 44:71–73, 2002

Thorburn KM: Self-mutilation and self-induced illness in prison. J Prison Jail Health 4:40–51, 1984

Toch H, Adams K: The prison as dumping ground: mainlining disturbed offenders. J Psychiatry Law 15:539–553, 1987

U.S. Department of Health and Human Services: Public welfare, part 46: protection of human subjects. Code of Federal Regulations, title 45, sec. 305(a) [45 CFR 46.305(a)] (2005)

U.S. Drug Enforcement Administration: Benzodiazepines. Available at: http://www.usdoj.gov/dea/concern/benzodiazepines.html. Accessed March 17, 2009.

Vlach DL, Daniel AE: Commentary: evolving toward equivalency in correctional mental health care—a view from the maximum security trenches. J Am Acad Psychiatry Law 35:436–438, 2007

Warchol G: Workplace violence, 1992–96 (BJS Special Report, NCJ 168634). Washington, DC, Office of Justice Programs, Bureau of Justice Statistics, U.S. Department of Justice, 1998

Winchel RM, Stanley M: Self-injurious behavior: a review of the behavior and biology of self-mutilation. Am J Psychiatry 148:306–316, 1991

Yarvis RM: Correctional psychiatry, in Psychiatry, Vol 3. Edited by Michels R, Cooper AM, Guze SB, et al. Philadelphia, Lippincott-Raven, 1996–1997, pp 1–16

Zgourides GD: Paruresis: overview and implications for treatment. Psychol Rep 60:1171–1176, 1987

CHAPTER 5

Conducting Mental Health Assessments in Correctional Settings

Humberto Temporini, M.D.

The number of individuals in custody in the United States has increased consistently over the past two decades. At year-end 2007, more than 1.5 million individuals were incarcerated in federal and state correctional facilities, while local jails housed 780,581 men and women in different stages of the criminal justice process. Such a number indicates that approximately 1 in every 132 persons in the United States was held in custody at that time (West and Sabol 2008). This large number of incarcerated individuals is far from being a representative, random sample of the general population of the United States. The differences range from simple demographics, such as race and gender, to more complex issues, such as socioeconomic status and education. For example, males account for approximately 93% of incarcerated individuals, and black males represent almost 40% of all men serving a prison sentence (West and Sabol 2008). In contrast, the U.S. Census Bureau (2009) indicates that as of 2007, males made up 49.3% of the U.S. population, and black men represented approximately 12% of all U.S. males. Homelessness, which has been related to factors as diverse as age, education, marital status, substance abuse, and mental illness, is between 7.5 and 11 times more prevalent among jailed individuals than among the general population (Greenberg and Rosenheck 2008). Correctional populations also report lower educational attainment than do community samples. For example, 41.3% of individuals incarcerated in either jails or prisons, compared with 18.3% of the general population, reported not completing high school (Harlow 2003). Finally, incarcerated individuals are more likely to have had prior incarcerations and a higher prevalence of traumatic experiences (Gibson et al. 1999).

In sum, individuals in custody do not represent a random sample of the community; male sex, minority status, lower educational achievement, homelessness, and prior correctional experience are overrepresented in correctional settings. In this chapter, I explore the prevalence rates of psychiatric disorders in jails and prisons, and provide an overview of the specific issues that arise when conducting assessments in these settings.

PREVALENCE OF PSYCHIATRIC DISORDERS IN CORRECTIONAL SETTINGS

In the mid-1970s, data began to emerge suggesting that the rates of psychiatric illnesses among incarcerated individuals were higher than those observed in community samples (Petrich 1976). Although these initial surveys contained a number of methodological problems that contributed to somewhat inaccurate reporting, they nonetheless set the stage for more rigorous approaches to studying this phenomenon. Interestingly, in 1973, only 13% of U.S. jails reported that they had established psychiatric services for inmates with mental illness (American Medical Association 1973). By the early 1990s, several lines of evidence indicated that compared with the general population, individuals in custody had disproportionately higher rates of mental illness (Teplin 1990). This increased prevalence has been observed in populations in both jail (Teplin 1994; Trestman et al. 2007) and prison (Diamond et al. 2001; Gunter et al. 2008), and it has been attributed to various factors, such as transinstitutionalization (the transfer of individuals with mental illness from hospitals to the criminal justice system), the criminalization of substance abuse, and the use of mandatory minimum sentences. Evidence also indicates that the prevalence of mental illness in correctional settings shows a different pattern in men than in women. Chapter 17, "Female Offenders in Correctional Settings," contains a review of the specific issues related to mental health assessment and treatment of female inmates. The following discussion focuses on the prevalence of mental illness in male prisoners, who represent approximately 87% of the population in jails (Sabol and Minton 2008) and 93% of the population in prisons (West and Sabol 2008).

Psychotic Disorders

Both the lifetime and current prevalence rates of psychotic disorders in correctional settings appear to be significantly higher than those found in large epidemiological studies conducted in the community. Individuals with a diagnosis of schizophrenia, for example, are more likely to be arrested for trespassing, theft, property destruction, assault, battery, drug possession, or drug sales. In addition, risk factors that increase the likelihood of arrest in this population include minority status, nonadherence to prior interventions, and prior incarceration (Prince et al. 2007). Table 5–1 summarizes the current and lifetime prevalence rates of psychotic disorders in epidemiological studies done in jails and prisons.

TABLE 5–1. Current and lifetime prevalence of psychotic disorders among incarcerated males

Study	Assessment method	Current	Lifetime
Guy et al. 1985 (N=96)	Psychiatric interview	11.5%	—
Teplin 1994[a] (N=728)	NIMH DIS-III	2.98%	3.82%
Powell et al. 1997[a] (N=213)	NIMH DIS-III-R	2.8%	3.8%
Trestman et al. 2007[b] (N=307)	SCID-IV	1.3%	1.6%
Gunter et al. 2008 (N=264)	MINI-Plus	3.0%	8.7%

Note. —=not assessed
MINI-Plus=Mini-International Neuropsychiatric Interview—Plus; NIMH-DIS-III=National Institute of Mental Health Diagnostic Interview Schedule Version III; NIMH-DIS-III-R=National Institute of Mental Health Diagnostic Interview Schedule Version III-R; SCID-IV=Structured Clinical Interview for DSM-IV.
[a]Investigated schizophrenia only.
[b]Investigated the prevalence of psychiatric illness among inmates not identified as acutely mentally ill.

In 2006, a widely publicized report from the Office of Justice Programs of the U.S. Department of Justice indicated that 17.5% of a representative sample of inmates in U.S. jails (N=6,214) acknowledged experiencing symptoms compatible with delusions at least once over the 12 months prior to the assessment, and that 13.7% described experiencing hallucinations over the same period (James and Glaze 2006). The same report indicated that 11.8% of a representative sample of state prison inmates (N=12,846) reported symptoms compatible with delusions, and that 7.9% reported the presence of hallucinations at some point in the prior 12 months. The report has several limitations that may have contributed to such elevated rates. For example, the rates are based solely on face-to-face inmate reports to interviewers from the U.S. Census Bureau. The assessment used a modified version of the Structured Clinical Interview (SCID; Spitzer et al. 1992) that did not take into account the severity of the reported symptoms, the length of time symptoms lasted, the relationship of symptoms to substance abuse or medical conditions, or the possibility of willful misrepresentation. In spite of these caveats, the numbers still appear considerably higher than those in general population samples. In a large community sample (N=9,282), the lifetime prevalence of reported visual hallucinations was 6.3% and that of auditory hallucinations was 4%. Only 0.8% of the community sample reported persecutory delusions (Kessler et al. 2005).

Results from the National Comorbidity Survey indicated a lifetime prevalence rate of nonaffective psychosis in males in the general population of 0.8% and a 12-month (current) prevalence rate of 0.5% (Kessler et al. 1994). Interestingly, the results of the National Comorbidity Survey Replication (Kessler and Merikangas 2004) suggest that the lifetime prevalence rate may be 0.5%, lower than in the earlier study (Kessler et al. 2005).

Substance Use Disorders

The term *substance use disorders* refers to either substance abuse or dependence. Substance use increases the risk of criminal involvement, incarceration, reoffense, and poor institutional adjustment. Inmates with a history of substance abuse tend to have increased numbers of disciplinary sanctions and suicide attempts (Peters et al. 1998). The rates of substance abuse among incarcerated individuals (see Table 5–2) are dramatically higher than those in community samples.

Results from the National Epidemiologic Survey on Alcohol and Related Conditions (NESARC) indicate that the 12-month prevalence rate of drug use disorders (i.e., abuse or dependence of any drug except alcohol) in men in the community is approximately 2.8%. The lifetime

TABLE 5–2. Prevalence of substance use disorders among incarcerated males

Study	Assessment method	Any substance		Alcohol only		All substances (except alcohol)	
		Current	Lifetime	Current	Lifetime	Current	Lifetime
Teplin 1994 (*N*=728)	NIMH DIS-III	29.1%	61.95%	19.09%	51.11%	15.26%	32.37%
Peters et al. 1998 (*N*=400)	SCID-IV	56.4%	73.7%	34.5%	53.9%	36.8%	59.4%
Lo 2004 (*N*=503)	ADAM	46%	61%	25%	38%	34%	44%
Gunter et al. 2008 (*N*=264)	MINI-Plus	74.6%	91.3%	45.8%	77.7%	63.3%	76.9%

Note. ADAM=Arrestee Drug Abuse Monitoring interview schedule; NIMH DIS-III=National Institute of Mental Health Diagnostic Interview Schedule Version III; MINI-Plus=Mini-International Neuropsychiatric Interview—Plus; SCID-IV=Structured Clinical Interview for DSM-IV.

prevalence rate of drug use in the same population is 13.8% (Compton et al. 2007). Based on the same survey results, the 12-month prevalence rate for alcohol use disorder (i.e., alcohol abuse or dependence) in males in the general population is approximately 12.4%. The lifetime prevalence rate of alcohol use disorder in the same group is approximately 42% (Hasin et al. 2007). Chapter 7, "Evaluating and Treating Substance Use Disorders," provides additional information regarding the prevalence of substance use disorders in the inmate population.

Mood Disorders

Major depressive disorder, bipolar disorder, and other affective disorders are more prevalent in samples of incarcerated individuals than in general population samples. This information is relevant given the relationship between some affective disorders, such as bipolar disorder, and incarceration. For example, men with bipolar disorder tend to have a higher prevalence of criminal behavior than do men with unipolar depression or psychiatrically healthy matched controls (Modestin et al. 1997). In addition, 26% of men identified as having bipolar disorder using the Mood Disorders Questionnaire had a history of arrests and incarceration for reasons other than driving while intoxicated. The rate of lifetime arrests for the individuals who were not identified as having bipolar disorder was approximately 5% (Calabrese et al. 2003). Table 5–3 outlines the lifetime and point prevalence rates of affective disorders in correctional settings.

NESARC results indicate that the current (12-month) prevalence rate of major depressive disorder in men in the community is 3.56%, whereas the lifetime prevalence rate in the same group is 9.01% (Hasin et al. 2005). The same survey indicated that the current prevalence rate of bipolar I disorder in men in the community is 1.8% and that the lifetime rate is 3.2% (Grant et al. 2005).

Anxiety Disorders

The prevalence of anxiety disorders, including posttraumatic stress disorder (PTSD), is higher among incarcerated individuals than among their community counterparts. This fact is relevant for mental health professionals working in correctional settings given the association between specific anxiety disorders, such as PTSD in men, and suicidal ideation (Cougle et al. 2009). Table 5–4 notes the specific prevalence rates of anxiety disorders in male inmates.

Data from the National Comorbidity Survey Replication indicate that in men in the community, the 12-month prevalence rate of anxiety disorders is 14.3% and the lifetime prevalence rate is 25.4%. With regard to specific diagnoses among males in the community, the 12-month and life-

TABLE 5–3. Prevalence of affective disorders among incarcerated males

Study	Assessment method	Any disorder		MDD		Bipolar disorder	
		Current	Lifetime	Current	Lifetime	Current	Lifetime
Teplin 1994 N=728	DIS-III	—	—	3.42%	5.09%	1.18%	2.17%
Powell et al. 1997 N=307	DIS-III-R	—	—	10.3%	15.5%	5.2%	5.6%
Trestman et al. 2007 N=307	SCID-IV	15.8%	24.3%	—	21.2%	—	1.3%
Gunter et al. 2008 N=264	MINI-Plus	33.3%	53.0%	16.7%	22.7%	22%[a]	45.1%[a]

Note. —=not applicable; DIS-III=Diagnostic Interview Schedule Version III; DIS-III-R=Diagnostic Interview Schedule, Version III-R; MDD=major depressive disorder; MINI-Plus=Mini-International Neuropsychiatric Interview—Plus; SCID-IV=Structured Clinical Interview for DSM-IV.

[a]Recorded as prevalence rate of mania/hypomania.

TABLE 5–4. Prevalence of anxiety disorders among incarcerated males

Study	Assessment method	Any disorder		Panic disorder		GAD		PTSD	
		Current	Lifetime	Current	Lifetime	Current	Lifetime	Current	Lifetime
Teplin 1994 N=728	DIS-III	11.62%	21.02%	—	—	—	—	—	—
Powell et al. 1997 N=213	DIS-III-R	—	—	—	—	3.8%	5.6%	21%	32.5%
Trestman et al. 2007 N=307	SCID-IV	28.2%[a]	37.6%[a]	—	15%	—	—	5.7%	20%
Gunter et al. 2008 N=264	MINI-Plus	36.4%	—	4.9%	—	18.2%	—	10.2%	—

Note. —=not applicable; DIS-III=Diagnostic Interview Schedule Version III; DIS-III-R=Diagnostic Interview Schedule Version III-R; GAD=generalized anxiety disorder; MINI-Plus=Mini-International Neuropsychiatric Interview—Plus; PTSD=posttraumatic stress disorder; SCID-IV=Structured Clinical Interview for DSM-IV.
[a]Except PTSD.

time prevalence rates, respectively, are 1.6% and 3.1% for panic disorder, 1.9% and 4.2% for generalized anxiety disorder, and 1.8% and 3.6% for PTSD (National Comorbidity Survey 2007). In community samples, the most common causes for PTSD in men were having witnessed death or severe injury, and having been exposed to combat (Kessler et al. 2005). Although incarcerated men also reported witnessing severe injury or death as the most frequent antecedent trauma to PTSD, combat exposure was rarely mentioned (Gibson et al. 1999). In contrast, incarcerated men reported rape (25%) and physical assault (17%) as the second and third most common antecedent traumatic events. These two events were reported much less frequently in community samples of men with PTSD: approximately 7% reported physical assault and 5% reported rape as the most upsetting trauma type experienced. Overall, both sexual and physical abuses were reported as more common antecedents to PTSD among inmates than among men in the general population.

Personality Disorders

Maladaptive and pervasive patterns of behavior that interfere with one's functioning are highly prevalent in correctional settings. Impulsivity, proneness to anger, irritability, and a disregard for societal norms not only can have a negative impact on an individual's life but also can result in arrests and incarceration (Trestman 2000). In addition, antisocial and borderline personality disorders show a high degree of comorbidity with substance abuse, which further increases the likelihood of criminal behavior (Zlotnick et al. 2008). Given these findings, the fact that the prevalence rates of some personality disorders are significantly higher in jails and prisons than in community settings, and even in clinical settings, is not surprising. Table 5–5 summarizes the prevalence of different personality disorders in correctional environments.

General population samples show that personality disorders are relatively common. NESARC results indicate that the most prevalent personality disorder in a representative sample of the population is obsessive-compulsive personality disorder (7.88%). The prevalence of antisocial personality disorder among nonincarcerated men is approximately 5.5% (Grant et al. 2004). Borderline personality disorder shows a similar prevalence, with 5.6% of men in the study sample meeting the DSM-IV diagnostic criteria (Grant et al. 2008). In spite of these relatively high rates, the proportion of individuals in custody meeting the diagnostic criteria for personality disorder is much higher, as highlighted in Table 5–5.

TABLE 5–5. Lifetime prevalence of personality disorders among incarcerated males

Study	Assessment method	Antisocial PD	Borderline PD
Teplin 1994 N=728	DIS-III	49.21%	—
Powell et al. 1997 N=213	DIS-III-R	46.9%	—
Trestman et al. 2007 N=307	SCID-IV	39.5%	12.9%
Black et al. 2007 N=198	SCID-IV	—	26.8%
Gunter et al. 2008 N=264	MINI-Plus	37.1%	—

Note. —= not applicable; DIS-III=Diagnostic Interview Schedule Version III; DIS-III-R=Diagnostic Interview Schedule Version III-R; MINI-Plus=Mini-International Neuropsychiatric Interview—Plus; PD=personality disorder; SCID-IV=Structured Clinical Interview for DSM-IV.

MENTAL HEALTH SERVICES IN CORRECTIONAL SETTINGS

The provision of medical care to prisoners while incarcerated is a constitutional right in the United States (*Estelle v. Gamble* 1976). Access to medical care for inmates in prisons is protected under the Eighth Amendment of the U.S. Constitution, which prohibits cruel and unusual punishment. The U.S. Supreme Court has held that the deliberate indifference by prison officials to inmates' serious medical needs is unconstitutional (*Estelle* 1976). In contrast to prisoners' care, medical care for jail detainees is guaranteed under the Fourteenth Amendment to the U.S. Constitution. For more details on the constitutional underpinnings that guarantee medical and mental health care for inmates, see Chapter 3, "Legal Issues Regarding the Provision of Care in a Correctional Setting."

Although the U.S. Supreme Court has not yet specifically equated psychiatric care to medical care, the Fourth Circuit Court of Appeals has held that constitutionally required care includes psychiatric and psychological care (*Bowring v. Godwin* 1977). In the landmark case of *Ruiz v. Estelle* (1980), a federal district court in Texas outlined the following six minimum requirements that must be met for a mental health treatment program to be considered constitutionally acceptable:

1. Screening and evaluation to identify those needing mental health care
2. A treatment plan for identified problems that consists of more than segregation or close supervision
3. Qualified mental health staff sufficient to treat the population
4. Accurate, complete, and confidential records of the mental health treatment provided
5. Suicide prevention and treatment program
6. Appropriate use of behavior-altering medications, with appropriate supervision and periodic evaluations

The National Commission on Correctional Health Care (NCCHC) publishes guidelines, updated regularly, describing appropriate standards used in the evaluation and treatment of incarcerated persons (http://www.ncchc.org/pubs/index.html). In 2000, the American Psychiatric Association (APA) published the guidelines for psychiatric services in jails and prisons. These guidelines assume compliance with NCCHC standards, and divide mental health services in correctional settings into identification, treatment, and discharge planning.

OPPORTUNITIES FOR IDENTIFICATION AND ASSESSMENT OF MENTAL ILLNESS

The APA guidelines for psychiatric services in jails and prisons suggest using a three-step process to properly assess the presence of mental health symptoms:

1. Screening upon arrival at the booking area of the facility
2. Mental health intake within 2 weeks of arrival
3. Comprehensive mental health evaluation done within an appropriate time frame depending on urgency and severity

In addition, the APA guidelines describe the need for mechanisms to allow postclassification referral to mental health care services and recommend using a brief mental health assessment. I describe the specifics of these five various types of assessments in the following subsections.

Booking Mental Health Screen

Clinical Case 5–1

After her arrest for a high-speed chase, Ms. S was brought to the county jail. Upon arrival at the booking area, Ms. S asked to call Justice

Scalia of the U.S. Supreme Court, indicating that she was going to be late to her meeting with the solicitor general. When the jail staff declined her request, Ms. S became agitated and was placed in a single cell while waiting for processing. Ms. S's behavior worsened as time passed. She became loud, used profanity, and was sexually inappropriate. Mental health staff were called to evaluate Ms. S. In the course of the assessment, Ms. S reported that she had stopped using olanzapine 3 months prior to the arrest, after deciding that she could manage her symptoms by drinking chamomile tea. Ms. S was scheduled for a comprehensive psychiatric evaluation, which was done a day later. She agreed to restart medication but continued expressing her concern over not showing up to her meeting with the solicitor general and Justice Scalia.

From the moment that an inmate arrives at the booking area of a jail or the receiving area of a prison, he or she interacts with correctional officers, as well as medical and mental health staff. Depending on the jurisdiction and the particulars of the case, an inmate may be brought to the jail directly from the community after arrest, from a local lockup, or from court. The correctional staff in booking interviews the inmate and gathers appropriate information. A mental health screen, called the *receiving* or *booking mental health screen,* typically takes place at this stage. Such a screen has multiple purposes:

1. Identification of individuals with severe mental illness who may require immediate psychiatric attention
2. Suicide prevention
3. Continuation of care (e.g., psychiatric medications)
4. Identification of psychiatric problems that require further assessment and treatment on a nonemergency basis

In jail settings, individuals being booked are often under a great deal of stress, because incarceration typically occurs shortly after arrest. Recently booked inmates can present with high levels of agitation, anger, and even violent behavior. In addition, underlying mental health problems may surface in this context, giving rise to overt psychiatric symptoms that require prompt intervention. Immediate attention should be considered in rapidly escalating situations, such as when an inmate in the booking area displays disorganized or bizarre behavior or attempts suicide. In such cases, mental health staff should evaluate the individual promptly and, if appropriate, consider transfer to a setting with a higher level of care that would ensure the safety of both inmates and staff. Individuals with serious impairment who meet the criteria for inpatient psychiatric hospitalization are typically admitted to a jail psychiatric unit, transferred to outside mental health agencies, or placed under special observation, such as suicide watch, pending further evaluation and treatment.

Because substance use is frequently observed in recently incarcerated individuals, medical staff need to engage in prompt identification, assessment, and treatment of drug and alcohol intoxication and withdrawal symptoms. Questionnaires addressing recent substance use, toxicology screens, and monitoring of vital signs are key to the proper management of alcohol and drug intoxication or withdrawal.

Inmates with overt psychiatric symptoms may be easy to identify, as was Ms. S in Clinical Case 5–1. Although most inmates do not present in such dramatic fashion, they may require further assessment and rapid mental health treatment. Screening tools are usually used in this setting to accomplish the task. An optimal screening tool should

- accurately identify those inmates who require psychiatric care or further assessment (sensitivity), and separate them from those who do not (specificity);
- be used effectively by staff with no formal mental health training, such as technicians and correctional officers; and
- be quick and easy to use.

Brief mental health screens take one of two approaches: they focus on either 1) making a diagnosis or 2) identifying severe symptoms that cause significant impairment while de-emphasizing the need for a diagnosis (Lurigio and Swartz 2006). Examples of tools that focus on diagnosis are the Composite International Diagnostic Interview—Short Form (Kessler et al. 1998), Mini-International Neuropsychiatric Interview (Sheehan et al. 1998), and Referral Decision Scale (Teplin and Swartz 1989). These instruments provide a provisional diagnosis, on the basis of which the inmate can then be referred for further assessment. One drawback, however, is that the mere presence of a provisional Axis I disorder does not necessarily imply that the individual must be referred to mental health services on an emergency basis. For example, if an inmate screens positive for a simple phobia, such as fear of spiders or needles, should this individual be referred automatically for a more thorough mental health assessment or provided with instructions on how to contact mental health services if his or her needs change?

Another problem with diagnosis-based screening tools is that they require additional training, because the interviewer must either skip or include entire sections depending on the interviewee's responses to specific questions. Although this practice may be basic for mental health professionals, it adds a level of complexity when the screen is used by less trained individuals, such as correctional officers.

A different approach to mental health screens is the use of tools that help identify severe symptoms and functional impairment. These tools are preferred in correctional settings because they tend to focus less on making a diagnosis, which may or may not require further clinical assessment, and more on identifying those individuals who are most in need of services. Funded by grants from the National Institute of Justice, two brief screens have been developed for use with correctional populations.

The first, the Correctional Mental Health Screen (CMHS; Ford at al. 2007), uses separate yes-no questions for men and women. The version for women (CMHS-W; see Table 5–6) consists of eight questions, whereas the version for men (CMHS-M; see Table 5–7) contains 12 questions about current and past indicators of serious mental disorders. The screens can be administered in 3–5 minutes. Men who answer "yes" to six or more questions and women who answer "yes" to five or more questions should be referred for further mental health assessment. According to Ford at al. (2007), the screens correctly classified at least 75% of inmates as to whether they had a previously undetected mental illness. The CMHS-W questionnaire is the first mental health screen developed and validated specifically for women in correctional settings.

The second screen, the Brief Jail Mental Health Screen (BJMHS; Steadman et al. 2005), comprises eight questions to be answered "yes" or "no" (see Table 5–8), and it can be administered in approximately 2–3 minutes. The tool has six questions about current mental disorders and two questions about history of hospitalizations and medications for psychiatric problems. Inmates who answer "yes" to two or more questions about current symptoms, or "yes" to either of the two questions regarding past history, should be referred for further assessment. In validation studies, the BJMHS was able to accurately detect almost 74% of all men with previously undetected mental illness, but was not as effective in assessing women. Nonetheless, it remains a solid and useful tool in the screening process.

A positive screen for mental illness is not the only way that inmates can be referred for further assessment and treatment. In fact, gross psychopathology is usually easily identified by correctional officers and booking staff. For example, most staff can recognize the need for further mental health assessment in an inmate who displays overly bizarre behavior, such as fecal smearing, inappropriate sexual conduct, severe agitation, or self-injurious behavior. For those cases, as well as for inmates who have been identified as mentally ill through the screening process, staff must arrange for a follow-up assessment within 24 hours.

TABLE 5–6.   Correctional Mental Health Screen—Female Version

1. Do you get annoyed when friends and family complain about their problems? Or do people complain that you are not sympathetic to their problems?

2. Have you tried to avoid reminders of, or to not think about, something terrible that you experienced or witnessed?

3. Some people find their mood changes frequently—as if they spend every day on an emotional rollercoaster. For example, switching from feeling angry to depressed to anxious many times a day. Does this sound like you?

4. Have there been a few weeks when you felt you were useless, sinful, or guilty?

5. Has there been a time when you felt depressed most of the day for at least two weeks?

6. Do you find that most people will take advantage of you if you let them know too much about you?

7. Have you been troubled by repeated thoughts, feelings, or nightmares about something terrible that you experienced or witnessed?

8. Have you ever been in the hospital for non-medical reasons, such as a psychiatric hospital?

Note.   Five (5) or more "yes" answers to the above questions warrant referral for further mental health assessment.
Source.   Reprinted from Ford J, Trestman R, Wiesbrock V, et al.: "Development and Validation of a Brief Mental Health Screening Instrument for Newly Incarcerated Adults." *Assessment* 14:279–299, 2007.

Medication at Booking

During booking assessments, inmates sometimes report that they are under psychiatric care by an outside provider. Individuals with prior correctional experience, or those with competent legal counsel, often arrive at jail with medication containers, prescriptions, or pharmacy printouts. In those cases, nursing staff should verify that the medications are current. If so, the staff should consult with a physician to evaluate if the medication is appropriate for the inmate, considering the jail setting and the presenting symptoms. In addition, the inmate should be scheduled for an intake mental health assessment and subsequent psychiatric consultation.

A more complicated, but nonetheless more common, issue involves what to do when an inmate reports that he or she is taking a certain psy-

TABLE 5–7.   Correctional Mental Health Screen—Male Version

1. Have you ever had worries that you just can't get rid of?

2. Some people find their mood changes frequently—as if they spend every day on an emotional rollercoaster. Does this sound like you?

3. Do you get annoyed when friends and family complain about their problems? Or do people complain that you are not sympathetic to their problems?

4. Have you felt like you did not have any feelings, or felt distant or cut off from other people or from your surroundings?

5. Has there ever been a time when you felt so irritable that you found yourself shouting at people or starting fights or arguments?

6. Do you often get in trouble at work or with friends because you act excited at first but then lose interest in projects and don't follow through?

7. Do you tend to hold grudges or give people the silent treatment for days at a time?

8. Have you ever tried to avoid reminders, or to not think about, something terrible that you experienced or witnessed?

9. Has there ever been a time when you felt depressed most of the day for at least two weeks?

10. Have you ever been troubled by repeated thoughts, feelings, or nightmares about something you experienced or witnessed?

11. Have you ever been in the hospital for non-medical reasons, such as a psychiatric hospital?

12. Have you ever felt constantly on guard or watchful even when you didn't need to, or felt jumpy and easily startled?

Note.   Six (6) or more "yes" answers to the above questions warrant referral for further mental health assessment.

Source.   Reprinted from Ford J, Trestman R, Wiesbrock V, et al.: "Development and Validation of a Brief Mental Health Screening Instrument for Newly Incarcerated Adults." *Assessment* 14:279–299, 2007.

chiatric medication but has no documentation to this effect. In these cases, the inmate should be referred for further mental health assessment. Mental health staff, usually nurses or social workers, should attempt to verify the inmate's account by contacting his or her provider or the pharmacy that dispensed the medication. If the medication is verified, nursing staff should then consult with the jail prescriber regarding the necessity and appropriateness of the requested medication. If the staff cannot verify the inmate's account, he or she should be referred for

TABLE 5–8. Brief Jail Mental Health Screen

1. Do you currently believe that someone can control your mind by putting thoughts into your head or taking thoughts out of your head?

2. Do you currently feel that other people know your thoughts and can read your mind?

3. Have you currently lost or gained as much as two pounds a week for several weeks without even trying?

4. Have you or your family or friends noticed that you are currently much more active than you usually are?

5. Do you currently feel like you have to talk or move more slowly than you usually do?

6. Have there currently been a few weeks when you felt like you were useless or sinful?

7. Have you *ever* been in a hospital for emotional or mental health problems?

8. Are you currently taking any medication prescribed for you by a physician for any emotional or mental health problems?

Note. Two or more "yes" answers to items 1–6 and/or one "yes" answer to items 7–8 warrants referral for further mental health assessment.
Source. Reprinted from Steadman H, Scott J, Osher F, et al.: "Validation of the Brief Jail Mental Health Screen." *Psychiatric Services* 56:816–822, 2005. Used with permission.

further mental health evaluation to determine the appropriate level of care and intervention required.

Intake Mental Health Screen

All inmates should undergo an intake mental health screen within 14 days of booking. Unlike the booking screening, this evaluation is typically done by mental health staff. The intake screen is a fairly comprehensive assessment that includes questions about current symptoms, past psychiatric history, suicide potential, social history, and educational history. The APA guidelines recommend that an institution use a standardized questionnaire to maintain consistency across different evaluators (American Psychiatric Association's 2000). The results become part of the inmate's medical and mental health record. The outcome of the screen determines whether the inmate is referred for further mental health assessment. Individuals identified as not requiring further evaluation should receive information about how to contact mental health staff if they develop symptoms or changes in their condition.

If the inmate requires further mental health evaluation, assessment, or care, the staff performing the mental health screen should consider obtaining appropriate collateral information, such as relevant medical records or information from family members when feasible and appropriate.

In jail settings, the intake mental health screen provides an opportunity to assess whether the individual is eligible for participation in programs that provide an alternative to further criminal detention. Mental health and drug courts, as well as other jail diversion programs, have been established to minimize the incarceration rates of people with severe mental illness (Draine and Solomon 1999). Many programs use detention facilities as the first point of contact to identify a person with mental illness who may be eligible for diversion (Council of State Governments 2002). Finally, some jurisdictions have mechanisms in place that allow correctional mental health staff to obtain information directly from community mental health agencies about the inmates under their care. For example, through an automated information system, the Cook County Jail (Illinois) electronically transfers its jail census on a daily basis to mental health clinics in the Chicago area. Clinic staff review the lists to see if they can identify any of their clients. The goal is to notify these clinics when one of their clients is in custody, to aid in the continuation of treatment while in custody (Council of State Governments 2002).

In addition to providing an opportunity to identify and refer inmates for further evaluation and treatment, the intake mental health screen also gives inmates an opportunity to request further care. Approximately 11% of a large sample of U.S. federal inmates ($N= 2,674$) requested mental health services during the intake mental health screen. Individuals with a history of prior mental health treatment, concurrent medical conditions, and prior head injury were more likely to request mental health services. Of note, men in the study were 60% more likely to request mental health services than women. The most commonly reported problems underlying the request were difficulty sleeping, "nervousness," depression, and racing thoughts (Diamond et al. 2008).

Comprehensive Mental Health Evaluation

The comprehensive mental health evaluation is a standard mental health evaluation geared to individuals in a correctional setting. This assessment, which typically consists of a face-to-face interview and a review of records and collateral sources, usually results in a diagnosis and treatment plan. The evaluation is usually performed by a psychiatrist or other licensed and qualified mental health professional, and it should be documented in the inmate's mental health record. The time frame of the evaluation should be based on the level of urgency according to the specific institution's policy and procedures. In addition to the basic sections of a typical psychiatric evaluation (e.g., a history of present illness, past psychiatric and substance abuse history, social and family histories), this assessment should include inquiries specific to the setting. For example, for pretrial detainees, upcoming court appearances may generate significant anxiety, which can exacerbate a preexisting psychiatric condition. The time of sentencing, the separation from family members, and the potential loss of social standing associated with incarceration, among many other situational stressors, can cause significant psychiatric morbidity.

Postclassification Referral

Clinical Case 5–2

After 3 months in a county jail, Mr. G was offered a plea agreement of 30 years to life for several charges of production of child pornography. Mr. G, a mild-mannered software engineer, was housed in a protective custody area within the facility. The deputies noticed that Mr. G had stopped exercising during recreation and that he had not requested shaving utensils for several days. Approximately a week later, Mr. G stopped leaving his cell. The deputies noticed that he had not been eating and that the logs reflected he had not showered in at least 8 days. Mental health staff was notified at this point and visited Mr. G at his cell door due to his refusal to attend the interview. The clinician noticed that Mr. G was malodorous, had little energy or motivation, and appeared to have lost a significant amount of weight. Mr. G was scheduled for a psychiatric evaluation, at which time he reluctantly agreed to a trial of sertraline to target his obvious depressive symptoms.

Individuals assessed as not needing psychiatric care after being screened for mental illness may later experience a new onset or recurrence of symptoms. *Postclassification referral* describes the mechanism by which these inmates are brought to the attention of the mental health staff. Self-referral is the most common referral mechanism, and correctional environments usually have a system in place that allows inmates to request mental health attention. Inmate manuals, provided to all newly admitted individuals, should describe how to access mental health care on a nonemergency basis by recommending that the inmate file a written request. In emergency cases, inmates are encouraged to notify custody staff, who in turn notify mental health staff. Inmates who request emergency mental health care due to potential danger to themselves or others, as well as inmates who are unable to care for themselves, should be placed under observation (possibly constant observation) pending the outcome of the mental health evaluation.

In addition to providing a mechanism for inmate self-referrals, correctional staff are encouraged to notify mental health staff of behavioral changes observed in particular inmates. A simple six-question screening tool was developed to assist officers in this task (Birmingham and Mullee 2005). A "yes" answer to at least two of the six questions below suggests that the inmate may suffer from a serious mental illness and should be referred for further evaluation.

1. Is the inmate excessively isolating himself from staff and other inmates?
2. Is the inmate's behavior persistently erratic and/or bizarre?
3. Are the sleeping and eating patterns of the inmate causing concern?
4. Has there been a sudden unexplained change in the inmate's presentation, such as stopping work for no obvious reason?
5. Has the inmate's personal hygiene appeared strange, changed suddenly, or deteriorated?
6. Does the inmate have any other symptoms that are likely to suggest a mental illness?

An inmate's relatives and acquaintances are another source of mental health referrals. Calls from concerned family members, attorneys, and court staff regarding deterioration in the inmate's mental status should be noted in the inmate's mental health record. For example, an inmate may send a farewell letter to his or her mother, or a spouse may notice oddities in an individual's behavior a few weeks after incarceration. These types of communications are exceedingly informative and should trigger prompt evaluation by mental health staff.

Consultation referrals from other services, such as internal medicine, provide another opportunity to assess not previously identified mental illness. For example, an inmate may present with a substantial decrease in self-care that interferes with the management of a medical condition, such as refusing wound dressing changes or not leaving his or her cell for blood glucose checks. Inmates who refuse medical treatment are often referred to mental health services for further assessment. Also, inmates may present to medical providers with absurd or bizarre complaints, such as a male inmate who requests a pregnancy test or an individual who complains of having a radio receiver in his or her brain. These individuals may have suffered psychotic decompensation since their intake screens or may lack insight into their illness. Medical staff should refer these inmates for mental health assessment rather than dismiss the complaint or assume that the individual is willfully providing an implausible story for secondary gain.

Brief Mental Health Assessment

When an inmate screens positive for mental health symptoms during the booking or intake screen, or is referred to mental health services through one of the mechanisms described above, a brief mental health assessment is the next step. This assessment usually serves as a second-level triage and should be tailored to explore the complaint or concern that prompted the referral. The APA (2000) guidelines recommend that the brief mental health screen occur within 72 hours of the referral. In addition, the assessment should be performed by a mental health professional and recorded in the inmate's medical record.

The brief assessment may result in a referral for a comprehensive mental health evaluation, but a more rapid intervention may be required if the clinician deems it necessary. For example, if an inmate expresses suicidal ideation during a brief assessment, the clinician should refer the inmate immediately for further evaluation while taking steps to ensure the inmate's safety, which in most settings involves increasing the level of observation (e.g., initiating constant observation). In these cases, the brief assessment commonly turns into a comprehensive mental health evaluation. Although psychologists and psychiatrists can perform brief assessments of inmates, their role is typically indirect in the provision of this service. Psychiatrists and psychologists can develop policy and procedures involving the brief assessment, or they can supervise other mental health clinicians in this role.

TELEPSYCHIATRY IN CORRECTIONAL SETTINGS

The National Library of Medicine defines *telepsychiatry* as the use of electronic communication and information technologies to provide or support clinical psychiatric care at a distance (American Psychiatric Association 1998). This definition includes many communication modalities, but the most applicable to psychiatry is the use of live, interactive two-way audiovideo communication (videoconferencing) (Antonacci et al. 2008). Over the past decade, the use of telepsychiatry has played a significant role in psychiatric assessments and treatment in correctional settings. By 2001, correctional services in 26 states used some form of telemedicine, with provision of mental health care being one of the most common applications (Larsen et al. 2004).

The results from the use of telepsychiatry in correctional settings have been encouraging. Evidence indicates that telepsychiatry can deliver treatment whose results do not differ significantly from the gold standard of in-person evaluation (O'Reilly et al. 2007). Studies of incarcerated populations show no difference between telepsychiatry and face-to-face therapy in measures of perceptions of the therapeutic relationship, postsession mood, or general satisfaction with services (Morgan et al. 2007). In addition, the use of telepsychiatry appears to improve the safety and security of the institution and staff due to decreased inmate movement and increase the availability of specialized providers familiar with the setting (Ax et al. 2007), and decrease wait times and improve follow-ups (Leonard 2004).

Telepsychiatry in a correctional setting involves the use of adequate policy and procedures. When endorsing telepsychiatry, the institution must consider issues such as model of care (i.e., consultative vs. ongoing and single-provider treatment vs. collaborative or multidisciplinary team treatment), role and responsibilities of the telepsychiatrist and mental health staff, provision of services after hours, and inclusion of information in the medical record (Shore et al. 2007).

Although the benefits of telepsychiatry appear clear, the importance of having a clinician on site should not be disregarded. The vast majority of research in telepsychiatry indicates that it is well accepted, but that does not rule out the possibility of individuals refusing the evaluation, leaving or attempting to leave the office, or making threats of self-harm or harm to others. In those cases, the presence of an on-site clinician becomes paramount because hospitalization or other changes in level of care might be required. Finally, should the inmate require involuntary hospitalization, administrative issues may become evident if the telepsychiatry provider is located in a different state and does not have the appropriate license to mandate inpatient admission. In those cases, an on-site clinician must become involved to minimize delays and ensure prompt transfer of the inmate to the appropriate site.

PROFESSIONAL ROLES AND RESPONSIBILITIES

Mental health assessments and subsequent treatment in correctional settings require coordination of services and responsibilities. Psychiatrists, psychologists, nursing staff, social workers, and correctional officers participate in this process with roles that may overlap depending on issues of availability, financial constraints, and licensing requirements. Although the role and responsibilities of correctional psychiatrists are described in detail in various chapters throughout this book, the roles of other personnel are described below.

Psychologists

Jails and prisons employ psychologists more frequently than any other mental health professionals. A survey of 830 correctional psychologists employed in the United States found that the largest proportion of their work time was spent in administrative duties, closely followed by direct treatment and performing assessments (Boothby and Clements 2000). Psychologists working in jails and prisons conduct crisis, individual, and group psychotherapy, as well as perform psychological evaluations for the courts or for classification purposes. In this environment, psychologists frequently train correctional staff in the recognition and management of inmates who may require special management, such as those with mental illness or disruptive behavior. Finally, psychologists may refer inmates for further psychiatric evaluation (Fagan and Ax 2003). In certain jurisdictions, psychologists may be eligible to prescribe psychoactive medication upon completing special training.

Nursing Staff

As in other environments, nurses in correctional settings are the frontline staff when it comes to inmate contact (Weinstein et al. 2005). Nurses have a variety of essential duties, including dispensing medications, patient education, and identification of signs and symptoms of mental illness.

Medication administration, also known as "pill call," is typically done on a daily basis in the housing unit where the inmate resides. At this time, nurses have an invaluable opportunity for monitoring changes in inmates' symptoms and presentation, as well as ensuring medication compliance. During this task, nurses are at the forefront of custody staff efforts to curtail medication trafficking, by ensuring that the individual inmate takes the medication as prescribed, without "cheeking" and passing it to others or saving it for later use. Medication refusals are recorded and communicated to medical and/or mental health staff to ensure appropriate follow-up.

Nurses also play essential roles in the management of inpatient psychiatric units in correctional settings. Daily monitoring, assessments of suicidality, supportive individual and group therapy, and medication monitoring are common tasks that nurses perform in these units.

Social Workers

Just as they do in the community, social workers in correctional psychiatry settings have a variety of roles that range from direct patient care to liaison with outside agencies on behalf of their clients. Social workers' direct care delivery is most commonly done through counseling and other therapeutic modalities, such as individual and group therapy. In addition, social workers can mobilize appropriate resources to aid inmates with community reinsertion by engaging in appropriate discharge planning.

Substance abuse treatment, recommendations for participation in vocational and educational programs within the facility, and overall advocacy are other essential roles that social workers play in this setting.

Correctional Officers

Although not formally trained in mental health assessments or therapeutic interventions, correctional officers are the staff members who spend the largest amount of time with inmates. Correctional staff, such as officers and counselors, have a distinct mission in this setting: to confine inmates and ensure that the institution is run safely and securely. This role may seem to conflict with that of mental health professionals, which consists of providing care to the same population. The difference in roles may result in significant conflict between these groups. Correctional line staff often consider mental health staff gullible, easily manipulated, and overall "soft." On the other hand, correctional officers are frequently perceived by mental health staff as being intransigent, harsh, and punishment oriented (Appelbaum et al. 2001).

In spite of these differences, both sides can work well together. Consultation between correctional and mental health staff, which is often informal, is an essential tool in the management of psychiatrically ill inmates (Dvoskin and Spiers 2004). Seeking information about an inmate from correctional officers or simply responding to the concerns of correctional officers is an example of this form of consultation. The use of treatment teams that include correctional staff is a more elaborate way of interdisciplinary collaboration that has been successfully adopted by several jurisdictions in the United States, including the Federal Bureau of Prisons (Holt 2001). In these teams, mental health staff and correctional officers work together to ensure that both treatment and security decisions are made in unison, taking into account custody and treatment variables. Another way to foster the relationship between both sides is the provision of cross-discipline training (Dvoskin and Spiers 2004). Mental health staff can also improve the relationship by providing tools for correctional officers to identify and manage offenders who are difficult or mentally ill beyond typical disciplinary ones, such as write-ups. In addition, mental health staff are set to gain a deeper understanding of the correctional officer culture by attending security trainings.

Correctional officers can effectively participate in inmates' mental health care by providing observation and appropriate intervention (Appelbaum et al. 2001). Given the amount of time that officers spend with inmates, they are usually the first to observe changes in inmates' behavior that correlate with the presence of psychiatric symptoms. Clear changes in an individual's self-care, the onset of bizarre or disorganized behavior, or a surge in irritability can easily be detected by properly trained officers, who can then make a referral for a mental health assessment. In addition, correctional officers can encourage inmate participation in mental health programming and medication compliance, thus providing appropriate intervention.

CONCLUSION

Whether due to transinstitutionalization, the criminalization of substance abuse, or the use of mandatory minimum sentences, the number of individuals in jails and prisons in the United States has grown significantly over the past two decades. Accompanying this increase, the prevalence of serious mental illness in correctional settings surpasses that observed in epidemiological studies in the community. Correctional mental health professionals come in contact with this reality on a daily basis, because jails and prisons have become de facto treatment centers. Therefore, the importance of adequate assessments tailored to this population is higher than ever. Mental health clinicians of different disciplines and correctional staff must work together to appropriately accomplish the often difficult, frequently thankless, and always rewarding task of providing care to those behind bars.

SUMMARY POINTS

- Psychiatric illnesses are more prevalent in correctional settings than in community samples.
- The assessment of psychiatric illnesses in correctional settings is best approached in a team fashion, using valuable input from correctional officers.
- The use of brief screening instruments that require minimal additional training enhances the staff's ability to detect serious psychopathology.
- Telepsychiatry is a useful modality in the assessment and management of inmates with mental disorders.

REFERENCES

American Medical Association: Medical Care in U.S. Jails. Chicago, American Medical Association, 1973

American Psychiatric Association: Telepsychiatry via videoconferencing resource document, July 1998 (APA Resource Document Reference No 98-0021). Available at: http://archive.psych.org/edu/other_res/lib_archives/archives/199821.pdf. Accessed June 16, 2009.

American Psychiatric Association: Psychiatric Services in Jails and Prisons: A Task Force Report of the American Psychiatric Association, 2nd Edition. Washington, DC, American Psychiatric Association, 2000

Antonacci DJ, Bloch RM, Saeed SA, et al: Empirical evidence on the use and effectiveness of telepsychiatry via videoconferencing: implications for forensic and correctional psychiatry. Behav Sci Law 26:253–269, 2008

Appelbaum K, Hickey J, Packer I: The role of correctional officers in multidisciplinary mental health care in prisons. Psychiatr Serv 52:1343–1347, 2001

Ax R, Fagan T, Magaletta P, et al: Innovations in correctional assessment and treatment. Crim Justice Behav 34:893–905, 2007

Birmingham L, Mullee M: Development and evaluation of a screening tool for identifying prisoners with severe mental illness. Psychiatr Bull R Coll Psychiatr 29:334–338, 2005

Black DW, Gunter T, Allen J, et al: Borderline personality disorder in male and female offenders newly committed to prison. Compr Psychiatry 48:400–405, 2007

Boothby J, Clements C: A national survey of correctional psychologists. Crim Justice Behav 27:716–732, 2000

Bowring v Godwin, 551 F.2d 44 (4th Cir. 1977)

Calabrese JR, Hirschfeld MA, Reed M, et al: Impact of bipolar disorder on a U.S. community sample. J Clin Psychiatry 64:425–432, 2003

Compton W, Thomas Y, Stinson F, et al: Prevalence, correlates, disability, and comorbidity of DSM-IV drug abuse and dependence in the United States: results from the National Epidemiologic Survey on Alcohol and Related Conditions. Arch Gen Psychiatry 64:566–576, 2007

Cougle JR, Keough ME, Riccardi CJ, et al: Anxiety disorders and suicidality in the National Comorbidity Survey-Replication. J Psychiatr Res 43:825–829, 2009

Council of State Governments: Criminal Justice/Mental Health Consensus Project. June 2002. Available at: http://www.consensusproject.org. Accessed March 18, 2009.

Diamond P, Wang E, Holzer C, et al: The prevalence of mental illness in prison. Adm Policy Ment Health 29:21–40, 2001

Diamond P, Magaletta P, Harzke A, et al: Who requests psychological services upon admission to prison? Psychol Serv 5:97–107, 2008

Draine J, Solomon P: Describing and evaluating jail diversion services for persons with serious mental illness. Psychiatr Serv 50:56–61, 1999

Dvoskin J, Spiers E: On the role of correctional officers in prison mental health. Psychiatr Q 75:41–59, 2004

Estelle v Gamble, 426 U.S. 97 (1976)

Fagan T, Ax R: Correctional Mental Health Handbook. Thousand Oaks, CA, Sage, 2003

Ford J, Trestman R, Wiesbrock V, et al: Development and validation of a brief mental health screening instrument for newly incarcerated adults. Assessment 14:279–299, 2007

Gibson L, Holt JC, Fondacaro K, et al: An examination of antecedent traumas and psychiatric comorbidity among male inmates with PTSD. J Trauma Stress 12:473–484, 1999

Grant BF, Hasin DS, Stinson FS, et al: Prevalence, correlates, and disability of personality disorders in the United States: results from the National Epidemiologic Survey on Alcohol and Related Conditions. J Clin Psychiatry 65:948–958, 2004

Grant BF, Stinson FS, Hasin DS, et al: Prevalence, correlates, and comorbidity of bipolar I disorder and Axis I and II disorders: results from the National Epidemiologic Survey on Alcohol and Related Conditions. J Clin Psychiatry 66:1205–1215, 2005

Grant BF, Chou SP, Goldstein RB, et al: Prevalence, correlates, disability, and comorbidity of DSM-IV borderline personality disorder: results from the Wave 2 National Epidemiologic Survey on Alcohol and Related Conditions. J Clin Psychiatry 69:533–545, 2008

Greenberg G, Rosenheck R: Jail incarceration, homelessness, and mental health: a national study. Psychiatr Serv 59:170–177, 2008

Gunter T, Arndt S, Wenman G, et al: Frequency of mental and addictive disorders among 320 men and women entering the Iowa prison system: use of the MINI-Plus. J Am Acad Psychiatry Law 36:27–34, 2008

Guy E, Platt JJ, Zwerling I, et al: Mental health status of prisoners in an urban jail. Criminal Justice and Behavior 12:29–53, 1985

Harlow CW: Education and correctional populations (NCJ 195670). Washington, DC, U.S. Department of Justice, Bureau of Justice Statistics, Office of Justice Programs, January 2003

Hasin D, Goodwin R, Stinson F, et al: Epidemiology of major depressive disorder: results from the National Epidemiologic Survey on Alcoholism and Related Conditions. Arch Gen Psychiatry 62:1097–1106, 2005

Hasin D, Stinson F, Ogburn E, et al: Prevalence, correlates, disability, and comorbidity of DSM-IV alcohol abuse and dependence in the United States: results from the National Epidemiologic Survey on Alcohol and Related Conditions. Arch Gen Psychiatry 64:830–842, 2007

Holt C: The correctional officer's role in mental health treatment of youthful offenders. Issues Ment Health Nurs 22:173–180, 2001

James D, Glaze L: Mental health problems of prison and jail inmates (NCJ 213600). Washington, DC, U.S. Department of Justice, Bureau of Justice Statistics, Office of Justice Programs, September 2006

Kessler RC, Merikangas KR: The National Comorbidity Survey Replication (NCS-R): background and aims. Int J Methods Psychiatr Res 13:60–68, 2004

Kessler RC, McGonagle KA, Zhao S, et al: Lifetime and 12-month prevalence of DSM-III-R psychiatric disorders in the United States: results from the National Comorbidity Survey. Arch Gen Psychiatry 51:8–19, 1994

Kessler R, Andrews G, Mroczek D, et al: The World Health Organization Composite International Diagnostic Interview Short-Form (CIDI-SF). Int J Methods Psychiatr Res 7:171–185, 1998

Kessler R, Birnbaum H, Demler O, et al: The prevalence and correlates of non-affective psychosis in the National Comorbidity Survey Replication (NCS-R). Biol Psychiatry 58:668–676, 2005

Larsen D, Hudnall Stamm B, Davis K, et al: Prison telemedicine and telehealth utilization in the United States: state and federal perceptions of benefits and barriers. Telemed J E Health 10 (suppl 2):S81–S90, 2004

Leonard S: The development and evaluation of a telepsychiatry service for prisoners. J Psychiatr Ment Health Nurs 11:461–468, 2004

Lo C: Sociodemographic factors, drug abuse, and other crimes: how they vary among male and female arrestees. J Crim Justice 32:399–409, 2004

Lurigio A, Swartz J: Mental illness in correctional populations: the use of standardized screening tools for further evaluation or treatment. Fed Probat 70:29–35, 2006

Modestin J, Hug A, Ammann R: Criminal behavior in males with affective disorders. J Affect Disord 42:29–38, 1997

Morgan R, Patrick A, Magaletta P: Does the use of telemental health alter the treatment experience? Inmates' perceptions of telemental health versus face-to-face treatment modalities. J Consult Clin Psychol 76:158–162, 2007

National Comorbidity Survey: National Comorbidity Survey (NCS) and National Comorbidity Survey Replication (NCS-R). 2007. Available at: http://www.hcp.med.harvard.edu/ncs. Accessed March 18, 2009.

O'Reilly R, Bishop J, Maddox K, et al: Is telepsychiatry equivalent to face-to-face psychiatry? Results from a randomized controlled equivalence trial. Psychiatr Serv 58:836–843, 2007

Peters R, Greenbaum P, Edens J, et al: Prevalence of DSM-IV substance abuse and dependence disorders among prison inmates. Am J Drug Alcohol Abuse 24:573–587, 1998

Petrich J: Rate of psychiatric morbidity in a metropolitan county jail population. Am J Psychiatry 133:1439–1444, 1976

Powell T, Holt J, Fondacaro K: The prevalence of mental illness among inmates in a rural state. Law Hum Behav 21:427–438, 1997

Prince J, Akincigil A, Bromet E: Incarceration rates of persons with first-admission psychosis. Psychiatr Serv 58:1173–1180, 2007

Ruiz v Estelle, 503 F.Supp. 1265, 1339 (S.D. Tex. 1980), aff'd in part, 679 F.2d 1115 (5th Cir. 1982)

Sheehan D, Lecrubier Y, Sheehan K, et al: The Mini-International Neuropsychiatric Interview (M.I.N.I.): the development and validation of a structured diagnostic psychiatric interview for DSM-IV and ICD-10. J Clin Psychiatry 59 (suppl 20):22–33, 1998

Shore J, Hilty D, Yellowlees P: Emergency management guidelines for telepsychiatry. Gen Hosp Psychiatry 29:199–206, 2007

Sabol W, Minton T: Jail inmates at midyear 2007 (NCJ 221945). Washington, DC, U.S. Department of Justice, Office of Justice Programs, Bureau of Justice Statistics, 2008

Spitzer RL, Williams JB, Gibbon M, et al: The Structured Clinical Interview for DSM-III-R (SCID), I: history, rationale, and description. Arch Gen Psychiatry 49:624–629, 1992

Steadman H, Scott J, Osher F, et al: Validation of the Brief Jail Mental Health Screen. Psychiatr Serv 56:816–822, 2005

Teplin L: The prevalence of severe mental disorder among male urban jail detainees: comparison with the Epidemiologic Catchment Area Program. Am J Public Health 80:663–669, 1990

Teplin LA: Psychiatric and substance abuse disorders among male urban jail detainees. Am J Public Health 84:290–293, 1994

Teplin L, Swartz J: Screening for severe mental disorders in jails: the development of the Referral Decision Scale. Law Hum Behav 13:1–18, 1989

Trestman R: Behind bars: personality disorders. J Am Acad Psychiatry Law 28:232–235, 2000

Trestman R, Ford J, Zhang W, et al: Current and lifetime psychiatric illness among inmates not identified as acutely mentally ill at intake in Connecticut's jails. J Am Acad Psychiatry Law 35:490–500, 2007

U.S. Census Bureau: Resident population by sex, race, and Hispanic origin for the United States: April 1, 2000 to July 1, 2007. Available at: http://www.census.gov/compendia/statab/tables/09s0006.pdf. Accessed March 18, 2009.

Weinstein H, Kim D, Mack A, et al: Prevalence and assessment of mental disorders in correctional settings, in Handbook of Correctional Mental Health. Edited by Scott CL, Gerbasi JB. Washington, DC, American Psychiatric Publishing, 2005

West H, Sabol W: Prisoners in 2007 (NCJ 224280). December 2008. Available at: http://www.ojp.usdoj.gov/bjs/pub/pdf/p07.pdf. Accessed March 18, 2009.

Zlotnick C, Clarke JG, Friedmann PD, et al: Gender differences in comorbid disorders among offenders in prison substance abuse treatment programs. Behav Sci Law 26:403–412, 2008

CHAPTER 6

Continuous Quality Improvement and Documentation

Amanda Ruiz, M.D.

Given that medical and mental health care within a correctional setting are held to a community standard, quality medical documentation and a sound continuous quality improvement (CQI) committee are important cornerstones of a strong correctional health care system. More medically defensible cases in the community are either settled or lost due to poor quality of medical records than to any other factor (Medical Insurance Exchange of California 2008). In this chapter I review the role of CQI in a correctional setting and provide practical guidelines for documentation useful in the provision of care to inmates.

CONTINUOUS QUALITY IMPROVEMENT

Terminology and Definitions

During the past several decades, significant gains have been made in the methods used to assess the quality of care provided by a health care system. CQI is a team-based management strategy that emphasizes the continual improvement of the process an organization (e.g., prison, jail) uses to deliver its product (client-focused health care.) Table 6–1 highlights key definitions important to understand in regard to CQI.

149

—

As an approach to quality management, CQI promotes the need for objective data to analyze and improve *processes* in relation to capacity or *outcomes* (Hughes 2007). Via an evidence-based team approach, CQI may increase staff cooperation, boost satisfaction, and unearth wasteful health care expenditures, which may be up to 30%–50% of costs in some facilities (National Commission on Correctional Health Care [NCCHC] 2008). CQI committees exist in community hospitals and private practices, as well as in correctional settings.

NCCHC has specified the maintenance of a CQI program as an essential standard for accreditation, an external peer-review process in which the NCCHC renders a professional judgment regarding health services provided and assists correctional facilities in their continued improvement. Specific to mental health, NCCHC (2008, p. 10) recommends that a CQI program complete the following significant reviews:

1. An annual review of the effectiveness of the CQI program by reviewing CQI studies, minutes of administrative meetings, results of mental health reviews and other pertinent data;
2. At least one process quality improvement study and one outcome quality improvement study each year; and
3. An annual review of deaths and serious incidents involving inmates with mental illness to identify trends and needed corrective actions.

Several different process and outcome studies may be undertaken. For example, the institution's CQI committee might examine the process by which inmates with a mental disorder and a substance use disorder are referred to a substance abuse treatment program and aftercare. Sample areas to explore in this situation might include the following:

- Are *all* the inmates with a mental disorder referred, or are they first screened for the presence of a substance use disorder and subsequently referred?
- Do delays occur between referral and evaluation?
- How many of the dual-diagnosis inmates are accepted into a substance use treatment program or aftercare?
- What circumstances were deemed most important in accepting inmates into the referral program?

In examining the outcome of a specified treatment, the CQI committee might consider, for example, whether the inmates referred for substance abuse treatment have a higher rate of adherence with their routine programming than do those inmates who are not referred for treatment.

TABLE 6–1. Continuous quality improvement terminology

Term	Definition
Continuous quality improvement	A team-based management strategy that identifies problems, implements and monitors corrective action and studies the effectiveness of the action. The team analyzes systems and measures process steps in relation to outcomes for health care (Hughes 2007).
Total quality management	An organizational approach involving organizational management, teamwork, defined processes, systems thinking, and charge to create an environment for improvement. This term is typically applied to industrial settings (Hughes 2007).
Quality assurance	Activities intended to improve the quality of care in either a defined medical setting or a program. Activities include assessment or evaluation of the quality of care; identification of problems or shortcomings in the delivery of care; designing procedures to overcome these deficiencies; and follow-up monitoring to ensure effectiveness of corrective steps. Quality assurance generally focuses on issues identified by regulatory or accreditation organizations, such as checking documentation, reviewing the work of oversight committees, and studying credentialing processes (National Library of Medicine 1980).
Clinical practice improvement	A clinician-led approach to quality improvement that develops evidence-based protocols to achieve desirable clinical outcomes at the lowest essential cost over the continuum of care. An improvement team determines a purpose, collects data, assesses findings, and then translates those findings into practice changes (Horn 2002).
Process study	Examination of the methods by which services are delivered. *Example:* Evaluation of the process by which administrative segregation inmates are screened for suicide risk.
Outcome study	Direct examination of whether treatment goals are achieved. *Example:* Measurement of time to relapse or rule violation reports following substance abuse treatment.

Five important components for a successful CQI program include the following:

1. Taking a practical, critical look at the system in place, with an eye toward identifying what needs to be reconfigured for efficiency. This strategy may include

    a. comparing an institution's own practices to those of nationally recognized guidelines, such as those of the American Psychiatric Association (2006), NCCHC (2008), American Correctional Association (2007), or National Guideline Clearinghouse (2009)[1]; and

    b. brainstorming or anonymously surveying team members for opinions and ideas (Winter 2008).

2. Developing a plan to improve the CQI program.

3. Implementing the plan in a timely manner, setting specific deadlines and designating persons responsible.

4. Tracking the status of identified issues, the success level of the plan put into operation, and necessary adjustments.

5. Repeating the plan at regularly scheduled intervals.

In practice, identifying a plan is easier than fixing it. Numerous obstacles have thwarted well-meaning attempts at CQI; however, a combination of strong leadership, foresight, and planning increases the likelihood that jails and prisons will be successful in their CQI efforts. Thriving CQI committees generally embrace a philosophy toward the provision of health care that includes the following beliefs:

- An opportunity for improvement exists in every process on every occasion.
- Negative outcomes can often be prevented.
- Facilities do not need to be "broken" in order to be "fixed."

Implementing this philosophy requires the involvement of multiple key players at the table, representing administration, custody, and health care. CQI committee members may include the warden; health care warden or captain; chief medical officer(s); health services administrator; and

---

[1]Specific National Guideline Clearinghouse guidelines that the reader may find of interest include practice parameters for the assessment and treatment of youth in juvenile detention and correctional facilities and various disease management guidelines.

managers or designated representatives from medical, mental health, nursing, dental, pharmacy, emergency response, death review, information technology, food services, central supply, personnel, and budgets. Given such a large group of persons, meetings may be limited to a bimonthly to quarterly basis, as needed, depending on the size of the facility. CQI meetings should be scheduled regularly, and taking attendance is advised. For maximum efficiency, participants are wise to come to the meeting prepared.

Recommended Documentation for Continuous Quality Improvement

Unlike peer review, which is discussed later in this chapter, CQI meetings and materials are generally not protected from legal discovery. To protect individual clinicians, neither physician nor inmate patient names need to be used when documenting chart reviews and resultant policy changes. A common misconception is that policy changes that result from CQI activity should not be documented for liability reasons. In truth, documentation is evidence of the institution's effort to continually improve systems and practice. Specifically, the designated health care manager or health services authority may set the agenda for the meeting and be responsible for producing minutes from the meeting. Another recommended strategy is to maintain a CQI log of actions taken and dates of policy changes subsequent to CQI and/or clinical chart review. The following case example demonstrates how a CQI audit can be used to improve the provision of care in a correctional setting.

> As a result of an audit of the urgent-care complaint list in the reception center, Jail X noted that in the last 30 days, 15 inmate patients had been seen for a chief complaint of seizure. A secondary chart review found that although 98% of these inmate patients had been identified as having a seizure disorder, a mental health disorder, or a substance abuse disorder that required treatment with an anticonvulsant medication, only 70% of them were evaluated by a clinician within 72 hours. A review of their medication administration records demonstrated that only 15% were provided any form of medication for any of the identified disorders.
>
> Upon analysis of these results, the CQI committee identified two major problems:
>
> 1. Of inmates referred for a comprehensive evaluation and medication, 30% were not receiving it; that is, too many persons were slipping through the cracks.
> 2. Inmates in need of urgent or emergent medication were not receiving an evaluation for medication in a timely manner.

As a result, the sheriff appointed the chief of medicine and the chief of mental health to work together to identify issues with screening and referral to the appropriate clinicians. He also instructed the chief nurse and the chief pharmacist to follow up on the medication administration issue and asked them to report their proposed solutions in 2 weeks. Two weeks later, the group met to report their findings and proposed solutions. Interviews with both medical and mental health staff identified high turnover among clinicians and problems with sign-outs as key issues. The medical and mental health chiefs proposed to institute policy changes to improve communication between shift changes so that inmates were not left unseen or without orders. The nurse and pharmacist noted that orders for anticonvulsants were best started in the urgent care itself, rather than waiting the 48- to 72-hour lag time for the medication administration record to be generated and the medication to be dispensed; this policy change was proposed as well. The changes were carefully noted, and plans were made to follow up on the new procedures and their efficacy in 6 months.

Continuous Quality Improvement Tools

Specific quality improvement tools may be used by team members to standardize the process of data collection. For example, process flow diagrams are "a visual representation of the flow of a particular process, showing the steps, tasks, operations, decisions, time taken, and sequence of events" (Winter 2008, p. 173). These diagrams allow all individuals in the process to see the chain of events and understand how each role fits into the whole; they also can be used to pinpoint flaws in the process and areas of waste. Other process improvement tools may include properly constructed guidelines and robust forms of decision support that focus on providing information, ideally at the "point of service" and in the context of a particular clinical situation (Goldfarb 1999). The consistent and reliable reproduction of reports is essential to productive quality management. Commonly used reports are described in Table 6–2 (Lundquist and Dronet 2010; Winter 2008).

PEER REVIEW

Standard Peer Review

Peer review is colleagues' "evaluation of a practitioner's professional performance, including identification of opportunities for improving the quality, necessity, and appropriateness-suitability of care" (Segen 2006). It is one of the most useful tools in the toolbox for motivating improved clinical practice; rules that are self-imposed by physicians are much more likely to be adopted (Ramsey 1993). Peer review is typically practiced as a confidential clinical review for a specific group of physicians. For exam-

TABLE 6–2. Common quality improvement tools

Tool	Purpose
Access to care/backlog report	Measures number of inmates who are 30 days past due for periodic reviews or follow-up; measures access to care.
Chart review/audit report	Measures specific processes or outcomes. For example, a random chart review may assess the number of inmates taking atypical antipsychotics who have been screened for weight gain and diabetes.
Utilization management report	Tracks trends in the use of medical and mental health services. For example, a report may analyze trends in the use of forced psychotropic medication or use of restraints.
Employee satisfaction review	Measures opinions and possible ideas of staff.
Medication administration record review	Tracks distribution of medications and adherence.
Suicide prevention and watch review	Reviews specifics in inmate management prior to a suicide attempt and may reveal opportunities for improvement.
Psychotropic medication utilization and medication error report review	Identify patterns of use that may be compared against expected standards. Error reports assist in detecting system errors and preventable inmate injuries.

ple, physicians will meet to review the facts of a select group of cases, the approach to care, the patient's response or lack thereof, and future recommendations. Properly employed, it is designed to be a learning forum as opposed to a punitive one.

Peer review findings are generally not discoverable. The philosophy underlying this protection is that physicians must be encouraged to be candid and vigorous in the performance evaluations of their peers, without fear that those evaluations would be used for improper purposes (e.g., medical malpractice lawsuits). However, physicians should be familiar with the specific laws in their jurisdiction that govern the confidentiality of the peer review process. For example, on March 6, 2008, the Florida Supreme Court upheld Amendment 7, which states that patients "have a right to have access to any records made or received in the course of business by a health care facility or provider relating to any adverse medical incident" ("Florida Peer Review" 2008). The high court ruled that the language in the amendment and the ballot measure "make it abundantly clear that the chief purpose of Amendment 7 was to do away with the legislative restrictions on a Florida patient's access to a medical provider's 'history of acts, neglects or defaults' because such history 'may be important to a patient.'" Medical providers have never been granted a substantive vested right in the secrecy of information contained in the limited medical records in question (Sorrel 2008). Similarly, in some state correctional systems, peer review evaluations and/or quality assurance reports have led to complaints against physicians to the medical board and the National Practitioner Data Bank (Union of American Physicians and Dentists 2007). Peer review is often part of a remedial plan in class action suits and is available to court monitors, who focus on whether the process is functioning appropriately, in contrast to using the findings for other purposes.

Peer review is facilitated by maintaining a standardized approach and a regular schedule. Random clinical cases for psychiatry or psychology peer review may be chosen at select intervals (i.e., monthly or quarterly) by appropriately trained staff. Several different models for peer review exist. In one model, one clinician may be asked to screen another clinician's charts according to selected criteria; then the reviewer sets aside charts that do not meet the listed criteria so that the clinicians can discuss them together during the peer review process. Learning and practice improvement result from the discussion of the results of these periodic screenings and problem solving during a private meeting between clinicians. Any clinicians who fail to meet the practice and documentation criteria should be informed of their deficiencies and the potential risks of poor documentation. A plan to more closely monitor their charting should be strongly considered to ensure inmate patient and institutional safety, as well as clinician defensibility. Table 6–3 lists items that commonly appear on peer review checklists for monitoring care provided.

TABLE 6–3. General chart review items

Description of chief complaint or reason for consultation

History of the present illness

Past medical history, habits, family history

Mental status examination (MSE)

1. Diagnosis substantiated by history and MSE
2. Appropriate recommendation or plan
3. Appropriate diagnostic studies
4. Recognition of complications of therapy
5. Abnormal findings addressed
6. Consultations addressed
7. Legible handwriting
8. Chart entries dated and signed or initialed

One understandable criticism of this type of peer review process is that the focus on the presence or absence of documentation is more in line with a quality assurance approach than with a CQI model. Establishing clear goals for improvement, with documentation training as necessary, helps to prevent the peer review process from becoming a laborious nonproductive process.

Multisource Feedback

Multisource feedback (MSF) is a newer concept in the drive to improve health care delivery and motivate positive clinician change. MSF is a questionnaire-based evaluation method in which ratees are evaluated on key performance behaviors not only by their peers, but also by their nonmedical coworkers and patients. For example, the College of Physicians and Surgeons of Alberta employs the Physician Achievement Review (PAR) program to give physicians feedback on their performance. Every 5 years, physicians distribute questionnaires to patients, physician colleagues, and nonphysician healthcare co-workers. Topics covered in the survey include medical competency, communication skills, and office management. Survey results give physicians a benchmark for good performance and identify opportunities for professional development and practice improvement (College of Physicians and Surgeons of Alberta 2009). A criticism of this program has been that it is not used with sufficient frequency to give physicians feedback in a timely manner so that change can be effected; positive and negative comments may lag years behind the action that prompted them, thus making it difficult for the physician to remember what worked and what did not. As a result, it is recommended that similar programs be implemented on a more frequent basis, such as quarterly.

MSF's strengths include assessing and providing guidance on six fundamental domains identified by the Accreditation Council for Graduate Medical Education as necessary for a physician to achieve competence (Lockyer 2003):

1. Patient care
2. Knowledge
3. Practice-based learning
4. Interpersonal and communication skills
5. Professionalism
6. Systems-based practice

Medical knowledge and practice-based learning and improvement may be better assessed by other tools, such as chart review/audit. Studies have shown that MSF can be a reliable, valid program for psychiatrists and physicians who will accept MSF data to contemplate or initiate change in their practice (Lipner et al. 2002; Sargeant et al. 2008; Violato et al. 2008).

Table 6–4 provides sample items that may be useful in an MSF review process.

DOCUMENTATION: PROMOTING APPROPRIATE CARE THROUGH WRITTEN COMMUNICATION

Reasons for Documentation

The medical record serves multiple purposes:

- Reflecting, as accurately as possible, the current evaluation and management of an inmate patient's illness(es)
- Tracking the course of an illness over time, its response to therapy, and future treatment possibilities
- Documenting the rationale for why care was provided or denied
- Communicating with immediate team members and others (e.g., consultants, colleagues from other disciplines, correctional officers, administrators)

TABLE 6–4. Sample multisource feedback items

Medical colleague questions

1. Communicates effectively with inmate patients
2. Verbally communicates effectively with other professionals
3. Effectively communicates in writing with other professionals
4. Accepts responsibility for inmate patient care
5. Is courteous to coworkers

Nonmedical colleague/supervisor questions

1. Accepts responsibility for professional actions
2. Participates effectively as a member of the health care team
3. Responds appropriately in emergency situations
4. Facilitates the learning of coworkers
5. Presents self in a professional manner

Inmate questions

1. Examined me appropriately for my illness
2. Explained medication and its side effects
3. Explained the results of my laboratory work and/or received my medical history
4. Spends an appropriate amount of time on visit
5. Provides adequate privacy

- Recording care provided that may assist if the standard of care is questioned (i.e., malpractice)
- Functioning as a legal document subject to review by medical review boards, and at times by the courts
- Serving as part of the basis for CQI reviews and assisting with performance improvement
- Verifying compliance with state and/or federal guideline requirements
- Recording mental status in individuals with maladaptive behaviors (to be considered in administrative hearings)
- Providing professional consultation or feedback for colleagues' consults

Guidelines for Documentation

Basic guidelines for charting and documentation are summarized in the following list (Mossman 2008; Roth 2005):

- Write legibly. A common misconception is that messy handwriting or an illegible signature protects the writer by obscuring the facts; this is not the case.
- Use dark blue or black ink when charting.
- Carefully consider each chart entry, because the information becomes a permanent part of the inmate patient's record.
- Draw a single line through any errors, write "error," and initial the change.
- Document responses from consultants and other providers. If a treatment course is chosen other than that suggested by the consultant or other providers, clearly explain why. A sample note in response to a pharmacist's recommendation to change a particular medication might read as follows: "The pharmacist recommends discontinuing the inmate patient's second-generation antipsychotic in favor of a first-generation agent. However, the inmate is stable on the current treatment and is at elevated risk of developing tardive dyskinesia due to age, ethnicity, and length of treatment. Will submit nonformulary item request."

Correctional Mental Health Care Documentation

Strong medical records promote effective communication. Many national organizations recommend documentation of pertinent inmate patient encounters in the medical record (American Psychiatric Association 2006; NCCHC 2008). Such encounters include, but are not limited to, progress notes regarding inmate patient encounters, orders for psychotropic medication, and documentation of consent or refusal. The documenter should also include the date and time of the clinical encounter as well as his or her signature and title. Collateral sources of information that are often relevant to documentation in a correctional setting may include observations and reports from correctional officers, inmate encounters with other medical and nursing personnel, and contacts from attorneys or family members regarding the inmate.

The most common recommended format for a progress note is the SOAPE note. This common acronym stands for Subjective, Objective, Assessment, Plan, and Education. Good progress notes are internally consistent. For example, the inmate diagnosis should comport with the medications prescribed. Notes do not need to be exhaustive, but they should be clear and state the reason for medical decision making. For instance, the education section of a typical progress note may state, "Have discussed the risks, benefits, and alternatives such as weight gain, sedation, and liver problems; inmate consents to treatment with antipsychotic

X at Y dosage." This statement indicates that the inmate was educated regarding his treatment, affirms that informed consent was obtained in a thoughtful manner, and notes the medication prescribed.

In practice, for each medication order, the clinician should write a short progress note that describes when and why the order was written, what medication(s) the inmate is currently taking, and the follow-up plan. In the event that no follow-up plan is recommended, the provider should clearly explain why he or she felt no further monitoring was necessary. Finally, the value of dating and timing all orders as well as signing all entries in a legible manner cannot be understated.

Documenting Involuntary Medication Administration

The administration of involuntary intramuscular medication involves particularly careful documentation and consideration due to the invasive nature of this treatment and potential risks to the patient. In the case of *Washington v. Harper* (1989), the U.S. Supreme Court considered Washington State's procedures for involuntarily medicating inmates. Walter Harper, an inmate in the Washington State prison system, repeatedly became violent when not taking an antipsychotic medication. He was transferred twice to the Special Offender Center (SOC), where he was forced to take psychiatric medications against his will. Upon his second transfer to this facility, Harper filed suit claiming that his due process rights were violated because the SOC failed to provide a judicial hearing prior to involuntarily medicating him. Rather than granting a judicial hearing, Washington State provided an internal institutional review process when considering the inmate's medication refusal. The U.S. Supreme Court held that a judicial hearing was not constitutionally required for involuntary medication administration and that Washington State's administrative procedures provided adequate due process. In particular, an internal and independent administrative review panel (consisting of a psychiatrist, a psychologist, and an SOC official) evaluates situations in which the treating psychiatrist orders involuntarily medication. In Washington State, approval of involuntary medication is given if the inmate suffers from a "mental disorder" and is gravely disabled or poses a likelihood of serious harm to self or others (*Washington v. Harper* 1989).

Many states have adopted review mechanisms similar to those of Washington State for considering medicating an inmate against his or her will. The clinician should be familiar with the exact procedure and criteria for involuntary medication provided in his or her jurisdiction and appropriately document justification for forced treatment. Common factors a prescriber may document when considering involuntary medication psychotropic medication include the following:

- The inmate's mental disorder
- Current signs and symptoms of the inmate's mental disorder
- The relationship of the mental disorder to a risk of harm to self or others
- The relationship of the mental disorder to the inmate's ability to meet basic needs (i.e., whether the inmate has become gravely disabled)
- The threat posed to self or others by not treating
- The clinical indications for use of involuntary medication
- The risks versus benefits of the treatment
- Other modalities attempted for less restrictive treatment

For example, involuntary intramuscular psychotropic medication may be prescribed to patients who meet their jurisdiction's criteria. Table 6–5 shows a weak note and a stronger note that document the emergency administration of psychotropic medication to an inmate.

TABLE 6–5. Sample progress notes regarding documentation of involuntary medication

Weak sample note

Inmate was medicated with Haldol 5 mg IM.

Stronger sample note

Subjective: Inmate S.T. is a 35-year-old with a history of bipolar disorder. Called to assess for agitated behavior, hitting cell wall, and not responding to redirection. Medical record review indicates inmate has not been adherent to treatment with Depakote 500 mg bid.

Objective: Awake and alert. Poor grooming, nails long, hair unkempt. Speech is loud, pressured. Mood is agitated, angry. "I know they are looking at me. I can hear them." Thought process: loose associations. Thought content: evidence of paranoid ideation and auditory hallucinations. Full examination not possible due to agitation. No spontaneous suicidal statements. Self-injurious behavior currently and poor impulse control observed. Insight: limited.

Provisional assessment: Bipolar disorder, manic.

Plan: 1) Prescribe Haldol 5 mg IM×1 to target acute agitation and danger to self. Inmate has no known contraindications to treatment. He has failed attempts at redirection and refuses oral meds. 2) Transfer to inpatient unit for stabilization. Signed by Dr. O.P.

Education: Inmate too agitated to discuss medication side effects at this time; recommend reassessment and discussion in 4–6 hours.

Note.   bid=twice daily; IM=intramuscular.

A common misconception is that angry or noncompliant inmates with no known mental illness may be treated with intramuscular psychotropic medication. In these cases, alternative strategies should be employed and their results clearly documented. Recording each step of an intervention along the way assists in missteps and adverse outcomes.

When *voluntary* intramuscular medication is to be administered, the recommended practice includes a discussion with the patient of the risks, benefits, and alternatives of treatment. Some facilities also require a signed consent for psychotropic medication as part of the informed consent process; the recommended practice is for the treating psychiatrist to document the rationale for treatment planning and medical decision making.

CONCLUSION

Practicing mental health care in a correctional setting can be challenging, especially in today's litigious society. Jails and prisons across the nation are grappling with court mandates, consent decrees, and externally imposed expectations, as opposed to driving health care in a proactive and self-directed manner. One of the best "defenses" is a good offense; the foundation of a strong correctional health care system involves good communication supported by solid proof of practice. This documentation includes the medical record, as well as logs relevant to CQI meetings and peer review.

To ensure that the skilled, responsible, and professional persons involved in inmate patient care decisions establish high standards both for themselves and the facility, management should consider positive strategies for reinforcement and private constructive criticism. Team spirit should be cultivated, and employees at all levels should receive recognition for positive efforts. Exemplary work should be both complimented and judiciously rewarded. Satisfied team members are productive ones.

SUMMARY POINTS

- Continuous quality improvement focuses on evaluating the processes and systems for identifying problems and their causes; intervention and continued monitoring are necessary to achieve and maintain gains.

- Peer reviews coupled with achievable goals can be effective means of educating clinicians and improving inmate patient care.

- Appropriate documentation of inmate patient encounters serves as evidence of efforts to provide appropriate care.

REFERENCES

American Correctional Association: Proposed standards: 4-ALDF-2A-21; 4-ALDF-2A-23. 2007. Available at: http://www.aca.org. Accessed March 21, 2009.

American Psychiatric Association: Practice guidelines: psychiatric evaluation of adults. May 2006. Available at: http://www.psychiatryonline.com. Accessed March 21, 2009.

College of Physicians & Surgeons of Alberta: Physician Achievement Review Program. Available at: http://www.cpsa.ab.ca. Accessed March 21, 2009.

Florida peer review after amendment 7: challenges and solutions to a national trend. Foley & Lardner LLP Newsletter, May 5, 2008. Available at: http://www.foley.com/publications/pub_detail.aspx?pubid=5012. Accessed March 21, 2009.

Goldfarb S: Utility of decision support, clinical guidelines, and financial incentives as tools to achieve improved clinical performance. Jt Comm J Qual Improv 25:137–144, 1999

Horn S: Clinical practice improvement: a new methodology to assess and improve quality. 2002. Available at: http://gateway.nlm.nih.gov/MeetingAbstracts/ma?f=102274218.html. Accessed March 21, 2009.

Hughes R: Tools and strategies for quality improvement and patient safety. Agency for Health Research and Quality. 2007. Available at: http://www.ahrq.gov/qual/nurseshdbk/docs/HughesR_QMBMP.pdf. Accessed March 21, 2009.

Lipner RS, Blank LL, Leas BF, et al: The value of patient and peer ratings in recertification. Acad Med 77(suppl):64–66, 2002

Lockyer J: Multisource feedback in the assessment of physician competencies. J Contin Educ Health Prof 23:4–12, 2003

Lundquist T, Dronet T: Continuous quality improvement, in Manual of Forms and Guidelines for Correctional Mental Health. Edited by Ruiz A, Dvoskin JA, Scott CL, et al. Washington, DC, American Psychiatric Publishing, 2010

Medical Insurance Exchange of California: Cost of malpractice. MIEC Newsletter, April 2008

Mossman D: Tips to make documentation easier, faster and more satisfying. Current Psychiatry 7(2):80, 84–86, 2008

National Commission on Correctional Health Care: Standards for Mental Health Services for Correctional Facilities. Chicago, National Commission on Correctional Health Care, 2008

National Guideline Clearinghouse. 2009. Available at: http://www.guideline.gov. Accessed March 21, 2009.

National Library of Medicine: Quality assurance. Pub Med. 1980. Available at: http://www.nlm.nih.gov/cgi/mesh/2009/MB_cgi?mode=&index=11306&field=all&HM=&ll=&PA=&form=&input=. Accessed January 22, 2009.

Ramsey CI: Use of peer ratings to evaluate physician performance. JAMA 269:1655–1660, 1993

Roth L: Writing progress notes: 10 dos and don'ts. Current Psychiatry 4(2):63–66, 2005

Sargeant P, Mann K, Vleuten C, et al: Directed self assessment: practice and feedback within a social context. J Contin Educ Health Prof 28:47–54, 2008

Segen JC: Concise Dictionary of Modern Medicine. New York, McGraw-Hill, 2006

Sorrel A: Florida Supreme Court lifts past peer review confidentiality. Am Med News, April 7, 2008. Available at: http://www.ama-assn.org/amednews/2008/04/07/gvsb0407.html. Accessed March 21, 2009.

Union of American Physicians and Dentists: Peer review and disciplinary hearing policies. State Doctors Newletter, May 2007. Available at: http://www.uapd.com/wiki/uapd/state_doctors_newsletter_may_2007?wikiPageId=1329087. Accessed March 21, 2009.

Violato C, Lockyer J, Fidler H: Assessment of psychiatrists in practice through multisource feedback. Can J Psychiatry 53:525–533, 2008

Washington v Harper, 494 U.S. 210, 110 S. Ct. (1989)

Winter SJ: Improving the quality of health care delivery in a corrections setting. J Correct Health Care 14:168–182, 2008

CHAPTER 7

Evaluating and Treating Substance Use Disorders

Tracy D. Gunter, M.D.
Sandra K. Antoniak, M.F.S., M.D.

The U.S. correctional system comprises a heterogeneous group of facilities and programs. Each facility and program is shaped by the community and judicial district that it serves and therefore has unique features. All correctional settings are confronted with high frequencies of substance use disorders among offenders, and ongoing substance use is both a significant public health problem and a risk factor for recidivism. Although correctional facilities are not under a constitutional mandate to provide treatment for substance use disorders, correctional settings may be ordered to provide treatment as part of the sentencing of an offender and may provide services based on the enormity of the need within the populations that they serve.

In this chapter, we provide an overview of the challenges raised by substance use disorders for jails and prisons. The goals of this brief overview of the evaluation and treatment of substance use disorders in the correctional setting are to describe the extent of the problem posed by substance use disorders, to familiarize the reader with the most current practice standards for the evaluation and treatment of substance use disorders in correctional institution settings, and to comment briefly on drug courts as a potential strategy for diverting some cases from confinement. In general, information in the chapter is grouped by facility type (jail or prison) within each section.

SCOPE OF THE PROBLEM

Substance use disorders are pressing national public health problems. In 2002, the total economic cost of substance use disorders (i.e., substance intoxication, withdrawal, abuse, and dependence) in the United States was estimated to be $180.9 billion and could be divided into three broad categories: health care costs, lost productivity, and crime-related costs (Harwood et al. 2004). Although the term *substance* commonly refers to illicit drugs, the definition also includes pharmaceuticals, alcohol, and inhalants. Despite the frequency of substance use disorders, not all substance use is pathological. Pathological substance use is characterized by the frequency of substance use and the degree of medical or psychosocial dysfunction experienced by the individual. For example, alcohol can be used in moderation by many individuals, and individuals who have experimented with cocaine or marijuana once do not meet criteria for a substance use disorder (American Psychiatric Association 2000). Substance use disorders, as defined by the *Diagnostic and Statistical Manual of Mental Disorders*, 4th Edition, Text Revision (American Psychiatric Association 2000), emphasize overall dysfunction and negative consequences (medical, social, occupational).

According to the Bureau of Justice Statistics (2009), over 7.3 million people (3.2% of the U.S. adult population) are involved in the criminal justice system. Of these, approximately 2.2 million are incarcerated in jails and prisons (Sabol and Couture 2008; Sabol and Minton 2008), and the remaining 5 million individuals are supervised by community corrections. Researchers have well documented the association between substance use disorders and criminal offending, as well as the rapid growth of correctional populations (Adams and Reynolds 2002; Bureau of Justice Statistics 2009; Ditton 1999; Greenfield 1998; James 2004; Kanato 2008; Karberg and James 2005; Peters et al. 2004). The net result is that correctional systems are responsible for managing increasing numbers of individuals with substance use disorders each year.

Substance use disorders are rampant in correctional settings. Although estimates vary, well over half of all incarcerated individuals have a significant substance use disorder (Peters et al. 2008). More than two-thirds of jail inmates (Karberg and James 2005) and approximately half of prisoners (53% state and 45% federal) meet full diagnostic criteria for a substance use disorder (Mumola and Karberg 2006). Peters et al. (2008)

noted that the lifetime prevalence of substance dependence (a specific category of substance use disorders) among individuals in prison was 74%, with 46% meeting criteria for drug dependence and 37% meeting criteria for alcohol dependence. Among inmates using drugs, marijuana was most commonly used, followed by cocaine or crack, and methamphetamine (James and Glaze 2006; Mumola and Karberg 2006). Although alcohol use disorders are not significantly less common than drug use disorders, they have received relatively less attention in recent years (Beck et al 2000; Jones and Hoffmann 2006).

Substance use disorders frequently co-occur with other mental health disorders. Among jail inmates, 68% of all inmates (Karberg and James 2005) and 76% of inmates with a self-reported mental health history met criteria for a substance use disorder (James and Glaze 2006). Of state and federal prisoners, 77% were noted to be "alcohol and drug involved" (Mumola 1999), and over two-thirds of those with self-reported mental health problems met criteria for at least one substance use disorder (James and Glaze 2006). Whereas over 40% of all incarcerated persons met criteria for both a mental health issue and a substance use disorder, less than one-fourth of inmates met criteria for a substance use disorder without another mental health concern (James and Glaze 2006).

ONGOING SUBSTANCE USE WHILE INCARCERATED

A common misperception is that jails and prisons are drug-free environments. Home-brewed alcohol (pruno), illicit drugs, and trafficked prescription medications are used by inmates to maintain their previous drug-using behavior, establish trade within the prison environment, or escape the unpleasantness of incarceration. The particular intoxicants found within secure settings vary by local custom, availability, and distribution systems.

Although anecdotal accounts of ongoing covert substance use by offenders while incarcerated are common, literature providing data on this issue in the United States is limited. It is well known that illicit substances are entering secure settings (Okie 2007). Drugs and paraphernalia are "muled" into correctional settings by individuals known to an inmate or as part of a tiered arrangement that separates those bringing in the contraband from the recipient. Unfortunately, corrections staff are occasionally an active part of the process or are otherwise complicit (Atchison 2008). Visitation areas and mailrooms are common sites for interdiction of substances smuggled into jails and prisons (Butler 2002).

Medical providers practicing in correctional settings may be unaware of the high potential for diversion and redistribution of pharmaceuticals and therefore may become unwitting participants in the drug trade. Most prescription medications that are diverted are used for their direct narcotic, hallucinogenic, stimulant, sedative, or hypnotic/anxiolytic effects, but virtually any drug with psychoactive properties can be used for intoxication, including low-potency antipsychotics, antiemetics, antidepressants, antiparkinsonian agents, and over-the-counter antihistamines and cold or allergy preparations. Inmates may feign symptoms to receive prescription or over-the-counter medications with psychoactive properties from medical practitioners. In general, practitioners should ask staff about substances that have been problematic in the particular facilities in which they are practicing. Special care should be taken when considering treatments for insomnia, pain, and attention-deficit/hyperactivity disorder, because commonly used treatments are frequently diverted.

In addition to smuggling intoxicants into a secure setting or diverting them from legitimate use within the setting, inmates sometimes produce intoxicating substances. Pruno is one example of "home brew" that has received particular attention over the years. Pruno production was described by San Quentin death row inmate Jarvis Masters in his 1992 poem "Recipe for Prison Pruno" (Masters 1997). The pruno production process involves heating and fermenting oranges, apples, canned fruit, sugar, ketchup, and bread. The taste and odor of pruno have been described as similar to vomitus and, according to contributors to Wikipedia (2009), the alcohol content can vary from 2% to 14%, depending on the ingredients and the time spent fermenting. In some facilities, local production of alcohol has become such an issue that certain food items have been banned from facility menus, but this is only a partial solution at best. The effective treatment of substance use disorders could result in decreased demand for intoxicants and therefore decreased production.

Covert substance use should be suspected even in long-term inmates who exhibit abrupt transient changes in mental status.

Clinical Case 7–1

Mr. Q, age 60 years, has been imprisoned for the last 5 years. He has never presented behavioral challenges, but officers began reporting increasing difficulty with his completing work details in the kitchen. He was sent to the prison infirmary after being found slumped over on a counter while trying to complete his work. On arrival at the infirmary, he was euphoric, his speech was slurred, and he did not recognize the nurse. Because he had had a stroke the year before, an emergency medical service was called to take him to the local emergency room. En route he was noted to have high blood pressure and a slowing respiratory rate.

At the emergency room, a computed tomographic scan of Mr. Q's brain was found to be normal. Urine studies indicated the presence of opiates and benzodiazepines. When he lost consciousness, he was given naloxone and flumazenil to reverse the effects of the opiate and benzodiazepine. He made a full recovery and was returned to the prison late that evening.

EVALUATION

Evidence-Based Principles in Evaluating Substance Use Disorders: Costs and Benefits

Incarceration provides a unique opportunity for intervention in the lives of offenders with substance use disorders. Standardized screening and assessment protocols aim to refine referral and placement decisions (Taxman et al. 2006). Timely identification of substance use disorders allows for informed allocation of resources to address the needs of high-risk offenders (Taxman et al. 2007). Standardized actuarial risk assessment tools have been used to increase equity and consistency in matching offenders with services; however, implementation of screening and assessment for the purpose of triaging offenders for treatment is not a universal practice (Taxman et al. 2007).

Correctional systems are increasingly adopting evidence-based practices in the evaluation of substance use disorders, with goals of effectively changing offender behavior, improving community safety, and decreasing recidivism, but barriers exist to the implementation of consistent evaluation protocols. These barriers might include inadequate resources to competently perform the tasks of evaluation and treatment, poor coordination between and among the agencies involved with the offender, insufficient training in efficient and effective screening and assessment strategies, and lack of standardized recording of the data obtained. All of these issues may lead to inaccuracies and inefficiencies (Moore and Mears 2003) that then further delay treatment and increase the perceived cost of effective assessment. Proper application of instruments suitable for the offender being examined and consistent documentation of answers are necessary for a valid analysis of each offender's needs (Mears et al. 2003).

A shift to evidence-based principles by correctional service providers may serve to bolster the perceived social and financial benefit of treatment for inmates with substance use disorders (Clawson et al. 2005). Meta-analyses of corrections data have provided the basis for the eight evidence-based principles listed in Table 7–1 (Clawson et al. 2005).

TABLE 7–1.   Eight evidence-based principles for effective interventions

1. Assess risks and needs using formal and informal strategies on an ongoing basis.

2. Engage the offender in the process of change using motivational interviewing.

3. Formulate interventions of sufficient intensity and duration and specific to the individual offender, taking into account factors such as gender, culture, temperament, relapse risk, and recidivism risk.

4. Implement evidence-based programming such as cognitive-behavioral skills building.

5. Use a structured approach that couples predictable consequences for negative behavior with positive reinforcement for progress to promote sustained behavioral change.

6. Actively identify, recruit, and use community resources capable of supporting the offender upon return to his or her neighborhood.

7. Maintain consistent quality practices and monitor outcomes.

8. Provide actionable feedback to offenders and staff in a timely manner.

Source.   Adapted from Clawson et al. 2005.

Screening

The screening process is focused on the identification of offender issues in need of further assessment and treatment, as well as offender eligibility for the facility resources available to meet those needs (Center for Substance Abuse Treatment 2005). Screenings are generally performed by trained nonprofessional staff and are limited to instruments that are succinct and easily administered during a brief encounter (Center for Substance Abuse Treatment 2005). A high degree of variability exists with respect to the type and quality of the instrument used for screening (Moore and Mears 2003). By its nature, the screening process is cursory, and the triaging of inmates for detoxification and treatment may be compromised unless both vigilance and efficiency are maintained (Moore and Mears 2003). The screening process should include the following domains: substance abuse (e.g., detoxification needs, substance abuse history, desire for treatment), criminal involvement (e.g., prior convictions, number of incarcerations, criminal thinking), physical health (e.g., infectious disease, pregnancy, acute conditions), mental health (e.g., suicidality, psychopathy, acute symptoms), and special considerations (e.g., literacy, housing, family issues) (Center for Substance Abuse Treatment 2005).

The Center for Substance Abuse Treatment (2005) identified three screening instruments deemed to be the most effective in identifying substance dependence: the combination of the Alcohol Dependence Scale (ADS; Skinner and Horn 1984) and the Addiction Severity Index (ASI)—Drug Use section, the Simple Screening Instrument for Substance Abuse (SSI-SA; Center for Substance Abuse Treatment 1994), and Texas Christian University's TCU Drug Screen II (TCUDS; TCU Institute of Behavioral Research 2006). These instruments outperformed several other screens, including the Michigan Alcoholism Screening Test (MAST)—Short Version, the Addiction Severity Index—Alcohol Use section, the Drug Abuse Screening Test (DAST), and the Substance Abuse Subtle Screening Inventory (SASSI), on key measures of positive predictive value, sensitivity, and overall accuracy (Peters et al. 2008). The TCU Drug Screen II (see Table 7–2) and Simple Screening Instrument for Substance Abuse (see Table 7–3) both performed well based on ease of administration, psychometric properties, and free availability in the public domain (Peters et al. 2008).

TABLE 7–2.   TCU Drug Screen II (TCUDS-II)

The TCUDS-II is a 15-item self-reported measure of substance use within the past year. Screened elements include frequency of substance use, history of treatment, substance dependence, and motivation for treatment.

Positive features

Highly effective in identifying substance-dependent prisoners.

High sensitivity (0.85) and accuracy (0.82) with good specificity (0.78) when compared with other screens tested on a correctional population.

Test-retest reliability is good (0.89–0.95) on correctional populations.

Easy to administer and score.

Available in the public domain.

Concerns

Validity has not been determined in correctional population with co-occurring disorders.

Concurrent screening for deception is indicated because deception is not adequately detected.

Note.   Instrument is available at http://www.ibr.tcu.edu/pubs/datacoll/Forms/ddscreen-95.pdf.
Source.   Peters et al. 2000, 2008; Richards and Pai 2003.

TABLE 7–3. Simple Screening Instrument for Substance Abuse (SSI)

The SSI is a 16-item self-reported measure of symptoms of substance dependence experienced within the last 6 months. Screened elements include alcohol and/or drug consumption, preoccupation and loss of control, adverse consequences, problem recognition, tolerance, and withdrawal.

The SSI is one of the most frequently used substance abuse screening instruments within state correctional systems (Moore and Mears 2003).

Positive features

Highly effective at identifying prisoners with substance dependence disorders.

Highest sensitivity (0.87) and overall accuracy (0.84) when compared with other screens tested on a correctional population.

Easy to administer and score.

Available in the public domain.

Concerns

Validity has not been determined in correctional population with co-occurring disorders.

Does not examine use patterns (e.g., quantity, frequency).

Note. Instrument is available at http://www.ncbi.nlm.nih.gov/books/bv.fcgi?rid=hstat5.table.33647.
Source. Center for Substance Abuse Treatment 2005; Mears et al. 2003; Peters et al. 2008.

Because screening instruments rely on self-report and the screening is occurring in a legal context, screening validity may be limited by offender reliability. Denial is common among those with substance use disorders, regardless of the context in which they find themselves, but legally involved individuals with substance use disorders face additional challenges. The legal context of pretrial or probationary hearings may discourage self-disclosure of symptoms of substance use disorders because of an offender's fear that admitting to substance use may have a negative impact on legal proceedings (Richards and Pai 2003). Collateral sources, such as booking records, presentencing investigations, treatment records, police reports, corrections reports, emergency medical reports, and drug test reports, should be used when available.

In addition to interview techniques and record review, analysis of hair or urine prior to the screening interview may increase offender self-report validity (Hamid et al. 1999). Many jails emphasize urine testing (Pretrial

Services Resource Center 1999; Wilson 2000). Slightly more than half of offenders in jail undergo drug testing, but the percentage varies based on local policy, resources, and perceived need. In one study, jails in larger jurisdictions more commonly tested inmates and staff than did those in smaller jurisdictions (Wilson 2000). The frequency and timing of testing depended on the facility's regulations: 69% of jails tested inmates based on presentation of signs and symptoms typical for drug use, 50% tested on a random basis, and 5% tested all inmates at intake (Wilson 2000).

Assessment

Assessments are typically performed by professional staff to define a clinical problem identified in the screening process and provide specific recommendations for treatment and disposition. Like the screening process, the assessment is often limited by time, space constraints, availability of trained staff, and financial resources (Center for Substance Abuse Treatment 2005). Ideally, assessment determines suitability for treatment, as well as the likelihood of benefit from treatment, and outlines positive and negative factors that may influence the course of substance use disorder treatment (Center for Substance Abuse Treatment 2005). Unfortunately, as a practical matter, assessment is frequently completed only after an offender is assigned to a treatment program (Moore and Mears 2003).

Many assessment tools are available. The choice of an assessment tool depends on the facility's needs and resources. Commonly used assessment tools include the Addiction Severity Index (ASI; McLellan et al. 1980, 1992), Stages of Change Readiness and Treatment Eagerness Scale (SOCRATES; Center for Substance Abuse Treatment 2005), and University of Rhode Island Change Assessment (URICA; DiClemente and Hughes 1990). Once the assessment is complete, then treatment planning begins. The paradigm of choice has been the American Society of Addiction Medicine Patient Placement Criteria (ASAM PPC; National Institute on Drug Abuse 2006).

The ASI (McLellan et al. 1980, 1992) is a 155-item structured interview that examines alcohol and drug dependence, frequency of use, and associated psychosocial factors (family and social relationships, employment, support status, and mental health status). It has high reliability (Brodey et al. 2004) and high correlation between objective indicators of addiction severity and diagnoses of alcohol and drug dependence. Validation and normative data are available for the criminal justice populations (McLellan et al. 1992). The ASI is somewhat lengthy and cumbersome to administer, requiring 45–90 minutes and rather extensive interviewer training. The alcohol and drug sections can be completed in much less time but may not have adequate reliability and validity without the remainder of the instrument (Carey 1997; Corse et al. 1995; McLellan et al. 2004).

SOCRATES focuses on alcohol abuse (Center for Substance Abuse Treatment 2005). It was developed to examine readiness to change through separate subscales corresponding to five stages of change (Prochaska and DiClemente 1992). Versions of SOCRATES are available for each gender and for collateral historians (Peters et al. 2008). SOCRATES was found to be highly reliable in correctional populations, with moderately good sensitivity and specificity; additionally, it is brief to administer and easy to score (Peters and Greenbaum 1996). However, it has only modest predictive validity and, unlike the ASI, it has not been tested in individuals with co-occurring disorders (Peters et al. 2008). SOCRATES is free and available in the public domain.

URICA (DiClemente and Hughes 1990) consists of a self-report survey that indicates the individual's readiness for change (i.e., precontemplation, contemplation, action, and maintenance). URICA is less specific with respect to alcohol or drug treatment than the SOCRATES, and its questions are asked in a general manner. URICA has good reliability and is able to discriminate readiness to change in individuals with alcohol dependence, but validity testing has been mixed (Peters et al. 2008). It is in the public domain.

Other assessment tools, such as the Psychiatric Research Interview for Substance and Mental Disorders (PRISM; Samet et al. 2004), might be selected if co-occurring mental health and substance use disorders are suspected. PRISM was developed to diagnose mental illness in individuals with substance use disorders (Samet et al. 2004). It is a semistructured interview that requires approximately 90 minutes to administer (Peters et al. 2008). It examines current and lifetime substance abuse and dependence, Axis I mental disorders, and borderline and antisocial personality disorders (Peters et al. 2008). It has excellent reliability for primary major depression and good to excellent reliability for substance dependence. However, it was found to have less reliability for low-prevalence substances of abuse and poor reliability for anxiety (Hasin et al. 2006). In addition to being time consuming to administer, the interview must be administered by highly trained professionals, so it has not been widely used or tested in criminal justice populations (Peters et al. 2008). The PRISM instrument and manual can be downloaded from a Web site (http://www.columbia. edu/~dsh2/prism). For further discussion of evaluation strategies in those with co-occurring or dual disorders, the reader is referred to Center for Substance Abuse Treatment 1995 and Peters et al. 2008.

The ASAM PPC (National Institute on Drug Abuse 2006) are intended to provide a structure to assist mental health care providers with appropriate placement of individuals in need of treatment for substance use disorders along the continuum of care ideally available in the community. These criteria are considered the most fundamental evidence-based treatment, but they assume availability of a range of resources not frequently found in correctional settings. Additional dimensions addressing the risk of criminal recidivism, and modifications of level of services to include jail- and prison-based programs, could be added to the ASAM PPC to facilitate applicability in the correctional setting (National Institute on Drug Abuse 2006). Table 7–4 summarizes the ASAM PPC, which can be purchased from the American Society of Addiction Medicine Web site (http://www.asam.org/PatientPlacementCriteria.html).

Challenges in Screening and Assessment

Several systems and administrative barriers exist that inhibit implementation of consistent screening and assessment protocols. The Urban Institute Justice Policy Center published "Drug Treatment in the Criminal Justice System: The Current State of Knowledge" (Mears et al. 2003) as one part of a four-part series that examined issues surrounding substance use disorders in U.S. prisons and jails. In the report, barriers to treatment for inmates with substance use disorders were grouped into two broad categories: 1) administrative and systems issues and 2) inappropriate use or interpretation of screening and assessment tools. Administrative barriers occurring at the systems level include inadequate time for evaluation and inappropriate handling of data (Moore and Mears 2003). Proper application of instruments suitable for each offender being examined and consistent documentation of answers are necessary for valid analysis of the offender's needs (Mears et al. 2003). Ideally, screening and assessment should be thought of as processes rather than single events, such that an inmate would be screened again with changes in his or her status. In this way, one could then match treatment interventions to a recent assessment of offender need and readiness for the intervention.

Social and political factors may also serve as barriers to the treatment of substance use disorders in incarcerated populations. These factors include a downward trend in the level of concern expressed by the public and policymakers, lack of coordination among agencies, and lack of commitment of financial and human resources to provide treatment for a condition largely viewed as self-inflicted (Mears et al. 2003). However, with a shift to evidence-based correctional principles with an outcome-based focus for reducing recidivism, both corrections agencies and the general public may see the social and financial benefit of treatment for inmates with substance use disorders (Clawson et al. 2005).

TABLE 7–4.   American Society of Addiction Medicine Patient
                  Placement Criteria

Assessment dimensions

Acute intoxication and/or withdrawal potential

Biomedical conditions and complications

Emotional, behavioral, and cognitive conditions and complications

Readiness to change

Relapse, continued use, or continued problem potential

Recovery/living environment

Levels of treatment services

Level 0.5: Early intervention

Level I: Outpatient treatment

Level II: Intensive outpatient/partial hospitalization treatment

Level III: Residential/inpatient treatment

Level IV: Medically managed intensive inpatient treatment

Source.   National Institute on Drug Abuse 2006.

TREATMENT

The U.S. Supreme Court ruled in *Marshall v. United States* (1974) that an individual has no constitutional right to rehabilitative treatment for substance use disorders at the public's expense after being convicted of a crime. Additionally, in *Pace v. Fauver* (1979), a federal district court ruled that a correctional facility's failure to provide rehabilitative treatment for alcoholism was not cruel and unusual punishment. Notwithstanding these rulings, treatment programs may be created within correctional settings for a variety of reasons, such as the need to satisfy judicial orders, a desire to take advantage of state or federal grant–funded initiatives, a response to class-action lawsuits, or the result of community-initiated collaborations designed to improve continuity of care.

In part because of the number of different ways programs may arise and the number of purposes they may serve, the availability of treatment services for substance use disorders in jails and prisons is variable and based on factors unique to each facility, such as staffing, availability of facilities, and financial resources. Programs are highly inconsistent with respect to where they are, what they do, who they serve, and how long they endure. Appreciating these variables is important while evaluating the literature on programs and their outcomes.

Despite the lack of a constitutional mandate to provide rehabilitative treatment for substance use disorders, correctional systems do have a mandate to treat medical and mental health problems, including complications of substance use disorders. Correctional facilities therefore evaluate for infectious diseases, such as hepatitis C and HIV; for mental health symptoms, including those related to substance ingestion and withdrawal; and for physical withdrawal from ingested substances.

Detoxification

Among offenders incarcerated in the nation's jails, substance ingestion is common just prior to arrest (James 2004), and an estimated 1 million arrestees are at risk for untreated alcohol and opiate withdrawal (Fiscella et al. 2004a). *Withdrawal* is defined as the physiological response to the cessation of substance ingestion (Fiscella et al. 2004b). Table 7–5 summarizes some commonly encountered drug withdrawal states.

Accurate and timely physical triage of individuals with substance use disorders is essential for identifying those inmates at greatest risk of withdrawal and those requiring medically supervised detoxification (Fiscella et al. 2004b). Although behavioral changes early in the course of incarceration may represent coping difficulties and challenges to authority, they may also be symptoms of impending withdrawal or other medical problems.

Clinical Case 7–2

Ms. B is a 23-year-old female who was arrested for possession of marijuana and carrying a concealed weapon without a permit. She told the arresting officer that she had been drinking all day with friends, but her Breathalyzer test at the scene yielded an approximate blood alcohol level of 0.07 µg/dL. While being booked into jail, she was drowsy and her speech was slurred. During this intake, her sixth in as many months, she reported ongoing psychiatric treatment for intermittent explosive disorder, panic disorder, and borderline personality disorder, but could not recall the names of any of her medications.

After intake, she was placed in her cell to "sleep it off" and fell asleep within minutes. The next morning, Ms. B reported that she was feeling anxious. Over the course of the day, she paced and required frequent redirection by staff to even minimally comply with the jail routine. Her agitation worsened throughout the day, and by the evening she was observed to be sweaty, shaky, and pale. She stated that "nothing feels real" and that she had a headache. She was sent back to her bunk to lie down but collapsed in the hallway. The emergency medical service was called, and she was transported to the local emergency room.

TABLE 7–5.   Withdrawal syndromes

Alcohol

Intoxication: Ataxia, slurred speech, disinhibition, odor of alcohol

Mild to moderate withdrawal: Tremors, nausea, anxiety, diaphoresis, disturbed sleep

Severe: Hallucinations, seizures, emesis, diarrhea

Benzodiazepines

Intoxication: Ataxia, slurred speech, sedation, nystagmus, drooling, disinhibition

Early- and middle-stage withdrawal: Anxiety, sleep disturbance, hypersensitivity to sensory stimuli, derealization, memory impairment, headache, myalgias, palpitations

Late-stage withdrawal: Seizure, depression, agoraphobia, increased suicidal ideation

Opioids

Intoxication: Sedation, miosis, bradycardia, pruritis

Mild to moderate: Lacrimation, rhinorrhea, perspiration, yawning, restlessness, insomnia, dilated pupils, anorexia, nausea, weakness, mydriasis, piloerection, myalgias, diarrhea, fatigue

Stimulants

Intoxication: Agitation, irritability, grandiosity, mydriasis, tremor, diaphoresis, rapid speech and movement

Mild to moderate withdrawal: Anxiety, agitation, depression, fatigue, hypersomnolence, hyperphagia

Severe withdrawal: Psychosis

Source.   Federal Bureau of Prisons 2000.

En route, she began experiencing continuous generalized tonic-clonic seizures. Blood was obtained, and an intravenous (IV) line was placed. Anticonvulsant medications were given in the IV, and Ms. B was intubated. After arrival in the emergency room, she received IV fluids and was extubated 12 hours later. Drug screen results were consistent with recent ingestion of tetrahydrocannabinol, antidepressants, and benzodiazepines. Upon awakening, Ms. B admitted to using escalating amounts of alprazolam over the last 2 months to "get the buzz but not the hangover" that she got from drinking. Collateral information obtained from her mother at the hospital indicated that Ms. B had been treated with risperidone, citalopram, trazodone, and alprazolam by her psychiatrist and had been unable to stop drinking.

Factors influencing triage for detoxification include the type of drug abused and the severity of its associated withdrawal syndrome, medical and psychiatric comorbidities, and the availability of local resources. Medical concerns of the individual inmate are frequently balanced against public safety concerns and security, or escape risks (National Institute on Drug Abuse 2006). Therefore, when clinical suspicion for complicated withdrawal is low, detoxification may be safely achieved in the general population of the facility under standard conditions. If complicated withdrawal (e.g., medical complications such as seizures) is possible, then the inmate should be triaged to an appropriate medical unit either within the facility or at a local hospital. Psychiatric conditions, such as depression and bipolar disorder, can increase the complexity of managing the withdrawing individual and may increase the already elevated risk of suicide (Center for Substance Abuse Treatment 2006). Table 7–6 summarizes risk factors for complicated withdrawal.

Each person with a substance use disorder experiences withdrawal differently based on individual physiological, psychological, and neurochemical characteristics. Vigilance and a high index of suspicion are necessary to detect early withdrawal symptoms and identify those who require additional medical supervision. In addition to asking questions of the offender, the evaluator should be alert to physical signs and symptoms of intoxication or withdrawal. For example, chemical odors (e.g., alcohol, or "cat urine" or ammonia in the case of methamphetamine) and stereotypic behaviors (ataxia, nystagmus, slurred speech) may indicate that an individual is acutely intoxicated (Center for Substance Abuse Treatment 2006). Table 7–7 summarizes the evaluation and treatment process for withdrawal from alcohol, benzodiazepines, and opiates.

Fatal withdrawal syndromes are associated primarily with benzodiazepines and alcohol. The health consequences of complicated alcohol withdrawal mandate that any offender who is acutely intoxicated at intake be treated as if he or she is at risk for complicated withdrawal until it can be safely excluded (Federal Bureau of Prisons 2000). Alcohol withdrawal syndrome can range in severity from mild (nausea, headache, malaise) to life threatening (seizures and delirium tremens) (Federal Bureau of Prisons 2000). Indicators of medically complicated withdrawal from alcohol include previous seizures during withdrawal and blood alcohol levels greater than 100 mg/dL in the context of withdrawal symptoms (Federal Bureau of Prisons 2000). Withdrawal commonly occurs within the first 6–72 hours following cessation of alcohol intake. Symptoms such as anxiety, irritability, and increased blood pressure and heart rate indicate impending withdrawal seizure. Symptoms may progress to tremor, fever, and diaphoresis, which should alert care staff that a com-

TABLE 7–6. Factors indicating need for medical attention during detoxification

Increased age

Co-occurring medical problems

Polydrug withdrawal

Temperature>101°F, chills

Symptoms of sympathetic activation: systolic blood pressure>180, heart rate>120, respiratory rate>20, tremors

Mental status changes: loss of consciousness, agitation, aggression, hallucinations

Escalating nausea, vomiting, or diarrhea

Unstable mental illness and suicidal ideation

Source. American Psychiatric Association 2000; Fiscella et al. 2002; Tetrault and O'Connor 2008.

plicated withdrawal course is possible and pharmacological intervention is indicated. If withdrawal is allowed to progress, changes in mental status, seizure, autonomic instability, hallucinations, seizure, and death could occur (Federal Bureau of Prisons 2000).

Although withdrawal from stimulants (cocaine or methamphetamine), hallucinogens, and inhalants does not often cause life-threatening withdrawal syndromes, psychological symptoms (anxiety, restlessness, fatigue) will be present. Cocaine or methamphetamine withdrawal may cause dysphoria or depression, hypersomnolence, and rarely psychotic symptoms (Nutt and Lingford-Hughes 2008). Even if withdrawal symptoms are not imminently life threatening, therapeutic support, frequent reassessment, and reasonable symptomatic treatment are necessary for treatment.

When an individual is dependent on more than one substance, the assessment of withdrawal symptoms is more complicated. Guidelines for management of withdrawal in the criminal justice setting have been established by the American Society of Addiction Medicine, the American Psychiatric Association, the Federal Bureau of Prisons, and the National Commission on Correctional Health Care (Fiscella et al. 2004a). Regardless of the etiology, the following symptoms warrant immediate attention from medical staff: temperature greater than 101°F (Federal Bureau of Prisons 2000), changes in blood pressure or pulse, dark or bloody stools, bloody vomitus, abdominal pain, hallucinations, suspected seizure activity, altered level of consciousness, sluggish pupils, and increasing psychomotor agitation (National Institute on Drug Abuse 2006).

TABLE 7–7.	Evaluation and treatment for common withdrawal syndromes

Alcohol

Evaluation

Examination by a health care professional is indicated for all inmates suspected of significant alcohol use, assessing for indications of dependence and including a targeted physical examination that includes vital signs and an evaluation of cardiovascular, neurological, and mental health status.

Medical history to include signs and symptoms of gastritis, gastric bleeding, trauma, liver disease, and pancreatitis.

Labs to include complete blood count, comprehensive blood chemistry panel, urine toxicology, and pregnancy test for women. Viral hepatitis serologies and HIV testing should be based on individual assessment.

Treatment

If dependence is suspected, give thiamine 100 mg orally or intramuscularly to prevent Wernicke's encephalopathy.

Mild withdrawal: Supportive therapy with close monitoring of vital signs and behavior.

Moderate withdrawal: Lorazepam or chlordiazepoxide taper.

Severe withdrawal: Consider hospitalization on the medical unit or community hospitalization.

Monitoring

Vitals every 4 hours to monitor for indication of worsening sympathetic activation.

Benzodiazepines

Evaluation

Examination by a health care professional is indicated for all inmates suspected of significant benzodiazepine use, assessing for indications of dependence and including a targeted physical examination that includes vital signs and an evaluation of cardiovascular, neurological, and mental health status.

Medical history to include previous history of withdrawal seizure, trauma, or liver disease.

Labs to include complete blood count, comprehensive blood chemistry panel, urine toxicology, and pregnancy test for women. Viral hepatitis serologies and HIV testing should be based on individual assessment.

Treatment

Substitution of an equivalent amount of long-acting benzodiazepine such as clonazepam for shorter-acting alprazolam or lorazepam.

Taper the dose by 10% every 3–5 days.

TABLE 7–7.	Evaluation and treatment for common withdrawal syndromes *(continued)*

Benzodiazepines *(continued)*

Monitoring

Vitals every 8 hours to monitor for indication of worsening sympathetic activation.

Stop treatment if excessive somnolence, slurred speech, or other indication of intoxication.

Opiates

Evaluation

Examination by a health care professional is indicated for all inmates suspected of significant opiate use, assessing for indications of dependence and including a targeted physical examination that includes vital signs and an evaluation of cardiovascular, neurological, and mental health status. The examiner should also look for stigmata of injection drug use, including scars, needle tracks, and abscesses.

Medical history and review of symptoms for conditions associated with chronic opiate use, such as malnutrition, tuberculosis infection and disease, trauma, skin infections, endocarditis, and sexually transmitted diseases.

Labs to include complete blood count, comprehensive blood chemistry panel, urine toxicology, and pregnancy test for women. Viral hepatitis serologies and HIV testing should be based on individual assessment.

Treatment

Supportive treatment is indicated except for pregnant women and persons with significant cardiovascular risk factors. Pregnant women should be treated with methadone because opiate withdrawal is associated with an increased risk of premature labor.

Methadone can be given in doses of 5–10 mg orally every 4–6 hours as needed to control objective signs of withdrawal.

Nonsteroidal anti-inflammatory drugs, antidiarrheals, antiemetics, and benzodiazepines can be used for additional symptomatic relief.

Once symptoms are stabilized, taper the dose by 10% per day.

Monitoring

Stop treatment if excessive somnolence, slurred speech, or other indication of intoxication.

Source.   Federal Bureau of Prisons 2000.

Elderly and pregnant inmates present unique difficulties during withdrawal. As a normal consequence of aging, individuals who are elderly are less likely to display signs such as increased heart rate and blood pressure, sweating, and tremor—signs that might signify imminent seizure activity in younger people—but these individuals are no less likely to have a seizure as a consequence of withdrawal. If a pregnant inmate requires detoxification, the fetus or infant should be considered. Drugs of abuse and medication used in the treatment of withdrawal can have adverse effects on the fetus if they cross the placenta and enter fetal circulation. Treatment, however, may prevent obstetric complications; for example, methadone treatment of a pregnant woman addicted to opiates should continue, because discontinuation of methadone increases the risk of premature labor and miscarriage (Federal Bureau of Prisons 2000).

Treatment Interventions

The increasing prevalence of substance use disorders among inmates in U.S. jails and prisons has prompted the correctional system to consider treatment needs that extend beyond stabilization of the acutely intoxicated individual requiring detoxification. Although studies have had mixed results (Young et al. 2004), most authors now conclude that coerced, or legally mandated, treatment is as effective a mode of treatment as voluntary treatment, particularly if one controls for internal motivation to change (Belenko 1999; Center for Substance Abuse Treatment 2005; National Institute of Justice 2006; National Institute on Drug Abuse 2006; Peters et al. 1999; Satel 2000; Satel and Farabee 2004; Sung et al. 2004; Young et al. 2004). Legally mandated treatment of offenders provides consequences for failing to complete treatment program objectives and tends to result in a longer time in treatment, which is then correlated with success after discharge (Taxman 1999). Thus, correctional providers maintain optimism that treatment within the secure setting, often occurring as a condition of the inmate's sentence, will be beneficial.

Public safety is a primary goal of any correctional system, and treatment providers must be willing to accept that mental health and substance use disorder treatment aims are, to some extent, secondary to the primary objective of the correctional system. Cooperative and collaborative efforts will most likely yield outcomes acceptable to both treatment and correctional professionals when measurable operational outcomes are identified, agreed upon, and emphasized (Wexler 2003). In the past, treatment providers have traditionally focused on assisting each inmate to cope with the realities of his or her life circumstances, without much regard for outcome measures such as recidivism and social reintegration (Wexler 2003).

Therapeutic communities within correctional settings can provide interventions to facilitate harm reduction and abstinence, but traditional models must be adapted to accommodate the unique features and limitations of the correctional setting (Center for Substance Abuse Treatment 2005; Peters et al. 2004). Motivation to enter treatment is frequently a major obstacle to obtaining treatment in the community (Marlowe et al. 1996), but interactions with corrections staff and treatment providers often positively influence the offender's readiness for change (Clawson et al. 2005). Programming such as the Texas Christian University Readiness Program improves attitudes and behaviors by assisting the inmate to gain insight into his or her substance dependence, enhancing self-esteem, identifying specific actions that will facilitate treatment, and developing individual strategies to potentiate treatment and maintain sobriety (Welsh and McGrain 2008). Targeting high-risk individuals with programs and services that adequately engage the offender increases the likelihood of successful treatment and decreased recidivism (Clawson et al. 2005). Incorporating the offender's culture, gender, motivational stage, and learning style into treatment planning increases the likelihood that he or she will respond to therapeutic intervention (Center for Substance Abuse Treatment 2005; Clawson et al. 2005). Other factors associated with successful treatment include therapeutic engagement, a therapeutic community setting, low offender hostility, high offender conformity, and program characteristics such as peer support and rapport with treatment staff (Welsh and McGrain 2008).

Treatment Issues in Jails

Substance abuse and dependence treatment in local jails presents a challenge for the U.S. criminal justice system. Each jail is a unique microenvironment reflective of the community in which the facility operates, and efforts to create standards and guidelines have largely been thwarted by the wide variability in size, funding, inmate population served, and local administrative styles. Jails are by definition short-term facilities, and the time available to engage in treatment activities is both limited and highly variable. The duration of incarceration may vary from hours, as in detoxification centers, to months. Additionally, an offender's security status may influence what type of programming will be both available and appropriate (Center for Substance Abuse Treatment 2005). The Center for Substance Abuse Treatment (2005) and the National Commission on Correctional Health Care (2002) have written general standards for substance abuse treatment in the jail setting.

Treatment during a brief length of stay (1 month or less) focuses on educating the inmate about community resources, making referrals to a community provider, and enhancing motivation for treatment (Center for Substance Abuse Treatment 2005). Jail programs frequently use tools to facilitate communication between the inmate and care providers; however, no long-term, large-sample studies have systematically collected outcome data.

Engaging inmates during a brief stay is challenging. Tools such as board games and exercises may assist offenders in identifying the consequences of substance abuse (Center for Substance Abuse Treatment 2005). If offenders will be in jail for 1–3 months, then coping skills and relapse prevention can be addressed (Center for Substance Abuse Treatment 2005). Evaluation of the family and social environment to which the inmate will return following release is vital, because unresolved family or partner conflicts and financial stressors place the inmate at increased risk for relapse following release. Cognitive skills training that focuses on the identification of maladaptive thoughts and behaviors can help inmates develop strategies to minimize criminal behavior following release (Clawson et al. 2005).

For an inmate whose jail stay exceeds 3 months, treatment can be similar to that in inpatient residential facilities. The emotional and behavioral context of the inmate's substance use or dependence can be explored in greater depth. Co-occurring mental health issues can be identified, and triggers for both substance abuse and mental health relapses can be explored (Center for Substance Abuse Treatment 2005). Reintegration into previously established social structures influences the offender's risk of relapse; therefore, completing family and social mapping may be necessary to identify factors that may influence the individual's ability to maintain sobriety after release (Clawson et al. 2005).

Treatment Issues in Prisons

The modalities for treatment of substance use disorders vary widely across state and federal facilities. The spectrum of treatments includes no services, drug detoxification and testing, drug abuse education, drug abuse counseling alone or in combination with drug abuse education, individual and/or group counseling, family therapy, milieu therapy, client-initiated or client-maintained services (such as Alcoholics Anonymous and Narcotics Anonymous), dedicated short- and long-term residential units, drug maintenance programs, and transitional services (James 2004; Mears et al. 2003; Mumola and Karberg 2006).

In general, each treatment modality has strengths and limitations and is preferentially used based on non-outcome-based criteria, such as the number of inmates who can participate, cost, and staffing concerns. For example, self-help programs such as Alcoholics Anonymous and Narcotics Anonymous are the most widely used treatment modalities, accommodating a large group setting and being primarily inmate driven, while costing very little and easing staffing pressure for the facility (James 2004; Mears et al. 2003; Mumola and Karberg 2006). At the other extreme, although research has demonstrated that intensive inpatient residential treatment programs reduce recidivism, only a small portion of inmates who meet criteria for substance dependence receive such treatment (Bhati et al. 2008; Mears et al. 2003). Regardless of modality, however, the best outcomes are achieved with services that address individual needs (Mears et al. 2003).

DRUG COURTS

With the advent of mandatory sentencing for drug violations and increased enforcement during the 1980s, the correctional system experienced an unprecedented surge in the number of people being convicted of drug-related offenses and receiving longer sentences (Fox and Huddleston 2003). Large, heavily populated jurisdictions were the most affected, and a cycle of arrest, incarceration, and rearrest overwhelmed limited criminal justice resources (National Institute of Justice 2006). Judge Herbert M. Klein noted that "putting more and more offenders on probation just perpetuates the problem. [...] The same people are picked up again and again until they end up in the state penitentiary and take up space that should be used for violent offenders" (Warren 2007, p. 14).

In the late 1980s, treatment-oriented drug courts were implemented as an alternative to traditional adjudication and incarceration of nonviolent substance-abusing offenders. Drug courts blend elements of community-based judicial supervision with elements of substance abuse treatment in programs designed to both facilitate treatment and maintain accountability. Successful completion of a drug court program may result in the dismissal of charges or a reduction in the severity of the sentence (Bureau of Justice Assistance 2004).

Voluntary participation in drug court is restricted to nonviolent offenders who have victimless drug-related charges, such as intoxication or possession of drugs or paraphernalia (Lessenger and Roper 2002). Following legal screening, the offender is assessed to predict the clinical likelihood that he or she would be successful in the treatment program. In the past, individuals with co-occurring mental illness could be excluded from drug court, having been deemed unlikely to benefit from the treatment program, but this is changing in some jurisdictions.

Judicial intervention in the form of a drug court program can provide the impetus for individuals with substance use disorders to obtain the help that they are unable, or unwilling, to obtain for themselves while in the community without judicial intervention. Drug courts blend judicial oversight with intensive drug treatment, with the goal of decreasing recidivism for the offender (Fox and Huddleston 2003) outside the setting of incarceration.

Treatment services that are available to drug courts depend on the communities in which they operate. In a study by Taxman and Bouffard (2002), slightly more than half of the courts reported that residential treatment services were available. Most courts tended to rely on a broker-age model in which the court referred clients to community services, but the content of programming remained largely unknown to the referring court. At the other end of the spectrum, some drug courts referred clients directly to services, perhaps consisting of nearby private and public providers (Taxman and Bouffard 2002).

The goals of treatment are to enhance offender strengths (coping mechanisms and competencies) and provide extrinsic structure (drug testing, treatment staffings, and monitoring) to reduce substance use and dependence by providing reinforcements (rewards or sanctions) that are relevant to the offender (Taxman and Bouffard 2002). Treatment is divided into three phases: stabilization (alcohol or drug detoxification and treatment and/or needs assessment), intensive treatment (individual and group therapy), and transition (graduation, social reintegration, and other aftercare activities) (Bureau of Justice Assistance 2004). These three consecutive phases are outlined in Table 7–8. The National Drug Court Professional Association and the Drug Court Office of the U.S. Department of Justice recommend comprehensive treatment, lasting for at least 1 year.

TABLE 7–8. Drug court treatment phases and durations

Phase I (1–3 months)
Client assessment and orientation

Assessment of readiness and development of a treatment plan

Phase II (6 months)
Treatment phase

Phase III (2–4 months)
Relapse prevention

Discharge planning

Education and vocational training

Anger and stress management

Source. Adapted from Belenko et al. 2007.

Current recommendations suggest that services should be based on empirical cognitive or behaviorally based treatment methods; however, little is known of the efficacy of these treatment methods in drug court populations (Belenko 2002; Taxman and Bouffard 2002; Turner et al. 2002). Although some controversy exists, most authors now conclude that offenders who are compelled to undergo drug or alcohol treatment have higher completion and lower attrition rates than those who enter treatment of their own accord, and longer time in treatment is associated with long-term success in most studies (Lessenger and Roper 2002; Satel and Farabee 2004).

Research indicates that drug courts reduce recidivism rates by 10%–70% for participating offenders compared with nonparticipating offenders (Warren 2007). In addition to the direct benefit to the offender, cost-benefit analyses indicate that drug courts provide savings to the taxpayer through decreased jail time, decreased probation costs, and lower recidivism rates (National Institute of Justice 2006; Warren 2007). The cost of treatment in the context of drug court is less than that in the community and is further defrayed by decreased law enforcement involvement (National Institute of Justice 2006). In theory, drug court programs reduce recidivism by reducing drug use and thereby its associated criminal activity (Butzin et al. 2002; Sung et al. 2004; Taxman and Bouffard 2002; Young et al. 2004).

Approximately 2,018 drug courts are operating in the United States (including all 50 states, the District of Columbia, Northern Mariana Islands, Puerto Rico, and Guam), and an additional 257 courts are planned (Bureau of Justice Assistance Drug Court Clearing House Project 2009). Drug courts serve an estimated 70,000 offenders at any given point in time (Huddleston et al. 2005). The drug court model of a "problem-solving" court has been used to address other issues, such as domestic violence and nonviolent law-breaking behavior occurring in the context of chronic mental illness. A consensus opinion among drug court experts is that the degree to which drug courts incorporate evidence-based practices determines how well drug courts reduce recidivism (Warren 2007).

CONCLUSION

Substance use disorders are pressing but treatable problems facing both the general population and the correctional setting. Offenders with substance use disorders typically have more medical and mental health problems than those without substance use disorders and therefore need multimodal assessment and treatment. Because correctional facilities have limited financial and human resources with which to evaluate and treat inmates with substance use disorders, efficiency in assessment and treatment must be combined with effectiveness in reaching outcomes of mutual benefit to both the treatment and correctional communities in order for the programs to succeed. The need for ongoing research in substance use disorders in correctional settings cannot be understated. Although correctional systems are moving toward evidence-based practices and clinical practice guidelines, very little evidence is currently available to assist in moving forward.

SUMMARY POINTS

- Substance use disorders are common in correctional settings and frequently co-occur with other medical and mental health issues.
- A high level of suspicion should be maintained for complicated withdrawal, and prompt referral to medically supervised settings should be considered if changes in mental status or vital signs occur. Substance use may continue within secure settings, so staff should remain aware of issues related to intoxication and withdrawal.
- Screening and evaluation are essential to matching offenders with appropriate treatment services, but such activities are often underfunded and understaffed.
- Therapeutic communities and other treatment modalities translate well to the correctional system when all stakeholders agree on security issues and treatment outcomes early in the process.
- Drug court programs are growing in number because of their demonstrated effectiveness in reducing recidivism, facility overcrowding, and costs in appropriately selected cases. A number of initiatives are under way to involve individuals with dual diagnoses, who were previously excluded from drug court programming, in modified drug court treatment.

REFERENCES

Adams D, Reynolds L: Bureau of Justice Statistics 2002: at a glance (NCJ 194449). Washington, DC, U.S. Department of Justice, Office of Justice Programs, Bureau of Justice Statistics, 2002

American Psychiatric Association: Diagnostic and Statistical Manual of Mental Disorders, 4th Edition, Text Revision. Washington, DC, American Psychiatric Association, 2000

Atchison D: Former prison guards sentenced. Daily Home Online, August 18, 2008

Beck A, Bonczar T, Ditton P, et al: Correctional populations in the United States, 1997 (NCJ 177614). Washington, DC, U.S. Department of Justice, Office of Justice Programs, Bureau of Justice Statistics, 2000

Belenko SR: Research on drug courts: a critical review 1999 update. National Drug Court Institute Review 2(2):1–58, 1999

Belenko SR: The challenges of conducting research in drug treatment court settings. Subst Use Misuse 37:1635–1664, 2002

Belenko SR, DeMatteo D, Patapis N: Drug courts, in Handbook of Forensic Mental Health With Victims and Offenders. Edited by Spring DW, Roberts AR. New York, Springer, 2007, pp 385–425

Bhati A, Roman J, Chalfin A: To treat or not to treat: evidence on the prospects of expanding treatment to drug-involved offenders (NCJ 222908). Washington, DC, Justice Policy Center, Urban Institute, 2008

Brodey BB, Rosen CS, Brodey IS, et al: Validation of the Addiction Severity Index (ASI) for Internet and automated telephone self-report administration. J Subst Abuse Treat 26:253–259, 2004

Bureau of Justice Assistance: Defining drug courts: the key components (NCJ 205621). Washington, DC, U.S. Department of Justice, Office of Justice Programs, Bureau of Justice Assistance, 2004

Bureau of Justice Statistics: Corrections statistics. Last revised May 29, 2009. Available at: http://www.ojp.usdoj.gov/bjs/correct.htm. Accessed June 10, 2009.

Bureau of Justice Assistance Drug Court Clearing House Project: summary of drug court activity by state and county. Washington, DC, Bureau of Justice Assistance, 2009

Butler R: Mailroom scenario evaluation, final report (NCJ 199048). Rockville, MD, National Institute of Justice, 2002

Butzin CA, Saum CA, Scarpitti FR: Factors associated with completion of a drug treatment court diversion program. Subst Use Misuse 37:1615–1633, 2002

Carey KB: Reliability and validity of the time-line follow-back interview among psychiatric outpatients: a preliminary report. Psychol Addict Behav 11:26–33, 1997

Center for Substance Abuse Treatment: Treatment improvement protocol 11: simple screening instruments for outreach for alcohol and other drug abuse and infectious diseases (SMA 95-3058). Rockville, MD, Substance Abuse and Mental Health Services Administration, 1994

Center for Substance Abuse Treatment: Treatment improvement protocol 9: assessment and treatment of patients with coexisting mental illness and alcohol and other drug abuse (SMA 95-3061). Rockville, MD, Substance Abuse and Mental Health Services Administration, 1995

Center for Substance Abuse Treatment: Treatment improvement protocol 44: substance abuse treatment for adults in the criminal justice system (SMA 05-4056). Rockville, MD, Substance Abuse and Mental Health Services Administration, 2005

Center for Substance Abuse Treatment: Treatment improvement protocol 45: detoxification and substance abuse treatment (SMA 06-4131). Rockville, MD, Substance Abuse and Mental Health Services Administration, 2006

Clawson E, Bogue B, Joplin L: Implementing evidence-based practices in corrections: using an integrated model to implement evidence-based practices in corrections. Washington, DC, National Institute of Corrections, 2005

Corse SJ, Hirschinger NB, Zanis D: The use of the Addiction Severity Index with people with severe mental illness. Psychiatr Rehabil J 19:9–18, 1995

Czuchry M, Sia TL, Dansereau DF, et al: Downward Spiral: A Cognitive Intervention From the CETOP Project. Ft Worth, TX, Texas Christian University, Institute of Behavioral Research, 1998

DiClemente CC, Hughes SO: Stages of change profiles in outpatient alcoholism treatment. J Subst Abuse 2:217–235, 1990

Ditton P: Mental Health and Treatment of inmates and probationers (NCJ 174463). Washington, DC, U.S. Department of Justice, Office of Justice Programs, Bureau of Justice Statistics, 1999

Federal Bureau of Prisons: Clinical practice guidelines for detoxification of chemically dependent inmates. Washington, DC, Federal Bureau of Prisons, 2000

Fiellin DA, O'Connor PG, Holmboe ES, et al: Risk for delirium tremens in patients with alcohol withdrawal syndrome. Subst Abus 23:83–94, 2002

Fiscella K, Pless N, Meldrum S, et al: Alcohol and opiate withdrawal in U.S. jails. Am J Public Health 94:1522–1524, 2004a

Fiscella K, Pless N, Meldrum S, et al: Benign neglect or neglected abuse: drug and alcohol withdrawal in U.S. jails. J Law Med Ethics 32:129–136, 2004b

Fox C, Huddleston W: Drug courts in the U.S. Issues of Democracy 8:13–19, 2003

Greenfield L: Alcohol and crime: an analysis of national data on the prevalence of alcohol involvement in crime (NCJ 168632). Washington, DC, U.S. Department of Justice, Office of Justice Programs, 1998

Hamid R, Deren S, Beardsley M, et al: Agreement between urinalysis and self-reported drug use. Subst Use Misuse 34:1585–1592, 1999

Harwood H, Bouchery E, Group L: The Economic Costs of Drug Abuse in the United States, 1992–2002 (NCJ 207303). Washington, DC, Executive Office of the President, Office of National Drug Control Policy, 2004

Hasin D, Samet S, Nunes E, et al: Diagnosis of comorbid psychiatric disorders in substance users assessed with the Psychiatric Research Interview for Substance and Mental Disorders for DSM-IV. Am J Psychiatry 163:689–696, 2006

Huddleston CW III, Freeman-Wilson K, Marlowe DB, et al: Painting the current picture: a national report card on drug courts and other problem solving court programs in the United States. Alexandria, VA, U.S. Department of Justice, Office of Justice Programs, Bureau of Justice Systems, 2005

James D: Profile of jail inmates, 2002 (NCJ 201932). Washington, DC, U.S. Department of Justice, Office of Justice Programs, Bureau of Justice Statistics, 2004

James D, Glaze L: Mental health problems of prison and jail inmates (NCJ 213600). Washington, DC, U.S. Department of Justice, Office of Justice Programs, Bureau of Justice Statistics, 2006

Jones GY, Hoffmann NG: Alcohol dependence: international policy implications for prison populations. Subst Abuse Treat Prev Policy 1:33, 2006

Kanato M: Drug use and health among prison inmates. Curr Opin Psychiatry 21:252–254, 2008

Karberg J, James D: Substance dependence, abuse, and treatment of jail inmates, 2002 (NCJ 209588). Washington, DC, U.S. Department of Justice, Office of Justice Programs, Bureau of Justice Statistics, 2005

Lessenger J, Roper G: Drug courts: a primer for the family physician. J Am Board Fam Pract 15:298–303, 2002

Marlowe D, Kirby K, Bonieskie L, et al: Assessment of coercive and noncoercive pressures to enter drug abuse treatment. Drug Alcohol Depend 42:77–84, 1996

Marshall v United States 414 U.S. 417 (1974)

Masters J: Recipe for prison pruno, in Finding Freedom: Writings From Death Row. Junction City, CA, Padma, 1997, pp 63–65

McLellan AT, Luborsky L, Woody GE, et al: An improved diagnostic evaluation instrument for substance abuse patients: the Addiction Severity Index. J Nerv Ment Dis 168:26–33, 1980

McLellan AT, Kushner H, Metzger D, et al: The fifth edition of the Addiction Severity Index. J Subst Abuse Treat 9:199–213, 1992

McLellan AT, Cacciola JS, Alterman AI: The ASI as a still developing instrument: response to Mäkelä. Addiction 99:411–412, 2004

Mears D, Winterfield L, Hunsaker J, et al: Drug treatment in the criminal justice system: the current state of knowledge. Washington, DC, Urban Institute Justice Policy Center, 2003

Moore G, Mears D: Voices from the field: practitioners identify key issues in corrections-based drug treatment (NCJ 222807). Washington, DC, Urban Institute Justice Policy Center, 2003

Mumola C: Substance abuse and treatment, state and federal prisoners, 1997 (NCJ 172871). Washington, DC, U.S. Department of Justice, Office of Justice Programs, Bureau of Justice Statistics, 1999

Mumola C, Karberg J: Drug use and dependence, state and federal prisoners, 2004 (NCJ 213530). Washington, DC, U.S. Department of Justice, Office of Justice Programs, Bureau of Justice Statistics, 2006

National Commission on Correctional Health Care: The Health Status of Soon-to-be-Released Inmates, Vols 1 and 2. Chicago, IL, National Commission on Correctional Health Care, 2002

National Institute of Justice: Drug courts: the second decade (NCJ 211081). Washington, DC, U.S. Department of Justice, Office of Justice Programs, 2006

National Institute on Drug Abuse: Principles of drug abuse treatment for criminal justice populations: a research-based guide. 2006. Available at: http://www.nida.nih.gov/PODAT_CJ. Accessed March 23, 2009.

Nutt D, Lingford-Hughes A: Addiction: the clinical interface. Br J Pharmacol 154:397–405, 2008

Okie S: Sex, drugs, prisons, and HIV. N Engl J Med 365:105–108, 2007

Pace v Fauver 470 F.Supp. 456 D.N.J. (1979)

Peters RH, Greenbaum PE: Texas Department of Criminal Justice/Center for Substance Abuse Treatment Prison Substance Abuse Screening Project. Milford, MA, Civigenics, 1996

Peters RH, Haas AL, Murrin M: Predictors of retention and arrest in drug courts. National Drug Court Institute Review 2:33–60, 1999

Peters RH, Greenbaum PE, Steinberg ML, et al: Effectiveness of screening instruments in detecting substance use disorders among prisoners. J Subst Abuse Treat 18:349–358, 2000

Peters RH, Matthews CO, Dvoskin JA: Treatment in prisons and jails, in Substance Abuse: A Comprehensive Textbook. Edited by Lowison J, Ruiz P, Millman R, et al. Philadelphia, PA, Lippincott Williams & Wilkins, 2004, pp 707–722

Peters RH, Bartoi MG, Sherman PB: Screening and Assessment of Co-occurring Disorders in the Justice System. Delmar, NY, Center for Mental Health Services National GAINS Center, 2008

Pretrial Services Resource Center: Integrating drug testing into a pretrial services system: 1999 update (NCJ 176340). Washington, DC, U.S. Department of Justice, Office of Justice Programs, Bureau of Justice Assistance, 1999

Prochaska JO, DiClemente CC: The transtheoretical approach, in Handbook of Psychotherapy Integration. Edited by Norcross JC, Goldfried MR. New York, Basic Books, 1992, pp 300–334

Richards H, Pai S: Deception in prison assessment of substance abuse. J Subst Abuse Treat 24:121–128, 2003

Sabol W, Couture H: Prison inmates at midyear 2007 (NCJ 221944). Washington, DC, U.S. Department of Justice, Office of Justice Programs, Bureau of Justice Statistics, 2008

Sabol W, Minton T: Jail inmates at midyear 2007 (NCJ 221945). Washington, DC, U.S. Department of Justice, Office of Justice Programs, Bureau of Justice Statistics, 2008

Samet S, Nunes E, Hasin D: Diagnosing comorbidity: concepts, criteria, and methods. Acta Neuropsychiatrica 16:9–18, 2004

Satel S: Drug treatment: the case for coercion. National Drug Court Institute Review 3:1–56, 2000

Satel S, Farabee D: The role of coercion in drug treatment, in Substance Abuse: A Comprehensive Textbook. Edited by Lowison J, Ruiz P, Millman R, et al. Philadelphia, PA, Lippincott Williams & Wilkins, 2004, pp 690–706

Skinner HA, Horn JL: Alcohol Dependence Scale: Users Guide. Toronto, ON, Canada, Addiction Research Foundation, 1984

Sung HE, Belenko S, Feng L, et al: Predicting treatment noncompliance among criminal justice–mandated clients: a theoretical and empirical exploration. J Subst Abuse Treat 26:315–328, 2004

Taxman FS: Unraveling what works. National Drug Court Institute Review 2:93–134, 1999

Taxman FS, Bouffard J: Treatment inside the drug treatment court: the who, what, where, and how of treatment services. Subst Use Misuse 37:1665–1688, 2002

Taxman FS, Thanner M, Weisburd D: Risk, need, and responsivity (RNR): it all depends. Crime Delinq 52:28–51, 2006

Taxman FS, Cropsey KL, Young DW, et al: Screening, assessment, and referral practices in adult correctional settings: a national perspective. Crim Justice Behav 34:1216–1234, 2007

TCU Institute of Behavioral Research: TCU Drug Screen II. 2006. Available at: http://www.ibr.tcu.edu/pubs/datacoll/Forms/ddscreen-95.pdf. Accessed March 25, 2009.

Tetrault JM, O'Connor PG: Substance abuse and withdrawal in the critical care setting. Crit Care Clin 24:767–788, 2008

Turner S, Longshore D, Wenzel S, et al: A decade of drug treatment court research. Subst Use Misuse 37:1489–1527, 2002

Warren RK: Evidence-based practice to reduce recidivism: implications for state judiciaries. 2007. Available at: http://nicic.org/Downloads/PDF/Library/022843.pdf. Accessed March 23, 2009.

Welsh W, McGrain P: Predictors of therapeutic engagement in prison-based drug treatment. Drug Alcohol Depend 96:271–280, 2008

Wexler H: The promise of prison-based treatment for dually diagnosed inmates. J Subst Abuse Treat 25:223–231, 2003

Wikipedia: Pruno. Available at: http://en.wikipedia.org/wiki/Pruno. Accessed March 24, 2009.

Wilson D: Drug use, testing, and treatment in jails (NCJ 179999). Washington, DC, U.S. Department of Justice, Office of Justice Programs, Bureau of Justice Statistics, 2000

Young D, Fluellen R, Belenko S: Criminal recidivism in three models of mandatory drug treatment. J Subst Abuse Treat 27:313–323, 2004

CHAPTER 8

Managing the Disruptive or Aggressive Inmate

Steven J. Helfand, Psy.D.

Susan Sampl, Ph.D.

Robert L. Trestman, Ph.D., M.D.

The disruptive/aggressive inmate presents unique management challenges within jail and prison environments. Maintaining facility safety and order, and reducing the likelihood of maladaptive inmate behaviors require collaborative management strategies. The inmate who is disruptive is often quite different from the inmate with serious and persistent mental illness. Indeed, the disruptive inmate often triggers debates about mad versus bad behavior, behavioral versus mental health issues, and Axis I versus Axis II disorder. Although such categorization reflects efforts to understand the etiology of the behaviors, it does little to foster the needed coordination and collaboration among mental health, medical, and custody disciplines to safely reduce and extinguish the behaviors. Staff need to work together to determine how best to manage situations that span the gamut from typical physical assault and nontraditional assault (e.g., throwing feces or urine, spitting), to disruptive behavior (flooding or setting fires, failing to exit the cell), to self-harm (threatening to mutilate or actually mutilating oneself through cutting or insertion), to inappropriate or aggressive sexual and emotional abuse (public masturbation, lewd comments, coercive sex).

Many of these extreme behaviors are specific to the context of being housed within a correctional environment. Although no clear evidence exists to suggest that such behaviors occur in direct response to abuses of authority by officers, these behaviors may at times be viewed as tools of last resort for achieving a sense of control within restrictive environments (Skeem et al. 2005). As discussed in more detail subsequently, inmates who consistently engage in physical aggression toward peers and staff without engaging in other disruptive behaviors appear best managed by consistent institutional rules and restrictive settings, which may include concurrent mental health intervention. In this chapter, we focus on those inmates who engage in maladaptive behaviors, including sexual abuses and nontraditional physical assault, for which traditional correctional practices such as segregation are not optimally effective.

Correctional professionals use a clear set of directives that dictate responses to inmate misbehavior. Disruptive and aggressive behaviors by incarcerated offenders are frequently associated with mental health disorders. For example, prison and jail inmates with mental health problems are approximately two to three times more likely to be physically and verbally assaultive than inmates without mental health problems (James and Glaze 2006). Aggressive behavior by inmates may be associated with a wide variety of mental health disorders, including personality disorders, psychosis, bipolar mania, dementia, depression, traumatic brain injury, mental retardation, and substance abuse disorders (Lewis 2000). Determining the etiology of aggressive behaviors is needed before choosing a treatment strategy focused on the inmate, a correctional strategy focused on the officer and system responses, or both. Apparently, however, many correctional institutions do not perform an adequate assessment and consequently move forward with ineffective treatments for aggressive inmates (Gontkovsky 2002).

Mental health personnel are armed with an understanding of psychological principles and interventions developed primarily for use in community settings. In addition, correctional professionals utilize systems of offender classification and management to address and contain offenders demonstrating disruptive and aggressive behaviors. Although these traditional responses and tools are effective for the majority of inmates, these approaches have been found to have limitations (Byrne and Hummer 2007). The focus of this chapter is on the minority of inmates who create the disproportionate majority of institutional disruptions. Such disruptions are poorly tolerated in correctional settings. They often lead to program or visit cancellations for the cell block or entire facility; if allowed to continue, they may set a negative tone throughout the institution or the larger correctional system. Management of these inmates demands flexibility in institutional directives and in treatment strategies. The mental health professional has the duty not only to treat the individual inmate patient but also to provide educated consultation to the system to assure that the management style of the correctional institution and correctional officers focuses on adapted and potentially successful interventions that do not require the inmate to be tolerant of confinement conditions that are perceived as disrespectful or inhumane. The consequences of failure include staff division and conflict. Potential negative staff relationships are even more likely to occur in today's age of outsourcing correctional health care services. In this chapter, we explore various categories of disruptive inmate behaviors and detail tools and strategies for joint management among disciplines to target a range of inmate misconduct.

STANDARDS OF CARE

Management of disruptive inmates is supported by current standards of care. The National Commission on Correctional Health Care's (2008, p. 5) mental health standards speak to clinical autonomy in which "custody and administrative staff support and do not interfere with the implementation of clinical decisions" (Standard MH-A-03). The delivery of mental health care is seen as a "collaborative effort between custody, administrative and mental health staff," ideally achieved through cooperation. These standards also refer to "behavioral consultation," which involves consultation between mental health personnel and other facility staff on inmate mental health needs and the disciplinary process. The American Correctional Association (2004, p. 61) mandates crisis intervention and management of acute psychiatric episodes (Standard 4-ALDF-4C-27). The American Psychiatric Association (2000, p. 46) more specifically states that for jails, "special observation, seclusion, or restraint capability must exist." Although local statutes may vary, on-site or off-site service delivery provisions must be built into policies for managing inmate misconduct. Standards that support collaborative strategies are critical to reaching the joint goals of safety and security on the one hand and adaptive functioning of inmates on the other. In addition, local settlement agreement and consent decree requirements often include strong collaboration requirements for managing disruptive inmates. These requirements typically include, for example, mental health staff consultation prior to disciplinary proceedings and clinical intervention by mental health staff prior to a planned use of force (e.g., *State of Connecticut Office of Protection and Advocacy for Persons With Disabilities v. Choinski et al.*, often referred to as *OPA v. Choinski et al.*, 2004). Features of these legal requirements should be considered in policy development to manage the disruptive inmate.

SELF-INJURIOUS BEHAVIORS

Self-injury in correctional settings is typically defined as deliberate self-harm that excludes clear cases of tattooing, piercing, autoerotic intent, and suicidal intent (Favazza 1998). *Self-mutilation*, and more broadly *self-injurious behavior*, refers to the behavior of intentional self-harm without conscious intent to die (Feldman 1988; Walsh and Rosen 1988). Self-injurious behaviors may include cutting, scratching, burning, insertion, ingestion, asphyxiation, enucleation, amputation, evisceration, and other creative damage to one's body. Although the intent may not be suicidal, suicide may be an unintended outcome, as is lifelong injury or disability.

In addition to potential developmental and psychological factors that may contribute to the etiology of these behaviors, some empirical evidence supports a biological component to the etiology (Pies and Popli 1995; Simeon and Hollander 2001). Based on a review of pharmacotherapy for treatment of aggressive behaviors, Goedhard et al. (2006) reported that medications of multiple drug classes have demonstrated benefit in many cases of self-injurious behavior (see "Role of Skills Training and Medication Management," later in chapter). In general, the effective medications have serotonin receptor– or opiate receptor–mediated function and are also effective in reducing impulse dyscontrol in disorders as diverse as psychosis, mental retardation, autism, and severe personality disorder.

Not so long ago, most prison systems treated self-injury as "destruction of state property" and therefore administered discipline (e.g., time in segregated housing, suspension of privileges). Although this approach is no longer common, mental health providers have an obligation to discern self-injurious behavior from suicidal behavior and take actions not only for safety reasons, but also to extinguish self-injurious behaviors and help create more adaptive coping strategies. Hillbrand et al. (1994) found that within a forensic psychiatric institution, male patients who self-mutilated were more likely than non-self-mutilators to engage in outwardly directed aggressive behavior. In a study of Japanese male inmates with a mean age of 24 years, Matsumoto et al. (2005) found that compared with males who did not self-cut, male self-cutters more frequently self-reported overt violent tendencies toward people or objects. Self-injury can thus be conceptualized as part of the continuum of disruptive behaviors rather than as a distinct disorder. The operational challenges are to distinguish self-injury from a suicide attempt, to maintain safety, and to extinguish self-injurious behavior and replace it with more adaptive coping.

Self-injury has a variety of etiologies: as a symptom of depression, as an effort to regulate one's mood or affective experience, as a means of decreasing dissociation, as a tool to achieve a desired external outcome, or as a part of a psychotic disorder (Briere and Gil 1998; Jeglic et al. 2005). Understanding the etiology helps clinicians develop an integrated treatment plan that may include a behavioral management plan, use of appropriate psychotropic medication, and/or supportive therapies. Prior to developing a management strategy, the clinician needs to assess for all possible functions of self-injury (Jeglic et al. 2005).

Prevalence and Types of Self-Injurious Behavior

Based on a review of the literature, Brooker et al. (2002) reported that an estimated 30% of all offenders engaged in some self-harm behavior during incarceration. In the literature, Shea (1993) found reported prevalence rates of 6.5% to 25% among male prisoners. In contrast, the rate of self-harm appears to be much lower among the general population, with two studies finding a 4% rate of self-injurious behavior within non-clinical, nonforensic samples (Briere and Gil 1998; Klonsky et al. 2003). The variability in the prevalence rates can be due to different definitions of self-injurious behavior across various populations, as well as the absence of a self-injury registration process (Lohner and Konrad 2006).

Inmates may engage in varying types of self-injury based on a variety of factors, including motivation, opportunity, environment or conditions of confinement, history, and perceived consequences. Boiko and Lester (1995) postulated that inmates who self-injure believe that 1) the action itself is easy; 2) the desired goal (e.g., admission to the hospital) is easily obtained; and 3) afterward, the inmate will retain the ability to conduct activities that he or she considers important. Self-injury and other disruptive inmate behaviors are used as tools. Because incarceration limits the range of tools available to the inmate to control the environment (e.g., simply asking for a transfer to another unit or facility is unlikely to be successful), maladaptive strategies are often employed. Although most inmates use the same method of self-injury repeatedly (Boiko and Lester 1995), some "up the ante" by increasing the risk of harm if their goals are not achieved. Regardless of the type of self-injury or other maladaptive behaviors, they all share similarities with regard to intent and motivation, and ultimately the same management strategies are employed.

As multiple factors influence behavior, Linehan et al. (2006) suggested a typology for self-injurious behavior to include categories of nonsuicidal intentional self-injury (nonsuicidal habitual self-injury, nonsuicidal nonha-bitual self-injury) and of suicide attempts (ambivalent suicide attempt, suicide attempt without ambivalence, failed suicide). More extensive dis-cussions of the typology of self-injurious behavior are available (e.g., Favazza 1998; Meunier and Sellborn 2001). Such typologies focus on the intent of the action and support the use of a targeted evaluation to assess each self-injurious action (see "Behavioral Management and Intervention," later in the chapter).

Intent and Motivation for Self-Injury

Self-harm may be thought of as a crude but often effective form of prob-lem solving (Jeglic et al. 2005). In both clinical and nonclinical com-munity samples, self-harm is frequently associated with childhood abuse, particularly sexual abuse (Briere and Gil 1998; Favaro et al. 2007), and with mental health disorders, especially affective or personality disorders (Briere and Gil 1998; Klonsky et al. 2003; Welch 2001). In the commu-nity, self-injury may be motivated by psychotic delusion, occur as a ste-reotypical behavior secondary to developmental disabilities, or be a coping mechanism for stress reduction. Within correctional settings, de-lusion-driven or stereotypical self-injury is less common than self-injury in the service of stress reduction or situational problem solving. Approx-imately one-fourth of inmates with mental health problems report a his-tory of past physical or sexual abuse (James and Glaze 2006); some of these individuals may demonstrate the self-harm as an attempt to cope with the residual emotional effects of trauma. Self-injurious behaviors attributed to organic or psychiatric impairment are usually repetitive, not related to its antecedents or consequences, and easily identifiable (Favazza 1998).

Self-injury in correctional institutions is often intended to meet needs that are frustrated within the restrictive correctional environment (Shea 1993). The motivation from a secondary-gain perspective of stress reduc-tion and coping is typically to get or to avoid. Because behavioral princi-ples indicate that the tendency to avoid is stronger than the tendency to approach, self-injurious behavior may persist when linked to correctional stressors such as threats, gangs, undesired transfers, and disciplinary con-sequences such as restrictive housing. Inmate interactions with correc-tions staff must also be considered because the staff control, among other things, time and provision of meals, showers, recreation time, and access to off-unit activities. In our experience, inmates periodically cite stressful relations with officers as sources of misbehavior. Opportunities to escape or avoid within a correctional institution are extremely limited, and legitimate escape-avoidance strategies such as requesting relocation or taking a long walk are typically refused, occasionally leading to aggression or self-injury (Livingston and Beck 1997). Quite simply, the coping strategy of self-injury works to meet an inmate's needs and may also serve a pain- or anxiety-reducing function, because the consequences of the behavior are extremely reinforcing, and the escape-avoidance behavior then becomes added to a repertoire of possible adaptive responses (Livingston and Beck 1997).

Situational factors frequently may trigger disruptive inmate behavior. Such common factors include "Dear John" or "Dear Jane" letters and news of a relative's death or illness. Similarly, relationships within jails and prisons often develop among inmates, especially within female prison settings. Jealousies and breakups of these relationships may trigger disruptive and aggressive behaviors. In a qualitative study of 15 women who engaged in potentially lethal self-injury, institutional transfers, losses of a girlfriend, and outside problems were identified as primary risk factors for suicide and self-harm (Borrill et al. 2005). From another perspective, male inmates have hurt themselves to facilitate a move from the unit due to gambling debt. The inability to verbalize, be heard, or cope through previously available means, such as substance use or coping skills requiring freedom in the community, often leads to reliance on more primitive and aggressive actions.

In a study of young Scottish offenders with a mean age of 18.6 years, the majority of self-injurious inmates reported that anticipated confrontation with their peers was the major precipitant to self-injurious behavior; self-injury occurred in the service of avoidance (Power and Spencer 1987). Martinez (1980) observed that the intentional component of self-injury becomes clear when examining antecedents and consequences. Livingston and Beck (1997) proposed that self-injurious behavior is one possible response to bullying; by self-injuring, the inmate is able to communicate distress to staff without having to be specific about the cause.

Understanding antecedents, contexts, and consequences is central to success when seeking to manage and extinguish maladaptive self-injurious behaviors within jails and prisons. A confounding issue is that given the dangerous consequences of self-injurious behaviors, the inmate essentially forces the health services staff to respond with actions that further reinforce the target problem (Martinez 1980). Such inadvertent reinforcement may include time out of the cell, provision of desired medications such as analgesics (Martinez 1980), change of housing unit, interaction with staff and other inmates, or a trip out of the facility to a local hospital. If these are the desired consequences, typical institutional responses make the maladaptive behaviors more likely to recur. Self-injurious behavior is one of the few available behaviors that will reliably obtain staff attention (Karten 1992). Inmates tend to engage in maladaptive behavior until their demands are met. Repeated self-injurious behavior suggests that an inmate has found a useful tool for environmental control. The inmate may not have considered or cannot easily implement more adaptive strategies for coping (Franklin 1988). Karten (1992) uniquely proposed that self-cutting may be an example of a higher level of problem-solving ability for prison inmates because it is typically effective in solving perceived problems such as segregation placement.

Past data indicate that 24%–50% of all self-injurious acts in correctional institutions can be attributed to manipulation (Franklin 1988; Power and Spencer 1987), with the intent of accomplishing a goal other than suicide (Franklin 1988). Dear et al. (2000) defined a manipulative motive as either attention seeking (e.g., "wanted staff to take me more seriously") or changing one's circumstances (e.g., "wanted to get transferred off the unit"). By having inmates self-report through semistructured interview within 48 hours of a self-injury, Power and Spencer (1987) determined that manipulation accounted for 28% of self-injuries. A review of psychiatric records among a mentally ill prison population resulted in an estimated manipulation rate of 50% (Franklin 1988). A more recent study found that 24.3% of male and female prisoners reported motives classified as manipulative (Dear et al. 2000); however, the authors of that study also concluded that manipulative motivations did not always equate with low suicidal intent or low lethality. Based on a study of 49 German inmates, Lohner and Konrad (2006) concluded that self-injury may not always be independent of setting and context, and that intent should be assessed along with lethality and an appreciation of the setting and context. Caution is clearly advised: lethality of the behavior is not directly tied to intent, and the risk of significant self-harm or death in individuals who are manipulative is substantial (Jeglic et al. 2005). Although helpful in conceptualizing motivational factors of self-injury, the use of words such as *manipulation* by staff is potentially dangerous to inmate safety and is not generally helpful in resolving issues of self-injury (Karten 1992).

Within an institution's population, self-injury may occur in clusters and appear to be contagious. Inmates who copy self-injurious behaviors tend to have the most limited social skills (Martinez 1980). Of note, many who self-injure while incarcerated have no history of self-injury prior to incarceration (Martinez 1980; Meunier and Sellborn 2001), suggesting that the behavior is acquired during confinement or meets confinement-specific needs. That said, in our experience, most inmates do not have the will to engage in more than superficial self-injury. Further, our experience argues against the concern that making special behavioral contingencies and arrangements with particular inmates may lead to "everyone doing it." Few inmates have the will, for example, to swallow a razor blade to get different cell mates. Nontraditional management strategies (discussed in the section "Behavioral Management and Intervention" below) are employed only for extreme and rare behaviors.

With regard to the motivational features of those who self-injure, mutilators in prison score significantly higher on the Minnesota Multiphasic Personality Inventory (MMPI) subscales that measure somatic concerns, subjective distress, alienation, and immature defenses (Shea 1993). Self-injurious behaviors may occur as part of a depressive presentation, as a tool to achieve a desired gain, in an effort to regulate mood or affect, or as a function of a psychotic presentation (Jeglic et al. 2005). Shea (1993) reported that male prisoners who self-injure are more likely to withdraw, ruminate, and externalize blame than those who do not self-injure. The construct of externalizing versus internalizing symptoms may be useful in understanding disruptive behaviors. Inmates may perceive that consequences simply happen rather than derive from their own behaviors. Such externalizing tendencies must be considered when targeting individuals' problem-solving skills. Snow (2002), in a content analysis study of 143 self-injuring prisoners in England and Wales, found that those who self-injured without intent to die described precipitating factors related to negative emotions and the desire to reduce anger and frustration, whereas suicide attempters reported specific events or experiences that served as triggers.

MMPI profiles suggest that mutilators may exhibit immature coping strategies, despondency, and poorly focused hostility and rebellion toward authority figures (Shea 1993). This connection with immature coping strategies is helpful in understanding the combination of self-injury and assaultive behaviors such as the throwing of feces at staff as described in Clinical Case 8–1 later in this chapter.

Personality Disorder

The aggression and violence of a subset of patients with personality disorder cause significant challenges in forensic, community, and correctional environments (Daffern and Howells 2007). High rates of borderline personality disorder are common in jails and prisons; Trestman et al. (2007) found a male prevalence rate of 12.9% and female prevalence rate of 23.2% in Connecticut jails. Although individuals clearly vary, the criteria for borderline personality disorder include impairment in interpersonal skills, impulsivity and emotional lability, and an elevated risk for self-destructive behavior. Staff responses commonly include irritation, frustration, and anger (Trestman 2000). Staff should be educated that these behaviors are not personal, but rather are multidetermined and require reasoned and planned intervention rather than emotional reactions.

When inmates engage in repeated suicide threats, the risk of staff frustration and burnout is extremely high (Holton 2003). Incarceration seriously limits an inmate's options for solving problems proactively, leading inmates to rely on new, and sometimes self-destructive, strategies to restore their sense of freedom and power (Martinez 1980). Clinicians can seek to address these needs through management strategies.

Linkage to Other Disruptive Behaviors

In an early study of state prison inmates, Panton (1962), using the MMPI, found that self-cutters tended to have an MMPI profile that showed impulsivity and a tendency toward compulsive behaviors when other more overt means of expressing hostility were blocked. This study serves as a useful guide to understanding maladaptive behaviors that often co-occur with self-injury, including feces smearing and flooding of the cell with water. In a study of hospitalized forensic patients, Hillbrand et al. (1994) found that self-mutilating patients were significantly more verbally and physically aggressive toward people and objects than were non-self-mutilating controls. This finding again appears to support the inclusion of (nonsuicidal) self-injury on the continuum of externalizing disorders that includes aggressive behaviors. Furthermore, Hillbrand et al. (1994) found support for the premise that self-mutilation is a facet of generalized behavioral dyscontrol, allowing for the use of similar management strategies for most, if not all, of the behaviors discussed in this chapter. According to Hillbrand et al. (1994), self-mutilation is consistent with an impulse control disorder in that the individual fails to resist an impulse, experiences tension prior to the act, and feels pleasure or gratification following the act. This gratification is often inadvertently provided in correctional settings.

Hunger Strikes

A hunger strike in its various forms is an example of passive self-injury (Boiko and Lester 1995). In the literature, hunger strikes are typically considered a type of self-harm behavior (e.g., Marasco et al. 1995). Therefore, hunger strikes are firmly within the continuum of disruptive behaviors, and clinicians can use behavioral management strategies comparable to those outlined in the section "Behavioral Management and Intervention" below. Certainly, a hunger strike or threat of such is an age-old means of protest by inmates against those in charge (Miller 1987). Food has a long history of being used by correctional officials to modify behavior. That inmates would also use food as a strategy to modify the behaviors of others is quite understandable, because food does not require any specific tools or setting.

Inmate hunger strikes are of concern for a number of reasons. Hunger strikes pose a risk of "contagion" to other inmates, who may wish to gain a share of the attention and control that the hunger-striking inmate appears to be getting. Additionally, the responsibility to maintain the safety of the hunger-striking inmate can drain valuable staffing resources. Even before the risk of imminent death presents itself, severe caloric restriction may lead to significant psychological changes, including persecutory and grandiose delusions, confusion, and hallucinations (Fessler 2003), potentially diminishing the inmate's competence to reevaluate his or her hunger strike. For these reasons, hunger strikes are considered to be serious disruptive behaviors. Providing forced nourishment is fraught with legal hurdles, and even if medical care is received, many inmates may require restraint because they often remove intravenous or feeding tubes. In parallel with medical staff who monitor and treat the physical consequences of reduced food intake, mental health professionals play a role in cessation of the behavior through consultation and development of behavioral management plans that reward adaptive behaviors.

Violence

The role of mental health staff is often unclear when institutional violence occurs within jails and prisons. The management of violent behaviors such as fighting, assault with a weapon, assault on staff, sexual assault, and even intimidation has traditionally been the role of correctional staff under the rubric of public and institutional safety.

A good argument can be made for mental health staff involvement in the disciplinary process for inmates who are already considered to have mental illness. This type of intervention is supported by the results of litigation and provides an opportunity for the mental health service to adjust treatment and to provide consultation to correctional staff. The settlement agreement reached in *OPA v. Choinski et al.* (2004) alludes to a role for mental health staff in addressing violence among inmates who are seriously mentally ill by requiring the management of "disciplinary problems through collaboration between mental health staff and correctional staff in devising an intervention that both maintains security and the smooth operation of the institution and promotes treatment goals."

Certainly, those inmates who engage in repetitive misconduct, including violence, can be referred to mental health services. Inmates displaying new-onset aggression should be assessed for medical or psychiatric conditions that may underlie this behavioral change, and undergo appropriate diagnosis and treatment to facilitate behavioral improvement (Lewis 2000). Aggressive and disruptive behaviors tend to be associated with the following factors: limited social and familial support, multiple incarcerations, lower education, and a history of violence (Berg and DeLisi 2006). Some aggressive inmates lack anger management skills. In DiGiuseppe and Tafrate's (2003) meta-analysis of 57 studies of cognitive-behavioral interventions for adults with anger problems, the average overall effect size was 0.71; that is, 76% of individuals receiving the anger-focused treatment improved. The authors found no significant main effect based on the specific type of cognitive-behavioral intervention employed. Incarcerated offenders have also benefited from anger-focused cognitive-behavioral interventions (Stermac 1987; Vannoy and Hoyt 2004). As a general rule, clinical intervention is most useful with impulsive aggression as opposed to premeditated violence and other acts determined to be under the inmate's behavioral control.

BEHAVIORAL MANAGEMENT AND INTERVENTION

Depending on their history and institutional factors, inmates may engage in a variety of behaviors in an attempt to meet their needs: fire setting, flooding, swallowing of objects, self-mutilation, feces smearing, urine throwing, insertion, refusal to leave the cell, barricading their cell door with a mattress, hunger strikes, violence, feigning of seizures, and various other maladaptive behaviors. Traditional correctional responses or consequences typically include use of force, cell extraction, disciplinary sanctions, loss of commissary or canteen privileges, restrictive housing placement, restraints within the cell, removal of personal items, meal modifications, and transfer to another facility or unit. Traditional mental health interventions include transfer to the infirmary or outside hospital, therapeutic restraints when permitted by law, involuntary medication when permitted by law, continuous or staggered observation, and crisis intervention prior to a planned use of force.

When inmate maladaptive behaviors are understood as part of a spectrum of behavioral dyscontrol, interventions can be planned accordingly. For each act of self-injury, the clinician should perform a targeted evaluation that looks at motivation, intent, lethality, and context, to distinguish suicide attempts from other self-injurious behavior. This evaluation should include asking the inmate directly whether his or her motivation was to seek relief or to seek reward, so that interventions can be tailored. Reviewing the action itself is important because the majority of suicide attempters in prison cut their wrists as opposed to hanging or overdosing, which are more common methods among suicide completers, and self-injury may indicate that an inmate is dissatisfied with his or her current situation but not clearly committed to suicide (Daniel and Fleming

2005). Appropriate and successful treatment of self-injury requires an understanding of the function of the behavior (Jeglic et al. 2005). The self-injurer can then be identified and receive attention using specific management strategies. For other repetitive disruptive behaviors, a similar targeted review is advised. A particularly important practice is to perform a functional assessment of ways that the system itself may be an inadvertent reinforcer (Webb 2001a). Conceptualizing interventions for disruptive behaviors as behavioral management plans draws attention to the need for collaboration among all health services staff and correctional personnel. This strategy is in line with standards, the trend in legal mandates, and evolving best practices for addressing the disruptive inmate within correctional settings.

A behavioral management plan should be conceptualized as any planned set of interventions that utilizes positive reinforcement to increase desired behaviors and/or restricts punishment to extinguish unwanted behavior. This simple approach deriving from the most basic of behavioral psychology concepts should be the basis for all plans and should be readily understandable to all parties. In some situations, extinguishing unwanted behaviors may best be achieved by ignoring (i.e., not rewarding) them. More commonly, however, behavioral management plans should include provisions for rapid response and brief medical treatment as required. This response should occur without peripheral banter, and the positive reinforcement of staff attention for adaptive behavior should be integral to the plan. In this manner, timely and individually developed behavioral plans can reduce morbidity and extinguish behaviors, resulting in a safer environment for all (Jeglic et al. 2005). To enhance collaboration and increase the likelihood of success, correctional officers should be involved in the development and implementation of plans for targeted behaviors (Webb 2001b).

The maintenance of a behavior is the product of reinforcing stimuli, such as social attention from staff (Webb 2001a). An initial step in behavioral management is to develop adaptive target behaviors and to have an agreed-upon plan to reinforce target behaviors when they occur. Inmates who self-injure or are seriously disruptive respond poorly to delayed gratification or reinforcement; behavioral plans are more likely to be effective when they are short-term and have clear operational definitions (Martinez 1980). The plan should be jointly authored by all stakeholders (including the inmate when possible) so that language is clear, consistent, and understandable by all. A joint approach to plan development is required to reduce the risk of a staff member's inadvertently undoing efforts to manage the behavior. Adaptive behaviors should be reinforced with reinforcers similar to those obtained through maladaptive behaviors. These may include cell or unit changes or eases in current restrictions (see Table 8–2 later in this chapter). This process will lead to generalization and enhance tolerance of gratification delay.

The first step in developing a behavioral management plan is to determine the cause of a target behavior. If a behavior is not driven by psychotic or developmental disability factors, the management team should work to understand the intent and purpose. The behavior may be driven by anxiety and resulting avoidance or by anger and resulting efforts to exert control. When developing a management plan, the team should attempt to help the inmate recognize potential options. This effort entails helping the inmate to accept responsibility and some control, which can ultimately include the ability to slow things down and modulate his or her behaviors. The management team may consider nontraditional ways that are contingent on the absence of maladaptive behaviors. When the inmate adjusts his or her own behavior in the context of the individually developed behavioral management plan, everyone, including the inmate, can recognize that the behavior is manageable.

Mental health and correctional staff share the goals of reducing the use of force, cell extractions, involuntary medications, therapeutic and custody restraint, staff injury, and temporary transfer. These shared goals can foster buy-in and a collaborative spirit around these emotionally taxing disruptive behaviors. A next step is to discuss the benefits of having inmates decrease their maladaptive behaviors, increase their adaptive behaviors, rely on verbalization of needs, and rely more on perceived collaboration than resistance. Other positive results include the building of trust across agencies and disciplines, and increasing appropriate utilization of inpatient cells and/or outside hospitalization. Table 8–1 outlines key behavioral plan components to manage maladaptive behavior.

Inmates who repeatedly engage in the behaviors discussed in this chapter show remarkable resilience and often have the time to outplan and outlast staff. Consider the following two examples of behaviors and typical outcomes.

> An inmate in restrictive housing broke his ceramic toilet and cut his wrist with a piece of porcelain. He then threatened to cut staff. He began to bang his head and flood his cell. He was given a burst of pepper spray but then put his mattress against the door. This led to a cell extraction in which two officers were injured. The inmate was taken to the medical clinic, where his wounds were dressed. He was admitted to the infirmary and placed in full stationary restraints under continuous observation.

> An inmate was in his cell bleeding from a self-inflicted wound to his forearm. He claimed to have used his toenail, which he swallowed when staff

TABLE 8–1. Key behavioral plan components to manage maladaptive behavior

Determine cause and function of maladaptive behavior.

Develop desired target behaviors.

Discuss benefits of decreasing maladaptive behaviors and increasing adaptive behaviors.

Use clear operational definitions.

Implement behavioral plans with short-term goals.

Include all stakeholders in the plan, including officers and the inmate.

Appoint senior mental health staff member and senior custody staff member as management plan leaders responsible for overseeing the creation of the plan and making adjustments as indicated.

arrived. He barricaded the door with his mattress, placed a wet towel around his head, spread soap on the cell floor, and covered the window with toilet paper. He yelled at staff, "I'm going to make you do some overtime." He was eventually placed in escort restraints, taken to a shower, issued a safety gown, and admitted to the infirmary for observation.

Inmates who repeatedly behave in such ways desire a transfer, attention, avoidance of restrictive housing, the feeling of control and autonomy, medication, and other things to meet their perceived needs. The management team's challenge is determining how to meet these inmates' needs without compromising safety and security. Typically, correctional systems assert that if inmates' demands are met, everyone will behave in the same way, the system will fail, and the inmates will be in control. Instead, when the correctional system does not modify responses for these dysfunctional few, these inmates will retain perceived control with each reinforced behavior. If no successful intervention occurs, the maladaptive behaviors continue, or may escalate, with resulting accusations of failure among increasingly fractured disciplines.

Collaborative behavioral management plans engage the disruptive inmate in developing a constructive plan, thus providing a sense of control, a forum for verbal expression, trust, consistency, access to mutually agreed-upon reinforcers, cognitive skills training, and other therapeutic programming upon cessation of the target behaviors. With the disruptive inmate, successful management plans require flexibility. Correctional institutions generally rely on rigid rules for all inmates for the sake of consistency. This strategy works for the vast majority of inmates; however, a few inmates will try to control things through disruptive behaviors unless an institution can use flexibility to disrupt a rigid pattern.

Many of the aggressive and disruptive behaviors described in this chapter occur in restrictive housing settings or in efforts to avoid such placements. The placement is typically for a specified time period (e.g., 15 days, 30 days) or, in cases of administrative segregation programs, sequential stages that may last for many months. Some inmates' lack of frustration tolerance, impulsiveness, and inability to employ adaptive problem solving leads to continued disruptive behaviors and increased lengths of stay in these units. The designated amount of time in isolation or restrictive housing in this fixed approach works for most inmates; however, it clearly is not a deterrent for the few who engage in the extreme behaviors discussed in this chapter. The typical consequences such as use of force, transfer, restraints, and removal of personal items do not work with these maladaptive inmates.

A strategy that may reduce reinforcement of disruptive behaviors is to keep the inmate in place subsequent to the undesired behavior. Early recommendations were to never return a self-injuring inmate to the original cell (Martinez 1980). Recent experience, however, reflects that inmates can self-injure in any setting and that a lack of transfer actually may limit the reinforcement and be more likely to extinguish the behaviors. The challenge is to keep the inmate safe in a nonrewarding environment other than the infirmary or an outside hospital. Appelbaum (2007) suggested that the ability to utilize therapeutic restraints without transferring an inmate to an infirmary or hospital may have some advantages when managing inmates who are self-injurious or who demonstrate other severe disruptive behaviors. An alternative strategy is to use infirmary and/or outside hospital placements as a planned respite for a period of adaptive functioning and in the absence of the targeted maladaptive behaviors. The rationale is that if things continue without flexibility, the inmate will continue to control such transfer through behaviors that are dangerous to self and others. By making such transfer contingent on a defined period of adaptive functioning, the management team has put in place a paradoxical intervention: the desired reward is achieved with inmate-initiated behaviors opposite those that he or she previously utilized. Therapeutic leverage has thereby been created to hold inmates accountable for behavioral dyscontrol. Although nontraditional (when coupled with on-unit precautions such as observation to ensure safety), this strategy is effective for changing the inmate's behavior set and establishing his or her internal sense of control.

Behavioral management plans should begin with very short-term expectations of behavioral control (e.g., 2 hours, 1 shift, or even 1 adaptive day). As the inmate demonstrates control, these time frames should be expanded as agreed upon. Management plans should also reward the inmate's verbalization of needs rather than behavioral displays. Creativity is to be encouraged to identify potential rewards, such as those listed in Table 8–2. The plan should also identify inmate-specific antecedents or triggering events that have historically led to disruptive behaviors. These antecedents might include feeling ignored by staff, craving attention from staff or peers, receipt of unpleasant information, feeling disrespected, threats on the units, and boredom. Wherever possible, management plans should focus on rewards because impulsively disruptive inmates have reduced concern about future negative consequences. In cases of extreme physical risk, negative consequences such as removal of preferred (but unsafe) items may be appropriate as long as a contingency has been devised for returning such items within a time frame achievable given the history and level of impulsivity (e.g., hours or days). The guiding principle should be that the plan must be attainable based on a review of factors specific to the inmate.

For these behavioral management plans to be most effective in extinguishing undesired behaviors, some methods are to be avoided. The plan should not be a standing unit practice that is untailored to the individual inmate. These individualized plans should be neither developed nor controlled solely by correctional or mental health staff. They also should not include elements that would violate constitutional and local rights, such as the withholding of food, and should not be simple placements in restrictive housing units without clear modification of consequences and provision of an attainable reward structure.

TABLE 8–2. Potential rewards for behavioral management plans

A systematic reduction in restrictive housing time

Walking around the unit

Walking outside

An extra shower

Additional recreation

One-to-one session with a staff member

Group programming

Access to magazines, books, or art supplies

Property items such as a radio, word games, or grooming products

Staggered segregation schedules, such as weekends in the general population

Utilization of infirmary or hospital as an inmate-initiated respite secondary to the absence of disruptive behaviors as indicated

---

Cognitive-behavioral skills training is recommended for treating in-carcerated offenders. Incorporation of a skills training component into the management of the inmate is recommended once the acutely dangerous behaviors cease. In a review article, Lipsey et al. (2007) reported that this approach, particularly when implemented with high fidelity, is particularly effective with offenders who are at the greatest risk for recidivism. Offenders treated using targeted cognitive-behavioral approaches have made significant positive changes, including reduced depression (Wilson 1990), reduced vengeful attitudes (Holbrook 1997), and improved self-esteem along with reduced anxiety and aggressive traits (Valliant and Antonowicz 1991). Incarcerated women treated with cognitive-behavioral therapy for substance use disorders and posttraumatic stress disorder reported high levels of client satisfaction with this intervention and significantly reduced posttraumatic stress disorder symptoms (Zlotnick et al. 2003). Dialectical behavior therapy (DBT) has also been found effective in reducing the severity and frequency of self-injurious behaviors (Linehan 2000). Manual-based cognitive-behavioral therapy that focuses on dangerous behaviors is being used increasingly within correctional environments, with corrections-specific adaptations. Milkman and Wanberg (2007) reviewed some promising research regarding a variety of manual-guided cognitive-behavioral interventions used to treat offenders with mental health and/or substance abuse disorders: Aggression Replacement Training (Goldstein and Glick 1987), criminal conduct and substance abuse treatment, strategies for self-improvement and change, reasoning and rehabilitation, relapse prevention therapy, Moral Reconation Therapy (Little and Wilson 1988), and Thinking for a Change (Bush et al. 1997).

DBT has also been recognized as a promising treatment for forensic populations (Berzins and Trestman 2004; McCann et al. 2000). DBT was originally developed to treat outpatients diagnosed with borderline personality disorder (Linehan 1993; Linehan et al. 1991). DBT has been shown to significantly reshape maladaptive cognitions and reduce the incidence of self-destructive behaviors (i.e., self-mutilation, suicidal and parasuicidal behaviors) and has become the first empirically supported treatment for borderline personality disorder (Linehan et al. 1991, 1994). With its clear hierarchy of treatment targets and behavior modification (through functional analysis), DBT is well suited for treatment of many problems characterized by behavior dyscontrol.

A number of investigators have reported findings supporting the use of DBT in correctional populations. The authors of a pilot study employing DBT to treat 30 female prisoners reported significantly increased self-esteem, as well as reduced impulsivity and dissociation, among the 14 treatment and follow-up assessment completers (Nee and Farman 2005). In the United Kingdom, Evershed et al. (2003) compared eight forensic hospital patients who received 18 months of DBT with nine patients who received treatment as usual. Those in the DBT condition showed reduced violence-related aggression and reported reduced hostility, cognitive anger, expressed anger, and angry disposition.

A small but growing body of evidence suggests that in some cases, medication may help reduce self-injurious behavior. The anticonvulsants lamotrigine (Pinto and Akiskal 1998) and divalproex (Frankenburg and Zanarini 2002; Hollander et al. 2001), the atypical antipsychotics olanzapine (Hough 2001) and clozapine (Chengappa et al. 1999), and high doses of the selective serotonin reuptake inhibitor (SSRI) fluoxetine (Rinne et al. 2002) and the opiate antagonist naltrexone (Roth et al. 1996) have shown promise in treating self-mutilating patients with a diagnosis of borderline personality disorder. Furthermore, in patients with mental retardation or autism spectrum disorders, naltrexone has fairly consistently demonstrated beneficial reduction of self-injurious behavior (Petty and Oliver 2005; Symons et al. 2004). In general, any use of medication should be integrated into a thoughtful multidisciplinary treatment plan (Goedhard et al. 2006).

Clinical Case 8–1

Mr Z, a 28-year-old male who has been incarcerated for 4 years, has been engaging in disruptive and dangerous behaviors for the past 4 months, prompting over 15 transfers to the mental health infirmary and two transfers to the county's forensic hospital. These behaviors began shortly after the inmate was placed in a 15-month segregation program due to chronic fighting. Recent incidents include the following: 1) Mr. Z stated that he had AIDS and was going to give it to the officers, and he threw feces at the officers during transport to the shower. 2) Mr. Z became acutely disruptive and flooded his cell; ripped his mattress; covered his door with wet tissue paper; threw feces at the door; stood on his bunk and masturbated; and kicked the cell door window, causing it to crack, and then removed broken glass from the window and cut his legs. 3) He smeared feces on the wall of his cell; tied a sheet around his neck; and then set toilet paper and the mattress on fire, causing a facility lockdown.

A behavioral management plan was jointly developed for Mr. Z to include the following:

1. *Identification of problematic behaviors:* Fecal smearing, superficial cutting (and other acts of self-harm without intent to die), threatening behavior, flooding, public indecency, fire setting, and destruction of property

2. *Primary goals:* Short-term goals—reduce the maladaptive behaviors by 50% over the next 2 weeks. Long-term goals—eliminate the maladaptive behaviors; maintain in housing unit or restrictive housing unit; eliminate utilization of infirmary hospitalization secondary to maladaptive behaviors; and eventual return to general population.

3. *Highlights of plan:* Upon transfer to restrictive housing, the following will be in place:

   • Inmate will be placed in cell nearest to officers' station.

   • Inmate will remain on continuous observation for 2 days upon arrival, with review thereafter.

   • Inmate will receive institutional clothing upon removal from continuous observation.

   • Inmate will be allowed reading materials.

   • If no maladaptive behavior is demonstrated Monday through Friday, inmate will be housed in the infirmary for the weekend at his request. This opportunity will be offered four times contingent on available bed space.

   • For each day that inmate is off continuous observation, one day of restrictive housing time will be waived.

   • Upon completion of 90 consecutive days with no instances of maladaptive behavior, inmate may be transferred to general population.

   • Upon transfer to general population and continued adaptive behaviors, inmate will be assisted by warden in presenting favorably to parole board.

Mr. Z engaged in cutting and fecal smearing behaviors for 3 days after his transfer to the restrictive housing unit. He received medical treatment for his wounds on the unit, and he was moved as needed to a clean cell that was kept open next to his cell during this period. He was removed from continuous observation after 6 days. Shortly thereafter, he used his first infirmary placement as a reward for 5 days of adaptive behavior. He was removed from the segregation program after a total of 108 days. He has not engaged in any of the targeted maladaptive behaviors for 6 months, although he has been in restrictive housing for two 15-day periods without incident secondary to fighting.

INAPPROPRIATE SEXUAL BEHAVIORS

Because inappropriate sexual behaviors share some features of the disruptive behaviors discussed thus far, they are quite amenable to the behavioral management strategies put forth in this chapter. Several features, how-ever, warrant a separate discussion. The purpose of this section is not to focus on preventing community recidivism of sexual offenders, but rather to focus on understanding and reducing sexual behaviors within jails and prisons. Sexual behavior within correctional institutions, with the exception of private masturbation, negatively impacts the assurance of safety and security in corrections and leads to victimization of other in-mates and staff. Inappropriate sexual behavior within correctional insti-tutions affects the physical and mental well-being of staff and inmates and presents a public health risk to those inside and outside the facility (Potter and Tewksbury 2005).

Inmate-on-Inmate Sexual Behavior

The rates of reported sexual behaviors in correctional institutions vary greatly. The Prison Rape Elimination Act of 2003 (PREA; P.L. 108-79) ini-tially contained an estimate that 13% of inmates had been sexually vic-timized; however, based on initial data from a PREA study of 40,419 inmates in local jails, Beck and Harrison (2008) reported a rate of in-mate-on-inmate sexual victimization of 1.6%. Groth and Burgess (1980) identified five motivational patterns offered by inmates to explain their behavior: conquest and control, revenge and retaliation, sadism and deg-radation, sexual conflict, and status affiliation. Similarly, Chonco (1989) indicated that sexual assault may be used to gain status, to make certain in-mates stay away from others, for revenge, for domination of other inmates, and to release tension. Deprivation has also being tied to inappropriate sexual behaviors within correctional institutions (Potter and Tewksbury 2005).

Fagan et al. (1996) suggested that a male inmate who sexually assaults others is likely to be older and larger in stature than victims, identify him-self as heterosexual, have a history of childhood sexual or physical abuse, have poor problem-solving skills, and demonstrate exhibitionistic and voyeuristic tendencies. The PREA's mandatory reporting requirements are expected to provide a better understanding of sex offenders within jails and prisons. Institutional sex offenders tend to have higher status within the institution, often holding prestigious jobs such as a unit boss or a janitor in a captain's office. They tend to work around correctional staff, have a good view of facility operations, and have the ability to watch potential targets and current victims. They often have a strong rapport with staff and the ability to facilitate cell changes and job assignments for themselves or others. Staff may inadvertently reinforce or encourage sex-ual assaults due to difficulty discerning consensual from coercive sexual incidents (Potter and Tewksbury 2005). This often leads to a perceived variable reinforcement schedule in which the absence of discipline may serve as a reward and bolster a perception of acceptance and enjoyment on the part of the victim.

Generally, the tools utilized by inmates to sexually assault other inmates are thought to include such manipulative techniques as protection from (more) violent sexual assault, threats and intimidation, and pure force (Groth and Burgess 1980). Research on community sex offending shows consistency in the modus operandi regarding victim preference (Sjostedt et al. 2004), and our experience indicates consistency in institutional offending patterns regarding victim type, offense type, and victim grooming patterns. Setting up a victim for a sex offense is commonly referred to as *grooming;* it involves targeting, watching, finding points of vulnerability, and ingratiation. Perpetrators of inmate-on-inmate sexual behaviors often present themselves as a friend, mentor, and teacher of the rules and ways of the institution. Common means of ingratiation are to offer protection from assault, including sexual assault; to give advice; and to discourage relations with other dangerous inmates. A likely practice would be to gain access to the potential victim as a cell mate, begin commuting together to meals and recreation, and begin confiding seemingly personal information. As this relationship becomes established, the content of discussion may shift to sexual practices. Queries such as "How does your girl like it?" and "Have you ever had sex with a man?" represent a testing of limits and an expectation of information exchange.

Within jails and prisons, the strength of grooming often has to do with debt (E. Redden, personal communication, July 2008). This debt may be for a service or favor provided, such as protection, or for items of value, including food, commissary items, and health products. The premise is that the provision of something special leads to an expectation of reciprocity. With the decrease of tobacco and drugs in many correctional settings, food remains readily available and has taken on a high value. Adults find themselves in a position of having to negotiate private time and space when housed together in a jail or prison. The institutional sex offender attempts to violate presumed personal space, for example, by staring while the victim is using the toilet or sitting next to the victim on his bunk. The correctional sex offender begins to physically intrude upon and muscle the victim in an effort to break the victim's sense of control.

Levels of inappropriate sexual behaviors appear to follow a hierarchy, beginning with consensual behavior and proceeding through begging, exploitation, coercion, sexual harassment, and forcible rape, with most behaviors falling within the exploitation and coercion levels (E. Redden, personal communication, July 2008; see Table 8–3 for definitions). A re-

TABLE 8–3. Definitions of sexual relations/behaviors in correctional institutions

Consensual relations	Dealings that reflect equal power and an understanding of the consequences for both parties
Begging	Behavior that involves repeatedly asking for and ultimately engaging in sexual behaviors with the victim
Exploitation	Taking advantage of an inmate's weakness (e.g., drug addiction)
Coercion	Behavior that wears the victim down emotionally until he or she sees no other option than to comply
Sexual harassment	Outright physical groping and assault of another
Rape	A forcible violation of another

view of prison vernacular suggests that all these levels exist within jails and prisons. Consensual sexual activity in prison was the best predictor of sexual coercion; 27% of men who admitted to consensual sexual activity within prison admitted to coercion, whereas only 3% of men who denied consensual sexual relations admitted to coercion (Warren et al., in press). Typically, the victim has some vice or debt that he or she would not wish to share with correctional officials, and reporting of the sexual assaults is often humiliating to the victim and may be perceived as snitching. Because these assaults have a flavor of entrapment, victims often may not view the sexual behavior as rape. Additionally, because the perpetrators are well aware of rape kits and forensic evidence, most sexual assaults in correctional institutions involve oral, manual, and dry intercourse.

Prison Rape Elimination Act

The PREA, signed into law by President George W. Bush on September 4, 2003, applies to all federal and state prisons, jails, juvenile facilities, police lockups, private facilities, and community correctional settings such as residential and parole settings. It established zero tolerance for sexual behavior between inmates or between inmates and staff. Under the PREA (2003) and in accordance with the rules of virtually all correctional institutions, all sexual contact between inmates and others is prohibited and can be classified as inappropriate sexual behavior. The act was founded on the premise that sexual assault and rape do occur in correctional settings and that acceptance of sexual behavior leads to continuances of rape and/or violence. The act supports the elimination, reduction, and prevention of sexual assault within the correctional system and created a national commission to develop standards and accountability measures. It mandates several national data collection activities whereby all states complete and report staff and inmate survey data. The act also provides funding for program development and additional research.

Exhibitionism

The existing research on exhibitionism within correctional settings has been sparse. Although few studies have reviewed the features of male inmates who engage in exhibitionism while incarcerated, the literature is filled with case studies (e.g., Evans 1970; Russell 1972) that are psychodynamically geared. These reports are helpful in conceptualizing individuals' behaviors and providing treatment, but they do not address the scope of this aggressive and disruptive behavior. Most research focuses on community offending and preparation for release.

In a fairly comprehensive study, Shiver (2003) examined the exhibitionistic behavior of 73 incarcerated subjects. Although many inmates receive disciplinary action for exhibitionism, the response tends to be minimal and is often not taken seriously by inmates, thus perpetuating the behaviors. Shiver opined that inmates and employees may actually view the behavior as humorous. We have observed that responses to exhibitionism vary across setting, shift, closeness to end of shift, gender, and officer pairing. Punishment occurs on a variable ratio schedule, thus strengthening the behaviors; the inmates often perceive the absence of punishment as acceptance or even as desire on the part of correctional staff. Those who expose themselves in corrections frequently have cognitive distortions that include the belief that the victims want to see their penis and gain pleasure from the exposure. The cognitive distortions are reinforced by the institutions' inconsistent responses. Over time, both employees and inmates may become desensitized to exhibitionism within correctional settings (Shiver 2003).

An understanding of why exhibitionism occurs in correctional settings is helpful to managing such behavior. Certainly, some exhibitionists are driven purely by anger. These inmates tend to resist treatment and behave inappropriately if they attend individual or group sessions. Others appear to act impulsively when the opportunity arises. Some exhibitionists lack the relational and social skills to interact with female staff and use their exposing behavior as a literal foot-in-the-door trick as a subject upon which to initiate banter when they are released from restrictive housing. Of concern is that inmates' exhibitionism can inadvertently become fueled by the institution and lead to similar offending upon release.

Treatment and Management of Inappropriate Sexual Behaviors

From a safety and management perspective, institutions need to implement some form of containment strategy for inappropriate sexual behaviors. The fact that such behaviors are not tolerated must be made clear to all correctional employees and inmates, and disciplinary interventions must be consistent across staff members, shifts, units, and institutions. Mental health staff should be available for referrals of those inmates who are exhibitionistic or who otherwise engage in repetitive inappropriate sexual behaviors that do not require enhanced containment. With regard to mental health treatment, repeat offenders who threaten the safety and security of the institution should have a behavioral management plan put in place. The preferred treatment options derive from the principles of cognitive-behavioral therapy. The decision to use a therapeutic approach as opposed to a psychoeducational intervention should be based on the offender's level of denial. Group treatment is the standard setting because peers effectively challenge patterns of denial and cognitive distortions. For inmates who are habitually disruptive through inappropriate sexual behaviors, treatment should be mandated as part of a management plan. Coupled with housing, use of an integrated management and treatment plan can be effective in presenting a unified front of zero tolerance and an expectation of adaptive skills building.

Treatment for sex offenses has been based historically on the concepts of extinguishment, sublimation of deviant sexual arousal, and aversive therapies. In correctional environments, the latter two are not practical. With those inmates who are chronically disruptive, the use of coercion in treatment through the placing of external pressure to control behavior is an option to be considered with a mandated management plan. Coercion occurs in the form of incapacitating the sex offender, thus rendering him or her quite restricted in terms of his or her ability to engage in illegal sexual acts, and also ensures that some sort of treatment is received (Burdon and Gallagher 2002). In jails and prisons, restrictive housing units or other undesirable locations can be utilized to contain the inmate, and treatment adherence can be set as a condition for changing housing location and receipt of privileges. Also, with exhibitionists, embarrassment (e.g., a phone call to the exhibitionist's mother or laughing during the exposure) may have a place in treatment to extinguish the behaviors.

The treatment structure for sex offending typically includes targeting denial, empathy, and relapse prevention. Cognitive-behavioral models also include attention to cognitive distortions, emotion management, and interpersonal skills development.

Examples of cognitive distortions, which the offender uses to minimize and justify offending behaviors, include the following: helping the victim get a block change, a job, or food; acting as a mentor; and blame attributions, such as "He was stupid and got what was coming." For those who expose themselves, misperception of cues, such as watching the female officer doubling back on a staggered observation tour, may be misperceived as desire or reflective of a relationship. Certainly, minimization as a cognitive distortion within corrections is represented by statements such as "Everyone does it" and "They love to see it."

When targeting cognitive distortions, the clinician should explore with the inmate the role of deviant thoughts in behavior, provide guidance for adjusting thoughts, assist in the recognition of inappropriate thoughts, and allow the inmate to challenge such thinking (Moster et al. 2008). In prison, one effective technique is to have the inmate depict the offense and allow the group members to challenge distortions. Incident reports can be used by the mental health staff to demonstrate collaboration and address denial and distortions. Other strategies include placing those who deny that they are sex offenders in psychoeducational groups where they can speak hypothetically and change their offense stories over time. The role of emotions in regard to offending should be explored; related homework assignments might include a mapping of feelings at the time of inappropriate sexual behaviors. Once the disruptive institutional sex offender has undergone treatment within the context of a behavioral plan, preparation for long-term housing with the general population of the institution must focus on relapse plans, including the ability to identify high-risk situations (e.g., new female officer on unit) and develop readily accessible plans.

Role of Medication

Although rarely used in practice, chemical castration relies on hormonal drugs, such as medroxyprogesterone acetate (Depo-Provera), to lower the physiological arousal of the offender (Burdon and Gallagher 2002). The use of SSRIs may aid in controlling the compulsive quality of the behavior, and these drugs may be useful as an adjunctive treatment (Kafka 1991). Many SSRI-compliant exhibitionists are successful in reducing or eliminating their offending behaviors; however, effectiveness is contingent on continued use (Burdon and Gallagher 2002). For offenders who are in denial, the use of SSRIs is not a viable adjunctive treatment to consider until the offender has engaged in treatment and admitted to all inappropriate sexual behavior patterns.

Clinical Case 8–2

Ms. C is a 39-year-old female incarcerated for 2 years, with three previous 1- to 5-year incarcerations. She is currently showing improved behavior and functioning; however, previous disruptive behaviors included the following:

- Inmate developed a coercive sexual relationship with cell mate, threatening to harm cell mate when she complained to staff or did not comply.
- Inmate fought lockups by screaming obscenities, spitting, and attempting to punch and bite staff members.
- Inmate became verbally aggressive and physically agitated, threatening to kill herself, upon planned transfer to restrictive housing, leading to transfer to the inpatient mental health unit.
- Inmate demanded a feminine hygiene product while in the restrictive housing unit, and became enraged that it was not provided as quickly as she wanted. She pulled the fire sprinkler head loose, thus flooding her cell and adjoining cells with foul water.

A behavior management plan was developed for Ms. C to include the following:

Identification of problematic behaviors

Sexual coercion, suicide threats contingent upon undesired transfer, threatening and assaultive behavior, flooding, and destruction of property.

Functional analysis

Analysis of problem incidents suggests primary motivators of need for control and for proximity to positive sources of attention.

Management plan

- When Ms. C is threatening suicide, maintain safety within the restricted housing unit through one-to-one observation and safety gown, without transfer to mental health unit.
- Keep Ms. C separate from inmates at risk for victimization.
- Extinguish attention-seeking maladaptive behaviors by limiting staff attention to these behaviors. Provide regularly scheduled brief positive interaction (twice weekly for 15 minutes) with mental health staff.
- Provide reading materials.

- Upon completion of 90 consecutive days with no instances of maladaptive behavior, inmate may be transferred to general population.

Ms. C threatened suicide on two additional occasions, when frustrated by staff procedures, and was maintained on the restricted housing unit. She also escalated verbal aggression in an apparent attempt to engage staff members. She appeared to value the interaction with the mental health staff. She has not engaged in any of the targeted maladaptive behaviors for 10 weeks and is nearing anticipated transfer to the general population.

CONCLUSION

Inmates who engage in disruptive and aggressive behaviors within jails and prisons create serious challenges for both custody and treatment staffs. The good news is that offenders who exhibit behavioral dyscontrol, are self-injurious or impulsively aggressive, or demonstrate problem sexual behavior are apt to seek mental health services (Morgan et al. 2007). Correctional settings provide an opportunity to shape adaptive functioning and promote effective coping. Collaboration among the mental health and custody staff, building on the strengths of each discipline, is critical to such change.

To effectively manage and reduce the occurrence of disruptive and aggressive behaviors such as self-injury, feces smearing, flooding, and problem sexual behaviors, correctional professionals must develop a reasoned and flexible behavioral management plan. The potential success of these plans leads to a change in the status quo, which in turn produces a sense of greater control and empowerment for the staff involved in the planning and implementation of innovative, flexible, and successful interventions. Recommended tools include creativity, adjunctive medication, and facility control techniques. Working together to address disruptive behaviors may allow mental health and correctional staff to succeed in effective management rather than fail in fractured relationships and frustration. Flexibility in the treatment of inmates by individual officers is paramount for reducing inmate acting out and facilitating a more favorable impression than has historically been represented. All too often, we have seen that the reinforcement of disruptive behaviors leads to more disruptive behaviors. In a healthy parallel, the success of eliminating disruptive and aggressive behaviors through joint behavioral management plans reinforces the collaborative process and makes correctional systems more likely to continue to develop such effective approaches. Success in use of the approach with a self-injurer will typically generalize to acceptance of the approach for other behaviors.

While seeking to have inmates expand their adaptive functioning, staff in correctional facilities should anticipate the parallel process of increasing their own response sets through flexibility. In fact, staff should model flexibility for the inmate within the context of developing and maintaining management plans. In our experience, most inmates do not want to be in distress and often go to extreme measures to avoid experiencing such feelings. One goal of mental health staff is to eliminate the distress experienced in the correctional system by developing skills for the inmates and for the institutions. Managing the disruptive behaviors of extreme inmates is an attainable challenge for all staff working in jails and prisons. The large majority of disruptive inmates can be helped to gain greater control of themselves in an attempt to ensure safety and security and to promote adaptive functioning within a difficult environment.

SUMMARY POINTS

- Determining the etiology of disruptive or aggressive behavior is needed to choose a treatment strategy focused on the inmate and/or a correctional strategy focused on the officer and system.
- Correctional standards of care encourage consultation by mental health staff and collaborative efforts between custody and mental health staff in the delivery of mental health services.
- Each act of self-injury should be assessed for motivation, intent, lethality, and context.
- Incarceration limits an inmate's options for solving problems proactively, which may lead to maladaptive behaviors.
- The goals of behavioral management plans must be attainable based on a review of inmate-specific factors.
- Cognitive-behavioral therapies, such as dialectical behavior therapy, are well suited for treatment of many problems characterized by behavioral dyscontrol.
- The Prison Rape Elimination Act of 2003 established zero tolerance for inmate-on-inmate sexual behavior and inmate–staff sexual behavior.
- Treatment of institutional sex offenses should incorporate cognitive-behavioral interventions that address cognitive distortions, emotion management, and interpersonal skills development.
- Effective management and reduction of disruptive behaviors require multidisciplinary involvement and flexibility in institutional practices.

REFERENCES

American Correctional Association: Performance-Based Standards for Adult Local Detention Facilities, 4th Edition. Alexandria, VA, American Correctional Association, 2004

American Psychiatric Association: Psychiatric Services in Jails and Prisons: A Task Force Report of the American Psychiatric Association, 2nd Edition. Washington, DC, American Psychiatric Association, 2000

Appelbaum KL: Commentary: the use of restraint and seclusion in correctional mental health. J Am Acad Psychiatry Law 35:431–435, 2007

Beck AJ, Harrison PM: Sexual victimization in local jails reported by inmates, 2007 (NCJ 221946). Washington, DC, U.S. Department of Justice, Office of Justice Programs, Bureau of Justice Statistics, 2008

Berg MT, DeLisi M: The correctional melting pot: race, ethnicity, citizenship, and prison violence. J Crim Justice 34:631–642, 2006

Berzins LG, Trestman RL: The development and implementation of dialectical behavior therapy in forensic settings. International Journal of Forensic Mental Health 3:95–105, 2004

Boiko IB, Lester D: Self-aggression among Russian prisoners. Correct Soc Psych J Behav Tech Methods Ther 41:67–70, 1995

Borrill J, Snow L, Medlicott D, et al: Learning from "near misses": interviews with women who survived an incident of severe self-harm in prison. Howard Journal of Criminal Justice 44:57–69, 2005

Briere J, Gil E: Self-mutilation in clinical and general population samples: prevalence, correlates, and functions. Am J Orthopsychiatry 68:609–620, 1998

Brooker C, Repper J, Beverley C, et al: Mental Health Services and Prisoners: A Review. Sheffield, UK, Mental Health Task Force, 2002

Burdon W, Gallagher C: Coercion and sex offenders: controlling sex-offending behavior through incapacitation and treatment. Crim Justice Behav 29:87–109, 2002

Bush J, Glick B, Taymans J: Thinking for a Change: Integrated Cognitive Behavior Change Program (NIC Accession No 016672). Washington, DC, U.S. Dept of Justice, National Institute of Corrections, 1997

Byrne J, Hummer D: In search of the "tossed salad man" (and others involved in prison violence): new strategies for predicting and controlling violence in prison. Aggress Violent Behav 12:531–541, 2007

Chengappa KN, Ebeling T, Kang JS, et al: Clozapine reduces severe self-mutilation and aggression in psychotic patients with borderline personality disorder. J Clin Psychiatry 60:477–484, 1999

Chonco NR: Sexual assaults among male inmates: a descriptive study. Prison J 69:72–82, 1989

Daffern M, Howells K: Antecedents for aggression and the function analytic approach to the assessment of aggression and violence in personality disordered patients within secure settings. Personality and Mental Health 1:126–137, 2007

Daniel AE, Fleming J: Serious suicide attempts in a state correctional system and strategies to prevent suicide. J Psychiatry Law 33:227–247, 2005

Dear GE, Thomson DM, Hills AM: Self-harm in prison: manipulators can also be suicide attempters. Crim Justice Behav 27:160–175, 2000

DiGiuseppe R, Tafrate R: Anger treatment for adults: a meta-analytic review. Clinical Psychology: Science and Practice 10:70–84, 2003

Evans DR: Exhibitionism, in Symptoms of Psychopathology: A Handbook. Edited by Costello C. New York, Wiley, 1970, pp 560–573

Evershed S, Tennant A, Boomer D, et al: Practice-based outcomes of dialectical behaviour therapy (DBT) targeting anger and violence, with male forensic patients: a pragmatic and non-contemporaneous comparison. Crim Behav Ment Health 13:198–213, 2003

Fagan TJ, Wennerstrom D, Miller J: Sexual assault of male inmates: prevention, identification, and intervention. J Correction Health Care 3:49–65, 1996

Favaro A, Ferrara S, Santonastaso P: Self-injurious behavior in a community sample of young women: relationship with childhood abuse and other types of self-damaging behaviors. J Clin Psychiatry 68:122–131, 2007

Favazza AR: The coming of age of self-mutilation. J Nerv Ment Dis 186:259–268, 1998

Feldman MD: The challenge of self-mutilation: a review. Compr Psychiatry 29:252–269, 1988

Fessler DMT: The implications of starvation induced psychological changes for the ethical treatment of hunger strikers. Psychiatric Ethics 29:243–255, 2003

Frankenburg FR, Zanarini MC: Divalproex sodium treatment of women with borderline personality disorder and bipolar II disorder: a double-blind, placebo-controlled pilot study. J Clin Psychiatry 63:442–446, 2002

Franklin RK: Deliberate self-harm: self-injurious behavior within a correctional mental health population. Crim Justice Behav 15:210–218, 1988

Goedhard LE, Stolker JJ, Heerdink ER, et al: Pharmacotherapy for the treatment of aggressive behavior in general adult psychiatry: a systematic review. J Clin Psychiatry 67:1013–1024, 2006

Goldstein AP, Glick B: Aggression Replacement Training: A Comprehensive Intervention for Aggressive Youth. Champaign, IL, Research Press, 1987

Gontkovsky ST: The psychology of aggression: a critique of correctional approaches to treating violent behavior. Adm Policy Ment Health 29:525–528, 2002

Groth AN, Burgess AW: Male rape: offenders and victims. Am J Psychiatry 137:806–819, 1980

Hillbrand M, Krystal JH, Sharpe KS, et al: Clinical predictors of self-mutilation in hospitalized forensic patients. J Nerv Ment Dis 182:9–13, 1994

Holbrook MI: Anger management training in prison inmates. Psychol Rep 81:623–626, 1997

Hollander E, Allen A, Lopez RP, et al: A preliminary double-blind, placebo-controlled trial of divalproex sodium in borderline personality disorder. J Clin Psychiatry 62:199–203, 2001

Holton SMB: Managing and treating mentally disordered offenders in jails and prisons, in The Correctional Mental Health Handbook. Edited by Fagan TJ, Ax RK. Thousand Oaks, CA, Sage, 2003, pp 101–122

Hough DW: Low-dose olanzapine for self-mutilation behavior in patients with borderline personality disorder. J Clin Psychiatry 62:296–297, 2001

James DJ, Glaze LE: Mental health problems of prison and jail inmates (NCJ 213600). Washington, DC, U.S. Department of Justice, Office of Justice Programs, Bureau of Justice Statistics, 2006

Jeglic EL, Vanderhoof HA, Donovick PJ: The function of self-harm behaviors in a forensic population. Int J Offender Ther Comp Criminol 49:131–142, 2005

Kafka MP: Successful antidepressant treatment in nonparaphilic sexual addictions and paraphilias in men. J Clin Psychiatry 52:60–65, 1991

Karten SJ: The relationship of borderline personality disorder, problem solving ability, and anxiety to self-cutting behavior of prison inmates. Dissertation Abstracts International 52:4977, 1992

Klonsky ED, Oltmanns TF, Turkheimer E: Deliberate self-harm in a nonclinical population: prevalence and psychological correlates. Am J Psychiatry 160:1501–1508, 2003

Lewis CF: Successfully treating aggression in mentally ill prison inmates. Psychiatr Q 71:331–343, 2000

Linehan MM: Cognitive-Behavioral Treatment of Borderline Personality Disorder. New York, Guilford, 1993

Linehan M: The empirical basis of dialectical behavior therapy: development of new treatments versus evaluation of existing treatments. Clin Psychol (New York) 7:113–119, 2000

Linehan MM, Armstrong HE, Suarez A, et al: Cognitive-behavioral treatment of chronically parasuicidal borderline patients. Arch Gen Psychiatry 48:1060–1064, 1991

Linehan MM, Tutek DA, Heard HL, et al: Interpersonal outcome of cognitive behavioral treatment for chronically suicidal borderline patients. Am J Psychiatry 151:1771–1776, 1994

Linehan MM, Comtois KA, Brown MZ, et al: Suicide Attempt Self-Injury Interview (SASII): development, reliability, and validity of a scale to assess suicide attempts and intentional self-injury. Psychol Assess 183:303–313, 2006

Lipsey MW, Landenberger NA, Wilson SJ: Effects of Cognitive-Behavioral Programs for Criminal Offenders. Campbell Systematic Reviews, August 9, 2007. Available at: http://db.c2admin.org/doc-pdf/lipsey_CBT_finalreview.pdf. Accessed March 27, 2009.

Little G, Wilson D: Moral Recognition Therapy: a systematic step-by-step treatment system for treatment-resistant clients. Psychol Rep 62:135–151, 1988

Livingston M, Beck G: A cognitive-behavioral model of self-injury and bullying among imprisoned young offenders. Issues in Criminological and Legal Psychology 28:45–49, 1997

Lohner J, Konrad N: Deliberate self-harm and suicide attempt in custody: distinguishing features in male inmates' self-injurious behavior. Int J Law Psychiatry 29:370–385, 2006

Marasco M, Cocco G, Pinacchio W, et al: Self-mutilation acts in prison: 3-year time trends (1992–1994) in the male district prison "Nuovo Complesso" Rebibbia-Rome (Italy). International Medical Journal 2:203–207, 1995

Martinez ME: Manipulative self-injurious behavior in correctional settings: an environmental treatment approach. Journal of Offender Counseling, Services and Rehabilitation 4:275–283, 1980

Matsumoto T, Yamaguchi A, Asami T, et al: Characteristics of self-cutters among male inmates: association with bulimia and dissociation. Psychiatry Clin Neurosci 59:319–326, 2005

McCann RA, Ball EM, Ivanoff A: DBT with an inpatient forensic population: the CMHIP forensic model. Cogn Behav Pract 7:448–456, 2000

Meunier GF, Sellborn M: Incarcerated self-mutilators: taxonomy and treatment. Correctional Psychologist 33:1–6, 2001

Milkman H, Wanberg K: Cognitive-behavioral treatment: a review and discussion for corrections professionals (NIC Accession No 021657). Washington, DC, National Institute of Corrections, 2007

Miller WP: The hunger-striking prisoner. J Prison Health 6:40–60, 1987

Morgan RD, Steffan J, Shaw LB, et al: Needs for and barriers to correctional mental health services: inmate perceptions. Psychiatr Serv 58:1181–1186, 2007

Moster A, Wnuk DW, Jeglic EL: Cognitive behavioral therapy interventions with sex offenders. J Correction Health Care 14:109–121, 2008

National Commission on Correctional Health Care: Standards for Mental Health Services in Correctional Facilities. Chicago, National Commission on Correctional Health Care, 2008

Nee C, Farman S: Female prisoners with borderline personality disorder: some promising treatment developments. Crim Behav Ment Health 15:2–16, 2005

Panton JH: The identification of predispositional factors in self-mutilation within a state prison population. J Clin Psychol 18:63–67, 1962

Petty J, Oliver C: Self-injurious behaviour in individuals with intellectual disabilities. Curr Opin Psychiatry 18:484–489, 2005

Pies RW, Popli AP: Self-injurious behavior: pathophysiology and implications for treatment. J Clin Psychiatry 56:580–588, 1995

Pinto O, Akiskal H: Lamotrigine as a promising approach to borderline personality. J Affect Disord 51:333–343, 1998

Potter RH, Tewksbury R: Sex and prisoners: criminal justice contributions to a public health issue. J Correction Health Care 11:171–190, 2005

Power KG, Spencer AP: Parasuicidal behavior of detained Scottish young offenders. Int J Offender Ther Comp Criminol 31:227–235, 1987

Prison Rape Elimination Act of 2003, Pub. L. No. 108-79, 117 Stat. 972. Available at: http://www.spr.org/pdf/PREA.pdf. Accessed March 27, 2009.

Rinne T, van den Brink W, Wouters L, et al: SSRI treatment of borderline personality disorder: a randomized, placebo-controlled clinical trial for female patients with borderline personality disorder. Am J Psychiatry 159:2048–2054, 2002

Roth AS, Ostroff RB, Hoffman RE: Naltrexone as a treatment for repetitive self-injurious behavior: an open-label trial. J Clin Psychiatry 57:233–237, 1996

Russell DH: Treatment of adult exhibitionists. Int J Offender Ther Comp Criminol 16:121–124, 1972

Shea S: Personality characteristics of self-mutilating male prisoners. J Clin Psychol 49:576–585, 1993

Shiver J: A correlational study of exhibitionistic behavior in a male correctional institution. Dissertation Abstracts International 63:4885, 2003

Simeon D, Hollander E (eds): Self-Injurious Behaviors: Assessment and Treatment. Washington, DC, American Psychiatric Press, 2001

Sjostedt G, Langstrom N, Sturidsson K, et al: Stability of modus operandi in sexual offending. Crim Justice Behav 31:609–623, 2004

Skeem JL, Miller JD, Mulvey E, et al: Using a five-factor lens to explore the relation between personality traits and violence in psychiatric patients. J Consult Clin Psychol 73:454–465, 2005

Snow L: Prisoners' motives for self-injury and attempted suicide. British Journal of Forensic Practice 4:18–29, 2002

State of Connecticut Office of Protection and Advocacy for Persons With Disabilities v Choinski, Gomez, Lantz. May 12, 2004. Available at: http://www.aclu.org/prison/gen/14734lgl20040512.html#attach. Accessed March 27, 2009.

Stermac L: Anger control treatment for forensic patients. J Interpers Violence 1:446–467, 1987

Symons FJ, Thompson A, Rodriguez MC: Self-injurious behavior and the efficacy of naltrexone treatment: a quantitative synthesis. Ment Retard Dev Disabil Res Rev 10:193–200, 2004

Trestman RL: Behind bars: personality disorders. J Am Acad Psychiatry Law 28:232–235, 2000

Trestman RL, Ford J, Zhang W, et al: Current and lifetime psychiatric illness among inmates not identified as acutely mentally ill at intake in Connecticut's jails. J Am Acad Psychiatry Law 35:490–500, 2007

Valliant PM, Antonowicz DH: Cognitive behaviour therapy and social skills training improves personality and cognition in incarcerated offenders. Psychol Rep 68:27–33, 1991

Vannoy SD, Hoyt WT: Evaluation of an anger therapy intervention for incarcerated adult males. Journal of Offender Rehabilitation 39:39–57, 2004

Walsh BW, Rosen PM: Self-Mutilation: Theory, Research, and Treatment. New York, Guilford, 1988

Warren JI, Jackson S, Loper AB, et al: Risk markers for sexual predation and victimization in prison (in press).

Webb LR: Addressing severe behavior problems in a "super-max" prison setting. 2001a. Available at: http://www.nicic.org. Accessed March 27, 2009.

Webb LR: Dealing with the problematic inmate: applying effective strategies in a correctional setting. 2001b. Available at: http://www.nicic.org. Accessed March 27, 2009.

Welch SS: A review of the literature on the epidemiology of parasuicide in the general population. Psychiatr Serv 52:368–375, 2001

Wilson GL: Psychotherapy with depressed incarcerated felons: a comparative evaluation of treatments. Psychol Rep 67 (3 pt 1):1027–1041, 1990

Zlotnick C, Najavits LM, Rohsenow DJ, et al: A cognitive-behavioral treatment for incarcerated women with substance abuse disorder and posttraumatic stress disorder: findings from a pilot study. J Subst Abuse Treat 25:99–105, 2003

CHAPTER 9

Toward a Better Understanding of Suicide Prevention in Correctional Facilities

Lindsay M. Hayes

According to available records, during the late evening of March 18, the Nathan County Sheriff's Department received information regarding a disturbance at the residence of 43-year-old James Cooper.[1] When Nathan County Sheriff Jack Buck and other personnel arrived at the scene, Mr. Cooper was observed wielding a gun and pointing it at himself and others. The weapon was eventually confiscated without injury, and Mr. Cooper was transported to the Nathan County Detention Facility (NCDF), arriving at approximately 9:00 P.M. Although not criminally charged, Mr. Cooper was known to suffer from mental illness and, according to NCDF documents (including the jail docket), was being held for "mental." Approximately 30 minutes later, at 9:30 P.M., Mr. Cooper was ob-

---

[1]To ensure complete confidentiality, names of the victim, staff, and jail facility have been changed.

served to be attempting suicide by hanging in a holding cell. He had tied one end of his shirt to the bunk bed and the other end around his neck. Mr. Cooper was rescued by jail staff and placed in a straitjacket. He continued his self-destructive behavior by repeatedly banging his head against the cell wall. Mr. Cooper was eventually transported to a local hospital for medical treatment and returned to the facility at approximately 11:00 P.M. He was again rehoused in the holding cell in a straitjacket and without his clothes. He was observed to be crying and again engaging in self-destructive behavior by banging his head against the wall. Mr. Cooper then was able to remove his straitjacket and began banging it against the cell door. Jail staff entered the cell and briefly chained Mr. Cooper to his bunk by waist chains and leg irons. The inmate eventually calmed down, was permitted to smoke a cigarette, and fell asleep. According to jail logs, Mr. Cooper was given a blanket at approximately 2:30 A.M. (on March 19), his clothing was returned at 12:00 A.M., and he was observed at 20-minute intervals between 2:00 A.M. to 5:15 A.M. (although these observations were not documented). Despite continuous suicidal behavior, he was never placed on suicide precautions by jail staff.

Later in the morning of March 19, Mr. Cooper was transported by sheriff's deputies to the county mental health center (CMHC) for evaluation of his need for civil commitment to a state hospital. The preevaluation screening form completed by the examining psychologist noted Mr. Cooper's prior outpatient treatment at the CMHC, history of or present danger to self ("high-risk behavior" and "self-mutilation"), depressive-like behaviors ("sadness," "crying," and "weight loss or gain"), "beating head against wall in admitted tantrum," recent fighting with his father, and substance abuse. The examining psychologist was unaware of Mr. Cooper's suicide attempt in the county jail the previous day. Following the assessment, the psychologist completed a certificate of examining physician/ psychologist, although the psychologist's recommendation appeared unclear. A prescription for daily doses of paroxetine was also written. Mr. Cooper was then returned to the county jail and, apparently due to the unclear recommendation on the certificate of examining physician/psychologist, was released from custody the following day (March 20).

On March 25, the Nathan County Chancery Court received from the CMHC a resubmitted certificate of examining physician/psychologist regarding Mr. Cooper that clearly recommended civil commitment. The resubmitted form included boxes checked off in the areas of "grossly disturbed behavior/faulty perception," "substantial likelihood of physical harm as manifested by recent threat or attempt to physically harm him/ herself or others," and "failure to provide necessary care for him/herself." According to a clinical note written by the CMHC examining psychologist on March 25, "Apparently the public officials misunderstood our possibly ambiguously stated intentions for him to be held until a comprehensive evaluation could be accomplished in a hospital setting. I further learned that the report that we sent was possibly incomplete. I immediately contacted Sheriff Buck and the Chancery Clerk by telephone to review our recommendations. I also faxed them a copy of the completed physician and psychologist recommendations."

During the late evening of March 29, the Nathan County Sheriff's Department again received information regarding a disturbance involving Mr. Cooper in the community. Sheriff Buck and other personnel again responded to the scene, and observed Mr. Cooper wielding a knife. The weapon was eventually confiscated without injury, and Mr. Cooper was transported to the county jail by Sheriff Buck, arriving at approximately 11:35 P.M. Mr. Cooper was not criminally charged and, according to jail documents, was again being held for "mental." Mr. Cooper was again placed in a holding cell and observed periodically, although not placed on suicide precautions by jail staff.

At approximately 3:20 P.M. on March 31, Mr. Cooper was rehoused from the holding cell to the general population section of the jail. He was allowed to take a shower and was given all his clothing and a box of personal items. According to jail staff, who did not consult with any mental health staff prior to rehousing Mr. Cooper, the rationale for the transfer was that his "state of mind was good" and they needed to utilize the holding cell for observation of another mentally ill detainee. When commenting later about Mr. Cooper's transfer to general population, the chief jailer stated, "We treated him like any other inmate when we moved him to the back of the jail."

On April 1, Mr. Cooper attended the Nathan County Chancery Court proceeding for his civil commitment to a state hospital for mental health examination and treatment. The commitment order was signed by Mr. Cooper, his attorney, and the court, stating, in part, that Mr. Cooper was a "danger to himself and others." According to his attorney, "James Cooper agreed to and signed the commitment order, and the order was entered by the chancellor at approximately 11:00 A.M. Sheriff Buck was aware that Mr. Cooper had agreed to be committed and was present when the chancellor signed the order. James Cooper was to be kept in custody at the Nathan County Detention Facility until an opening became available at the state mental hospital." The inmate was subsequently returned to his cell.

Several hours later, at approximately 8:16 P.M. on April 1, Mr. Cooper was again observed banging his head against the wall of his cell. He appeared agitated to jail staff, was observed to be crying, and requested his psychotropic medication and a cigarette. Although the officer believed that Mr. Cooper's head banging was an attempt to commit suicide, no effort was made to ensure his safety from further self-destructive behavior. Instead, at approximately 8:30 P.M., Mr. Cooper was given his medication and a cigarette (a.k.a. "smoke therapy"), and the lights in his cell were turned off. According to jail records, Mr. Cooper was not seen again for approximately 2½ hours, when he was found at approximately 11 P.M. hanging by a laundry bag cord that was tied to the upper bunk in his cell. The officer eventually entered the cell and cut the cord away from the victim's neck but did not initiate cardiopulmonary resuscitation. A medical emergency was called. and paramedics arrived approximately 10 minutes later. Mr. Cooper was subsequently pronounced dead.

SCOPE OF THE PROBLEM

Across the country, suicide is a leading cause of death in jails, where well over 400 inmates take their lives each year (Hayes 1989). The rate of suicide in county jails is estimated to be approximately four times greater than that of the general population (Mumola and Noonan 2007). Overall, most jail suicide victims are young white males who are arrested for nonviolent offenses and intoxicated upon arrest. Many are placed in isolation and are found dead within 24 hours of incarceration (Davis and Muscat 1993; Hayes 1989). The overwhelming majority of victims hang themselves with either bedding or clothing. Most victims are not adequately screened for potential suicidal behavior upon entrance into jail (Hayes 1989).

Research specific to suicide in urban jail facilities provides certain disparate findings. Most victims of suicide in large urban facilities are arrested for violent offenses and are dead within 1–4 months of incarceration (DuRand et al. 1995; Marcus and Alcabes 1993). Due to the extended length of confinement prior to suicide, intoxication is not always the salient factor in suicides in urban jails as it is in other types of jail facilities. Suicide victim characteristics such as age, race, gender, method, and instrument remain generally consistent in both urban and nonurban jails.

The precipitating factors of suicidal behavior in jail are well established (Bonner 1992, 2000; Winkler 1992). The two primary causes for jail suicide are theorized to be that 1) jail environments are conducive to suicidal behavior and 2) the inmate is facing a crisis situation. From the inmate's perspective, certain features of incarceration enhance suicidal behavior: fear of the unknown, distrust of authoritarian environment, lack of apparent control over the future, isolation from family and significant others, shame of incarceration, and the dehumanizing aspects of incarceration. In addition, certain factors are prevalent among inmates facing a crisis situation that could predispose them to suicide: recent excessive drinking and/or use of drugs, recent loss of stabilizing resources, severe guilt or shame over the alleged offense, current mental illness, prior history of suicidal behavior, and approaching court date. Some inmates simply are (or become) ill equipped to handle the common stresses of confinement. As the inmate reaches an emotional breaking point, the result can be suicidal ideation, attempt, or completion. During initial confinement in a jail, this stress can be limited to fear of the unknown and isolation from family, but over time (including stays in prison), the stress may become exacerbated and include loss of outside relationships, conflicts within the institution, victimization, further legal frustration, physical and emotional breakdown, and problems of coping within the institutional environment (Bonner 1992).

Although suicide is well recognized as a critical problem within jails, the issue of prison suicide has not received comparable attention, primarily because the number of jail suicides far exceeds the number of prison suicides. Suicide ranks third, behind natural causes and AIDS, as the leading cause of death in prisons (Mumola and Noonan 2007). Although the rate of suicide in prison is considerably lower than in jail, it still remains greater than in the general population (Hayes 1995). Most research on prison suicide has found that the vast majority of victims are convicted of personal crimes, are housed in single cells (often some type of administrative confinement), and have histories of prior suicide attempts and/or mental illness (Daniel and Fleming 2006; He et al. 2001; Patterson and Hughes 2008; Salive et al. 1989; White and Schimmel 1995). Although normally serving long sentences, most victims commit suicide in the early stages of their prison confinement (New York State Department of Correctional Services 2002), as well as during earlier stages of disciplinary confinement (Way et al. 2007). Precipitating factors in prison suicide may include new legal problems, marital or relationship difficulties, and inmate-related conflicts (Kovasznay et al. 2004).

An inmate suicide is emotionally devastating to the victim's family and can be financially devastating to the correctional facility (and its personnel). Many inmate suicides result in litigation against a state or local jurisdiction alleging that the death was caused by the negligence and/or deliberate indifference of facility personnel. Although the plaintiff's burden to demonstrate liability in these cases remains high (Cohen 2008), several federal court jury awards have well exceeded $1 million (*Sanville v. Scaburdine* 2002; *Woodward v. Myres* 2003).

COMPREHENSIVE SUICIDE PREVENTION PROGRAMMING

The literature is replete with examples of how jail and prison systems have developed effective suicide prevention programs (Cox and Morschauser 1997; Goss et al. 2002; Hayes 1995, 2006; White and Schimmel 1995). New York experienced a significant drop in the number of jail suicides following the implementation of a statewide comprehensive prevention program (Cox and Morschauser 1997). Texas saw a 50% decrease in the number of county jail suicides, as well as almost a sixfold decrease in the rate of these suicides from 1986 through 1996, much of it attributable to increased staff training and a state requirement for jails to maintain suicide prevention policies (Hayes 1996). One researcher reported no suicides during a 7-year time period in a large county jail after the development of suicide prevention policies based on the following principles: screening; psychological support; close observation; removal of dangerous items; clear and consistent procedures; and diagnosis, treatment, and transfer of suicidal inmates to the hospital as necessary (Felthous 1994).

Comprehensive suicide prevention programming has also been advocated nationally by such organizations as the American Correctional Association, American Psychiatric Association, and National Commission on Correctional Health Care. These groups have promulgated national correctional standards that are adaptable to individual jail, prison, and juvenile facilities. Although the American Correctional Association standards are the most widely recognized throughout the United States, they provide severely limited guidance regarding suicide prevention, simply stating that institutions should have a written prevention policy that is reviewed by medical or mental health staff. The American Correctional Association's (2004) broad focus on the operation and administration of correctional facilities precludes these standards from containing needed specificity.

Both the American Psychiatric Association and National Commission on Correctional Health Care standards, however, are much more instructive and offer the recommended ingredients for a suicide prevention program: identification, training, assessment, monitoring, housing, referral, communication, intervention, notification, reporting, review, and critical incident debriefing (American Psychiatric Association 2000; National Commission on Correctional Health Care 2003, 2008). Consistent with national correctional standards, the eight components discussed below (and outlined in Table 9–1) encompass a comprehensive suicide prevention policy.

TABLE 9–1.	Components of a comprehensive suicide prevention policy

1. Staff training
2. Intake screening and assessment
3. Communication
4. Housing
5. Levels of observation
6. Intervention
7. Reporting
8. Follow-up and morbidity-mortality review

Staff Training

The essential component of any suicide prevention program is properly trained correctional staff, who form the backbone of any jail or prison facility. Very few suicides are actually prevented by mental health, medical, or other health professional staff, because suicides are usually attempted in inmate housing units, often during late evening hours or on weekends, when inmates are generally outside the purview of program staff. These incidents, therefore, must be thwarted by correctional staff who have been trained in suicide prevention and have developed an intuitive sense about the inmates under their care. Correctional officers are often the only staff available 24 hours a day; thus, they form the front line of defense in preventing suicides. However, as is true with medical and mental health personnel, correctional staff cannot detect, assess, or prevent a suicide without training. Bluntly stated, lives will be lost and jurisdictions will incur unnecessary liability from these deaths if administrators do not create and maintain effective training programs.

All staff (including correctional, medical, and mental health personnel) should receive 8 hours of initial suicide prevention training, followed by 2 hours of refresher training each year. At a minimum, initial suicide prevention training should include, but not be limited to, the following:

- Reasons why correctional environments are conducive to suicidal behavior
- Staff attitudes about suicide
- Potential predisposing factors to suicide
- High-risk suicide periods
- Warning signs and symptoms

- Identification of suicide risk despite the denial of risk
- Liability issues
- Critical incident stress debriefing (CISD)
- Recent suicides and/or serious suicide attempts within the facility or agency
- Components of the facility's or agency's suicide prevention policy

In addition, all staff who have routine contact with inmates should receive standard first aid, cardiopulmonary resuscitation (CPR), and automated external defibrillator training. All staff should also be trained in the use of various emergency equipment located in each housing unit. In an effort to ensure an efficient emergency response to suicide attempts, mock drills should be incorporated into both initial and refresher training for all staff. Table 9–2 highlights the important components of staff training for suicide prevention.

Intake Screening and Assessment

Screening and assessment of inmates when they enter a facility is critical to a correctional facility's suicide prevention efforts. Although mental health and medical communities have not agreed on a single set of risk factors that can be used to predict suicide, they agree on the value of screening and assessment in preventing suicide (Cox and Morschauser 1997; Hughes 1995). Intake screening for all inmates and ongoing assessment of inmates at risk are critical because research consistently indicates that two-thirds or more of all suicide victims communicate their intent sometime before death and that any individual with a history of one or more suicide attempts has a much greater risk for suicide than those who have never made an attempt (Clark and Horton-Deutsch 1992; Maris 1992). Although ideation, prior attempt(s), and/or other forms of suicidal behavior are indicative of current risk, other factors such as recent significant loss, limited prior incarceration, lack of social support systems, and various "stressors of confinement" can also be strongly related to suicide (Bonner 1992).

Intake screening may be contained within the medical screening form or as a separate form and should include inquiry regarding past suicidal ideation and/or attempts; current ideation, threat, and plan; prior mental health treatment/hospitalization; recent significant loss (job, relationship, death of family member or close friend, etc.); history of suicidal behavior by family member or close friend; suicide risk during prior confinement; and arresting or transporting officer(s)' belief that inmate is currently at risk. The process should also include referral procedures to mental health and/or medical personnel for assessment.

TABLE 9–2. Staff suicide prevention training

1. Suicide risk factors
2. Suicide risk factors inherent in the correctional environment
3. Analysis of staff attitudes about suicide
4. Identification of high-risk suicide periods
5. Identification of suicide warning signs and symptoms
6. Identification of suicidality despite verbal denial of risk
7. Liability issues
8. Critical incident stress debriefing
9. Discussion about completed suicides and suicide attempts in the facility
10. Discussion about sound suicide prevention practices and the facility's written suicide prevention policy

---

Following the intake process, if any staff hear an inmate verbalize a desire or intent to commit suicide, observe an inmate engaging in any self-harm, or otherwise believe an inmate is at risk for suicide, a procedure must be in place to allow the staff member to take immediate steps to ensure that the inmate is continuously observed until appropriate assistance is obtained. Important topics covered by a suicide screening form are outlined in Table 9–3.

Communication

Certain behavioral signs exhibited by an inmate may be indicative of suicidal behavior, and detection of these signs and communication of their presence to others may prevent a suicide. A communication breakdown between correctional, medical, and mental health personnel is a common factor found in the reviews of many inmate suicides (Anno 1985; Appelbaum et al. 1997; Hayes 1995). Three stages of communication are important in preventing inmate suicides: 1) communication between the arresting or transporting officer and correctional staff; 2) communication among facility staff (including correctional, medical, and mental health personnel); and 3) communication between facility staff and the suicidal inmate.

In large measure, suicide prevention begins at the point of arrest. During initial contact, what an individual says and how he or she behaves during arrest, transportation to the jail, and booking are crucial in detecting suicidal behavior. The arrest itself is often the most volatile and emotional time for the arrestee. Arresting officers should pay close attention to the

---

TABLE 9–3.   Topics of a suicide risk screening form

---

1. Past suicidal ideation and/or attempts
2. Current suicidal ideation
3. Current suicide threat
4. Current suicide plan
5. Current suicidal intent
6. Prior mental health treatment/hospitalization
7. Recent significant loss (job, relationship, death of family member or close friend, etc.)
8. Suicide risk during prior confinement
9. Arresting/transporting officer(s) view of inmate's current risk

---

arrestee during the arrest, because suicidal behavior, anxiety, and/or hopelessness of the situation might be manifested. Prior behavior can also be confirmed by onlookers such as family and friends. Any pertinent information regarding the arrestee's well-being must be communicated by the arresting or transporting officer to facility staff. As noted in the previous subsection, the intake screening form should document whether the arresting or transporting officer believes that the inmate is currently at risk for suicide. Also, facility staff must make an effort not to create barriers of communication between themselves and the inmate's inner circle of family and friends, because this group often has pertinent information regarding the current and prior mental health status of the inmate.

Because an inmate can become suicidal at any point during incarceration, correctional officers must maintain awareness, share information, and make appropriate referrals to mental health and medical staff. At a minimum, facility officials should ensure that appropriate staff are properly informed of the status of each inmate placed on suicide precautions. Multidisciplinary team meetings, to include correctional, medical, and mental health personnel, should occur on a regular basis for the team members to discuss the status of an inmate on suicide precautions. In addition, the authorization of suicide precautions for an inmate, any changes to those precautions, and observation of an inmate placed on suicide precautions should be documented on designated forms and distributed to appropriate staff.

Facility staff must also use various communication skills with the suicidal inmate, including active listening, staying with the inmate if they suspect immediate danger, and maintaining contact through conversation, eye contact, and body language.

Most importantly, correctional staff should trust their own judgment and observation of risk behavior, and avoid being misled by others (including mental health staff) into ignoring signs of suicidal behavior. Because correctional staff have the unique opportunity to observe inmate behavior over an extended period of time (e.g., an 8-hour shift, several days), they are generally in the best position to identify signs and symptoms of suicidal behavior. Mental health staff generally spend only a brief amount of time assessing an inmate's risk for suicide, and an inmate may deny or mask symptoms. For example, correctional staff sometimes place an inmate on suicide precautions after observing suicidal behavior. The inmate is then referred to mental health staff for assessment. The inmate denies any suicidal ideation, and the clinician does not observe any self-harm behavior, so the inmate is released from suicide precautions and returned to his or her housing unit. The inmate again begins to engage in suicidal behavior that is observed by an officer. Should the officer discount these observations based on the recent conclusion by mental health staff that the inmate is not suicidal? The appropriate response would be for the officer to again place the inmate on suicide precautions, document his or her observations of the suicidal behavior, refer the inmate to mental health staff for further assessment, and share his or her observations with the clinician.

Housing

Although considerable energy is often devoted to the areas of staff training, identification, assessment, and observation, less thought is given to the physical plant environment and location. Decisions regarding the location of cells designated to house suicidal inmates should be based on the ability to maximize staff interaction with those inmates. To every extent possible, suicidal inmates should be housed in the general population, mental health unit, or medical infirmary, if available, but always located close to staff. Although suicidal inmates are often housed in segregation due to better staffing ratios and the ability to better control inmate movement, this environment tends to be punitive and antitherapeutic, further escalating the inmate's sense of alienation and despair. Nor surprisingly, a disproportionate number of suicides take place in segregation units (Patterson and Hughes 2008; Way et al. 2007). Suicidal inmates should not be placed in segregation unless all other viable housing options have been exhausted.

Inmates placed on suicide precautions are frequently housed in unsafe cells. Many cells contain protrusions (i.e., anchoring devices) conducive to suicide by hanging, which is the method of choice in the overwhelming majority of inmate suicides (Hayes 1989). One study indicated that air vent grates were used in over 50% of prison suicides by hanging (He et al. 2001). Based on the first national study on juvenile suicides, Hayes (2009) reported that doorknobs/hinges (21%), air vent grates (20%), bunk frames/holes (20%), and window frames (15%) were the anchoring devices used in most youth deaths. Finally, telephones with cords of varying length located inside holding cells have been shown to be dangerous in facilitating hanging attempts (Hayes 2003a; Quinton and Dolinak 2003).

Although creating a "suicide-proof" cell environment is impossible, a correctional facility should be able to ensure that any cell used to house a potentially suicidal inmate is free of all obvious protrusions (Atlas 1989; Hayes 2003b). As a federal appeals court once stated, "It is true that prison officials are not required to build a suicide-proof jail. By the same token, however, they cannot equip each cell with a noose" (*Tittle v. Jefferson County Commission* 1992).

Levels of Observation

With regard to suicide attempts in correctional facilities, the promptness of the emergency response is often driven by the level of observation afforded the inmate. Medical experts warn that brain damage from asphyxiation caused by a suicide attempt can occur within 4 minutes, and death often takes place within 5–6 minutes (American Heart Association 1992). Standard correctional practice requires that "special management inmates," including those housed in administrative segregation, disciplinary detention, and protective custody, be observed at intervals not exceeding every 30 minutes, with mentally ill inmates observed more frequently (American Correctional Association 2004). Inmates held in medical restraints and "therapeutic seclusion" should be checked by medical personnel every 15 minutes (National Commission on Correctional Health Care 2008) and be under continuous observation of correctional staff.

Consistent with national correctional standards and practices, two levels of supervision are generally recommended for suicidal inmates: close observation and constant observation. *Close observation* is reserved for the inmate who is not actively suicidal but who expresses suicidal ideation (e.g., expressing a wish to die, without a specific threat or plan) or an inmate who has a recent prior history of self-destructive behavior. Staff should observe such an inmate at staggered intervals not to exceed every 15 minutes (e.g., 5, 10, 7 minutes). Because death from asphyxiation can occur within minutes, supervising a suicidal inmate on close observation status is effective only if the observations are at staggered time intervals and the cell is suicide resistant (i.e., free of all obvious protrusions). *Constant observation* is required for the inmate who is actively suicidal, either threatening or engaging in suicidal behavior. Staff should observe such an inmate on a continuous, uninterrupted basis.

In some jurisdictions, an intermediate level of observation is used, with monitoring at staggered intervals that do not exceed every 5 minutes. A suicidal inmate should never be placed on a 30-minute observation level, because such a time frame provides little protection for the individual. Other aids (e.g., closed-circuit television, inmate companions or watchers) can be used as a supplement to, but never as a substitute for, these observation levels. Finally, mental health staff should assess and interact with (not merely observe) suicidal inmates on a daily basis.

Intervention

Many correctional officials cling to the misguided belief that suicide prevention begins when the inmate is initially screened for suicide risk during the intake process and ends when he or she is discharged from a level of observation by mental health personnel. Suicide prevention, however, is a multidimensional issue and includes effective intervention following incidents of self-injury. More importantly, following a suicide attempt, the degree and promptness of the staff's intervention often foretell whether the victim will survive. A study of inmate suicides in a large state prison system found that first responders failed to initiate lifesaving measures in approximately 30% of the cases (Patterson and Hughes 2008). National correctional standards and practices generally acknowledge that a facility's policy regarding intervention should be threefold (National Commission on Correctional Health Care 2008): 1) all staff who come into contact with inmates should be trained in standard first aid, CPR, and automated external defibrillator procedures; 2) any staff member who discovers an inmate engaging in self-harm should immediately survey the scene to assess the severity of the emergency, alert other staff to call for medical personnel, and begin standard first aid and/or CPR as necessary; and 3) staff should never presume that the inmate is dead but rather should initiate and continue appropriate lifesaving measures until relieved by arriving medical personnel. Finally, medical personnel should ensure that all equipment used in responding to an emergency within the facility is in working order on a daily basis.

Reporting

In the event of a completed or attempted suicide, all appropriate correctional officials should be notified through the chain of command. Following the incident, the victim's family should be immediately notified, as well as appropriate outside authorities. All staff who came into contact with the victim prior to the incident should be required to submit a statement including their full knowledge of the inmate and incident.

Follow-Up and Morbidity-Mortality Review

An inmate suicide can be extremely stressful for staff. Attendant staff may feel ostracized by fellow personnel and administration officials. After a death, reasonable guilt is sometimes displayed by the officer, who wonders, "What if I had made my cell check earlier?" When crises occur and staff are affected by the traumatic event, they should receive appropriate assistance. One form of assistance is *critical incident stress debriefing*. A CISD team, consisting of professionals trained in crisis intervention and traumatic stress awareness (e.g., police officers, paramedics, firefighters, clergy, mental health personnel), offers affected staff an opportunity to process their feelings about the incident, develop an understanding of critical stress symptoms, and develop ways of dealing with those symptoms (Meehan 1997; Mitchell and Everly 1996). For maximum effectiveness, the CISD process or other appropriate support services should occur within 24–72 hours of the critical incident.

Every completed suicide, as well as each suicide attempt of high lethality (i.e., requiring emergency room treatment), should be examined through a morbidity-mortality review process. If resources permit, clinical review through a psychological autopsy is also recommended (Aufderheide 2000; Sanchez 2006). Ideally, the morbidity-mortality review should be coordinated by an outside agency to ensure impartiality. The review, separate and apart from other formal investigations that may be required to determine the cause of death, should include a critical inquiry of 1) the circumstances surrounding the incident; 2) institutional procedures relevant to the incident; 3) all relevant training received by involved staff; 4) pertinent medical and mental health services/reports involving the victim; 5) possible precipitating factors leading to the suicide or attempt; and 6) recommendations, if any, for changes in policy, training, physical plant, medical or mental health services, and operational procedures.

Quality assurance documents (i.e., morbidity-mortality reviews) generated as a result of an inmate death or injury are *not* always protected from disclosure provisions of applicable state and/or federal laws. Therefore, to better ensure that the review process is conducted with the full candor of all participants, as well as to increase the likelihood of protecting such documents from future disclosure, each morbidity-mortality review should be initiated at the request of the agency's legal counsel. In addition, any documents generated during the review should *not* be kept in an inmate's institutional or medical file. Rather, the documents should be kept separately in a quality assurance file and each page clearly labeled as follows: "Attorney-Client Privilege: This Quality Assurance Document Was Attorney Requested and Prepared in Anticipation of Possible Litigation."

GUIDING PRINCIPLES FOR SUICIDE PREVENTION

More times than not, staff do an admirable job of safely managing inmates identified as suicidal and placed on suicide precautions. After all, few inmates successfully commit suicide while on suicide watch. What staff continue to struggle with is the ability to prevent the suicide of an inmate who is not easily identifiable as being at risk for self-harm. Kay Redfield Jamison, a prominent psychologist and author, has best articulated the point by stating that if "suicidal patients were able or willing to articulate the severity of their suicidal thoughts and plans, little risk would exist" (Jamison 1999, p. 150). With this in mind, the following guiding principles to suicide prevention are offered:

1. *View the assessment of suicide risk not as a single event but as an ongoing process.* Because an inmate may become suicidal at any point during confinement, suicide prevention should begin at the point of arrest and continue until the inmate is released from the facility. In addition, once an inmate has been successfully managed on, and discharged from, suicide precautions, he or she should remain on a mental health caseload and be assessed periodically until released from the facility.

2. *View screening for suicide during the initial booking and intake process as something similar to taking one's temperature: it can identify a current fever but not a future cold.* The shelf life of behavior that is observed and/ or self-reported during intake screening is time limited, and far too much weight is often placed on this initial data collection stage. Following an inmate's suicide, the morbidity-mortality review process often focuses exclusively on whether the victim threatened suicide during the booking and intake stage, a time period that could be far removed from the date of suicide. If the victim answered in the negative to suicide risk during the booking stage, the participants of the review process often express a sense of relief and come to the misguided conclusion that the death was not preventable. Although the intake screening form remains a valuable prevention tool, the more important determination of suicide risk is the *current* behavior expressed or displayed by the inmate.

3. *Determine the inmate's prior risk of suicide.* Prior risk is strongly related to future risk. If an inmate was placed on suicide precautions during

a previous confinement in the facility or agency, that information should be made accessible to both correctional and health care personnel when determining whether the inmate might be at risk during the current confinement.

4. *Do not rely exclusively on the direct statements of an inmate who denies being suicidal and/or having a prior history of suicidal behavior, particularly when his or her behavior, actions, or history suggests otherwise.* Often, despite an inmate's denial of suicidal ideation, the individual's behavior, actions, or history speaks louder than his or her words. Consider the two examples below:

> In Washington State, an inmate being booked into a county jail informed the intake officer that she had a history of mental illness and had attempted suicide 2 weeks earlier, but "will not hurt herself in jail." Jail records indicated that the inmate threatened suicide during a recent prior confinement in the facility. The inmate attended a court hearing 2 days later, and the escort officer noticed that she appeared despondent, was crying, and appeared worried about her children. She was not referred to mental health staff or placed on suicide precautions. The inmate committed suicide the following day.

> In Michigan, police were called to the home of a man who accidentally shot and killed a friend during a domestic dispute with his estranged wife. On arrival of the police, the suspect placed a handgun to his head and clicked the trigger several times. He also encouraged the officers to shoot him. Following 5 hours of negotiations, the suspect surrendered without incident. He was transported to the county jail and denied being suicidal during the intake screening process. The inmate was not referred to mental health staff or placed on suicide precautions. He committed suicide the following day.

It is not surprising that these preventable deaths often escape detection. For example, the booking area of a jail facility is traditionally both chaotic and noisy—an environment where staff feel pressure to process a high number of arrestees in a short period of time. Two key ingredients for identifying suicidal behavior—time and privacy—are at a minimum. The ability to carefully assess the potential for suicide by asking each inmate a series of questions, interpreting his or her responses (including gauging the truthfulness of a denial of suicide risk), and observing his or her behavior is greatly compromised by an impersonal environment that lends itself to something quite the opposite. As a result, the clearly suicidal behavior of many arrestees and the circumstances that may lend themselves to potential self-injury go undetected.

In yet another example, a suicidal inmate sent to the hospital for an assessment may appear to be stable in front of an emergency room physician and even deny suicide risk, only to be discharged from the hospital and returned to the correctional facility, where he or she reverts to the same self-injurious behavior that prompted the initial referral. Given such a scenario, correctional staff should not assume that the hospital physician was cognizant or even appreciative of this cyclical behavior. On the contrary, regardless of the hospital physician's observations and/or recommendations, as well as the inmate's denial of risk, whenever staff hear an inmate verbalize a desire or intent to commit suicide, observe an inmate engaging in suicidal behavior, or otherwise believe an inmate is at risk for suicide, they should take immediate steps to ensure the inmate's safety.

5. *Arrange for meaningful preservice and annual suicide prevention training for all health care and correctional staff.* Although implementing suicide precautions for an inmate who verbally threatens suicide requires little training, identifying suicidal behavior of inmates who are unwilling or unable to articulate their feelings or who deny any ideation requires both comprehensive preservice and annual training. Simply stated, correctional staff, as well as medical and mental health personnel, cannot detect, assess, or prevent a suicide for which they have little, if any, useful training. Suicide prevention training must provide timely, long-lasting information that reflects the current knowledge base. Training should not be scheduled simply to comply with an accreditation standard. A workshop that is limited to an antiquated videotape or to recitation of the current policies and procedures might demonstrate compliance (albeit wrongly) with an accreditation standard, but it is not meaningful or helpful to the goal of reducing inmate suicides. Without regular suicide prevention training, staff often make wrong or ill-informed decisions, demonstrate inaction, become complacent, or react contrary to standard correctional practice, thereby incurring unnecessary liability.

6. *Promote and maintain communication among correctional, medical, and mental health staff.* Many preventable suicides result from poor communication among staff. Communication problems are often caused by lack of respect, personality conflicts, and other boundary issues. Simply stated, facilities that maintain a multidisciplinary approach avoid preventable suicides.

7. *Avoid creating barriers that discourage inmates from accessing mental health services.* Often, certain management conditions of a facility's policy on suicide precautions (e.g., automatic clothing removal/issuance of safety garment; lockdown; lack of visiting, telephone, and shower access) appear punitive to an inmate, as well as excessive and unrelated to his or her level of suicide risk. As a result, an inmate who becomes

suicidal and/or despondent during confinement may be reluctant to seek out mental health services, and may even deny the existence of a problem, if he or she knows that loss of basic amenities is an automatic outcome. As such, these barriers should be avoided whenever possible, and decisions regarding the management of a suicidal inmate should be based solely on the individual's level of risk.

For example, an inmate who is on suicide precautions for attempting suicide the previous day is naked except for a suicide smock, is given only finger foods, and is on lockdown status. He is housed with another inmate who is also on suicide precautions. Neither has been allowed out of the cell to shower. The mental health clinician approaches the cell and opens the food slot. The foul smell is immediate. The clinician leans down and asks the inmate, within hearing distance of everyone else on the cell block, "How are you feeling today? Still feeling suicidal? Can you contract for safety?" When the inmate responds, the clinician cannot know whether the response is based on suicidal ideation or influenced by the current environment. Most importantly, these circumstances complicate the clinician's job of conducting an accurate suicide risk assessment.

Although suicidal inmates need to be safely managed, health care and correctional personnel also need to make better decisions to avoid what appear to be punitive responses to self-injurious behavior. These measures are often taken to discourage inmates perceived as manipulative from threatening or engaging in self-harm, but they may inadvertently discourage suicidal inmates from coming forward for help.

At a minimum, inmates on suicide precautions should receive showers, access to telephone calls, legal and family visits, and other routine privileges commensurate with their classification status. Some would argue that telephone calls and legal and family visits might precipitate a suicide attempt; however, allowing these activities for an inmate on suicide precautions enables staff to monitor the inmate's reaction to negative news.

8. *Base decisions regarding the management of a suicidal inmate on the individual's clinical needs, not simply on the resources that are said to be available.* For example, if an acutely suicidal inmate requires continuous, uninterrupted observation from staff, he or she should not be monitored via closed-circuit cameras simply because that is the only option the system chooses to offer. A clinician should never feel pressured by correctional staff, however subtle that pressure may be, to prematurely downgrade, discharge, and/or change the management plan for a suicidal inmate because additional staff resources (e.g., overtime) are required to maintain the desired level of observation.

9. *Be aware of inmates perceived to be manipulative.* Some inmates threaten suicide or even feign a suicide attempt to avoid a court appearance or bolster an insanity defense; gain cell relocation, transfer to the local hospital, or simply preferential staff treatment; or seek compassion from a previously unsympathetic spouse or other family member. Some inmates simply use manipulation as a survival technique. Although the prevailing theory is that any inmate who would go to the extreme of threatening suicide or even engaging in self-injurious behavior has at least an emotional imbalance that requires special attention, too often the conclusion is that the inmate is simply attempting to manipulate his or her environment and, therefore, that such behavior should be ignored and not reinforced through intervention. Sometimes, however, a "feigned" suicide attempt goes further than anticipated and results in death. Recent research indicates that staff should not assume that inmates who appear manipulative are not also suicidal—those two behaviors are not mutually exclusive (Dear et al. 2000). Although no easy solutions exist to the management of manipulative inmates who threaten suicide or engage in self-injurious behavior for a perceived secondary gain, the critical issue is not how staff label the behavior, but how they react to it. The reaction (i.e., intervention) must include a multidisciplinary treatment plan.

10. *Be especially vigilant about the potential for suicidal behavior by inmates housed in special units.* As previously noted, few suicides take place when inmates are managed on suicide precautions. Rather, most suicides take place in various forms of (often locked down) special housing units (e.g., intake/booking, classification, disciplinary/administrative segregation, mental health) of the facility. One effective prevention strategy is to create more interaction between inmates and correctional, medical, and mental health personnel in these housing areas by increasing rounds of medical and/or mental health staff, in which these personnel walk up to each cell, attempt to briefly converse with the inmate, and observe his or her behavior; requiring regular follow-up of all inmates released from suicide precautions; increasing rounds of correctional staff; and avoiding lockdown due to staff shortages (and the resulting limited access of medical and mental health personnel to the units).

11. *Avoid interpreting a lack of inmates on suicide precautions as meaning that no suicidal inmates are currently in the facility or as representing a barometer of sound suicide prevention practices.* Correctional facilities contain suicidal inmates every day; the challenge is to find them. The goal should not be to have *no* inmates on suicide precautions; rather, the goal should be to identify, manage, and stabilize suicidal inmates.

12. *Avoid using the terms "watch closely" or "keep an eye on him" when describing an inmate who is of concern but not placed on suicide precautions.* For example, when a correctional facility receives a telephone call from an inmate's family member who states, "Please watch my husband closely; he sounded very depressed on the phone and might do something stupid," the typical response is, "Sure, we'll watch him closely" or "We'll keep an eye on him." Such casual statements rarely result in increased observation. If there is concern that an inmate may be at risk for suicide, the inmate should be on suicide precautions or at least referred immediately to a mental health clinician for a thorough assessment.

13. *Create and maintain sound suicide prevention programming.* Such programming should include the eight essential components described earlier in this chapter (see Table 9–1). It should also include a comprehensively written suicide prevention policy that is reviewed and adhered to by all correctional, medical, and mental health personnel in the facility. Some jurisdictions maintain suicide prevention committees that regularly review recent suicides and serious suicide attempts, develop corrective action plans, review and revise policies, develop and implement auditing tools to measure effectiveness of suicide prevention practices, and collaborate on and design meaningful training programs.

14. *Avoid the obstacles to prevention.* Experience has shown that negative attitudes often impede meaningful suicide prevention efforts. Obstacles to prevention often embody a state of mind that unconditionally implies that inmate suicides cannot be prevented (e.g., "If someone really wants to kill themselves, there's generally nothing you can do about it"). Of the numerous ways to overcome these obstacles, the most powerful is to demonstrate prevention programs that have effectively reduced the incidence of suicide and suicidal behavior within correctional facilities. As one administrator offered, "When you begin to use excuses to justify a bad outcome, whether it be low staffing levels, inadequate funding, physical plant concerns, etc., issues we struggle with each day, you lack the philosophy that even one death is not acceptable. If you are going to tolerate a few deaths in your jail system, then you've already lost the battle" (Hayes 1998, p. 6).

CONCLUSION

Hundreds of inmates continue to commit suicide in jail and prison facilities each year. Despite increased general awareness of the problem, research that has identified precipitating and situational risk factors, emerging correctional standards that advocate increased attention to suicidal inmates, and demonstration of effective strategies, prevention remains piecemeal and inmate suicides continue to pose a serious public health problem within correctional facilities. Although not all inmate suicides are preventable, many are, and the challenge for those who work in the correctional system is to conceptualize the issue as demanding a continuum of comprehensive suicide prevention services aimed at the collaborative identification, continued assessment, and safe management of inmates at risk for self-harm.

SUMMARY POINTS

- Suicide assessment is an ongoing process.
- Suicide risk screening at intake is important, but *current* behavior is more significant.
- Prior suicide risk is strongly related to future risk.
- A clinician cannot rely exclusively on an inmate's denial of suicidality. Behavior, actions, and history are extremely important.
- Meaningful preservice and annual suicide prevention training should be provided to all health care and correctional staff.
- Communication among correctional, medical, and mental health staff is critical.
- Staff must avoid creating barriers that discourage inmates from accessing mental health services.
- Basic decisions regarding the management of a suicidal inmate should be based on the individual's clinical needs, not simply on the resources that are said to be available.
- An inmate who appears manipulative may also be suicidal.
- Most suicides occur in special housing units and not while inmates are on suicide precautions.
- A lack of inmates on suicide precautions does not mean that a facility currently has no suicidal inmates in the facility or that sound suicide prevention practices are in place.
- Comprehensive suicide prevention training must be in place.

REFERENCES

American Correctional Association: Performance-Based Standards for Adult Local Detention Facilities, 4th Edition. Lanham, MD, American Correctional Association, 2004

American Heart Association, Emergency Cardiac Care Committee and Subcommittees: Guidelines for cardiopulmonary resuscitation and emergency cardiac care. JAMA 268:2172–2183, 1992

American Psychiatric Association: Psychiatric Services in Jails and Prisons: A Task Force Report of the American Psychiatric Association, 2nd Edition. Washington, DC, American Psychiatric Association, 2000

Anno B: Patterns of suicide in the Texas Department of Corrections, 1980–1985. J Prison Jail Health 5:82–93, 1985

Appelbaum K, Dvoskin J, Geller J, et al: Report on the Psychiatric Management of John Salvi in Massachusetts Department of Corrections Facilities: 1995–1996. Worcester, MA, University of Massachusetts Medical Center, 1997

Atlas R: Reducing the opportunity for inmate suicide: a design guide. Psychiatr Q 60:161–171, 1989

Aufderheide D: Conducting the psychological autopsy in correctional settings. J Correction Health Care 7:5–36, 2000

Bonner R: Isolation, seclusion, and psychological vulnerability as risk factors for suicide behind bars, in Assessment and Prediction of Suicide. Edited by Maris R, Berman A, Maltsberger J. New York, Guilford, 1992, pp 398–419

Bonner R: Correctional suicide prevention in the year 2000 and beyond. Suicide Life Threat Behav 30:370–376, 2000

Clark D, Horton-Deutsch S: Assessment in absentia: the value of the psychological autopsy method for studying antecedents of suicide and predicting future suicides, in Assessment and Prediction of Suicide. Edited by Maris R, Berman A, Maltsberger J. New York, Guilford, 1992, pp 144–182

Cohen F: The Mentally Disordered Inmate and the Law, 2nd Edition. Kingston, NJ, Civic Research Institute, 2008

Cox J, Morschauser P: A solution to the problem of jail suicide. Crisis 18:178–184, 1997

Daniel A, Fleming J: Suicides in a state correctional system, 1992–2002: a review. J Correction Health Care 12:24–35, 2006

Davis M, Muscat J: An epidemiologic study of alcohol and suicide risk in Ohio jails and lockups, 1975–1984. J Crim Justice 21:277–283, 1993

Dear G, Thomson D, Hills A: Self-harm in prison: manipulators can also be suicide attempters. Crim Justice Behav 27:160–175, 2000

DuRand C, Burtka G, Federman E, et al: A quarter century of suicide in a major urban jail: implications for community psychiatry. Am J Psychiatry 152:1077–1080, 1995

Felthous A: Preventing jailhouse suicides. Bull Am Acad Psychiatry Law 22:477–488, 1994

Goss J, Peterson K, Smith L, et al: Characteristics of suicide attempts in a large urban jail system with an established suicide prevention program. Psychiatr Serv 53:574–579, 2002

Hayes L: National study of jail suicides: seven years later. Psychiatr Q 60:7–29, 1989

Hayes L: Model suicide prevention programs, part III. Jail Suicide/Mental Health Update 8:1–7, 1998

Hayes L: Prison suicide: an overview and guide to prevention. Prison J 75:431–456, 1995

Hayes L: Jail standards and suicide prevention: another look. Jail Suicide/Mental Health Update 6:9–11, 1996

Hayes L: A jail cell, two deaths, and a telephone cord. Jail Suicide/Mental Health Update 11:1–8, 2003a

Hayes L: Suicide prevention and protrusion-free design of correctional facilities. Jail Suicide/Mental Health Update 12:1–5, 2003b

Hayes L: Juvenile suicide in confinement: a national survey. Washington, DC, U.S. Department of Justice, Office of Juvenile Justice and Delinquency Prevention, 2009

He XY, Felthous AR, Holzer CE 3rd, et al: Factors in prison suicide: one year study in Texas. J Forensic Sci 46:896–901, 2001

Hughes D: Can the clinician predict suicide? Psychiatr Serv 46:449–451, 1995

Jamison K: Night Falls Fast: Understanding Suicide. New York, Knopf, 1999

Kovasznay B, Miraglia R, Beer R, et al: Reducing suicides in New York State correctional facilities. Psychiatr Q 75:61–70, 2004

Marcus P, Alcabes P: Characteristics of suicides by inmates in an urban jail. Hosp Community Psychiatry 44:256–261, 1993

Maris R: Overview of the study of suicide assessment and prediction, in Assessment and Prediction of Suicide. Edited by Maris R, Berman A, Maltsberger J. New York, Guilford, 1992, pp 3–22

Meehan B: Critical incident stress debriefing within the jail environment. Jail Suicide/Mental Health Update 7:1–5, 1997

Mitchell J, Everly G: Critical Incident Stress Debriefing: An Operations Manual for the Prevention of Traumatic Stress Among Emergency Services and Disaster Workers, 2nd Edition. Ellicott City, MD, Chevron Publishing, 1996

Mumola C, Noonan M: Deaths in custody statistical tables. Washington, DC, U.S. Department of Justice, Office of Justice Programs, Bureau of Justice Statistics, July 2007

National Commission on Correctional Health Care: Correctional Mental Health Care: Standards and Guidelines for Delivering Services, 2nd Edition. Chicago, National Commission on Correctional Health Care, 2003

National Commission on Correctional Health Care: Standards for Health Services in Jails, 8th Edition. Chicago, National Commission on Correctional Health Care, 2008

New York State Department of Correctional Services: Inmate Suicide Report, 1995–2001. Albany, NY, New York State Department of Correctional Services, 2002

Patterson RF, Hughes K: Review of completed suicides in the California Department of Corrections and Rehabilitation, 1999 to 2004. Psychiatr Serv 59:676–682, 2008

Quinton R, Dolinak D: Suicidal hangings in jail using telephone cords. J Forensic Sci 48:1151–1152, 2003

Salive M, Smith G, Brewer T: Suicide mortality in the Maryland state prison system, 1979 through 1987. JAMA 262:365–369, 1989

Sanchez H: Inmate suicide and the psychological autopsy process. Jail Suicide/ Mental Health Update 15:5–11, 2006

Sanville v Scaburdine, U.S. District Court, Eastern District of Wisconsin, Case No. 99-C-715, 2002

Tittle v Jefferson County Commission, 966 F.2d 606 (11th Cir. 1992)

Way BB, Sawyer DA, Barboza S, et al: Inmate suicide and time spent in special disciplinary housing in New York State prison. Psychiatr Serv 58:558–560, 2007

White T, Schimmel D: Suicide prevention in federal prisons: a successful five-step program, in Prison Suicide: An Overview and Guide to Prevention. Edited by Hayes L. Washington, DC, National Institute of Corrections, U.S. Department of Justice, 1995, pp 46–57

Winkler G: Assessing and responding to suicidal jail inmates. Community Ment Health J 28:317–326, 1992

Woodward v Myres, U.S. District Court, Northern District of Illinois, Case No. 00-C-6010, 2003

CHAPTER 10

Assessment of Malingering in Correctional Settings

Michael J. Vitacco, Ph.D.
Richard Rogers, Ph.D., ABPP

Mental health professionals working in correctional settings are often asked to perform clinical assessments in which the determination of malingering is a critical component. To assist in this diagnostic endeavor, clinicians have an array of standardized measures at their disposal. However, a general awareness of assessment methods is insufficient. Instead, correctional psychiatrists and psychologists must possess in-depth theoretical knowledge of malingering and a conceptually sound understanding of its assessment.

In this chapter, we provide a substantive update from our chapter in the first edition of this book. We summarize recent advances, including new findings from the third edition of *Clinical Assessment of Malingering and Deception* (Rogers 2008) and recent studies on the validity and effectiveness of malingering screens (Vitacco et al. 2007), and provide in-depth knowledge on how models of malingering are applicable to the correctional environment. We also provide practical recommendations based on recent research aimed at improving assessments of malingering within correctional settings.

Rogers (1997) developed a general model for understanding why some examinees are honest and forthcoming whereas others engage in various forms of deception. Four principles of this model are germane to the frequent deception observed in correctional settings: agency, confidentiality, social control, and value imposition (see examples in Table 10–1). In a correctional setting, deception is likely to occur when referred inmates perceive situations as antagonistic or feel that clinicians are not working in their best interest.

MISCLASSIFICATION OF MALINGERING IN CORRECTIONAL SETTINGS

According to the *Diagnostic and Statistical Manual of Mental Disorders*, 4th Edition, Text Revision (DSM-IV-TR; American Psychiatric Association 2000, p. 739), malingering should be "strongly suspected if any combination of the following is noted":

1. Medicolegal context of presentation
2. Marked discrepancy between the person's claimed stress or disability and the objective finding
3. Lack of cooperation during the diagnostic evaluation and in complying with the prescribed treatment program
4. The presence of antisocial personality disorder

The four indicators lack empirical support. Although the marked discrepancy mentioned in criterion 2 is promising, it is too impermissibly vague to be clinically applicable. For instance, an inmate denying any psychological problems might paradoxically be considered a possible malingerer.

The lack of empirical support for the DSM-IV-TR indicators leads to a large number of false positives if the indicators are used to diagnose malingering. Rogers (1997) reported that "for every malingerer correctly identified, nearly four times as many bona fide patients were miscategorized as malingerers" (p. 9). A close examination of the DSM-IV-TR criteria suggests that a large majority of inmates would at some time be considered to be malingering. As noted by Gerson (2002), the DSM indicators were never intended to be used to diagnose or classify malingering. Unfortunately, the criteria present in DSM-IV-TR almost ensure their misuse. Correctional clinicians must be aware of misuses of malingering criteria and should be concerned that mislabeling an inmate as deceptive has potentially devastating consequences for an inmate who is denied needed treatment after being misclassified as malingering.

TABLE 10–1. Correctional situations that increase the risk of inmate deception
Clinicians appear to be working more for the institution than for the patients (*agency*).
Patients' disclosures can potentially be used against them (*lack of confidentiality*).
Clinicians are perceived as restricting patients' freedoms and even imposing sanctions (*social control*).
Clinicians do not respect patients' autonomy but seek to induce mainstream values (*value imposition*).

EXPLANATORY MODELS OF MALINGERING AND THEIR USE IN CORRECTIONAL SETTINGS

Rogers (1990, 2008) described three models—pathogenic, criminological, and adaptational—that are useful for generating hypotheses explaining potential motivations for malingering. Table 10–2 summarizes key aspects of the three models.

According to the *pathogenic model*, which provided the earliest explanation, underlying psychopathology is the primary motivation for malingering. The pathogenic model predicts that as the malingerer's functioning continues to deteriorate, the voluntary feigning of symptoms will gradually be replaced by genuine involuntary symptoms. Although the pathogenic model is still useful to understanding malingering in a very small minority of cases, it has fallen into disfavor and has been replaced by two markedly contrasting perspectives: the criminological (DSM-IV-TR) and adaptational models.

The *criminological model*, consistent with DSM-IV-TR, assumes that malingering is a deliberate antisocial act, which is often associated with antisocial personality disorder. In devising this list, the DSM-IV-TR work group made a fundamental error on the first two indicators. In criminal-forensic and correctional settings, antisocial personality disorder and forensic contexts are common characteristics; therefore, they cannot discriminate between malingered and genuine presentations (Rogers 2008). Kucharski et al. (2006) confirmed that use of antisocial personality disorder as an indicator of malingering would result in a large number of false-positive errors. Their findings underscore the point that being placed in a correctional setting cannot be used to diagnose malingering.

The criminological model has not been adequately validated and lacks specificity. As noted by Rogers and Vitacco (2002), reliance on this model

TABLE 10–2. Explanatory models for malingering

Model	Description	Cons	Pros
Pathogenic	Views psychopathology as the primary motivation for malingering	Has fallen out of favor in recent years for better-validated models	Continues to be relevant in explaining malingering in a small number of cases
Criminological	Views malingering as stemming from antisocial attitudes	Can lead to countertransference and a large number of false positives	Is applicable when the goal of the malingering is to frustrate staff or in some instances of medication seeking
Adaptational	Views malingering as a generally normative reaction to a difficult situation	Results in small possibility of misinterpreting malingerer's motives	Has empirical support and decreases the chance for inappropriate cynicism

would lead to an unacceptable false-positive rate. A further problem of the criminological model is its potential for unintended but corrosive effects on professional–inmate relationships. Its misplaced emphasis on antisocial acts can cause psychiatrists and other clinical staff to have a problematic level of cynicism toward inmates that may lead to the minimization or outright dismissal of legitimate mental health complaints. As reported by Rogers and Vitacco (2002), clinicians commit an *ad hominem fallacy* if they infer that most inmates with antisocial personality disorder, because of their criminal backgrounds, are misrepresenting their reports. In such instances, personal feelings and biases about inmates may override objective findings and assessment data. Moreover, overreliance on the criminological model may create countertransference, a related obstacle to effective clinical practice. Negative feelings about being fooled and misled can interfere with professional duties. Countertransference is sometimes expressed via nonclinical descriptive terms such as *liar, fraud,* or *faker* when referring to inmates who are possibly malingering. We encourage correctional psychiatrists and psychologists to be aware of their countertransference and avoid nonclinical and potentially derogatory terms.

The criminological model is applicable in a minority of cases—those in which malingering is simply one component of deceptive acts aimed to achieve antisocial objectives. In institutional settings, such cases are especially evident when the deception is goal directed, with one objective being to frustrate staff or test staff–patient boundaries. The following vignette illustrates such a case.

Clinical Case 10–1

Mr. W, a 27-year-old male, was sentenced to 15 years for drug possession and delivery. Once in the institution, he began reporting a variety of atypical Axis I symptoms, including vivid visual hallucinations. He also claimed insomnia as a consequence of his severe symptoms. His efforts were rewarded with psychotropic and sleep medications. His antisocial and narcissistic motivations became transparent when he was 1) overheard bragging about his ability to con staff and 2) observed selling his medications to other inmates. Psychological assessment and observations revealed that his psychotic symptoms were fabricated. Once all medications were discontinued and he was confronted about his malingering, Mr. W queried, "What took you so long to figure this out?"

The *adaptational model* (Rogers and Cavanaugh 1983) assumes that malingering is a response to adverse and adversarial situations. For example, a pretrial detainee may malinger a mental disorder as an attempt to delay the trial (e.g., by being found incompetent to stand trial) or to avoid a conviction (e.g., through an insanity acquittal). For those being sentenced, malingering may be motivated by a desire to be moved to a mental health unit that is both more calming and less dangerous. The stakes for malingering may be very high, such as for sex offenders facing a potential lifelong civil commitment (Novak et al. 2007) or California's three-strikes law, which results in very lengthy prison sentences (Jaffe and Sharma 1998). In these circumstances, individuals may view malingering as the best or only opportunity to extricate themselves. As an extreme example, an individual may malinger a psychotic disorder or severe cognitive impairment to avoid the death penalty. The following vignette provides an example of the adaptational model in the context of malingering.

Clinical Case 10–2

Mr. D, a 36-year-old male, was placed in jail awaiting trial after being charged with assault and battery that allegedly occurred during a fight at a local tavern. He has a lengthy history of arrests for a variety of offenses, including assaults, most of which occurred when he was intoxicated. Given his lengthy history of arrests, the defendant faces punishment as a habitual offender, which will likely result in a 10-year enhanced sentence. He sees malingering as his only opportunity to avoid a lengthy incarceration. He claims that at the time of the offense, he was experiencing command hallucinations ordering him to harm the victim. In this unsophisticated attempt at malingering, the defendant described intense tactile and visual hallucinations. His responses to these putative hallucinations were overly dramatic, with fearful screams. On psychological testing, the defendant's unsophisticated efforts at malingering were readily detected.

In contrast to the other two models, the adaptational model has empirical support and several advantages. In a naturalistic study by Walters (1988), inmates were able to alter their test results based on their desired outcome. For instance, they were able to feign severe impairment to obtain a single cell or better adjustment if their goal was parole. An advantage of the adaptational model is that it may assist in perspective taking in attempting to understand a feigning inmate and his or her predicament. Perspective taking may serve to minimize countertransference and its negative effects on assessment and treatment. In most instances, the adaptational model is preferred over other models for the understanding and assessment of malingering in a correctional context.

DETECTION STRATEGIES FOR THE ASSESSMENT OF MALINGERED MENTAL DISORDERS

The clinical interview forms the core of assessment procedures for psychiatrists and other mental health professionals (Jackson and Vitacco, in press). Correctional psychiatrists and other clinicians can integrate common detection strategies into their interviews. To do so, mental health professionals must be knowledgeable about detection strategies and their implementation. However, we wish to caution clinicians that the use of detection strategies via clinical interviews is only a first step in the detection of feigning. If interviews suggest feigning, the inmate should be referred for a more thorough assessment with standardized instruments. Therefore, the evaluation of malingering in correctional settings should be considered a multistep process that includes 1) clinical interviews, 2) well-validated screens of potential feigning, and 3) comprehensive assessment of both malingering and genuine disorders. (For a comprehensive review of detection strategies, see Rogers 2008.)

Common strategies for detecting feigned mental disorders include the following:

1. *Rare symptoms.* Malingerers are often unaware of which symptoms occur very infrequently among patients with genuine disorders. The rare symptoms strategy can be used when a patient reports highly infrequent symptoms (e.g., "thought extraction," whereby an inmate claims his or her ideas are being routinely stolen by some external force). This strategy has consistently yielded high effect sizes between feigned and genuine samples.
2. *Improbable symptoms.* Approximately one-third of malingerers dramatically overplay their presentations and present improbable symptoms that have a bizarre or fantastic quality. Resnick (2007) listed improbable symptoms as a key strategy for detecting feigned psychotic disorders (see also Pollock 1998). An example of an improbable symptom would be a pretrial defendant's claim that Satan is hovering above the judge's bench and lip-synching the judge's statements. Unlike rare symptoms, these symptoms often have an absurd quality.
3. *Symptom combinations.* Many malingerers do not consider which common symptoms are unlikely to occur together. For example, grandiose beliefs and purging are an unlikely symptom combination. This strategy is sophisticated because malingerers are unlikely to know which symptom groupings are unusual.
4. *Symptom severity.* Persons with genuine disorders experience symptoms on a continuum ranging from mild to moderate or even severe.

Individuals feigning mental disorders often report most symptoms in the severe or extreme range. However, some individuals with legitimate mental disorders sometimes use this approach, commonly referred to as "gilding the lily," to ensure they receive treatment. Inmates may rightly or wrongly surmise that only the most severe disorders are likely to receive treatment.

5. *Indiscriminant symptom endorsement.* During clinical interviews, when queried broadly about psychopathology, some malingerers report symptoms from practically every diagnostic category. Because of comorbidity, the description of many symptoms is not, by itself, indicative of malingering. Rather, the pervasive reporting of symptoms characterizes the strategy of indiscriminant symptom endorsement.

6. *Obvious versus subtle symptoms.* As noted by Rogers (2008), obvious symptoms have a clear connection to the presence of a disorder. In contrast, subtle symptoms may or may not be considered part of a mental disorder. Considering each type can be an effective method to detect malingering; malingerers often overreport both to varying degrees.

7. *Reported versus observed symptoms.* Malingerers may demonstrate marked disparities between observed presentations and self-reports. The self-reports tend to be more pathological than the clinical observations. This detection strategy is especially effective in inpatient or correctional settings where a patient or inmate is under frequent observation. As a note of caution, some individuals with mental disorders often have little to no insight regarding their diagnoses.

In addition to the seven previously described detection strategies, correctional professionals must be aware of additional strategies that are useful in the detection of malingering. As outlined by Rogers (2008), detection strategies are typically specific to a single domain: feigned mental disorders, feigned cognitive impairment, and feigned medical complaints. Staying with feigned mental disorders, additional strategies include the following:

- *Quasi-rare symptoms.* These symptoms and associated features are almost never observed in community (i.e., nonclinical) samples yet are found in some individuals with genuine mental disorders. Despite its potential for error (i.e., by miscategorizing genuine presentations as feigning), this strategy produces moderate to large effect sizes.
- *Spurious patterns of psychopathology.* By examining complex patterns of responses on well-established scales, a clinician can see if the pattern is very atypical for genuine patients. This strategy's application is cur-

rently limited to the Personality Assessment Inventory (Morey 1991) and requires large data sets for its development and validation.

• *Erroneous stereotypes*. This strategy identifies likely malingerers based on their extreme reporting of common misperceptions about mental disorders. Their reporting of erroneous stereotypes is far greater than the level of reporting by those with genuine disorders.

SCREENING MEASURES DESIGNED TO DETECT MALINGERED PSYCHOPATHOLOGY

Mental health staff who work on correctional admission units are often inundated with new inmates with a variety of mental health complaints. Clinicians may not have time to conduct comprehensive assessments of response styles on every inmate who enters the institution. A recent trend in correctional practice is the use of screens for malingered presentations. As noted by Smith (2008), three measures have garnered the most research: the Miller Forensic Assessment of Symptoms Test (M-FAST; Miller 2001), the Structured Inventory of Malingered Symptomatology (SIMS; Widows and Smith 2005), and the M Test (Beaber et al. 1985). The following subsections provide a synopsis of these three screens, with an outline of their respective advantages and disadvantages in correctional or clinical practice.

Miller Forensic Assessment of Symptoms Test

The M-FAST (Miller 2001) is a brief 25-question structured interview designed to screen for malingered mental disorders. It consists of a total score and seven individual scales. Recently, a confirmatory factor analytic study of the M-FAST (Vitacco et al. 2008) concluded that the test was best understood by a single, parsimonious factor labeled "spurious presentation," created by summing all 25 items. On the basis of this and other research, the total score on the M-FAST adequately captures blatant attempts at malingering.

Strengths

• The M-FAST relies on well-established detection strategies in screening for malingered presentation.
• It had large to very large effect sizes when tested in two studies (Jackson et al. 2005; Vitacco et al. 2007) using known-group designs.
• Strong reliability was reported for both total and scale scores (Miller 2001; Vitacco et al. 2007).
• Interview format makes for easy administration and avoids any problems that an inmate may have with reading comprehension.

Weaknesses

- Three of the seven scales possess only one item, thus limiting their effectiveness. As noted, however, the total M-FAST score is the most effective in screening for malingering.
- Confirmatory factor analytic results by Vitacco et al. (2008) indicate that the M-FAST lacks detection strategies when an inmate engages in subtle efforts at malingering. Detection strategies for subtle efforts are available in more comprehensive measures (e.g., the Structured Interview of Reported Symptoms [Rogers et al. 1992a]).
- Given its interview format and established detection strategies, the M-FAST is sometimes misused by clinicians as a comprehensive measure of malingering. By design, the M-FAST should only be used to screen for malingering; elevated scores indicate that a more in-depth evaluation is needed. Its misuse as more than a screen constitutes substandard practice.

Structured Inventory of Malingered Symptomatology

The SIMS (Widows and Smith 2005) is a 75-item paper-and-pencil measure designed to assess various aspects of malingering. The SIMS has five overlapping scales designed to assess different areas of malingering: Low Intelligence, Affective Disorders, Neurological Impairment, Psychosis, and Amnesia.

Strengths

- Various studies (Edens et al. 2007; Lewis et al. 2002; Smith and Burger 1997; Vitacco et al. 2007) found that the SIMS total score demonstrates good ability to classify likely malingerers.
- As noted by Vitacco et al. (2007), several individual scales performed exceptionally well in a known-group design.
- The SIMS is well validated with both simulation and known-group designs (see Edens et al. 2007; Rogers et al. 2005).
- The SIMS was found useful as a screen for malingering in adolescent offenders (Rogers et al. 1995).
- The inventory is easy to read and can be administered in small groups, which is advantageous on admission units with scarce professional resources.

Weaknesses

- The self-report format may lead to missing important interpersonal components of an inmate's feigned presentation.
- The usefulness of SIMS as a screen for feigned cognitive impairment has not been sufficiently studied, despite the inclusion of scales that purportedly screen for feigned low intelligence and neurological impairment. Further research is needed on the ability of SIMS scales to detect feigned neuropsychological deficits.
- Clinical utility of the SIMS is hindered by its positive relationship with genuine psychopathology (Edens et al. 1999). Some items may not distinguish between genuine and feigned presentations.

M Test

The M Test (Beaber et al. 1985) is a 33-item true-false test designed to detect malingered mental disorders, with a specific focus on psychotic symptoms. The M Test contains three scales: C (confusion), S (genuine symptoms associated with schizophrenia), and M (bogus symptoms). The M Test has been in use for over 20 years.

Strengths

- Extensive research is available on the validity and utility of the M Test (see Smith 2008).
- A revised scoring system was developed that demonstrates moderate utility (see Rogers et al. 1992b).
- Quick and simple administration is advantageous for small group administration in busy correctional settings.

Weaknesses

- The self-report format of the M Test may lead to missing important interpersonal components of an inmate's feigned presentation.
- Reported high false-positive rates (Smith et al. 1993) and varied utility estimates (Smith 2008) minimize its usefulness as a screen for malingering.
- Recent research on the M Test has been limited. One published study (Miller 2005) found the M Test to be less effective for screening for malingering than the M-FAST.

INSTRUMENTS FOR COMPREHENSIVE EVALUATIONS OF MALINGERING

Space allotment prevents adequate discussion of all the measures designed for the detection of malingering. In this chapter, we focus on one fully structured interview, the Structured Interview of Reported Symptoms (SIRS; Rogers et al. 1992a), and two multiscale inventories, the Minnesota Multiphasic Personality Inventory, 2nd Edition (MMPI-2; Butcher et al. 1989), and the Personality Assessment Inventory (PAI; Morey 1991). In the first edition of this book, we also considered the Millon Clinical Multiaxial Inventory–III (MCMI-III; Millon et al. 1997). Given the relative absence of recent studies, we do not discuss the MCMI-III in this text. Psychiatrists and psychologists should choose measures other than the MCMI-III when the issue of malingering is being considered.

Structured Interview of Reported Symptoms

The SIRS (Rogers et al. 1992a) is a structured interview designed specifically for the assessment of feigning and related response styles. The SIRS consists of eight primary scales and relies on empirically validated strategies, many of which were described in the earlier section on detection strategies. A confirmatory factor analysis of the SIRS (Rogers et al. 2005) found that its underlying scales were represented by two dimensions: spurious and plausible detection strategies. *Spurious strategies,* by their presence, indicate feigned disorders; these items are rarely reported by genuine patients. In contrast, *plausible strategies* are found in both genuine and feigned samples; they are distinguished by the matter of degree. In other words, spurious strategies focus on the content of the clinical presentation (e.g., rare symptoms), whereas plausible strategies focus on the magnitude of the presentation (e.g., symptom severity).

Strengths

- The SIRS can be administered and interpreted by psychologists and psychiatrists.
- The SIRS is a highly reliable measure that has been extensively validated (see Rogers 2001, 2008) using a variety of research designs with clinical, correctional, and forensic samples. An extensively updated SIRS manual is due to be published in late 2009.
- The SIRS scales consistently differentiate between honest responders and feigners. In many studies (see Rogers 2008), the SIRS has been used as the gold standard for research on feigned mental disorders.

Weaknesses

- By design, the SIRS is intended to be an important component in the assessment of feigned mental disorders; however, it should be used in conjunction with other validated methods.
- Recent data suggest that the SIRS may be less effective with highly traumatized and dissociative inpatients. In such cases, additional data and the use of the relatively new SIRS Traumatic Index are essential to minimize false positives.

Minnesota Multiphasic Personality Inventory, 2nd Edition

The MMPI-2 (Butcher et al. 1989) is a 567-item true-false instrument designed to assess psychopathology and response styles. For these purposes, it is the most widely researched multiscale inventory (Greene 2008). The MMPI-2 employs standardized and specialized scales for the assessment of feigned psychopathology. In the most comprehensive study of the MMPI-2 and malingering, Rogers et al. (2003) conducted an extensive meta-analysis that included 65 MMPI-2 feigning studies. An important finding of the meta-analysis was the lack of consensus on cut scores for different MMPI-2 feigning scales. In general, the wide range of cut scores diminishes the clinical usefulness of the MMPI-2 because it reflects a divergence of research findings. To reduce false positives, clinicians should only use cut scores in the upper ranges (Rogers 2003). Several MMPI-2 validity scales yield only modest effect sizes. Despite these concerns, the MMPI-2 is frequently employed as part of a formal battery to detect feigned mental disorders and feigned cognitive impairment (Greve et al. 2006).

Strengths

- An extensive database exists on the effectiveness of specific MMPI-2 validity scales (Rogers et al. 2003).
- The validity scales represent several well-designed detection strategies.
- The scales have been tested on the feigning of specific disorders, such as schizophrenia, posttraumatic stress disorder, and depression.

Weaknesses

- Because only extreme elevations can be interpreted accurately, the MMPI-2 validity scales often miss likely feigners.

- Validity scales have substantial overlap with each other and with scales measuring psychopathology. Psychiatrists and psychologists should be aware that findings from overlapping may not be independent.
- The MMPI-2 requires a seventh-grade reading level and sustained ability to attend to content for 567 items, which may require up to 2 hours of concentration. Both factors limit its usability with a substantial majority of inmates. Moreover, the effects of learning disabilities, common to correctional populations, need full investigation as they relate to the detection of response styles.

Personality Assessment Inventory

The PAI (Morey 1991) is a 344-item multiscale inventory that has garnered significant attention as an assessment measure for psychopathology and malingering. Unlike the MMPI-2, the PAI has only three scales for assessing feigned mental disorders: Negative Impression Management, which was designed to capitalize on rare symptoms; the Malingering Index, which focuses on complex symptom patterns that are atypical of genuine patients; and the Rogers Discriminant Function, which is a strictly empirical approach that evaluates probable feigning using complex symptom patterns. For a detailed review of PAI malingering studies, see Sellbom and Bagby (2008).

Strengths

- The PAI has a simple reading level (grade 4) and is much shorter than the MMPI-2, making it easier than the MMPI-2 to administer to inmates.
- The PAI has been validated with both known-group and simulation designs (Edens et al. 2007; Hopwood et al. 2007; Kucharski et al. 2007).
- The PAI has demonstrated effectiveness in detecting several feigned mental disorders.

Weaknesses

- Like the MMPI-2, only extreme elevations on the PAI scales can be used to identify probable feigning with low false-positive rates. These extreme elevations miss the majority of feigners.
- The Malingering Index and Rogers Discriminant Function have been inconsistent across studies (Kucharski et al. 2007). Of particular importance, the Rogers Discriminant Function has produced only modest results in clinical-correctional settings that use known-group comparisons.

DETECTION STRATEGIES FOR THE ASSESSMENT OF MALINGERING COGNITIVE PROBLEMS

The principal purpose of this chapter is to examine detection strategies for feigned mental disorders. Although less frequent, inmates sometimes feign cognitive deficits to delay or avoid trial (Heinze and Purisch 2001; Vitacco et al., in press) or to reduce their punishments (Brodsky and Galloway 2003). Clinical staff should be cognizant of detection strategies for feigned cognitive impairments and be knowledgeable of clinical measures for their assessment.

Assessment of feigned cognitive impairment requires different strategies from those used to detect feigned mental disorders. However, both types of assessment require a comprehensive approach that differentiates genuine from feigned impairment (Goldberg 2001). As an example, one of us (Vitacco) recently evaluated an individual with a lengthy history of special education classes and documented cognitive dysfunction. On cognitive testing, he was found to be in the severely mentally retarded range, unable to identify even the most basic of objects. Additional testing indicated he was clearly feigning. In this case, the patient had clear, well-documented dysfunction but was presenting as much more impaired. Unlike most malingerers, this individual was feigning to avoid being discharged from the institution.

In a seminal article, Rogers et al. (1993) outlined different detection strategies used to assess feigned cognitive impairment. Because of the formal testing requirements, suspected cases should be referred for psychological consultations. Nonetheless, psychiatrists and other qualified mental health professionals should be knowledgeable about detection strategies and the Slick criteria (Slick et al. 1999), the latter of which provide a method to comprehensively understand and assess cognitive malingering. We present and discuss five detection strategies often used to detect feigned cognitive impairment.

1. *Floor effect.* Most genuine patients, even those with severe cognitive impairments, retain basic abilities. Malingerers frequently miss even the most basic of questions (Frederick et al. 2000). Vitacco et al. (in press) found basic questions on the SIRS useful as a screen for cognitive malingering. The floor effect strategy is used in a number of validated measures of cognitive malingering: the Rey 15-item test (Lezak 1983), the Test of Memory Malingering (Tombaugh 1996), and the Hiscock Digit Memory Test (Hiscock and Hiscock 1989).
2. *Symptom validity testing (SVT).* With multiple-choice responses, SVT evaluates whether the inmate is failing at "below-chance" levels. As

noted by Rogers (2008), SVT is the only detection strategy that provides definite evidence that an individual is feigning. Although SVT
can provide evidence of malingering, most inmates, even if they are
malingering, will not perform worse than chance on multiple-choice
tests. As such, below-chance performance will indicate malingering,
but the absence of such a finding does not indicate honest responding. SVT can be used to evaluate purported amnesia for a crime (Frederick et al. 1995), providing that all the alternatives have an equal likelihood of being selected (Rogers and Shuman 2000).

3. *Forced-choice testing. Forced-choice testing* is a general and overly ambiguous term that is usually referenced in regard to lower than expected results. This strategy can be confounded with poor effort and often does
not yield robust results. However, it has had some success as a strategy
used with the California Verbal Learning Test—Second Edition (Delis
and Kramer 2000).

4. *Performance curve.* Inmates feigning cognitive deficits often do not
take into account item difficulty when deciding which items to fail.
For malingerers, this performance often results in a flattened or nonexistent performance curve. The Validity Indicator Profile (Frederick
1997) employs this strategy with good success (Frederick et al. 2000).

5. *Magnitude of error (MOE).* Blau (2001) refers to MOE as a variant of
SVT. In reality, it is much more than SVT, in that MOE evaluates the
degree of inaccuracy in the responses. Persons feigning cognitive impairment do not take into account the different types of incorrect answers and may be detectable by MOE. Bender and Rogers (2004)
found MOE to be the most robust detector of malingering, even
when simulators were warned about this detection strategy (see also
Martin et al. 1998). These early promising results require further validation before MOE can be routinely used as a detection strategy for
cognitive malingering.

MANAGING MALINGERING CASES IN CORRECTIONAL SETTINGS

What should clinical staff do once an inmate has been thoroughly evaluated and classified as a malingerer? One option is to confront the malingerer with the diagnostic and test data in an attempt to alter the client's
presentation. The primary difficulty is doing this without sounding accu-
satory. Possibly a better alternative is to present the inmate with viable alternatives; for example, the clinician can raise concerns about the validity
of the test results and offer the inmate the option of retesting on psycho-

logical tests. Towers and Frederick (2002) presented a case study in which the individual achieved valid results on the second attempt. As a result, they changed the classification from malingering to malingering resolved. Towers and Frederick underscored the importance of allowing the inmate to "save face." As such, direct feedback must be done tactfully with the ultimate goal being positive behavior change. Another option is to ignore the malingering and hope the situation resolves on its own. This approach might be preferred with inmates who are angry and defensive. In such cases, direct feedback may further impair the professional relationship.

When an inmate has been classified as a malingerer, the clinician has to consider what to do about treatment. Before all treatment is discontinued, several issues warrant consideration. First, many malingerers also have genuine mental disorders; these constructs are not mutually exclusive. Second, some malingerers are already responding well to treatment (see Han 1997), despite their feigning presentation. Third, interventions that address the malingering might be sought to achieve a better allocation of clinical resources. Malingerers are often motivated to stymie effective treatment because their "improvement" might compromise their objectives.

FIVE RULES FOR THE EARLY CAREER CORRECTIONAL PSYCHIATRIST/PSYCHOLOGIST

In this section, we offer general rules for mental health professionals providing correctional services. Although the list is primarily for early career professionals, their more experienced colleagues may also benefit from a thoughtful consideration of these rules.

1. Use appropriate clinical terms in diagnostic evaluations and in communicating the results to other professionals. Do not use ambiguous terms such as *secondary gain* (Rogers and Reinhardt 1998) or *suboptimal effort* in descriptions of malingering. Play close attention to nonclinical terms and negative descriptions that suggest the possibility of countertransference.
2. Use only well-validated detection strategies for the assessment of malingering. When consultations from psychologists and other clinical staff are being used, it is imperative to understand the underlying detection strategy, its comparative effectiveness, and its known or potential error rates. Also, clinicians must be aware of the rules governing admittance of scientific evidence in their jurisdiction (see *Daubert v. Merrell Dow Pharmaceuticals* 1993).

3. Ensure that malingering screens, such as the M-FAST and SIMS, are used appropriately. Depending on the setting, correctional psychiatrists and psychologists may need to educate other clinicians who might attempt to "shortcut" assessments of malingering.

4. Determinations of malingering have far-ranging consequences for inmates; these determinations may affect pending legal issues as well as future interventions. Challenge the clinical staff to use the best-validated measures and to render classifications of malingering only when empirically supported by multiple methods.

5. Use perspective taking in the management of malingerers. With better understanding of the malingerer, a collaborative goal may focus on appropriate behavioral change (e.g., prosocial interactions and a discontinuation of feigning). If the malingerer is allowed to participate in treatment planning, his or her deliberate efforts to feign may be replaced by a more adaptive process.

CONCLUSION

The assessment and management of malingering in correctional settings can be a challenging experience for both early career and seasoned clinicians. Our primary goal in this chapter has been to provide correctional practitioners with a useful framework for understanding malingering with inmate populations. Professional collaboration is crucial for all professionals because it further develops expertise for the assessment of malingering, provides an effective mechanism for identifying countertransference issues, and allows for a systematic assessment that incorporates subjective interview-based findings with objective data from malingering screens and comprehensive measures.

Finally, correctional psychiatrists and psychologists need to recognize the significant limitations associated with DSM-IV-TR's description of malingering. Its screening indicators are faulty; reliance on them will likely lead to unacceptable error rates of approximately 80% for the classification of malingering (Gerson 2002; Rogers 2008). Instead, correctional psychiatrists and psychologists must use validated detection strategies and appropriate methods in determinations of malingering. Falling back on DSM-IV-TR indices, while simple, is unacceptable for correctional practice. We encourage psychiatrists to remain updated on advances in malingering practice by consulting the literature and receiving formal training.

SUMMARY POINTS

• DSM-IV-TR criteria should not be used to diagnose malingering because they result in an unacceptable number of false positives.

• Malingering should be assessed with well-validated instruments that employ empirically validated strategies.

• Using screens to determine which inmates need more comprehensive assessment is an effective way to save valuable resources in busy correctional settings.

• Cognitive malingering requires different evaluation measures and detection strategies than feigning psychopathology. However, determinations of cognitive malingering must be held to the same rigorous standards (e.g., multiple methods, well-validated instruments) as determinations of malingering of psychopathology.

• When managing malingerers in correctional settings, clinicians must be flexible and creative in their approach and take special precautions to avoid countertransference.

REFERENCES

American Psychiatric Association: Diagnostic and Statistical Manual of Mental Disorders, 4th Edition, Text Revision. Washington, DC, American Psychiatric Association, 2000

Beaber RJ, Marston A, Michelli J, et al: A brief test for measuring malingering in schizophrenic individuals. Am J Psychiatry 142:1478–1481, 1985

Bender SD, Rogers R: Detection of neurocognitive feigning: development of a multi-strategy assessment. Arch Clin Neuropsychol 19:49–60, 2004

Blau TH: Psychologist as an Expert Witness, 2nd Edition. Hoboken, NJ, Wiley, 2001

Brodsky SL, Galloway VA: Ethical and professional demands for forensic mental health professionals in the post-Atkins area. Ethics Behav 13:3–9, 2003

Butcher JN, Dahlstrom WG, Graham JR, et al: Minnesota Multiphasic Personality Inventory–2 Manual. Minneapolis, University of Minnesota Press, 1989

Daubert v Merrell Dow Pharmaceuticals, 509 U.S. 579, 589 (1993)

Delis D, Kramer J: Advances in the neuropsychological assessment of memory disorders, in Handbook of Neuropsychology, 2nd Edition, Vol 2: Memory and Its Disorders. Edited by Cermak LS. Amsterdam, Elsevier Science, 2000, pp 25–47

Edens JF, Otto R, Dwyer T: Utility of the Structured Interview of Malingered Symptomatology in identifying persons motivated to malinger psychopathology. J Am Acad Psychiatry Law 27:387–396, 1999

Edens J, Poythress N, Watkins-Clay M: Detection of malingering in psychiatric unit and general population prison inmates: a comparison of the PAI, SIMS, and SIRS. J Pers Assess 88:33–42, 2007

Frederick RI: Validity Indicator Profile Manual. Minnetonka, MN, NCS Assessments, 1997

Frederick RI, Carter M, Powell J: Adapting symptom validity testing to evaluate suspicious complaints of amnesia in medicolegal evaluations. Bull Am Acad Psychiatry Law 23:231–237, 1995

Frederick R, Crosby R, Wynkoop T: Performance curve classification of invalid responding on the Validity Indicator Profile. Arch Clin Neuropsychol 15:281–300, 2000

Gerson AR: Beyond DSM-IV: a meta-review of the literature on malingering. Am J Forensic Psychol 20:57–69, 2002

Goldberg KB: Update on neuropsychological assessment of malingering. Journal of Forensic Psychology Practice 1:45–53, 2001

Greene RL: Malingering and defensiveness on the MMPI-2, in Clinical Assessment of Malingering and Deception, 3rd Edition. Edited by Rogers R. New York, Guilford, 2008, pp 159–182

Greve K, Bianchini K, Love J, et al: Sensitivity and specificity of MMPI-2 validity scales and indicators to malingered neurocognitive dysfunction in traumatic brain injury. Clin Neuropsychol 20:491–512, 2006

Han S: Social rehabilitation of ex-malingerers from prison. International Medical Journal 4:73–75, 1997

Heinze MC, Purisch AD: Beneath the mask: use of psychological tests to detect and subtype malingering in criminal defendants. Journal of Forensic Psychology Practice 1:23–52, 2001

Hiscock CK, Hiscock M: Refining the forced-choice method for the detection of malingering. J Consult Clin Psychol 46:892–900, 1989

Hopwood C, Morey L, Rogers R, et al: Malingering on the Personality Assessment Inventory: identification of specific feigned disorders. J Pers Assess 88:43–48, 2007

Jackson RL, Vitacco MJ: Structured and unstructured interviews, in Coping With Psychology and Psychiatric Testimony. Edited by Faust J, Ziskin M. New York, Oxford University Press (in press)

Jackson R, Rogers R, Sewell K: Forensic applications of the Miller Forensic Assessment of Symptoms Test (MFAST): screening for feigned disorders in competency to stand trial evaluations. Law Hum Behav 29:199–210, 2005

Jaffe ME, Sharma KK: Malingering uncommon psychiatric symptoms among defendants charged under California's "Three Strikes and You're Out" law. J Forensic Sci 43:549–555, 1998

Kucharski L, Falkenbach D, Egan S, et al: Antisocial personality disorder and the malingering of psychiatric disorder: a study of criminal defendants. International Journal of Forensic Mental Health 5:195–204, 2006

Kucharski L, Toomey J, Fila K, et al: Detection of malingering of psychiatric disorder with the Personality Assessment Inventory: an investigation of criminal defendants. J Pers Assess 88:25–32, 2007

Lewis JL, Simcox AM, Berry D: Screening for feigned psychiatric symptoms in a forensic sample by using the MMPI-2 and the Structured Inventory of Malingered Symptomatology. Psychol Assess 14:170–176, 2002

Lezak M: Neuropsychological Assessment. New York, Oxford University Press, 1983

Martin RC, Franzen MD, Orey S: Magnitude of error as a strategy to detect feigned memory impairment. Clin Neuropsychol 12:84–91, 1998

Miller HA: Miller Forensic Assessment of Symptoms Test (M-FAST) Professional Manual. Odessa, FL, Psychological Assessment Resources, 2001

Miller HA: The Miller Forensic Assessment of Symptoms Test (M-FAST). Crim Justice Behav 32:591–611, 2005

Millon T, Davis R, Millon C: The Millon Clinical Multiaxial Inventory–III Manual, 2nd Edition. Minneapolis, MN, National Computer Systems, 1997

Morey LC: Personality Assessment Inventory. Tampa, FL, Psychological Assessment Resources, 1991

Novak B, McDermott B, Scott C, et al: Sex offenders and insanity: an examination of 42 individuals found not guilty by reason of insanity. J Am Acad Psychiatry Law 35:444–450, 2007

Pollock P: Feigning auditory hallucinations by offenders. The Journal of Forensic Psychiatry & Psychology 9:305–327, 1998

Resnick P: My favorite tips for detecting malingering and violence risk. Psychiatr Clin North Am 30:227–232, 2007

Rogers R: Models of feigned mental illness. Prof Psychol Res Pr 21:182–188, 1990

Rogers R (ed): Clinical Assessment of Malingering and Deception, 2nd Edition. New York, Guilford, 1997

Rogers R: Handbook of Diagnostic and Structured Interviewing. New York, Guilford, 2001

Rogers R: Forensic use and abuse of psychological tests: multiscale inventories. J Psychiatr Pract 9:316–320, 2003

Rogers R (ed): Clinical Assessment of Malingering and Deception, 3rd Edition. New York, Guilford, 2008

Rogers R, Cavanaugh JL: "Nothing but the truth"…A reexamination of malingering. J Psychiatry Law 11:443–460, 1983

Rogers R, Reinhardt VR: Conceptualization and assessment of secondary gain, in Psychologist's Desk Reference. Edited by Koocher GP, Norcross JC, Hill SS. New York, Oxford University Press, 1998, pp 57–62

Rogers R, Shuman D: Conducting Insanity Evaluations. New York, Guilford, 2000

Rogers R, Vitacco MJ: Forensic assessment of malingering and related response styles, in Forensic Psychology: From Classroom to Courtroom. Edited by Van Dorsten B. New York, Kluwer Academic Press, 2002, pp 83–104

Rogers R, Bagby RM, Dickens SE: Structured Interview of Reported Symptoms (SIRS) Professional Manual. Odessa, FL, Psychological Assessment Resources, 1992a

Rogers R, Bagby RM, Gillis JR: Improvements in the M Test as a screening measure for malingering. Bull Am Acad Psychiatry Law 20:101–104, 1992b

Rogers R, Harrell EH, Liff CD: Feigning neuropsychological impairment: a critical review of methodological and clinical considerations. Clin Psychol Rev 13:255–274, 1993

Rogers R, Hinds JD, Sewell KW: Feigning psychopathology among adolescent offenders: validation of the SIRS, MMPI-A, and SIMS. Paper presented at the annual meeting of the American Psychological Association, New York, August 1995

Rogers R, Sewell KW, Martin MA, et al: Detection of feigned mental disorders: a meta-analysis of the MMPI-2 and malingering. Assessment 10:160–177, 2003

Rogers R, Jackson R, Sewell K, et al: Detection strategies for malingering: a confirmatory factor analysis of the SIRS. Crim Justice Behav 32:511–525, 2005

Sellbom M, Bagby RM: Response styles on multiscale inventories, in Clinical Assessment of Malingering and Deception, 3rd Edition. Edited by Rogers R. New York, Guilford, 2008, pp 182–206

Slick D, Sherman E, Iverson G: Diagnostic criteria for malingered neurocognitive dysfunction: proposed standards for clinical practice and research. Clin Neuropsychol 13:545–561, 1999

Smith GP: Brief screening measures for the detection of feigned psychopathology, in Clinical Assessment of Malingering and Deception, 3rd Edition. Edited by Rogers R. New York, Guilford, 2008, pp 323–342

Smith GP, Burger GK: Detection of malingering: validation of the Structured Inventory of Malingered Symptomatology (SIMS). J Am Acad Psychiatry Law 25:183–189, 1997

Smith GP, Borum R, Schinka JA: Rule-out and rule-in scales for the M Test for malingering: a cross validation. Bull Am Acad Psychiatry Law 21:107–110, 1993

Tombaugh TN: The Test of Memory Malingering. North Tonawanda, NY, Multi-Health Systems, 1996

Towers K, Frederick R: Competence to be sentenced, in Forensic Mental Health Assessment: A Casebook. Edited by Heilbrun K, Marczyk G, DeMatteo D. New York, Oxford University Press, 2002, pp 85–95

Vitacco M, Rogers R, Gabel J, et al: An evaluation of malingering screens with competency to stand trial patients: a known-groups comparison. Law Hum Behav 31:249–260, 2007

Vitacco MJ, Jackson RL, Rogers R, et al: Detection strategies for malingering with the Miller Forensic Assessment of Symptoms Test: a confirmatory factor analysis of its underlying dimensions. Assessment 15:97–103, 2008

Vitacco MJ, Rogers R, Gabel J: An investigation of the ECST-R in male pretrial patients: evaluating the effects of feigning on competency evaluations. Assessment (in press)

Walters GD: Assessing dissimulation and denial on the MMPI in a sample of maximum security, male inmates. J Pers Assess 52:465–474, 1988

Widows MR, Smith GP: Structured Inventory of Malingered Symptomatology Professional Manual. Odessa, FL, Psychological Assessment Resources, 2005

CHAPTER 11

Trauma and Incarcerated Persons

Nancy L. Wolff, Ph.D.

Jing Shi, M.S.

> During my many years in prison, I have actually witnessed personally hundreds of serious stabbings, beatings, inmates set on fire, and countless actual killings. My question to you is what makes the trauma of seeing "man's inhumanity to man" first hand here in prison any different than that experienced by soldiers....Yes,...PTSD is certainly a legitimate concern of inmates. (Personal correspondence from an incarcerated man in a New Jersey prison, 2004)

Both men and women in prison have histories of interpersonal violence. They are likely to have experienced physical, sexual, psychological, and emotional victimization, either directly or indirectly, as children and adults, and while living in the community and in prison. In this chapter, we explore the concept of interpersonal trauma, its relationship with posttraumatic stress disorder (PTSD), and the associated consequences of trauma on health and criminality; the prevalence of interpersonal trauma and mental illness among incarcerated persons and its relationship to feelings of safety; and trauma treatment interventions and their implications.

INTERPERSONAL TRAUMA

Interpersonal trauma refers generally to harm by one person (the abuser) against another (the victim) (Krug et al. 2002). The harmful behavior may involve abuse, neglect, or maltreatment and may be directed at harming the victim physically, sexually, psychologically, or emotionally (see, e.g., Child Abuse Prevention and Treatment Act of 1974, P.L. 93-237). Behaviors that generate trauma are as varied as physical or sexual assault, bullying, verbal degradation, and abandonment (e.g., a parent leaving a child in a mall because he or she is no longer wanted, or a husband leaving a wife after she is diagnosed with breast cancer). In some situations of interpersonal trauma, the abuser has the intent to humiliate, shame, terrorize, or in some other way harm the victim's sense of safety, self-efficacy, and, ultimately, well-being.

People who experience trauma are representative of all age, race/ ethnicity, gender, and socioeconomic groups. Whether old or young, white or black, Hispanic or non-Hispanic, male or female, rich or poor, each individual experiences a traumatic event subjectively. More specifically, Allen (1995) argues that

> it is the subjective experience of the objective events that constitutes trauma....The more you believe you are endangered, the more traumatized you will be....Psychologically, the bottom line of trauma is overwhelming emotion and a feeling of utter helplessness. There may or may not be bodily injury, but psychological trauma is coupled with physiological upheaval that plays a leading role in the long-range effects. (p. 14)

How a person responds subjectively to an objective event will depend on factors related to the event itself (e.g., its setting, level of violence, motivation) and its frequency, the nature of the relationship between the abuser and the victim (e.g., the level of intimacy and dependence), and characteristics of the individual (e.g., history of abuse, psychological resilience). People experiencing the same objective event may respond very differently, because it may violate expected norms of conduct between people (e.g., caregiver and child, inmate and officer), because it may trigger past experiences of abuse, and because people vary in their ability to cope with the consequences of harm (Browne and Finkelhor 1986; Kendall-Tackett et al. 1993).

Interpersonal trauma is internalized differently by its victims. Some responses to the experience of interpersonal trauma are dissociation, affect dysregulation, chronic characterological changes (e.g., self-blame, sense of ineffectiveness and/or helplessness), somatization, hyperarousal, depression, and substance or alcohol abuse (Allen 1995; Chilcoat and Breslau 1998; Herman 1992; Lasiuk and Hegadoren 2006; Norris et al. 2002; Terr 2003). The cluster of behavioral reactions to traumatic events was first defined diagnostically as PTSD in the *Diagnostic and Statistical Manual of Mental Disorders*, 3rd Edition (DSM-III; American Psychiatric Association 1980). According to DSM-IV-TR, PTSD is an anxiety disorder, and the essential feature is "the development of characteristic symptoms following exposure to an extreme traumatic stressor involving direct personal experience...or witnessing an event that involves death, injury, or a threat to the physical integrity of another person" (American Psychiatric Association 2000, p. 463). The DSM-IV-TR diagnostic criteria for PTSD are outlined in Table 11–1.

Although the classification of PTSD as a mental disorder added legitimacy and specificity to the constellation of traumatic-stress-related symptoms, it did not accurately capture the dimensionality of the psychological response to long-term exposure to trauma. Herman (1992) argued that the symptoms of trauma vary along a spectrum from acute to complex reactions. At the one end of the trauma response spectrum, the individual experiences an acute stress reaction that self-corrects without intervention, whereas at the other end, the individual reacts with "complex" PTSD, and in between these two extremes is "classic" or "simple" PTSD (Herman 1992, p. 119). Complex PTSD, also referred to as *disorder of extreme stress not otherwise specified* (DESNOS), is associated with chronic victimization that results in personality adaptations that challenge the person's ability to bond with others and form a stable identity (American Psychiatric Association 2000). (*Note:* Complex PTSD/DESNOS is not recognized in DSM-IV-TR.) The DESNOS diagnosis classification has been found to be coupled with early childhood victimization, extreme reexperiencing of the traumatic events, and impaired characterological functioning (Ford 1999).

PREVALENCE OF INTERPERSONAL TRAUMA AND POSTTRAUMATIC STRESS DISORDER

General Population

Interpersonal violence involves a variety of situations, ranging from domestic violence and childhood victimization to victimization by strangers during the course of a crime. For the general population, the 6-month and lifetime prevalence rates for domestic violence are estimated at 6%– 15% and 28%–54%, respectively (Abbott et al. 1995; Eisenstat and Bancroft 1999; Tjaden and Thoennes 1998), whereas the lifetime rates for childhood victimization vary between 3% and 40% (Children's Bureau 2008; Ernst et al. 1993). Kessler et al. (1995) estimated the lifetime prevalence rates for exposure to (any) traumatic event at over 50%, with exposure varying by gender (61% for men and 51% for women). Not all individuals, however, will respond to trauma in ways that meet the criteria

TABLE 11–1.   DSM-IV-TR diagnostic criteria for posttraumatic stress disorder

A.   The person has been exposed to a traumatic event in which both of the following were present:

   (1) the person experienced, witnessed, or was confronted with an event or events that involved actual or threatened death or serious injury, or a threat to the physical integrity of self or others

   (2) the person's response involved intense fear, helplessness, or horror.   **Note:** In children, this may be expressed instead by disorganized or agitated behavior

B.   The traumatic event is persistently reexperienced in one (or more) of the following ways:

   (1) recurrent and intrusive distressing recollections of the event, including images, thoughts, or perceptions.   **Note:** In young children, repetitive play may occur in which themes or aspects of the trauma are expressed.

   (2) recurrent distressing dreams of the event.   **Note:** In children, there may be frightening dreams without recognizable content.

   (3) acting or feeling as if the traumatic event were recurring (includes a sense of reliving the experience, illusions, hallucinations, and dissociative flashback episodes, including those that occur on awakening or when intoxicated).   **Note:** In young children, trauma-specific reenactment may occur.

   (4) intense psychological distress at exposure to internal or external cues that symbolize or resemble an aspect of the traumatic event

   (5) physiological reactivity on exposure to internal or external cues that symbolize or resemble an aspect of the traumatic event

C.   Persistent avoidance of stimuli associated with the trauma and numbing of general responsiveness (not present before the trauma), as indicated by three (or more) of the following:

   (1) efforts to avoid thoughts, feelings, or conversations associated with the trauma

   (2) efforts to avoid activities, places, or people that arouse recollections of the trauma

   (3) inability to recall an important aspect of the trauma

   (4) markedly diminished interest or participation in significant activities

   (5) feeling of detachment or estrangement from others

   (6) restricted range of affect (e.g., unable to have loving feelings)

   (7) sense of a foreshortened future (e.g., does not expect to have a career, marriage, children, or a normal life span)

TABLE 11–1. DSM-IV-TR diagnostic criteria for posttraumatic stress disorder *(continued)*

D. Persistent symptoms of increased arousal (not present before the trauma), as indicated by two (or more) of the following:

    (1) difficulty falling or staying asleep

    (2) irritability or outbursts of anger

    (3) difficulty concentrating

    (4) hypervigilance

    (5) exaggerated startle response

E. Duration of the disturbance (symptoms in Criteria B, C, and D) is more than 1 month.

F. The disturbance causes clinically significant distress or impairment in social, occupational, or other important areas of functioning.

Specify if:

    Acute: if duration of symptoms is less than 3 months

    Chronic: if duration of symptoms is 3 months or more

Specify if:

    With Delayed Onset: if onset of symptoms is at least 6 months after the stressor

---

Source. Reprinted from American Psychiatric Association: *Diagnostic and Statistical Manual of Mental Disorders,* 4th Edition, Text Revision. Washington DC, American Psychiatric Association, 2000. Copyright 2000, American Psychiatric Association. Used with permission.

for PTSD. Overall, roughly 15%–24% of individuals who experience a potentially traumatic event will develop PTSD (Breslau et al. 1998). Although men are more likely to experience a traumatic event during their lifetimes, women are more likely to develop PTSD (Breslau 2002; Breslau et al. 1998; Bromet et al. 1998; Davidson et al. 1991; Helzer et al. 1987; Kessler et al. 1995).

Prison Population

Many incarcerated men and women have experienced interpersonal violence. Overall, half or more of incarcerated women reported experiencing at least one traumatic event in their lifetime (Browne et al. 1999; Sacks 2004). One-quarter to one-half of incarcerated women reported experiencing childhood abuse (Bloom et al. 2003; Fletcher et al. 1993; Greenfeld and Snell 1999; Harlow 1999), compared to 6%–24% of their male counterparts (Harlow 1999; McClellan et al. 1997). Comparatively,

childhood exposure to physical abuse is more likely than sexual abuse for
incarcerated males, but the two forms of victimization occur at roughly
equal rates for incarcerated females (Harlow 1999; McClellan et al.
1997).

Over the past three decades, efforts to measure the prevalence of
mental illness among correctional populations have increased. Epidemiological studies have found a prevalence of serious mental illness ranging
from 3% to 50% (Guy et al. 1985; Teplin 1983; Teplin et al. 1996). Evidence from the Epidemiologic Catchment Area study estimated that 56%
of those incarcerated reported having symptoms that met criteria for some
form of mental illness at some point in their lives (Regier et al. 1990). Another set of studies focusing on state prisons found that the prevalence
of mental illness in these settings ranged from 10% to 15% (Jemelka et
al. 1989, 2000). The Bureau of Justice Statistics estimated that over half of
the nation's combined prison (56%) and jail (64%) populations had a recent history or current symptoms of a mental health problem (James and
Glaze 2006).

In general, rates of mental disorder in prison are more than double
those found in the general population and are considerably higher for
female inmates than for male inmates. This gender-based difference in
the prevalence of mental illness in prison is attributed in part to the fact
that women in prison are five times more likely than men to report being
the victim of physical and/or sexual abuse or having a history of other
trauma (Chesney-Lind 1997; Ditton 1999; Dodge and Pogrebin 2001;
Hartwell 2001; Parke and Clarke-Stewart 2003). Rates of PTSD are three
times higher among incarcerated women than in a community sample of
women (Teplin et al. 1996). Female inmates with mental health problems, compared with those without mental health problems, were more
likely to have a substance abuse problem (74% vs. 54%) and to report
prior physical and sexual abuse (68% vs. 44%) (James and Glaze 2006).
Regular use of illegal drugs and alcohol was more typical in the lives of
previously abused inmates than in the lives of those who were not previously abused (Harlow 1999; McClellan et al. 1997). Abused male inmates,
compared with their female counterparts, were more likely to regularly
use alcohol and to have committed their index offense under the influence of alcohol, whereas abused female inmates, compared with their
male counterparts, were more likely to have been using illegal drugs at
the time of their index offense (Harlow 1999).

Prison Violence and Victimization

Victimization continues inside prison for many inmates. Correctional settings are known for their violence. Rates of violent victimization (inclusive

of robbery and sexual and physical assault) are higher in prison settings than in the general community. In the community, violent victimization rates are estimated at approximately 21 per 1,000 residents (Rand and Catalano 2007). By comparison, based on a sample of inmates drawn from three Ohio prisons, approximately 1 of every 10 inmates reported being physically assaulted in the previous 6 months, whereas 1 of every 5 inmates reported being a victim of theft during that same time frame. Combining all crimes together, 1 of every 2 inmates surveyed reported being a victim of crime over a 6-month period (Wooldredge 1998). Based on a sample of more than 7,000 inmates, Wolff et al. (2007a) estimated 6-month inmate-on-inmate physical victimization rates at 21% for both female and male inmates—a rate of victimization that is 10 times higher than the overall rate in the community.

Sexual victimization also occurs inside prison, with prevalence rates ranging from <1% to 41% (Gaes and Goldberg 2004). Two studies measured the prevalence of sexual victimization inside prison using state-of-the-art methods. The first study, conducted by Wolff et al. (2006), was based on inmate data collected at all prisons within a state system. Wolff et al. estimated inmate-on-inmate sexual assault rates over a 6-month period at 3.2% for female inmates and 1.5% for male inmates. Relative to their counterparts who had no sexual victimization prior to age 18, the likelihood of sexual victimization doubled for female inmates and more than doubled for male inmates who experienced sexual abuse prior to age 18 (Wolff et al. 2007c). Similar prevalence estimates were found in a national study of prison rape conducted by the Bureau of Justice Statistics. Based on a national prison sample, the 12-month prevalence rate for sexual assault between inmates was estimated at 1.3%, and at 3.3% if staff-on-inmate sexual assaults were included (Beck and Harrison 2007).

More generally, when abusive sexual contact (i.e., inappropriate touching of genitals, breasts, or buttocks) was included in the definition of sexual victimization, the 6-month rate increased to 21.2% for inmate-on-inmate victimization and to 7.6% for staff-on-inmate victimization (Wolff et al. 2006). Female inmates with a mental disorder had higher rates of sexual victimization perpetrated by other inmates than did their counterparts without mental disorder (Wolff et al. 2007b). Moreover, female inmates with a mental disorder had significantly higher rates of any sexual victimization in all race/ethnicity groups, ranging from 1.6 times higher for African American inmates to 2.4 times higher for non-Hispanic white inmates (Wolff et al. 2008). The risk of abusive sexual contact between inmates was significantly elevated (doubled) for female inmates who experienced sexual abuse prior to age 18 (Wolff et al. 2007c). The inmate-on-inmate 6-month physical victimization prevalence rate for female in-

mates was approximately 21% (Wolff et al. 2007a). Female inmates with
a mental disorder also had higher rates of physical victimization than
their counterparts without mental disorders (25% vs. 15%) (Blitz et al.
2008).

CONSEQUENCES OF INTERPERSONAL TRAUMA

Health

Interpersonal trauma is strongly associated with physical illnesses, mental illnesses, and substance abuse. In general, individuals who have experienced trauma have poorer general, physical, and mental health (Felitti
et al. 1998; Kendall-Tackett et al. 1993; Malinosky-Rummell and Hansen
1993; Resnick et al. 1997; Schnurr and Green 2004) and are higher than
average users of health care services (Deykin et al. 2001; Firsten 1991;
Kartha et al. 2008). Some of the adult physical health care problems associated with childhood trauma include gastrointestinal disorders (Leserman et al. 1996; Scarinci et al. 1994); chronic headaches (Felitti 1991);
chronic lower back pain and pelvic pain (Reiter and Gambone 1990;
Schofferman et al. 1993); and lung, heart, and liver diseases (Felitti et al.
1998).

Interpersonal trauma contributes to the development of mental disorders, most notably depression (Ballanger et al. 2004; Hegarty et al.
2004; Kramer et al. 2004; Widom et al. 2007). For people with PTSD, comorbid mental illness is common (Carlson et al. 2003). The vast majority
of men (88%) and women (79%) with lifetime PTSD have a history of at
least one additional mental disorder (Kessler et al. 1995). Other psychiatric disorders associated with PTSD include affective disorders, other
anxiety disorders, phobias, conduct disorders, somatization, and substance use disorders (Kendall-Tackett et al. 1993; Kessler et al. 1995).

Compared with their counterparts without PTSD, men and women
with a lifetime history of PTSD are more likely to report experiences of
drug abuse or dependence (Kessler et al. 1995). Childhood physical
abuse and sexual abuse have been linked to emotional problems and
substance abuse in adulthood (Kendall-Tackett et al. 1993; Malinosky-
Rummell and Hansen 1993). PTSD and substance abuse commonly co-
occur (Jacobsen et al. 2001), and recent evidence suggests a causal connection (Chilcoat and Breslau 1998). Compared to their nonabused
counterparts, abused and neglected females, but not their male counterparts, were found to have a significantly higher risk for substance abuse
(Widom and White 1997).

Criminality and Suicidality

The effects of interpersonal trauma are not limited to health consequences. Responses to trauma include anger, aggression toward others, and self-destructive and suicidal behaviors (van der Kolk et al. 1996). Self-destructive and suicidal ideation are elevated among people who have experienced childhood abuse (Brodsky et al. 2001; Browne and Finkelhor 1986; Dervic et al. 2006; Dube et al. 2001; van der Kolk et al. 1996; Windle et al. 1995). Research also shows a strong association among childhood interpersonal trauma, delinquency, and criminality (Dutton and Hart 1992; Ireland and Widom 1994; Malinosky-Rummell and Hansen 1993; McClellan et al. 1997; Siegel 2000; Siegel and Williams 2003; Smith and Thornberry 1995; Widom 1995; Widom and Maxfield 2001). Abuse in childhood is strongly correlated with adult victimization and criminality (Browne et al. 1999; Chesney-Lind 1997; Dutton and Hart 1992; Goodman et al. 2001; Ireland and Widom 1994; McClellan et al. 1997; Siegel and Williams 2003; Smith and Thornberry 1995; Widom 1989). Moreover, the literature shows that men and women have different patterns in their experiences of and reactions to interpersonal violence over the life cycle (Cutler and Nolen-Hoeksema 1991; McClellan et al. 1997; Widom and Maxfield 2001; Widom and White 1997).

Research shows variation in abuse patterns and responses between males and females. Overall, females are more likely than males to experience sexual assault, whereas males are more likely than females to experience physical assault (Breslau et al. 1998; Widom and Maxfield 2001). Females who experience childhood abuse or neglect or other forms of trauma are more likely to develop PTSD (Hegadoren et al. 2006) and engage in criminal activity than are control subjects without such experiences (Widom and Maxfield 2001). Childhood abuse increases the risk that females will be arrested for violent and nonviolent crimes later in life. Although the risk of criminal activity does not increase for males who have experienced childhood abuse, their frequency of criminal activity increases over that of their male counterparts without such experiences (Widom and Maxfield 2001). Rates of maltreatment of men tend to decline over the life cycle, whereas rates of maltreatment increase for women as they age (McClellan et al. 1997).

INCARCERATED PERSONS AND IN-PRISON INTERPERSONAL TRAUMA

We (Wolff et al. 2006) studied a sample of 7,528 inmates drawn from the population of 22,231 inmates housed at 12 male adult prisons and one female adult prison operated by a single state; the data throughout this section are based on our findings from that study. After exclusion of inmates younger than 18; inmates in prehearing custody, detention, death row, halfway housing, a sex offender treatment facility; and inmates too sick to participate in the survey, a total of 19,788 adult inmates (89% of the entire population) were eligible to participate, and subjects were randomly selected for participation in the survey. Data were collected from June 1 through August 31, 2005. Our recruitment protocol, consent procedures, and consent form were approved by the appropriate university and correctional agency research review boards and committees. The survey was administered using an audio-computer–administered survey instrument, available in English and Spanish. In-prison victimization was measured by one general question and a set of behavior-specific questions for each type of victimization (sexual or physical) and perpetrator (inmates or staff members).

Sexual victimization is defined as nonconsensual sexual acts, inclusive of sexual contact and/or penetration and oral contact (i.e., rape or sexual assault), and abusive sexual contacts, inclusive of intentional touching of specified areas of the body (Beck and Harrison 2007). As in other environments, consensual sex between two willing adults (who are also inmates) is not considered sexual victimization. However, if one of the two consenting adults is a staff member of the prison, then by law the sex is not consensual.

Community Interpersonal Trauma and Mental Disorder

In the study, we reviewed the relationship of community interpersonal trauma and in-prison personal trauma to mental disorders, and the findings are summarized below. Interpersonal trauma experienced in the community may be of three types—physical, sexual, and emotional—and may occur prior to or after turning age 18. The perpetrators of the trauma may be a family member, friend, acquaintance, or stranger. Table 11–2 shows the percentage of male and female inmates reporting that they experienced various types of interpersonal trauma in the community. The inmates are distinguished further by those reporting a mental disorder (reported) and not reporting a mental disorder (none reported). "Reporting" a mental disorder means that the respondent reported being treated at some point in his or her life for a particular mental disorder (e.g., schizophrenia, depression, PTSD, anxiety, phobia).

Both male and female inmates with a self-reported mental disorder were significantly more likely to report experiencing all forms of physical interpersonal trauma in the community than their counterparts without a reported mental disorder. Physical interpersonal trauma independent of mental disorder was most likely to occur when the person was younger than 18 years. Over one-half of the inmates with a mental disorder reported being hit with an object that left welts or caused bleeding and being beaten up. Nearly one-quarter or more of male and female inmates reporting a mental disorder reported being choked or burned with a hot object, with this trauma experienced most frequently when the person was younger than 18.

Sexual trauma was most likely to be experienced prior to age 18 by male and female inmates alike. However, all forms of sexual trauma were more commonly reported by female inmates than by male inmates, and by female inmates with mental disorder than by female inmates without a reported mental disorder. On average, twice as many female inmates reported experiencing sexual trauma in the community if they reported a mental disorder. Sex by force was reported by nearly 45% of female inmates with a mental disorder and 25% of those without a mental disorder.

Over one-half of the inmates with a mental disorder and over one-third of those without a mental disorder reported experiencing abandonment in the community, most often when they were children (younger than age 18). *Abandonment* is an abruption in an interpersonal relationship in which one person chooses not to meet key responsibilities expected as a part of parental, familial, or marital obligations. Examples in youth include being given up for adoption and being left in a mall or on a doorstep; abandonment in adulthood is most frequently associated with divorce or being ostracized from a family unit. Compared with their counterparts without a mental disorder, inmates with a mental disorder were more likely to report abandonment before and after turning age 18.

Prison Interpersonal Trauma and Mental Disorder

Six-month prevalence rates (expressed as percentages) for interpersonal trauma are shown for male and female inmates by mental disorder in Table 11–3. Interpersonal trauma is defined as bodily harm divided into categories of physical victimization (being hit, choked, assaulted, or threatened with a weapon) or sexual victimization (sexually threatening touching or forced or attempted oral, anal, or vaginal sexual assault) perpetrated by inmates (inmate-on-inmate) or staff (staff-on-inmate).

Interpersonal trauma is common inside prison, especially trauma that involves physical victimization. Nearly one-third or more of male and female inmates reported experiencing some form of interpersonal trauma during a 6-month period. Inmates with a mental disorder, independent of gender, were more likely to report all forms of interpersonal trauma than were their counterparts without a reported mental disorder. These differences between male inmates were always statistically significant, but the differences between female inmates were only rarely so

TABLE 11–2. Interpersonal trauma experienced in the community, by gender and mental disorder

	Percent reporting "yes" to type of trauma			
	Male inmates (N=6,964)		Female inmates (N=564)	
	Mental disorder		Mental disorder	
Type of interpersonal trauma	None reported (n=5,300[a])	Reported (n=1,568)	None reported (n=116[a])	Reported (n=321)
Physical				
Hit with object, left welts or caused bleeding	43.2*	59.3	37.9*	61.6
Before age 18	37.8*	52.0	28.1*	48.0
After age 17	13.0*	19.1	17.8*	31.3
Both before and after age 18	9.4*	13.9	9.0*	20.1
Beaten up	36.3*	56.7	44.1*	62.9
Before age 18	31.1*	49.9	24.9*	45.0
After age 17	13.6*	23.2	25.8*	36.9
Both before and after age 18	10.6*	18.4	10.5*	23.2
Threatened or harmed with a knife or gun	35.3*	43.4	28.6*	43.4
Before age 18	21.8*	29.4	13.0*	23.4
After age 17	22.4*	26.8	19.3*	28.6
Both before and after age 18	11.3*	14.7	6.8	10.0

TABLE 11–2. Interpersonal trauma experienced in the community, by gender and mental disorder *(continued)*

	Percent reporting "yes" to type of trauma			
	Male inmates (*N*=6,964)		Female inmates (*N*=564)	
	Mental disorder		Mental disorder	
Type of interpersonal trauma	None reported (*n*=5,300ᵃ)	Reported (*n*=1,568)	None reported (*n*=116ᵃ)	Reported (*n*=321)
Physical *(continued)*				
Choked or attempted to drown	14.2*	27.6	16.9*	34.1
Before age 18	12.4*	24.0	8.5*	22.9
After age 17	3.8*	9.2	10.3*	17.1
Both before and after age 18	3.0*	7.0	3.4*	8.2
Burned with hot object	10.6*	21.7	7.1*	23.4
Before age 18	8.1*	17.5	3.9*	14.6
After age 17	3.4*	5.6	3.4*	11.4
Both before and after age 18	2.0*	3.6	1.0*	4.4
Sexual				
Touched in sexually threatening way	6.9*	19.0	31.4*	61.1
Before age 18	6.0*	17.0	28.2*	50.0
After age 17	1.3*	4.6	7.7*	23.7
Both before and after age 18	0.9*	3.5	5.8*	16.4

TABLE 11–2. Interpersonal trauma experienced in the community, by gender and mental disorder (*continued*)

	Percent reporting "yes" to type of trauma			
	Male inmates (*N*=6,964)		Female inmates (*N*=564)	
	Mental disorder		Mental disorder	
Type of interpersonal trauma	None reported (*n*=5,300[a])	Reported (*n*=1,568)	None reported (*n*=116[a])	Reported (*n*=321)
Sexual (*continued*)				
Forced to touch someone else's genitals	4.3*	12.9	21.2*	45.6
Before age 18	3.7*	11.1	19.3*	37.3
After age 17	0.8*	2.7	7.7*	16.9
Both before and after age 18	0.6*	1.8	6.5*	12.2
Sex by force or with threat of harm	2.4*	8.5	24.5*	44.7
Before age 18	2.0*	8.0	17.5*	32.8
After age 17	0.5	0.9	11.3*	18.3
Both before and after age 18	0.4	0.7	6.3	9.4
Forced oral or anal sex	2.2*	6.8	19.3*	43.3
Before age 18	1.9*	6.4	14.3*	32.4
After age 17	0.4*	1.1	10.7	16.5
Both before and after age 18	0.3*	0.8	6.6	8.5

TABLE 11–2. Interpersonal trauma experienced in the community, by gender and mental disorder *(continued)*

	Percent reporting "yes" to type of trauma			
	Male inmates (*N*=6,964)		Female inmates (*N*=564)	
	Mental disorder		Mental disorder	
Type of interpersonal trauma	None reported (*n*=5,300[a])	Reported (*n*=1,568)	None reported (*n*=116[a])	Reported (*n*=321)
Emotional				
Abandoned	34.6*	50.1	35.8*	51.7
Before age 18	25.0*	40.1	29.0*	39.8
After age 17	18.0*	23.9	15.3*	22.9
Both before and after age 18	10.6*	16.4	11.1	15.0

Note. Estimates are based on weighted valid percentages.
[a]Sample size does not add up to the sample total due to nonresponse to question on mental disorder.
*Statistically significant difference between no reported mental disorder group and reported mental disorder group with chi-square test (*P*<0.05).

TABLE 11–3. Six-month prevalence estimates for interpersonal trauma, by gender and mental disorder (with confidence intervals)

Source of interpersonal trauma	Male inmates (N=6,964) Mental disorder		Female inmates (N=564) Mental disorder	
	None reported (n=5,300[a])	Reported (n=1,568)	None reported (n=116[a])	Reported (n=321)
Physical victimization				
Inmate-on-inmate[b]	18.1 (17.0–19.2)*	29.6 (26.9–32.3)	14.9 (10.3–19.6)*	24.9 (20.0–29.7)
Staff-on-inmate[c]	23.8 (22.6–25.1)*	29.4 (26.7–32.1)	6.9 (3.5–10.3)	9.5 (6.3–12.7)
Either inmate- or staff-on-inmate[d]	32.8 (31.4–34.2)*	43.9 (41.0–46.8)	17.3 (12.4–22.2)*	28.9 (23.8–34.0)
Sexual victimization				
Inmate-on-inmate	3.1 (2.6–3.6)*	8.3 (6.8–9.8)	18.5 (13.4–23.7)	23.4 (18.6–28.1)
Staff-on-inmate	7.0 (6.3–7.8)*	9.5 (7.9–11.1)	7.5 (4.0–11.0)	7.9 (5.1–10.8)
Either inmate- or staff-on-inmate	8.9 (8.1–9.7)*	15.1 (13.2–17.1)	20.9 (15.5–26.3)	27.2 (22.3–32.2)
Physical *or* sexual victimization[e]				
Inmate-on-inmate	19.4 (18.2–20.6)*	32.3 (29.6–35.1)	26.2 (20.4–32.0)	37.0 (31.6–42.5)
Staff-on-inmate	26.7 (25.4–28.0)*	32.0 (29.3–34.8)	12.2 (7.8–16.5)	13.5 (9.8–17.2)
Either inmate- or staff-on-inmate	35.7 (34.3–37.1)*	47.7 (44.8–50.6)	29.9 (23.8–36.0)*	42.4 (36.8–48.0)

TABLE 11–3. Six-month prevalence estimates for interpersonal trauma, by gender and mental disorder (with confidence intervals) *(continued)*

Source of interpersonal trauma	Male inmates (*N*=6,964)		Female inmates (*N*=564)	
	Mental disorder		Mental disorder	
	None reported (*n*=5,300[a])	Reported (*n*=1,568)	None reported (*n*=116[a])	Reported (*n*=321)
Physical *and* sexual victimization[e]				
Inmate-on-inmate	1.7 (1.4–2.1)*	5.4 (4.2–6.5)	7.3 (3.9–10.7)	11.0 (7.5–14.5)
Staff-on-inmate	4.1 (3.6–4.7)*	6.6 (5.3–7.9)	2.3 (0.2–4.4)	3.8 (1.8–5.8)
Either inmate- or staff-on-inmate	5.9 (5.2–6.5)*	11.1 (9.4–12.7)	8.4 (4.7–12.0)	13.6 (9.8–17.3)

Note. Estimates are based on weighted valid percentages.

[a]Sample size does not add up to the sample total due to nonresponse to question on mental disorder.

[b]Denotes inmate perpetrator and inmate victim.

[c]Denotes staff perpetrator and inmate victim.

[d]Denotes either inmate *or* staff perpetrator and inmate victim.

[e]Physical *or* sexual victimization includes unduplicated counts of inmates who reported either sexual victimization or physical victimization during the 6-month period. Physical *and* sexual victimization includes unduplicated counts of inmates reporting both physical and sexual victimization during the 6-month period. Together, they equal the number of unduplicated counts of inmates reporting victimization, either physical or sexual. Consequently, percentages for the specific forms of victimization (physical, sexual) add to the percentages of conjoint forms of victimization (physical *or* sexual and physical *and* sexual). Deviations are due to rounding error.

*Statistically significant difference between no reported mental disorder group and reported mental disorder group (*P*<0.05).

(due in large measure to the sample size). Physical victimization perpetrated by staff against male inmates was more common than against female inmates. Inmates were more likely than staff to be perpetrators of sexual victimization against female inmates, independent of reported mental disorder. Approximately 10% of male and female inmates reported experiencing sexual and physical victimization during a 6-month period. Although self-reports by inmates may include some cases of false allegations of victimization, this possibility does not eradicate the differences in staff victimization rates against male versus female inmates.

With two types of interpersonal trauma (physical and sexual) and two potential perpetrators (inmates and staff), different combinations of trauma and perpetrators are possible. Table 11–4 explores these combinations for male and female inmates with and without reported mental disorder. For example, of the 1,419 (20.3%) male inmates reporting inmate-on-inmate physical victimization during the 6-month period, 22% (4.46% of total) reported also experiencing sexual victimization by either other inmates or staff (13% by other inmates and 15% by staff) and 51% (10.35% of total) experienced physical victimization by a staff member. For male inmates reporting physical victimization (inmate- or staff-perpetrated), co-occurring sexual victimization was more likely for those reporting a mental disorder. Likewise, for male inmates reporting sexual victimization (inmate- or staff-perpetrated), conjoint inmate-perpetrated physical victimization was more frequently reported if the inmate also reported a mental disorder.

Given the smaller sample size for females, the patterns are less robust. However, approximately one-half (48%) of the 116 female inmates reporting inmate-on-inmate physical victimization also reported some type of sexual victimization perpetrated by another inmate or staff member. Of those female inmates reporting sexual victimization by either inmates or staff, the likelihood of also experiencing physical victimization increased if the woman also reported a mental disorder.

Prison and Community Interpersonal Trauma

People in prison may have experienced physical, sexual, or both types of interpersonal trauma in the community, in prison, or in both locations. The unique and overlapping experiences are shown in Figures 11–1 through 11–4. The ovals in these figures show the relative magnitudes of the types of victimization and their conjointness. Because it is infeasible to accurately represent the overlap of four proportions in a Venn diagram, we use combinations of three proportions: 1) sexually assaulted in prison ever, physically assaulted in prison ever, and physical victimization in the community prior to prison (Figures 11–1 and 11–2 for males and

TABLE 11–4. Six-month prevalence estimates of inmates with conjoint physical and sexual trauma by gender and mental disorder

| | Interpersonal trauma experience, 6-month period | | | | | |
| | Percentage also experiencing sexual trauma | | | Percentage also experiencing physical trauma | | |
Type of interpersonal trauma	Inmate-on-inmate[a]	Staff-on-inmate[b]	Either inmate- or staff-on-inmate[c]	Inmate-on-inmate[a]	Staff-on-inmate[b]	Either inmate- or staff-on-inmate[c]
MALE INMATES						
Physical victimization						
Inmate-on-inmate[a] (n=1,419[c])	**12.6**	**15.0**	**22.2**	—	50.8	—
No reported mental disorder (n=950)	9.7	14.4	19.6	—	50.4	—
Reported mental disorder (n=456)	18.6	16.1	27.7	—	50.9	—
Staff-on-inmate[b] (n=1,725[c])	**9.5**	**19.0**	**23.2**	41.8	—	—
No reported mental disorder (n=1,252)	7.5	17.6	20.7	38.2	—	—
Reported mental disorder (n=453)	14.8	23.0	30.1	51.2	—	—
Sexual victimization						
Inmate-on-inmate[a] (n=295[c])	—	**37.1**	—	**60.2**	**55.2**	**72.7**
No reported mental disorder (n=164)	—	40.0	—	55.7	56.9	69.2
Reported mental disorder (n=128)	—	31.9	—	65.8	52.4	77.2

TABLE 11–4. Six-month prevalence estimates of inmates with conjoint physical and sexual trauma by gender and mental disorder (continued)

| | Interpersonal trauma experience, 6-month period | | | | | |
| | Percentage also experiencing sexual trauma | | | Percentage also experiencing physical trauma | | |
Type of interpersonal trauma	Inmate-on-inmate[a]	Staff-on-inmate[b]	Either inmate- or staff-on-inmate[c]	Inmate-on-inmate[a]	Staff-on-inmate[b]	Either inmate- or staff-on-inmate[c]
MALE INMATES (continued)						
Sexual victimization (continued)						
Staff-on-inmate[b] (n=519[c])	**20.9**	—	—	**40.4**	**62.2**	**70.4**
No reported mental disorder (n=368)	17.6	—	—	36.8	59.1	68.4
Reported mental disorder (n=145)	27.8	—	—	49.7	70.5	76.6
FEMALE INMATES						
Physical victimization						
Inmate-on-inmate[a] (n=116[c])	**46.5**	**16.2**	**48.3**	—	**24.3**	—
No reported mental disorder (n=35)	48.8	18.0	48.8	—	30.6	—
Reported mental disorder (n=80)	44.8	15.6	47.4	—	21.8	—
Staff-on-inmate[b] (n=47[c])	**51.6**	**37.5**	**63.3**	**60.2**	—	—
No reported mental disorder (n=16)	48.7	33.1	58.0	65.8	—	—
Reported mental disorder (n=30)	53.1	39.9	66.2	57.2	—	—

TABLE 11–4. Six-month prevalence estimates of inmates with conjoint physical and sexual trauma by gender and mental disorder *(continued)*

Type of interpersonal trauma	Interpersonal trauma experience, 6-month period					
	Percentage also experiencing sexual trauma			Percentage also experiencing physical trauma		
	Inmate-on-inmate[a]	Staff-on-inmate[b]	Either inmate- or staff-on-inmate[c]	Inmate-on-inmate[a]	Staff-on-inmate[b]	Either inmate- or staff-on-inmate[c]
FEMALE INMATES *(continued)*						
Sexual victimization						
Inmate-on-inmate[a] (*n*=119)	—	21.1	—	44.9	20.3	49.3
No reported mental disorder (*n*=44)	—	27.7	—	39.4	18.2	41.6
Reported mental disorder (*n*=75)	—	17.4	—	47.5	21.7	53.1
Staff-on-inmate[b] (*n*=43)	57.9	—	—	43.6	41.3	53.7
No reported mental disorder (*n*=18)	68.2	—	—	35.7	30.5	44.2
Reported mental disorder (*n*=25)	50.7	—	—	49.4	49.1	60.5

Note. Estimates are based on weighted valid percentages.
[a]Denotes inmate perpetrator and inmate victim.
[b]Denotes staff perpetrator and inmate victim.
[c]Sample size does not add up to the sample total due to nonresponse to question on mental disorder.

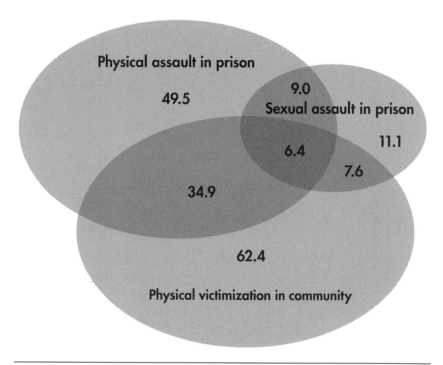

FIGURE 11–1. Proportional representation of physical and sexual assault inside prison and physical victimization in the community, male inmates.

females, respectively) and 2) sexually assaulted in prison ever, physically assaulted in prison ever, and sexual victimization prior to prison (Figures 11–3 and 11–4 for males and females, respectively).

As illustrated in Figures 11–1 and 11–2, relative to sexual victimization, physical victimization is more commonly experienced by males and females both in the community and in prison. Although both types of victimization were more frequently reported in the community than in prison, the relative prevalence between the two sites is an artifact of the longer reporting period for the community (ever in the community vs. ever in prison). The areas of overlap, however, are most noteworthy. An examination of co-occurring victimization by location indicates that 15% of female inmates, compared with 9% of male inmates, reported experiencing physical and sexual victimization inside prison, whereas 35% of male inmates, compared with 24% of female inmates, reported physical victimization in both locations. Gender differences are equally pronounced when comparing the overlap between types of victimization and loca-

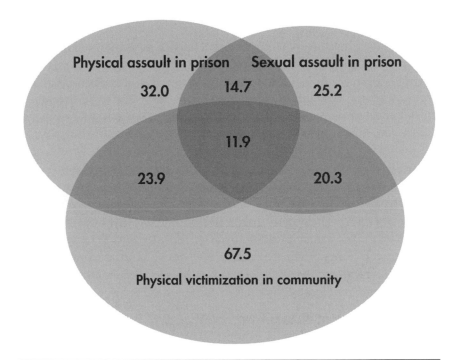

FIGURE 11–2. Proportional representation of physical and sexual assault inside prison and physical victimization in the community, female inmates.

tions. Approximately one-fifth of female inmates (20%) reported experiencing sexual assault inside prison and physical victimization prior to prison, compared to roughly 8% of male inmates. Female inmates were twice as likely as their male counterparts to experience sexual and physical assault in prison and physical victimization in the community (12% vs. 6%).

Regarding sexual victimization prior to prison (Figures 11–3 and 11–4), one in two female inmates reported experiencing sexual victimization in the community, compared with 1 in 10 male inmates. Female inmates reporting physical victimization inside prison were more likely than their male counterparts to report experiencing sexual victimization prior to prison (19% vs. 7%). Female inmates were five times more likely than their male counterparts to have experienced physical and sexual assault inside prison and sexual victimization in the community (11% vs. 2%).

Prison and Community Interpersonal Trauma and Mental Disorder

Community-based interpersonal trauma and reported mental disorder are associated with experiencing prison-based interpersonal trauma (see Table 11–5). In general, inmates, both male and female, were more likely to report prison-based physical victimization if they had experienced either physical or sexual victimization prior to age 18 and if they reported having a mental disorder. Approximately 70% or more of inmates with a mental disorder who reported physical victimization inside prison also reported experiencing physical victimization in the community prior to age 18, compared with about 50% of their counterparts without mental disorder (except staff–on–female inmate physical victimization, which was reported by 43%). These patterns are consistent for sexual victimization as well. Inmates, both male and female, who reported sexual victimization perpetrated by other inmates or staff in the past 6 months were more likely to have experienced physical or sexual victimization prior to age 18 and to have a reported mental disorder.[1]

Consequences of Interpersonal Trauma

Inmates were asked how often they experienced "problems" such as headaches, poor appetite, and disturbed or restless sleep; had difficulty caring about anything; had too little energy; worried about their safety; and had particular types of feelings (e.g., anxiety, hopelessness, helplessness). The percentages of inmates reporting that these problem experiences occurred once a week, a few times a week, or every day (referred to as "frequently") are shown in Table 11–6 by interpersonal trauma, mental disorder, and gender. In general, male inmates who experienced inter-

---

[1]Biased reporting of abuse may have occurred. We used an audio-computer–administered survey instrument to survey the inmate population, which is the most reliable method for collecting information about activities or events that are shaming or stigmatizing. Bias also may arise from the intent of inmates to make the facility and its staff members look bad. During the consent process, we stressed the importance of accurate reporting and its impact on the legitimacy of the data and survey. We surveyed respondents by units and rapidly over a 2- to 4-day period; staff did not have access to the survey questions; and the victimization questions were nested deep into a general survey focusing on quality of prison life. If inmates had systematically misreported victimization to malign the facility or staff, we would have expected to find much higher and clustered rates than those reported. We did find interprison differences in victimization rates, as well as in prison conditions, that were consistent with the "reputations" of the individual facilities.

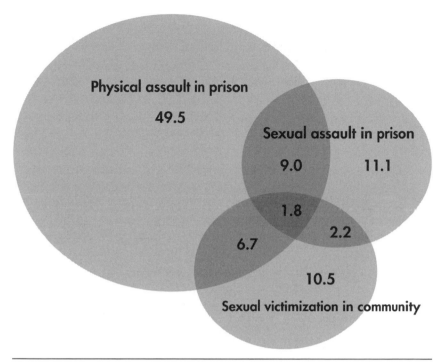

FIGURE 11–3. Proportional representation of physical and sexual assault inside prison and sexual victimization in the community, male inmates.

personal trauma (physical or sexual) during the past 6 months were more likely to report experiencing these problems than their counterparts without interpersonal trauma (indicated by "none") and if they reported a mental disorder (indicated by "yes"). More specifically, male inmates reporting any physical or sexual victimization and a mental disorder were significantly more likely than their counterparts without mental disorder to report that they frequently experienced headaches; felt tense or anxious, hopeless, and helpless; worried too much; and had difficulty caring about anything. Note, however, that male inmates who did not report any victimization in the past 6 months were also more likely to report these types of problems if they had a reported mental disorder than if they reported no mental disorder. In general, however, these inmates reported worrying less frequently about their safety than those inmates who experienced interpersonal trauma in the past 6 months, independent of reported mental disorder. Similar patterns were found for female inmates, although these differences rarely reached significance, perhaps because of the relatively small sample size. Approximately 80% of male and fe-

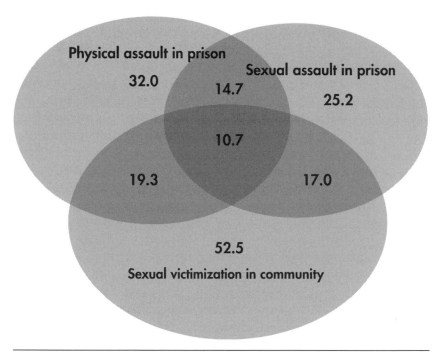

Physical assault in prison
32.0
14.7
Sexual assault in prison
25.2
10.7
19.3
17.0
52.5
Sexual victimization in community

FIGURE 11–4. Proportional representation of physical and sexual assault inside prison and sexual victimization in the community, female inmates.

male inmates reporting interpersonal trauma in the past 6 months said that they frequently had disturbed or restless sleep, felt tense or anxious, and felt they were worrying too much.

Correctional Health and Behavioral Health Treatment

Generally speaking, relative to inmates who did not report experiencing interpersonal trauma in the past 6 months, both male and female inmates reporting some form of victimization were more likely to report that they needed medical and mental health treatment in the past 6 months (see Table 11–7). However, independent of victimization status, male and female inmates with reported mental disorder were significantly more likely to report needing mental health treatment than their counterparts without mental disorder. Among males, a greater relative need for medical treatment was reported only by inmates with mental disorder (indicated by a significant difference). Overall, a reported mental disorder was a more reliable predictor of the need for mental health treatment than recent victimization experience for both male and female inmates.

TABLE 11–5. Percentage with prison- and community-based interpersonal trauma, by type of victimization, gender, and mental disorder

	Male inmates (N=6,964)		Female inmates (N=564)	
	Experienced at least once in past 6 months			
Source of interpersonal trauma	Yes	No	Yes	No
PRISON PHYSICAL VICTIMIZATION				
Inmate-on-inmate[a]	n=1,419	n=5,440	n=116	n=446
Prior physical victimization before age 18	67.4*	54.0	65.7*	49.5
No reported mental disorder	63.8*	51.0	58.5*	37.0
Reported mental disorder	75.2*	66.6	69.7	61.0
Prior sexual victimization before age 18	14.0*	8.7	56.1*	43.7
No reported mental disorder	10.8*	6.4	47.8*	30.0
Reported mental disorder	20.3	18.4	59.9	56.1
Staff-on-inmate[b]	n=1,725	n=5,131	n=47	n=516
Prior physical victimization before age 18	63.2*	54.5	61.9	52.0
No reported mental disorder	59.6*	51.3	43.1	40.0
Reported mental disorder	73.3*	67.5	72.1	62.2

TABLE 11–5. Percentage with prison- and community-based interpersonal trauma, by type of victimization, gender, and mental disorder (*continued*)

	Male inmates (*N*=6,964)		Female inmates (*N*=564)	
	Experienced at least once in past 6 months			
Source of interpersonal trauma	Yes	No	Yes	No
PRISON PHYSICAL VICTIMIZATION (*continued*)				
Staff-on-inmate[b] (*continued*)	*n*=1,725	*n*=5,131	*n*=47	*n*=516
Prior sexual victimization before age 18	10.8	9.5	53.2	45.6
No reported mental disorder	7.3	7.1	33.4	32.7
Reported mental disorder	20.6	18.4	63.8	56.3
PRISON SEXUAL VICTIMIZATION				
Inmate-on-inmate[a]	*n*=295	*n*=6,545	*n*=119	*n*=441
Prior physical victimization before age 18	64.0*	56.3	69.1*	48.4
No reported mental disorder	59.2	53.1	60.2*	35.6
Reported mental disorder	69.7	69.0	75.4*	59.4
Prior sexual victimization before age 18	27.2*	9.0	61.8*	41.9
No reported mental disorder	20.8*	6.7	51.0*	28.5
Reported mental disorder	35.1*	17.5	68.4*	53.3

TABLE 11–5. Percentage with prison- and community-based interpersonal trauma, by type of victimization, gender, and mental disorder *(continued)*

	Male inmates (*N*=6,964)		Female inmates (*N*=564)	
	Experienced at least once in past 6 months			
Source of interpersonal trauma	**Yes**	**No**	**Yes**	**No**
PRISON SEXUAL VICTIMIZATION *(continued)*				
Staff-on-inmate[b]	*n*=519	*n*=6,300	*n*=43	*n*=517
Prior physical victimization before age 18	66.6*	55.9	65.4	51.7
No reported mental disorder	63.2*	52.5	45.9	39.7
Reported mental disorder	74.5	68.6	79.2	61.6
Prior sexual victimization before age 18	15.6*	9.3	56.8	45.1
No reported mental disorder	13.0*	6.7	56.5*	30.8
Reported mental disorder	22.1	18.7	57.1	56.7

Note. Estimates are based on weighted valid percentages.
[a]Denotes inmate perpetrator and inmate victim.
[b]Denotes staff perpetrator and inmate victim.
*Statistically significant difference between victimization group and no victimization group with chi-square test (*P*<0.05).

TABLE 11–6. Personal well-being in the past 6 months by type of interpersonal trauma, gender, and mental disorder

Prison victimization experience in past 6 months

During the past 6 months, how often have you had (or been)...[c]	Male inmates (N=6,964)						Female inmates (N=564)					
	Any physical[a]		Any sexual[a]		None[b]		Any physical[a]		Any sexual[a]		None[b]	
	Reported mental disorder						Reported mental disorder					
	No n=1,724	Yes n=677	No n=467	Yes n=233	No n=3,364	Yes n=803	No n=41	Yes n=93	No n=50	Yes n=87	No n=166	Yes n=184
Headaches	45.9*	59.5	47.5*	58.5	31.3*	46.6	57.5	58.3	53.5	62.3	42.5*	57.3
A poor appetite	63.9*	72.7	64.1	70.6	45.5*	53.7	53.6	54.5	55.6	64.1	36.2*	54.7
Disturbed or restless sleep	79.9*	84.8	82.3	87.1	60.1*	72.0	68.9	81.0	62.0*	84.5	58.4*	70.0
Difficulty caring about anything	43.9*	55.2	46.0*	57.4	25.1*	37.1	39.2	43.3	32.3	47.7	15.1*	30.6
Too little energy	48.2*	62.8	53.2	60.0	29.3*	44.8	49.8	60.9	48.8	65.4	37.8*	48.7
Worried about your safety	68.8	71.0	72.7	72.9	43.6	42.9	51.0	63.2	38.0*	57.5	30.0	39.3
Feeling tense or anxious	68.1*	81.2	70.6*	82.4	47.6*	72.9	63.0*	85.0	54.0*	84.0	43.6*	74.9
Feeling of worrying too much	68.6*	79.5	67.7*	85.0	49.7*	67.0	57.4*	87.0	60.5*	82.8	57.4*	73.1

TABLE 11–6. Personal well-being in the past 6 months by type of interpersonal trauma, gender, and mental disorder *(continued)*

Prison victimization experience in past 6 months

During the past 6 months, how often have you had (or been)...[c]	Male inmates (N=6,964)						Female inmates (N=564)					
	Any physical[a]		Any sexual[a]		None[b]		Any physical[a]		Any sexual[a]		None[b]	
	Reported mental disorder						Reported mental disorder					
	No n=1,724	Yes n=677	No n=467	Yes n=233	No n=3,364	Yes n=803	No n=41	Yes n=93	No n=50	Yes n=87	No n=166	Yes n=184
Feeling of anger	70.3*	77.5	71.1	76.4	46.5*	56.5	56.3	69.2	46.3*	69.8	37.3*	51.1
Feeling hopeless	50.3*	63.9	53.1*	64.9	28.0*	46.1	47.2	58.2	46.2	60.6	26.6*	45.3
Feeling helpless	49.5	65.1	53.3*	67.0	28.4*	47.7	45.9	59.0	40.8*	61.8	29.2*	39.9

Note. Estimates are based on weighted valid percentages.

[a]"Any" denotes victimization perpetrated by either inmate or staff.

[b]"None" indicates no reported sexual or physical victimization during the past 6 months.

[c]Percentage of each group that reported experiencing the problem either once a week, a few times a week, or every day.

*Statistically significant difference between no reported mental disorder group and reported mental disorder group with chi-square test (P<0.05).

Virtually all male and female inmates (90% or more) reporting a need for medical treatment requested treatment, and the percentage of those receiving treatment ranged from 62% to 91%. Of those who received treatment, the vast majority of the male and female inmates rated the quality of care received as poor or fair, independent of victimization and mental disorder.

Requests for and receipt of mental health treatment varied by gender. Male inmates without a reported mental disorder but with recent victimization were very unlikely to report needing mental health treatment. Moreover, of those without self-reported mental disorder who identified a need, only 65%–70% requested treatment, and less than half of those requesting treatment received mental health treatment. Their counterparts with a reported mental disorder were more likely to identify needing mental health treatment (over 50%), requesting it (75%), and receiving it (80%). The quality of the mental health treatment received by male inmates was rated as poor or fair less often by those with reported mental disorder (ranging from 38% to 55%) than by those without a mental disorder (52%–71%).

Female inmates with and without a reported mental disorder were more likely than their male counterparts to report needing mental health treatment. Less than 30% of female inmates with a recent victimization experience but without a reported mental disorder identified a need for mental health treatment. Of those, roughly 91% requested treatment, and 75% or more of those requesting treatment received it. Most who had treatment (64%–73%) reported the quality as poor or fair. Of female inmates with reported victimization and mental disorder, over 60% said they needed mental health treatment during the past 6 months, three-quarters or more of these individuals requested treatment, virtually all (91%) received it, and over half thought the quality of care received was poor or fair.

TRAUMA INTERVENTIONS AND THEIR IMPLICATIONS

A two-step intervention strategy is suggested by our findings. The first step is *prevention* of prison-based interpersonal trauma. This requires a combination of classifying inmates in ways that minimize the exposure of vulnerable inmates to predators and sanctions for victimizing inmates, especially by correctional staff. Classification systems, in particular, need to account for the association of mental illness and history of prior victimization with future victimization. Simply asking people about prior victimization history as part of the classification process would be beneficial. Research clearly shows that people with mental illness, particularly

TABLE 11–7. Need, use, and ratings of medical and mental health treatment during the past 6 months by victimization status, gender, and mental disorder

During the past 6 months, have you needed…	Male inmates (N=6,964)						Female inmates (N=564)					
	Prison victimization experience in past 6 months[a]											
	Any physical		Any sexual		None		Any physical		Any sexual		None	
	Reported mental disorder						Reported mental disorder					
	No	Yes	No	Yes	No	Yes	No	Yes	No	Yes	No	Yes
	n=1,724	n=677	n=467	n=233	n=3,364	n=803	n=41	n=93	n=50	n=87	n=166	n=184
Medical treatment	68.4*	75.1	71.6*	81.7	54.1*	68.4	83.2	87.5	83.1	85.1	65.2	72.9
Treatment requested[b]	93.3	94.5	92.0	94.6	88.6	91.5	100.0	94.6	100.0	97.2	91.4	94.7
Treatment received[c]	80.1*	85.8	79.2	82.0	61.6*	91.3	72.5*	89.7	79.4	84.1	91.1	79.7
Treatment quality rated poor or fair[d]	83.3	81.2	83.2	79.9	69.6*	64.4	97.2	83.3	78.2	86.8	71.5	72.0
Mental health treatment	12.3*	54.1	14.2*	57.1	4.9*	50.0	28.0*	70.7	20.6*	62.5	13.4*	59.8
Treatment requested[b]	64.8*	75.3	71.1	75.3	59.5*	69.8	91.6	78.6	91.0	76.0	82.9	66.8
Treatment received[c]	47.0*	80.9	43.8*	79.0	86.4	87.9	75.1	93.6	83.6	92.0	90.4	90.0
Treatment quality rated poor or fair[d]	70.9*	55.0	63.5	49.6	52.1*	38.2	64.1	55.1	73.1	61.4	54.6	49.2

Note. Estimates are based on weighted valid percentages.

[a]"Any" denotes perpetrated by either inmate or staff. [b]Percentage among those who requested it. [c]Percentage among those who needed it.

[d]Percentage among those who received it.

*Statistically significant difference between no reported mental disorder group and reported mental disorder group with chi-square test (P<0.05).

serious mental illness, are at greater risk of victimization in the community (Teplin et al. 2005), in psychiatric settings (Frueh et al. 2005), and in prison (Wolff et al. 2007b).

Preventive classification must be combined with education, training, and investigative initiatives that 1) stress internal investigations of all reports of physical and sexual abuse of inmates and 2) explain what constitutes interpersonal trauma between inmates, inmates and correctional staff, inmates and administrative staff, inmates and medical and psychological staff, and inmates and other professional staff (e.g., teachers, social workers, custodial staff); how to avoid it; how to report it if it happens; and what the legal, classification, and therapeutic consequences are of being a predator. Information pamphlets and videos on interpersonal trauma should be available to inmates upon admission to a facility (analogous to the information protocols in place at most prisons regarding HIV and other infectious diseases). Officer and staff training is also required on the detection of and response to interpersonal victimization of inmates and the penalties associated with perpetrating or instigating abuse and not taking appropriate steps to prevent or report abuse of inmates. The goal of such training would be to eliminate accounts like the one cited below.

> I been jumped, attacked and brutally assaulted by Sgt. _____ and a group of officers. After beating me up for no reason and laughing about it, Sgt. _____ lied and gave me a threatening charge and had Officer _____ as a witness give a false statement....I did not resist but excessive force was used against me. I been badly assaulted and accused of a charge I did not do. I was badly hurt and refused medical treatment until my bruises were gone. My teeth were broken in the process. I reported all this to Special Investigation Division immediately, but they waited two weeks to investigate again all my black and blue marks from bruises were gone....I signed a paper stating I wanted to take a polygraph test to prove my innocence. I was transferred three days later to another prison before taking the test....I did nine months in adseg [short for administrative segregation, or solitary confinement].... (From a letter from an inmate, 2005)

Reasonable standards for investigation of abuse would include an impartial investigative team, a videotaped interview with the alleged victim within 24 hours of the abuse, the option of administering a polygraph test to the alleged victim and/or the perpetrator, and criminal penalties for proven allegations and administrative penalties for false allegations.

The second step of the intervention strategy is effective *diagnosis and treatment.* Trauma-related problems are underdiagnosed and undertreated in correctional facilities, and rarely are they taken into account when developing or modifying programming (Bloom et al. 2003; Morash et al. 1998). The prevalence and consequences of interpersonal trauma among male and female inmates suggest that ignoring it compromises the likely effectiveness of other related treatments for problems such as depression, anxiety, and substance use, as well as reentry initiatives focused on healthy and prosocial living in the community upon release. Interpersonal trauma is part of the problem and must be part of an integrated, multifaceted recovery strategy.

Any recovery-focused treatment approach must be informed by the comorbidity of interpersonal trauma (before prison and in prison), mental illness, and substance use, as well as by awareness that "gender makes a difference" (Bloom et al. 2003). Accordingly, efforts are advancing that encourage the development and implementation of gender-specific programming (American Correctional Association 1995; Balis 2007; Bloom et al. 2003; Morash et al. 1998; Sharp 2006). The literature is encouraging. Trauma-related psychological difficulties can be effectively treated (Harris and Fallot 2001). Moreover, an array of interventions are available (Rosenberg et al. 2001), although studies are ongoing regarding which are most effective in the community or correctional settings. The following are some general principles that can be used to choose among the possible interventions.

- *Treatment must be integrated.* Integrated treatment for comorbid conditions, such as mental illness and substance use problems, is considered superior to parallel, sequential, or single treatment models (Harris and Fallot 2001; Mueser et al. 2005).
- *Stepwise treatment of trauma-related difficulties is considered optimal* (Harris and Fallot 2001; Herman 1992). The first step focuses on safety and is achieved through recognition, education, and skill (i.e., cognitive, behavioral, and interpersonal) building that develops coping and life skills. These skills substitute for coping strategies that include the use of drugs or alcohol or other self-harming behaviors. The subsequent steps of trauma recovery address the experiences of trauma and their consequences, but only after stable and reliable functioning is achieved.
- *Environment matters.* Effective application of efficacious trauma processing therapies, such as exposure therapy or cognitive restructuring, requires safe and supportive environments (Bradley et al. 2005; Van Etten and Taylor 1998). Authoritative and punitively oriented settings, such as prisons, are not meant to be and are not healing. These environments are reminiscent in many ways of the community settings (typically involving the abuse of authority, power, and trust) in which trauma originally occurred (Bottoms 1999).

- *Continuity of care is vital to recovery.* Prison life and the return to the community from prison are stressful situations and, as a consequence, can trigger unhealthy coping mechanisms and relapse. It is important to remember that recovery is a lifelong process requiring maintenance and diligence (Drake et al. 2005; Rosenberg et al. 2001). (See Chapter 13, "Creating Wellness Through Collaborative Mental Health Interventions," for a discussion of "recovery" as a model and process.) As with recovery from substance and alcohol abuse, the coping skills developed as part of an integrated treatment approach must be practiced and reinforced to be useful in times of stress.

A number of gender-sensitive, integrated, skill-based (first-step) interventions exist that focus on trauma recovery and substance use problems among people with co-occurring mental illness (including serious mental illness) (Hien et al. 2004; Najavits et al. 2004; Rosenberg et al. 2001). The most well-known and researched models are Seeking Safety (Najavits 2003, 2009) and the Trauma Recovery and Empowerment Model (TREM; Fallot and Harris 2002). Both of these models are first-step therapies employing a manualized and integrated approach drawing heavily on cognitive-behavioral treatment for substance use problems and skill-building orientations to foster empowerment and safety. Although both models focus on trauma-related psychopathology, the underlying philosophies and contents are quite different.

Seeking Safety was designed for both individual and group modalities (Najavits 2003, 2009). The model integrates cognitive-behavioral treatment and psychoeducational principles. It is a present-focused cognitive-behavioral therapy designed to target trauma/PTSD and substance use disorders (Najavits 2009). The 25-session manual covers topics that address the cognitive, behavioral, interpersonal, and case management needs of persons with both substance use disorders and trauma/PTSD, and focuses on deficits found in the incarcerated population, including impulsiveness, social maladjustment, and emotional dysregulation.

TREM integrates empowerment, trauma education, and skill building. The goal of TREM is to build recovery skills that are grounded in healing and connecting trauma with self-harming behaviors such as substance use problems, interpersonal problems, and mental health symptoms. Although this treatment involves the provision of some psychoeducation, it mainly draws from psychodynamic and experiential techniques, along with the use of peer support. The intervention includes a clinician guide, a 33-session manual, and training videos (Fallot and Harris 2002).

The research, although limited, is growing and positive. Seeking Safety has shown positive outcomes in correctional settings both in a pilot study

(Zlotnick at al. 2003) and in a randomized controlled trial (Zlotnick et al. 2009), and a growing evidence base supports the efficacy of TREM (McHugo et al. 2005). No study has directly compared TREM and Seeking Safety and, as a consequence, no evidence exists on which model is best in a correctional (or community) setting or whether they work equally well for people with different types of co-occurring mental illness (e.g., serious mental illness).

CONCLUSION

Interpersonal trauma and its consequences are part of the life history of incarcerated persons, and often continue while these individuals are incarcerated. The challenge is to prevent further interpersonal trauma inside prison, through preventive interventions that include training and information strategies, and to treat such trauma effectively with integrated treatment interventions that recognize the overlap among trauma, mental illness, substance abuse, and behavioral problems. A dialogue among key stakeholders in the correctional and public health systems should be encouraged, focusing on procedures, training, and interventions to prevent and treat the consequences of interpersonal trauma within the incarcerated population. Creating safe prisons and prisons that provide effective treatments for complex trauma-related problems may be the smartest investment in future public safety and health.

SUMMARY POINTS

- Interpersonal trauma in childhood increases the likelihood of criminal justice involvement in adulthood among males and females.
- Compared with community samples, correctional populations have higher rates of mental illness and childhood victimization.
- Female inmates have higher rates of mental illness and childhood abuse relative to their male counterparts.
- Rates of sexual and physical victimization are higher in correctional settings than in community settings.
- Inside prison, physical victimization is more common than sexual victimization.
- Interpersonal trauma is strongly associated with physical illnesses, mental illnesses, and substance abuse.
- Community-based interpersonal trauma and reported mental disorder are associated with experiencing prison-based interpersonal trauma.

- Victimization and mental disorder predict the need for mental health treatment, with mental disorder being a stronger predictor.

- Our findings suggest a two-step safety intervention strategy. The prevention step seeks to reduce the likelihood of prison-based interpersonal trauma by incorporating historical interpersonal victimization into the inmate classification system and training officers and other staff to identify signs of potential victimization and to investigate reports or evidence of victimization. Effective diagnosis and treatment is the second step of the intervention strategy. Any recovery-focused treatment would be gender sensitive and informed by the comorbidity of interpersonal trauma, mental illness, and substance abuse.

REFERENCES

Abbott J, Johnson R, Koziol-McLain J, et al: Domestic violence against women: incidence and prevalence in an emergency department population. JAMA 273:1763–1767, 1995

Allen JG: Coping With Trauma: A Guide to Self-Understanding. Washington, DC, American Psychiatric Press, 1995

American Correctional Association: Public Correctional Policy on Female Offender Services. Lanham, MD, American Correctional Association, 1995

American Psychiatric Association: Diagnostic and Statistical Manual of Mental Disorders, 3rd Edition. Washington, DC, American Psychiatric Association, 1980

American Psychiatric Association: Diagnostic and Statistical Manual of Mental Disorders, 4th Edition, Text Revision. Washington, DC, American Psychiatric Association, 2000

Balis AF: Female prisoners and the case for gender-specific treatment and reentry programs, in Public Health Behind Bars: From Prisons to Communities. Edited by Greifinger RB. New York, Springer, 2007, pp 320–332

Ballanger JC, Davidson JR, Lecrubier Y, et al: Consensus statement update on posttraumatic stress disorder from the International Consensus Group on Depression and Anxiety. J Clin Psychol 65:55–62, 2004

Beck AJ, Harrison PM: Sexual victimization in state and federal prisons reported by inmates (NCJ 2194414). Washington, DC, U.S. Department of Justice, 2007

Blitz CL, Wolff N, Shi J: Physical victimization in prison: the role of mental illness. Int J Law Psychiatry 31:385–393, 2008

Bloom B, Owen B, Covington S: Gender-responsive strategies: research, practice, and guiding principles for women offenders. Washington, DC, U.S. Department of Justice, National Institute of Corrections, 2003

Bottoms AE: Interpersonal violence and social order in prisons, in Prisons. Edited by Tonry M, Petersilia J. Chicago, IL, University of Chicago Press, 1999, pp 205–281

Bradley R, Greene J, Russ E, et al: A multidimensional meta-analysis of psychotherapy for PTSD. Am J Psychiatry 62:214–227, 2005

Breslau N: Gender differences in trauma and posttraumatic stress disorder. J Gend Specif Med 5:34–40, 2002

Breslau N, Kessler RC, Chilcoat HD, et al: Trauma and posttraumatic stress disorder in the community: Detroit area survey of trauma. Arch Gen Psychiatry 55:626–632, 1998

Brodsky BS, Oquendo M, Ellis SP, et al: The relationship of childhood abuse to impulsivity and suicidal behavior in adults with major depression. Am J Psychiatry 158:1871–1877, 2001

Bromet E, Sonnega A, Kessler RC: Risk factors for DSM-III-R posttraumatic stress disorder: findings from the National Comorbidity Survey. Am J Epidemiol 147:353–361, 1998

Browne A, Finkelhor D: Impact of child sexual abuse: a review of the research. Psychol Bull 99:66–77, 1986

Browne A, Miller A, Maguin E: Prevalence and severity of lifetime physical and sexual victimization among incarcerated women. Int J Law Psychiatry 22:301–322, 1999

Carlson BE, McNutt LA, Choi DY: Childhood and adult abuse among women in primary health care: effects on mental health. J Interpers Violence 18:924–941, 2003

Chesney-Lind M: The Female Offender: Girls, Women, and Crime. Thousand Oaks, CA, Sage, 1997

Chilcoat MD, Breslau N: Posttraumatic stress disorder and drug disorders: testing causal pathways. Arch Gen Psychiatry 559:13–17, 1998

Child Abuse Prevention and Treatment Act of 1974, Pub. L. No. 93-237, 45 C.F.R. 1340. Available at: http://www.acf.hhs.gov/programs/cb/laws_policies/cblaws/capta/index.htm. Accessed April 4, 2009.

Children's Bureau: Maltreatment types of victims, 2006. Children's Bureau, U.S. Department of Health and Human Services, 2008

Cutler NJ, Nolen-Hoeksema S: Accounting for sex differences in depression through female victimization: childhood sexual abuse. Sex Roles 24:425–438, 1991

Davidson JR, Hughes D, Blazer DG, et al: Post-traumatic stress disorder in the community: an epidemiological study. Psychol Med 21:713–721, 1991

Dervic K, Grunebaum MF, Burke AK, et al: Protective factors against suicidal behavior in depressed adults reporting childhood abuse. J Nerv Ment Dis 194:971–974, 2006

Deykin EY, Keane TM, Kaloupek D, et al: Posttraumatic stress disorder and the use of health services. Psychosom Med 63:835–841, 2001

Ditton PM: Mental health and treatment of inmates and probationers (NCJ-174463). Washington, DC, U.S. Department of Justice, Bureau of Justice Statistics, 1999

Dodge M, Pogrebin MR: Collateral consequences of imprisonment for women: complications of reintegration. Prison J 81:42–54, 2001

Drake RE, Wallach MA, McGovern MP: Special section on relapse prevention: future directions in preventing relapse to substance abuse among clients with severe mental illnesses. Psychiatr Serv 56:1297–1302, 2005

Dube SR, Anda RF, Felitti VJ, et al: Childhood abuse, household dysfunction, and the risk of attempted suicide throughout the life span: findings from the Adverse Childhood Experiences Study. JAMA 286:3089–3096, 2001

Dutton D, Hart S: Evidence for long-term, specific effects of childhood abuse and neglect on criminal behavior in men. Int J Offender Ther Comp Criminol 36:129–137, 1992

Eisenstat S, Bancroft L: Domestic violence. N Engl J Med 341:886–892, 1999

Ernst C, Angst J, Foldenyi M: The Zurich study. Eur Arch Psychiatry Clin Neurosci 242:293–300, 1993

Fallot RD, Harris M: The Trauma Recovery and Empowerment Model (TREM): conceptual and practical issues in a group intervention for women. Community Ment Health J 38:475–485, 2002

Felitti VJ: Long-term medical consequences of incest, rape, and molestation. South Med J 84:328–331, 1991

Felitti VJ, Anda RF, Nordenberg D, et al: Relationship of childhood abuse and household dysfunction to many leading causes of death in adults: the Adverse Childhood Experiences (ACE) Study. Am J Prev Med 14:245–258, 1998

Firsten T: Violence in the lives of women on psych wards. Can Womens Stud 11:45–48, 1991

Fletcher BR, Shaver LD, Moon DG: Women Prisoners: A Forgotten Population. Portsmouth, NH, Greenwood Publishing Group, 1993

Ford JD: Disorders of extreme stress following war-zone military trauma: associated features of posttraumatic stress disorder or comorbid but distinct syndromes? J Consult Clin Psychol 67:3–12, 1999

Frueh BC, Knapp RG, Cusack KJ, et al: Patients' reports of traumatic or harmful experiences within the psychiatric setting. Psychiatr Serv 56:1123–1133, 2005

Gaes GG, Goldberg AL: Prison rape: a critical review of the literature (working paper). Washington, DC, National Institute of Justice, 2004

Goodman LA, Salyers MP, Mueser KT, et al: Recent victimization in women and men with severe mental illness: prevalence and correlates. J Trauma Stress 14:615–632, 2001

Greenfeld LA, Snell TL: Women offenders. Washington, DC, U.S. Department of Justice, Office of Justice Programs, Bureau of Justice Statistics, 1999

Guy E, Platt JJ, Zwerling I, et al: Mental health status of prisoners in an urban jail. Crim Justice Behav 12:29–53, 1985

Harlow CW: Prior abuse reported by inmates and probationers (NCJ 172879). Washington, DC, U.S. Department of Justice, 1999

Harris M, Fallot RD: Designing trauma-informed addictions services. New Dir Ment Health Serv 89:57–73, 2001

Hartwell SW: Female mentally ill offenders and their community reintegration needs: an initial examination. Int J Law Psychiatry 24:1–11, 2001

Hegadoren KM, Lasiuk GC, Coupland NJ: Posttraumatic stress disorder, part III: health effects of interpersonal violence among women. Perspect Psychiatr Care 42:163–173, 2006

Hegarty K, Gunn J, Chondros P, et al: Association between depression and abuse by partners of women attending general practice: descriptive, cross sectional survey. BMJ 328:621–624, 2004

Helzer JE, Robins LN, McEvoy L: Post-traumatic stress disorder in the general population: findings of the Epidemiologic Catchment Area survey. N Engl J Med 317:1630–1634, 1987

Herman JL: Trauma and Recovery: The Aftermath of Violence—From Domestic Abuse to Political Terror. New York, Basic Books, 1992

Hien DA, Cohen LR, Miele GM, et al: Promising treatments for women with comorbid PTSD and substance abuse. Am J Psychiatry 161:1426–1432, 2004

Ireland T, Widom CS: Childhood victimization and risk for alcohol and drug arrests. Int J Addict 29:235–274, 1994

Jacobsen LK, Southwick SM, Kosten TR: Substance use disorders in patients with posttraumatic stress disorder: a review of the literature. Am J Psychiatry 158:1184–1190, 2001

James DJ, Glaze LE: Mental health problems of prison and jail inmates (NCJ 213600). Washington, DC, U.S. Department of Justice, Bureau of Justice Statistics, 2006

Jemelka RP, Trupin E, Chiles JA: The mentally ill in prison: a review. Hosp Community Psychiatry 40:481–491, 1989

Jemelka RP, Rahman S, Trupin EW: Prison mental health: an overview, in Mental Illness in America's Prisons. Edited by Steadman HJ, Cocozza JJ. Seattle, WA, National Coalition for the Mentally Ill in the Criminal Justice System, 2000, pp 9–24

Kartha A, Brower V, Saitz R, et al: The impact of trauma exposure and posttraumatic stress disorder on healthcare utilization among primary care patients. Med Care 46:388–393, 2008

Kendall-Tackett KA, Williams LJ, Finkelhor D: Impact of sexual abuse on children: a review and synthesis of recent empirical studies. Psychol Bull 113:164–180, 1993

Kessler RC, Sonnega A, Bromet E, et al: Posttraumatic stress disorder in the National Comorbidity Survey. Arch Gen Psychiatry 52:1048–1060, 1995

Kramer A, Lorenzon D, Mueller G: Prevalence of intimate partner violence and health implications for women using emergency departments and primary care clinics. Womens Health Issues 14:19–29, 2004

Krug EG, Dahlberg LL, Mercy JA, et al (eds): World Report on Violence and Health, 2002. Geneva, World Health Organization, 2002. Available at: http://www.who.int/violence_injury_prevention/violence/world_report/en. Accessed April 4, 2009.

Lasiuk GC, Hegadoren KM: Posttraumatic stress disorder: development of the construct within the North American psychiatric taxonomy. Perspect Psychiatr Care 42:72–81, 2006

Leserman J, Drossman DA, Li S, et al: Sexual and physical abuse history in gastroenterology practice: how types of abuse impact health status. Psychosom Med 58:4–15, 1996

Malinosky-Rummell R, Hansen DJ: Long-term consequences of childhood physical abuse. Psychol Bull 114:68–79, 1993

McClellan DS, Farabee D, Crouch BM: Early victimization, drug use, and criminality: a comparison of male and female prisoners. Crim Justice Behav 24:455–467, 1997

McHugo GJ, Caspi Y, Kammerer N, et al: The assessment of trauma history in women with co-occurring substance abuse and mental disorders and a history of interpersonal violence. J Behav Health Serv Res 32:113–127, 2005

Morash M, Bynum TS, Koons BA: Women offenders: programming needs and promising approaches. Washington, DC, U.S. Department of Justice, 1998

Mueser KT, Drake RE, Sigmon SC, et al: Psychosocial interventions for adults with severe mental illnesses and co-occurring substance use disorders: a review of specific interventions. J Dual Diagn 1:57–82, 2005

Najavits LM: Seeking Safety: a new psychotherapy for posttraumatic stress disorder and substance use disorder, in Trauma and Substance Abuse: Causes, Consequences, and Treatment of Comorbid Disorders. Edited by Ouimette P, Brown PJ. Washington, DC, American Psychological Association, 2003, pp 147–170

Najavits LM: Seeking Safety: a model for trauma and/or substance abuse. 2009. Available at: http://www.seekingsafety.org. Accessed April 4, 2009.

Najavits LM, Sonn J, Walsh M, et al: Domestic violence in women with PTSD and substance abuse. Addict Behav 29:707–715, 2004

Norris FH, Friedman MJ, Watson PJ: 60,000 disaster victims speak, part I: an empirical review of the empirical literature, 1981–2001. Psychiatry 65:207–239, 2002

Parke RD, Clarke-Stewart KA: Effects of parental incarceration on young children, in Prisoners Once Removed: The Impact of Incarceration and Reentry on Children, Families, and Communities. Edited by Travis J, Waul M. Washington, DC, Urban Institute, 2003, pp 189–232

Rand M, Catalano S: Criminal victimization, 2006 (NCJ 219413). Washington, DC, U.S. Department of Justice, Bureau of Justice Statistics, 2007

Regier DA, Farmer ME, Rae DS, et al: Comorbidity of mental disorders with alcohol and other drug abuse: results from the Epidemiologic Catchment Area (ECA) study. JAMA 264:2511–2518, 1990

Reiter RC, Gambone JC: Demographic and historic variables in women with idiopathic chronic pelvic pain. Obstet Gynecol 75:428–432, 1990

Resnick HS, Acierno R, Kilpatrick DG, et al: Health impact of interpersonal violence, 2: medical and mental health outcomes. Behav Med 23:65–78, 1997

Rosenberg SD, Mueser KT, Friedman MJ, et al: Developing effective treatments for posttraumatic disorders among people with severe mental illness. Psychiatr Serv 52:1453–1461, 2001

Sacks JY: Women with co-occurring substance use and mental disorders (COD) in the criminal justice system: a research review. Behav Sci Law 22:449–466, 2004

Scarinci IC, McDonald-Haile J, Bradley LA, et al: Altered pain perception and psychosocial features among women with gastrointestinal disorders and history of abuse: a preliminary model. Am J Med 97:108–118, 1994

Schnurr PP, Green BL (eds): Trauma and Health: Physical Health Consequences of Exposure to Extreme Stress. Washington, DC, American Psychological Association, 2004

Schofferman J, Anderson D, Hines R, et al: Childhood psychological trauma and chronic refractory low-back pain. Clin J Pain 9:260–265, 1993

Sharp SF: It's not just men anymore: the criminal justice system and women in the 21st century. The Criminologist 31:2–5, 2006

Siegel JA: Aggressive behavior among women sexually abused as children. Violence Vict 15:235–255, 2000

Siegel JA, Williams LM: The relationship between child sexual abuse and female delinquency and crime: a prospective study. Journal of Research in Crime and Delinquency 40:71–94, 2003

Smith C, Thornberry TP: The relationship between childhood maltreatment and adolescent involvement in delinquency. Criminology 33:451–481, 1995

Teplin LA: Criminalization of the mentally ill: speculation in search of data. Psychol Bull 94:54–67, 1983

Teplin LA, Abram KM, McClelland GM: Prevalence of psychiatric disorders among incarcerated women: pretrial jail detainees. Arch Gen Psychiatry 53:505–512, 1996

Teplin LA, McClelland GM, Abram KM, et al: Crime victimization in adults with severe mental illness: comparison with the National Crime Victimization Survey. Arch Gen Psychiatry 62:911–921, 2005

Terr LC: Childhood traumas: an outline and overview. Focus 1:322–333, 2003

Tjaden P, Thoennes N: Prevalence, incidence, and consequences of violence against women: findings from the National Violence Against Women Survey. Research in Brief. Washington, DC, Office of Justice Programs, National Institute of Justice, 1998

van der Kolk BA, Pelcovitz D, Roth S, et al: Dissociation, somatization, and affect dysregulation: the complexity of adaptation of trauma. Am J Psychiatry 153:83–93, 1996

Van Etten ML, Taylor S: Comparative efficacy of treatments for posttraumatic stress disorder: a meta-analysis. Clin Psychol Rev 5:126–144, 1998

Widom CS: Child abuse, neglect, and violent criminal behavior. Criminology 27:251–271, 1989

Widom CS: Victims of childhood sexual abuse: later criminal consequences. Washington, DC, U.S. Department of Justice, 1995

Widom CS, Maxfield MG: An update on the "cycle of violence." 2001. Washington, DC, National Institute of Justice, 2001. Available at: www.ncjrs.gov/pdffiles1/nij/184894.pdf. Accessed April 4, 2009.

Widom CS, White HR: Problem behaviours in abused and neglected children grown up: prevalence and co-occurrence of substance abuse, crime and violence. Crim Behav Ment Health 7:287–310, 1997

Widom C, DuMont K, Czaja S: A prospective investigation of major depressive disorder and comorbidity in abused and neglected children grown up. Arch Gen Psychiatry 64:49–56, 2007

Windle M, Windle RC, Scheidt DM, et al: Physical and sexual abuse and associated mental disorders among alcoholic inpatients. Am J Psychiatry 152:1322–1328, 1995

Wolff N, Blitz CL, Shi J, et al: Sexual violence inside prison: rates of victimization. J Urban Health 83:835–848, 2006

Wolff N, Blitz C, Shi J, et al: Physical violence inside prison: rates of victimization. Crim Justice Behav 34:588–599, 2007a

Wolff N, Blitz C, Shi J: Rates of sexual victimization inside prison for people with and without mental disorder. Psychiatr Serv 58:1087–1094, 2007b

Wolff N, Shi J, Blitz C, et al: Understanding sexual victimization inside prisons: factors that predict risk. Criminol Public Policy 6:201–231, 2007c

Wolff N, Shi J, Blitz C: Racial and ethnic disparities in types and sources of victimization inside prison. Prison J 88:451–472, 2008

Wooldredge JD: Inmate lifestyles and opportunities for victimization. Journal of Research in Crime and Delinquency 35:480–502, 1998

Zlotnick C, Najavits LM, Rohsenow DJ, et al: A cognitive-behavioral treatment for incarcerated women with substance abuse disorder and posttraumatic stress disorder: findings from a pilot study. J Subst Abuse Treat 25:99–105, 2003

Zlotnick C, Johnson J, Najavits LM: Randomized controlled pilot study of cognitive-behavioral therapy in a sample of incarcerated women with substance use disorder and PTSD. Behav Ther 2009; doi:10.1016/j.beth.2008.09.004

CHAPTER 12

Pharmacotherapy in Correctional Settings

Kathryn A. Burns, M.D., M.P.H.

Since the early 1990s, the use of psychotropic medications in correctional settings has undergone a profound transformation. In the not so distant past, the tendency was to use psychotropic medications, and in particular antipsychotic medications, for their sedating side effects as a means of managing undesirable behavior. Courts presiding over correctional litigation cases viewed psychotropic medications as "dangerous drugs" prescribed to control thinking and behavior (*Ruiz v. Estelle* 1980). Scientific advances in understanding serious mental illnesses as biologically based brain disorders and prescriptive advances in targeting psychotropic medication toward amelioration or elimination of specific symptoms have reformed psychopharmacological practice in both civilian and correctional populations. Subsequent class-action correctional litigation has underscored that the availability of psychotropic medication is a necessary component of inmate mental health care. Inmates with serious mental illness have a constitutional right to treatment of their condition. Withholding treatment for serious mental illness constitutes cruel and unusual punishment, a violation of the U.S. Constitution's Eighth Amendment (Cohen 1998). Psychotropic medication is the medically accepted standard of care or treatment of choice for certain of the serious mental illnesses.

In this chapter, I address psychopharmacological principles in correctional settings, highlighting those aspects of care that are unique or deserving of special consideration in the correctional environment. I do not intend to imply that treatment with psychotropic medication is the sole requirement for appropriate mental health care of inmates; rather, psychotropic medication is one significant component of a comprehensive treatment plan. Other treatment plan components are based on the clinical condition being treated and the duration and conditions of confinement, but I do not discuss these because they are outside the scope of this chapter. Underlying this chapter are two assumptions: 1) that psychotropic medications will be prescribed only when they are clinically indicated and will not be used for disciplinary purposes and 2) that the correctional facility will have appropriately trained staff in sufficient numbers to periodically monitor clinical response and potential side effects when psychotropic medications are used.

PSYCHOPHARMACOLOGICAL PRACTICE PRINCIPLES REQUIRING SPECIAL CONSIDERATION IN CORRECTIONAL FACILITIES

Informed Consent

Correctional facilities, by their very nature, are inherently coercive environments. Nevertheless, the principles of informed consent remain applicable to inmates. The nature and purpose of treatment and the risks and benefits of potential types of treatment, including the risks and benefits of no treatment, should be explained such that the inmate can make an informed choice. The discussion itself and the inmate's consent to treatment should be documented in the medical record. This documentation may take the form of a detailed progress note or a specialized form that the inmate is asked to sign. Inmates also have a right to refuse treatment. Facility policies concerning their right to refuse treatment should conform to the rules and procedures of the jurisdiction in which the facility is located (American Psychiatric Association 2000).

Involuntary Medication: Ability to Force Medication

As in the civilian world, involuntary forcible administration of medication during an emergency is permissible if the drug is administered for medical reasons and for a limited duration of time, as may be specified by state rules and regulations. An *emergency* is generally defined in this case as significant property destruction or an imminent threat to the life or safety of the inmate or others. Emergency administration of medication may prevent the need for the application of physical restraints or may be used in conjunction with physical restraint to assist the inmate in regaining control of his or her thoughts and behavior. Procedures for the administration of medication during an emergency should conform to the pertinent requirements of the jurisdiction in which the facility is located.

In other, "nonemergency" situations, correctional settings also have the capacity to administer psychotropic medication to competent but refusing inmates, provided that the correctional facility follows certain procedural requirements. Correctional facilities have an obligation to protect the safety of other inmates in their custody, their own staff, and visitors, and they have an interest in maintaining order in the facility. Therefore, under certain circumstances, correctional facilities may override medication refusals in instances where an inmate has a mental disorder and poses a likelihood of serious harm to self or others or is gravely disabled (*Washington v. Harper* 1990).

In 1990, the U.S. Supreme Court upheld a prison policy in Washington State that provided the following rights to inmates facing involuntary medication: the right to a hearing on the issue; the right to notice of the hearing; the rights to attend the hearing, present evidence, and cross-examine witnesses; the right to representation by a lay adviser; the right to appeal the decision; and the right to periodic review of ongoing administration of involuntary medication (*Washington v. Harper* 1990). Under the Washington State policy, the involuntary medication hearing is presided over by a small committee, composed of medical/mental health professionals with no current treatment relationship with the inmate who must render a medical decision regarding the necessity of treatment with medication. Security factors may be considered, but the decision is primarily medical (Cohen 1998). Individual state laws may impose additional procedural requirements beyond these rights that were accepted as adequate by the *Harper* Court.

Medication Administration

Virtually all psychotropic medication doses are individually administered in correctional settings. Medication administration is the act in which a single dose of an identified medication is given to an inmate. Correctional systems have devised several different mechanisms to accomplish this goal. This process can include "pill call" or centralized "med pass," medication "delivery" processes, or a combination of various systems.

Larger correctional facilities that permit inmate movement (alone or with correctional escorts) have a centralized medication administration area in the medical clinic or infirmary. At scheduled medication administration times, inmates walk or are escorted to the centralized administration area to receive their medications. In this model, inmates generally wait in a single-file line under the supervision of a correctional officer until called up to a medication administration "window" by a health care worker, most often a nurse. The nurse checks the inmate's identity by looking at his or her identification; reviews the medication administration record to be certain which medications, as well as their doses and form (liquid, pill, injectable), are to be administered; and visually inspects the medication before handing it to the inmate. Medication ingestion is observed during this process, usually by the nurse administering the medication or the correctional officer supervising the inmates in line. The nurse who administers the medication immediately documents the transaction on the medication administration record.

Facilities using the pill-call line for medication administration must be mindful of the impact of the location, duration, and efficiency of the process on medication compliance. For example, if inmates are required to wait outdoors for medication and the weather is inordinately hot or otherwise inclement, some inmates will be tempted to skip one or more doses of medication to avoid the unpleasant weather. Similarly, if receiving each dose of medication requires standing in line for more than 15–20 minutes, many inmates may opt to forgo their medication. Some facilities have attempted to address these potential problems by building an awning over the pill-call line or by issuing medications indoors to provide protection from the elements for inmates waiting in line. Others have staggered the times at which small groups of inmates are called to the pill-call line. This may involve calling inmates to the line according to their assigned housing unit at staggered 5- or 10-minute intervals so the line never has more than 10–15 people.

In facilities where security concerns do not permit inmate movement to a centralized medication administration area, in segregation units, or in facilities that do not have a centralized medication administration area, medications are taken to the inmates' cells, pods, or cell blocks. Medications are administered in this delivery method by nursing staff or by correctional staff trained to do so. Certainly, the preferred practice is to have nursing staff administer all doses of prescription medication. Nurses can provide brief medication education during the administration process, are better able to answer questions posed by the inmate receiving the medication, and can make skilled observations of the effectiveness or potential side effects of the medication prescribed. However, some correctional facilities do not have around-the-clock nursing coverage and must use correctional officers to deliver medications, provided that the state pharmacy board in which the facility is located permits medication delivery by nonmedical staff. If so permitted, the officers delivering medications must receive training in the basics of medication delivery to ensure that the right inmate receives the correct medication at the right time and that the process is appropriately documented. In addition, the state pharmacy and nursing boards should be consulted to ensure that the prescription medications are appropriately packaged and labeled for delivery by nonmedical personnel to be consistent with state law.

Some facilities have developed a self-carry or keep-on-person medication administration procedure. This procedure allows some inmates to be given a specified amount of certain medications (generally medications for treatment of physical conditions) to maintain on their own and take as directed by prescription. Although any medication may be subject to a keep-on-person procedure, psychotropic medication prescriptions are generally not subject to self-carry programs. The purpose of this limitation is to reduce the possibility of hoarding, overdose, trading, and/or noncompliance that might not become evident until an adverse effect on mental state or adverse incident occurs. Inmates on self-carry medication programs pick up their supply of medication from the infirmary or clinic area at set intervals (often 30 days) and turn in any unused medication and/or the empty blister pack when the new supply is given to them.

Many correctional facilities, particularly large ones, often use a combination of medication administration practices. These may include delivery to inmates in lockdown settings, centralized administration for general population, and a self-carry program for certain medications and/or for inmates who may not be available to participate in a centralized pill-call process because of their involvement in work details where schedules conflict with the posted pill-call times.

In correctional settings, essentially all psychotropic medications are administered by staff (nursing staff or correctional officers trained in the appropriate delivery of medication) and recorded in real time. This practice provides valuable information about inmate medication compliance and staff observations of medication effectiveness that are not generally available in the community, where the only source of medication compliance information is self-report and where observations of effectiveness are more limited to infrequent contacts. *Medication compliance* is the degree of patient adherence to taking all doses of medication as prescribed. Effectiveness of psychotropic medication is difficult, if not impossible, to assess unless the patient has been 100% compliant with taking all doses of the medication as prescribed.

These major advantages are not without some challenges, however. Medication administration records are most often maintained for the current month (and sometimes recent past months) in a location separate from the inmate medical and mental health files and, therefore, are not always immediately or readily available during mental health clinic appointments with the inmate. In addition, the time involved and staff intensiveness of some medication administration processes may limit the number of med passes or pill calls that may be accomplished during the day. Fortunately, most psychotropic medications may be taken in once- or twice-daily doses based on their metabolism or half-life. Some medications may require more frequent delivery times, but this should be the exception, because increased frequency is often unnecessary based on metabolism, reduces inmate compliance due to the added burden of frequent dosing, and creates added work for nursing and correctional staff. Prescribers' capacity to order emergency ("stat") medications and/or as-needed ("prn") medications may be limited.

Prescribers of psychotropic medication must be familiar with the correctional facility's medication processes, procedures, and administration times. Such familiarity may assist in choosing among various alternative medications on the basis of recommended dosing schedules, be of assistance to medication administration staff, and permit accurate orders for laboratory testing, particularly trough serum levels of medications. Also, psychotropic medication prescribers must advocate for appropriate medication administration times, consistent with medication pharmacodynamics and actions. Some correctional facilities have attempted to eliminate bedtime ("hs," for "hour of sleep") medication administration for budgetary or other reasons. (Limiting medication administration to two passes instead of three saves nursing and correctional supervision time.) However, afternoon administration of medications prescribed for bedtime is problematic for a number of reasons, including daytime sedation when promoting nighttime sleep was intended. In this instance, inmates may attempt to "cheek" (fail to swallow) medications administered early and save them for use at bedtime, a practice that presents serious correctional management issues and may result in disciplinary measures for the inmate and potential medication order discontinuation. Physicians must be aware of these administrative decisions and provide appropriate education and advocacy to decision makers when necessary so as not to compromise patient care. Physicians should be able to advocate that first-dose morning medications be administered after 6:00 A.M. and that bedtime medications be administered after 8:00 P.M. in correctional facilities.

Clinical Case 12–1

Mr. J, a 42-year-old man with a long history of bipolar disorder that has been well controlled with lithium carbonate maintenance therapy, was booked into a county jail in March. His lithium dosage was continued at 600 mg twice daily. The jail's twice-daily medication administration times were 9:00 A.M. and 4:00 P.M.

Mr. J. was unable to make bond and was retained in the county jail awaiting trial. After 2 months, the treating psychiatrist in the jail ordered a serum lithium level. The morning dose of lithium was held, and the inmate's blood was drawn at approximately 10:30 A.M., 18½ hours after his last dose. The lithium level was reported as 0.3 mEq/L (the therapeutic range is 0.5–1.5 mEq/L). Although the patient was asymptomatic in terms of his mood, the treating psychiatrist decided to increase the lithium dosage based on the upcoming stress of trial and a subtherapeutic serum lithium level. The dosage was increased to 600 mg orally in the morning and 900 mg orally at "bedtime." A subsequent blood level was also reported as being 0.3 mEq/L, and the lithium dosage was increased again. The inmate was compliant with taking the increasing dosage of lithium and made no complaints about experiencing any side effects.

The jail was not air-conditioned, and in mid-July, the nurse passing out medications noted the inmate to be uncharacteristically confused, disoriented, tremulous, and unsteady on his feet. He was subsequently taken to the local medical hospital and found to have lithium toxicity. Contributing factors included dehydration and increasing dosages of prescribed medication based on the doctor's misinterpretation of serum lithium levels being low when the blood was actually drawn well beyond trough time. The prescriber not only was unfamiliar with medication administration times but failed to consider blood draw time and its impact on the results.

Heat Sensitivity

Persons taking many of the psychotropic medications, particularly antipsychotic and certain antidepressant medications, demonstrate an increased sensitivity to sunlight and are at higher risk of heat-induced syndromes: heatstroke, hyperthermia, and heat prostration. (Note that selective serotonin reuptake inhibitors, or SSRIs—one class of antidepressant medications discussed later in this chapter—are less problematic than tricyclic antidepressants in this regard.) Heatstroke is a very serious and potentially fatal medical condition. Signs and symptoms of heatstroke are summarized in Table 12–1. Sustained high body temperatures that occur in untreated heatstroke may result in brain or muscle damage, kidney failure, coma, and even death. The occurrence of heat-related prob-

TABLE 12–1.   Signs and symptoms of heatstroke

Muscle cramps and weakness

Nausea and vomiting

Dehydration

Increased heart rate

Hyperventilation

Hot, flushed skin (ashen color in severe cases)

Agitation

Elevated body temperature (fever)

lems for inmates taking psychotropic medications may be exacerbated in correctional facilities, where inmates may be assigned to outdoor work details and where living areas often have very limited (or nonexistent) means of cooling the temperature.

When psychotropic medications are prescribed, appropriate precautions to prevent the development of heat-related problems should be exercised. When outdoor temperatures are elevated, inmates taking these medications should avoid excessive exhausting activities, and when under direct sunlight, these inmates should wear protective clothing and sunscreen. Care should be taken both for inmate outdoor work assignments and for outdoor recreation activities. Additional water and break times must be provided. Inmate patients should be permitted and encouraged to drink 8–12 glasses of liquid per day. Indoor temperatures of housing units should be monitored during periods of warm or hot weather, and when the indoor temperature exceeds 85°F, consideration must be given to increasing ventilation (moving fans into the area), providing increased fluids and ice to the inmates, permitting additional showers to provide cooling, and possible transfer to another area of the institution that is more compatible with clinical status.

Correctional security, administrative, medical, and mental health staff must all be aware of the increased sensitivity of inmates taking psychotropic medication to heat-related problems, be able to recognize the signs and symptoms of heatstroke, and be able to respond rapidly to lower the inmates' body temperature.

Clinical Case 12–2

Mr. S is a 40-year-old inmate with a diagnosis of schizophrenia who is serving a 15-year sentence for assault. The symptoms of his schizophrenia have responded well to treatment with haloperidol, 5 mg/day at bedtime. Mr. S's illness had been very stable for the past 4 years. He had a job assignment in his housing unit as an aid to another inmate, his roommate, who was wheelchair bound. He fulfilled his job assignment responsibly and was very attentive to his fellow inmate. Security staff often asked Mr. S to run errands for them, to relay information between housing units or to other areas of the prison.

One summer evening, Mr. S suddenly began to behave in a bizarre manner: he stripped off all his clothing and began yelling incoherently. He was noted to be sweating profusely. He did not respond to officers' attempts to calm him down, and his roommate became frightened. Medical staff had gone off duty for the evening. Correctional staff moved Mr. S out of his cell into an observation area—a different cell, in which he was housed alone. The cell did not contain a sink or commode, but officers permitted Mr. S to come out of the cell regularly for bathroom breaks and water. Medical staff were consulted and believed the problems were secondary to an exacerbation of mental illness. They did not see Mr. S but recommended consultation with the psychiatrist. Without taking vital signs or physically assessing the inmate, the psychiatrist ordered an increased dosage of haloperidol, with which Mr. S was compliant.

Over the next 2 days, Mr. S became increasingly confused and disoriented. His responses to questions were incoherent. He had great difficulty following instructions from correctional staff during bathroom breaks. He displayed difficulty operating the water fountain, and his fluid intake was nil. Similarly, officers noted his meal trays were returned untouched. Neither medical nor mental health staff were notified of Mr. S's condition or lack of food and water intake. Cell block room temperatures were recorded as being between 90° and 94°F consistently throughout this time period. On the evening of the third day, Mr. S was discovered lifeless in his cell during routine rounds. Although cardiopulmonary resuscitation was initiated and emergency medical service was summoned, Mr. S could not be revived. An autopsy revealed dehydration as the cause of death.

Use of Benzodiazepines

Benzodiazepine use in correctional facilities should be restricted to medical detoxification from alcohol and/or benzodiazepines, prevention of withdrawal syndromes, and perhaps time-limited management of acute agitation, anxiety, or stress. Benzodiazepine use is strongly discouraged in correctional facilities due to the high abuse potential in a population estimated to have a prevalence rate for substance use disorders of 70%–90% (American Psychiatric Association 2000). Use of benzodiazepines in correctional facilities raises the possibility of drug seeking or manipulation to obtain the medication and may set up serious security problems with bartering, selling, or trading the medication. Inmates with legitimate need may become targets of intimidation or assault by others seeking the medication. Therefore, alternative, effective, but nonaddicting medications are more appropriate choices for managing anxiety in the correctional environment. (Specific suggestions for the treatment of documented anxiety disorders may be found later in this chapter.)

Medication Algorithms and Expert Consensus Guidelines

Psychotropic medication prescribing practices are becoming increasingly standardized through the issuance of expert consensus and evidence-based practice guidelines and the development of medication algorithms for the treatment of specific psychiatric disorders. Medication algorithms specify the conditions for which certain types of medications may be used, specify appropriate dosage levels, and provide alternative stepwise directions for changing or augmenting medication as clinically appropriate. One such medication algorithm project, the Texas Medication Algorithm Project, was started in 1996. This project includes treatment algorithms for schizophrenia, major depression, and bipolar disorder. A prospective comparison of the clinical outcomes and economic costs of using the medication algorithms versus "treatment as usual" within the public mental health outpatient system in Texas has been undertaken, and the results are currently under analysis (Kashner et al. 2006; Rush et al. 2003).

Correctional facilities may wish to consider adopting formal practice guidelines. Evidence-based expert consensus treatment guidelines offer a scientific and clinically sound basis for making treatment decisions and are consistent with the evolving community standard of care. Another potential advantage of adopting guidelines is that they help correctional systems achieve treatment consistency across institutions. In addition, use of evidence-based treatment algorithms is likely to result in short- and long-term cost savings, both of which result from improved patient outcomes and less need of more intensive (expensive) crisis and inpatient care. If formal treatment guidelines are not adopted, correctional facilities should consider developing a mechanism to access consultation if psychotropic medications are being prescribed above recommended dosing guidelines or for indications not formally approved by the U.S. Food and Drug Administration (FDA).

CORRECTIONAL FORMULARY CONSIDERATIONS

In this section, I discuss major classes of psychotropic medication. The discussions are not intended to be exhaustive. In general, the classes and types of psychotropic medication that should be available in the facility's formulary are highly dependent on the facility's size, mission, psychiatric illnesses encountered in the inmate population, and inmate length of stay. However, if a correctional facility houses inmates with serious mental illnesses, antipsychotic, antidepressant, and mood-stabilizing medications must be on the medication formulary. In addition, correctional policy must permit access to nonformulary medications on a case-by-case basis to ensure access to appropriate treatment for serious mental illness. Psychiatrists must be involved in the development of the institution's formulary. Involvement may take the form of simply recommending psychotropic medications for inclusion on the formulary in the case of individual facilities or representation on a pharmacy and therapeutics committee in the case of larger facilities or correctional systems. (Correctional formulary considerations are summarized in Table 12–2.)

Antipsychotic Medications

Antipsychotic medications must be available for use in the treatment of schizophrenia, psychotic disorders, and psychotic symptoms accompanying other diagnoses. They fall into two large classes: conventional (older or first-generation) antipsychotics and next-generation (also called atypical or second-generation) antipsychotic medications. Conventional antipsychotic medications include chlorpromazine (Thorazine), haloperidol (Haldol), fluphenazine (Prolixin), trifluoperazine (Stelazine), loxapine (Loxitane), thiothixene (Navane), and thioridazine (Mellaril). These medications were developed and released in the United States during the late 1950s through early 1970s. All of them have a high affinity for blockade of dopamine receptors in the brain, which is believed to be responsible for their ameliorative effects on hallucinations. However, the blockade of dopamine receptors throughout the brain also interferes with neurological processes involved in normal movement and is responsible for the side effects on movement observed when conventional medications are prescribed.

Side effects on movement include severe, involuntary, and painful muscle spasms (dystonia); tremors and rigidity (drug-induced parkinsonism); profound restlessness (akathisia); and the possible development, usually over time, of involuntary, uncontrolled movement of various muscle groups, but most often those around the face and mouth (tardive dyskinesia). Some of these movement disorders are preventable with or responsive to the concomitant administration of antiparkinsonian medications, including benztropine (Cogentin), amantadine (Symmetrel), and trihexyphenidyl (Artane). Unfortunately, particularly benztropine and trihexyphenidyl have some abuse potential in the correctional environment,

TABLE 12–2. Correctional formulary considerations[a]

Class	Type	Correctional formulary recommendations and notes
Antipsychotic medications	Conventional	Include several medications and various forms, including oral (tablets and liquids) and injectable (short- and long-acting) forms. Antiparkinsonian medications must also be available for administration with conventional antipsychotic medications.
	Next-generation	Include access to clozapine, in addition to two or more other atypical medications. Consider inclusion of several formulations, such as injectable and orally disintegrating tablets.
Antidepressant medications	Selective serotonin reuptake inhibitors	Include several medications of this type and several formulations.
	Miscellaneous	Consider inclusion of venlafaxine and nefazodone because they can also be efficacious in the treatment of some anxiety disorders.
Mood stabilizers	Lithium	Lithium is efficacious in the treatment of bipolar disorder and is inexpensive. Periodic monitoring of blood levels and renal and thyroid functioning is required.
	Anticonvulsant medications	Include divalproex, valproic acid, and carbamazepine because they are approved for the treatment of bipolar disorder.
Anxiolytics	Benzodiazepines	Include several types and formulations for management of detoxification and withdrawal prevention. Consider for time-limited use in management of acute agitation, anxiety, or stress.
	Miscellaneous	Consider inclusion of buspirone and hydroxyzine for management of anxiety.

[a]All correctional formulary policies must include a mechanism to access nonformulary medications on a case-by-case basis as clinically appropriate.

because they reportedly produce a type of high when ingested, and inmate access to other drugs of abuse is severely limited in this controlled environment. The potential for abuse and/or dealing of these medications can be minimized through the use of liquid preparations, but this leads to additional problems in storage, nursing preparation, administration times, and so forth. Not all patients who take conventional antipsychotic medications require antiparkinsonian medication, but it is often prescribed prophylactically to prevent the occurrence of a painful dystonic reaction that would negatively impact future medication adherence. Akathisia does not respond well to administration of a second medication and may necessitate discontinuation of the conventional antipsychotic medication. Tardive dyskinesia is similarly poorly responsive to treatment but may be ameliorated or resolve with discontinuation of the conventional antipsychotic medication. Other cases of tardive dyskinesia are permanent.

In any event, when conventional antipsychotic medications are prescribed, antiparkinsonian medications for the prevention or reversal of dystonia and treatment of drug-induced parkinsonism must be readily available. In addition, use of conventional antipsychotic medications requires the adoption and utilization of an instrument at regular intervals to examine for and document either the presence or absence of involuntary movements. One such instrument is the Abnormal Involuntary Movement Scale (Munetz and Benjamin 1988). The examination and documentation should occur at the initiation of treatment with antipsychotic medications and at 6-month intervals thereafter for the duration of treatment.

Advantages for including conventional antipsychotic medications on correctional formularies are that these medications are all available in generic, and hence relatively inexpensive, preparations and that many are available in multiple forms (tablet, liquid, short-acting injectable, and long-acting injectable preparations), although newer agents are increasingly available in multiple forms as well.

Next-generation, or atypical, medications have been developed and introduced since the 1980s. Antipsychotic medications in this group include clozapine (Clozaril), risperidone (Risperdal), olanzapine (Zyprexa), quetiapine (Seroquel), ziprasidone (Geodon), and aripiprazole (Abilify). As a group, these medications do not have as high an affinity for dopamine receptors in the brain and consequently have much less potential to impact normal movement or lead to the development of irreversible movement disorders. The exception is risperidone, which does have some dose-dependent impact on movement; larger dosages are more likely to cause movement side effects than smaller dosages.

Evidence suggests that the newer medications are at least as effective as the older medications in treating some psychotic symptoms and may be more effective than older medications in treating other symptoms, such as expressed aggression, hostility, and social withdrawal. Studies on the use of some of the next-generation antipsychotic medications in hospitalized patients have demonstrated a decreased use of seclusion and restraint, decreased expressions of aggression and hostility, and a decreased risk of suicide in patients treated with clozapine (Pinals and Buckley 1999). Although the studies have not been replicated specifically in correctional settings, there is no reason to believe the results are not generalizable to institutionalized populations. A decreased use of seclusion and restraint in correctional populations is clearly desirable from the standpoint of decreasing the possibility of staff and inmate injury both in the application of the restraint or seclusion and in the precipitating incidents for which restraint or seclusion may be an appropriate response (Burns 2003). More recent studies aimed at doing direct, head-to-head comparisons of safety and efficacy between conventional and next-generation antipsychotic medications, such as the Clinical Antipsychotic Trials of Intervention Effectiveness, have not yet demonstrated superiority of any particular agent or class of antipsychotic medication over another, although differences may accrue over time, and the studies may not have been ongoing for long enough at this point to make a determination about long-term effectiveness and tolerability (Meyer 2007).

One advantage of next-generation antipsychotic medication is that fewer unpleasant side effects may enhance medication compliance, which in turn leads to better symptom management and less need for transfer to more intensive (and hence more expensive) mental health care such as infirmary placement, specialized treatment units, or psychiatric inpatient care. These medications also result in less need for the concomitant prescription and administration of antiparkinsonian agents. A reduction in the use of such agents results in the dispensing of fewer medications at fewer times, which has an impact on nursing preparation and medication administration time, as well as security staff time.

A significant problem that has arisen among inmates is the abuse of quetiapine, presumably for its sedating effects. (This abuse also occurs in the community but at a lesser magnitude given the ready availability of other, more desirable drugs of abuse.) Inmates without serious psychiatric illness have frequently sought out quetiapine specifically through reporting psychotic or mood symptoms that are responsive only to quetiapine. In addition, because quetiapine is sometimes prescribed as a sedating agent for insomnia based on its side-effect profile rather than being prescribed for its primary, approved indication, some prescribers have unwittingly contributed to the abuse by indirectly fostering medication-seeking behavior for complaints of insomnia. The magnitude of quetiapine overutilization in correctional facilities and systems and the associated costs, both direct and indirect (nursing administration and psychiatric time), in conjunction with the associated security concerns (buying, selling, trading, and hoarding of the medication), have led to its exclusion from the correctional formulary in some places.

Although atypical antipsychotic medications demonstrate fewer side effects on normal movement and lower risk of developing tardive dyskinesia, epidemiological studies have demonstrated an increased risk of treatment-emergent metabolic adverse effects (hyperglycemia, diabetes, weight gain, and hyperlipidemia) in patients treated with these medications. In response to this observation, the FDA has requested that all manufacturers of atypical antipsychotic medications include a warning regarding hyperglycemia and diabetes mellitus in their product labeling. This step has obligated prescribers of these medications to monitor all patients for symptoms of hyperglycemia, with particular attention paid to patients with preexisting diabetes and those patients with risk factors for the development of diabetes, such as obesity or a positive family history. Measurements of weight, blood pressure, and fasting blood glucose and lipids are recommended for all patients at the initiation of treatment with atypical antipsychotic medications and at periodic intervals thereafter during treatment, in addition to regular monitoring for symptoms of hyperglycemia (e.g., polydipsia, polyuria, weight gain, weakness) (American Diabetes Association et al. 2004). If symptoms develop, fasting blood glucose testing must be undertaken and referral to specialized services considered. In some cases, hyperglycemia resolves with discontinuation of the atypical antipsychotic agent, but some patients require continued treatment of diabetes despite discontinuation of the medication.

Clinical Case 12–3

Ms. M, a 22-year-old woman, was received into the state prison system already taking olanzapine 30 mg/day and trazodone 150 mg hs, as prescribed by her community mental health care provider. Her admission health assessment indicated her height as 5 feet 4 inches and body weight as 265 pounds; her blood pressure was within normal limits. She denied any medical problems. The medical physician did not order any admission laboratory studies, based on the inmate's age and negative medical history. Records from the community provider were requested and received. The records indicated that Ms. M had been followed in community mental health and had a history of psychiatric inpatient care for exacerbations of schizoaffective disorder.

She had been stable for about a year while taking the olanzapine and trazodone. The community mental health records did not include any laboratory studies, but a notation in a recent progress note indicated that the inmate patient had expressed concern about gaining a lot of weight over the past year.

The prison psychiatrist continued the recommended medications at the same dosages but also requested a fasting blood sugar test. Her fasting blood sugar was 210 mg/dL. The psychiatrist worked in conjunction with the medical department to confirm the diagnosis of diabetes, and Ms. M was followed medically. Her antipsychotic medication was changed from olanzapine to aripiprazole. Although she experienced some transient psychotic symptoms during the antipsychotic medication transition, her diabetes improved and she started to lose weight.

Another serious side effect is the development of agranulocytosis (a potentially fatal decrease in white blood cell count) in some persons taking clozapine. The administration of clozapine requires a weekly and later biweekly or monthly complete blood count with differential to monitor for the potential development of agranulocytosis. In addition to the cost of the medication, weekly blood work presents an added expense to correctional systems and additional procedural challenges with respect to drawing the blood, sending and receiving results, and ensuring their availability to both the pharmacy and the prescribing physician. Patients receiving clozapine and pharmacies dispensing the medication must be registered with the national clozapine database, as mandated by the FDA, which may present additional procedural and administrative hurdles for correctional facilities. Nevertheless, in certain cases, access to clozapine is an absolute clinical necessity: it remains the only medication with demonstrated efficacy in treatment of persons with symptoms that have been refractory to other antipsychotic medications.

Ziprasidone use has been associated with the potential to prolong the QT interval in cardiac conduction beyond the interval prolongation noted with several other antipsychotic medications. The QT interval is the interval from the beginning of the QRS complex to the end of the T wave of one heartbeat on an electrocardiogram. Ziprasidone is therefore contraindicated in patients with a known history of QT prolongation, recent acute myocardial infarction, or uncompensated heart failure, or those who are receiving other QT-prolonging drugs. Prolongation of the QT interval may lead to cardiac arrhythmias and death (Burns 2003).

Most correctional facilities have older, conventional antipsychotic medications available, but some have either severely restricted or not added next-generation antipsychotic medications to their formulary because of the cost, particularly compared with the cost of conventional generic medications. Next-generation medications are far more expensive. This position, however, is no longer defensible in that the medically accepted standard of care dictates that both conventional and atypical antipsychotic medications be represented in correctional formularies. A permissible, and perhaps even desirable, practice for correctional systems or facilities is to implement some clinical prescribing guidelines or protocols to monitor and/or contain next-generation medication expense, in addition to ensuring utilization for clinically appropriate indications. For example, reserving the use of quetiapine for inmates with a documented history of psychiatric illness and good clinical response to quetiapine at the time of admission or prescribing it only after the inmate has had poor or inadequate response to trials of one or two other agents, including an older medication, is a clinically and fiscally sound recommendation. Potential disadvantages to offering *only* next-generation antipsychotic medications in correctional formularies include the cost of the medications themselves and the potential for metabolic side effects and their associated costs (monitoring, treatment, and associated morbidity). Previously, because of their relative newness, only limited non-pill-form preparations were available, but this is no longer the case; many of the next-generation agents are now available in multiple forms, including orally disintegrating tablets, extended-release tablets, oral solutions, and short-acting and long-acting preparations.

Antidepressant Medications

Accessibility to antidepressant medications for the treatment of major depression and other serious mental illnesses with an affective component is a must for correctional facilities housing inmates with serious mental illness. Many classes of antidepressant medication are available, and multiple medications are available within each class. Although clinical evidence exists to mandate the availability of antipsychotic medications in both conventional and atypical classes, similar evidence is not available for all classes of antidepressant medication. Some classes of antidepressant medication are contraindicated in correctional facilities.

Tricyclic antidepressants (TCAs), so named because of their biochemical structure, are the oldest class of antidepressant medication. They include amitriptyline (Elavil), desipramine (Norpramin), clomipramine (Anafranil), doxepin (Sinequan), imipramine (Tofranil), and nortriptyline (Pamelor). Although clinically efficacious, TCAs have fallen out of favor in civilian populations due to the risk of death in overdose and the availability of many other equally efficacious and safer antidepressants. In correctional settings, TCAs carry an additional risk: potential abuse based on their anticholinergic properties in a setting where other substances of abuse are more difficult to obtain. The abuse potential and the risk of death in overdose are therefore relative contraindications for use of TCAs in correctional settings. If TCAs are used, intensive monitoring to prevent stockpiling or hoarding for purposes of overdose is required. TCAs are inexpensive (a favorable asset for inclusion in correctional formularies) and may be considered, with appropriate monitoring safeguards, for treatment of patients who have failed to respond to adequate trials of other classes of antidepressant medication.

A second class of antidepressant medications, the monoamine oxidase inhibitors (MAOIs), so named for their mechanism of action on the enzyme monoamine oxidase, is also contraindicated in correctional settings. The MAOIs include isocarboxazid (Marplan), phenelzine (Nardil), and tranylcypromine (Parnate). Inhibition of monoamine oxidase can precipitate hypertensive crisis if certain foods containing tyramine are ingested. Hypertensive crisis can also be precipitated by the ingestion of certain over-the-counter medications for cold and flu symptoms. Because use of the MAOIs requires fairly rigid dietary monitoring and avoidance of some common over-the-counter medications, and because many other types of equally or more efficacious antidepressants are available, the use of MAOI antidepressants in correctional settings is contraindicated.

Selective serotonin reuptake inhibitors (SSRIs), a newer class of antidepressant medication, are very effective and have much lower toxicity than either TCAs or MAOIs, even in overdose. SSRIs include fluoxetine (Prozac), citalopram (Celexa), escitalopram (Lexapro), fluvoxamine (Luvox), paroxetine (Paxil), and sertraline (Zoloft). The SSRIs are generally more expensive than TCAs because many of the SSRIs are still under patent and thus generic forms are not available. However, the greater cost of procuring the SSRIs is far outweighed by their lower toxicity. For example, the cost of one completed suicide by TCA overdose is far more than the cost of procuring and administering an SSRI (Burns 2003).

Several other available antidepressant medications are biochemically distinct and do not fit neatly into any of the preceding classifications. These medications include amoxapine (Asendin), bupropion (Wellbutrin), mirtazapine (Remeron), venlafaxine (Effexor), nefazodone (Serzone), and trazodone (Desyrel). In general, these antidepressants have good safety profiles and are efficacious in the treatment of depression and sustaining remission. One side effect worthy of mention is male priapism associated with trazodone. Priapism is a sustained, painful erection of the penis, which may result in permanent sterility and which sometimes requires surgical intervention. Given the number of other antidepressant medication choices available, trazodone is generally not recommended for use by male inmates. In addition, restricting or limiting the use of bupropion may be worthwhile in correctional settings due to reports of inmates crushing and snorting it to attain a high not otherwise readily available to them in confinement.

In addition to their use in treating depressive and other affective disorders, antidepressants have demonstrated efficacy in the treatment of anxiety disorders, including posttraumatic stress disorder. Paroxetine, venlafaxine, and nefazodone are particularly helpful in this regard. Using antidepressant medications for the treatment of anxiety disorders reinforces the recommendation to severely restrict the use of benzodiazepines for this purpose in correctional facilities.

Many inmates without psychiatric illness are prescribed low dosages of antidepressant medication because of the sedating side effects and for complaints of trouble sleeping. Prescribing for side effect rather than targeted action is to be avoided primarily because of the limited psychiatric time resources available in most correctional facilities. Inmates taking medications for off-label purposes still require periodic examination for medication review and renewals, leaving clinicians with less time for treatment of inmates with serious mental illness. In addition, the abuse potential of some antidepressant medications in correctional facilities has previously been noted. Correctional settings are difficult places to sleep, but this problem should be managed in other ways, such as by reducing or eliminating caffeine consumption, increasing exercise, limiting sleep to a total of 6–10 hours in any 24-hour period, teaching relaxation exercises, and making earplugs available in the commissary for inmate purchase and use to block out loud snoring and other disruptive noise (Burns 2003).

Mood-Stabilizing Medications

Mood-stabilizing medications must be available on correctional formularies for the treatment of bipolar disorder, schizoaffective disorder, and other disorders with a recurrent or cyclical affective component. Lithium and some anticonvulsant medications fall into this classification. This class of psychotropic medication is the most intensive in terms of requirements for laboratory monitoring of serum levels of the medications themselves, as well as for monitoring for the development of untoward effects on other systems (e.g., liver metabolism, bone marrow production).

Lithium's efficacy in the treatment of bipolar disorder has been long recognized, and the medication is very inexpensive. The administration of lithium requires monitoring for therapeutic blood level (monthly for

3 months, then quarterly) and periodic monitoring of renal and thyroid functioning. In addition, a baseline electrocardiogram is recommended before instituting lithium treatment. Lithium can be fatal in overdose and also has a significant incidence of gastrointestinal distress as a side effect.

Anticonvulsants used in the treatment of bipolar and other disorders include divalproex (Depakote), valproic acid (Depakene), carbamazepine (Tegretol), clonazepam (Klonopin), lamotrigine (Lamictal), oxcarbazepine (Trileptal), and topiramate (Topamax). At this point in time, only divalproex, valproic acid, carbamazepine, and lamotrigine are approved by the FDA for treatment of bipolar disorder, although the other anticonvulsants are widely used off-label for this purpose (Bezchlibnyk-Butler and Jeffries 2009).

Divalproex and valproic acid are much less toxic in overdose situations than lithium but are not without potential complications on other body systems, namely, the liver and bone marrow. Use of these agents requires baseline and quarterly liver function tests and a complete blood count with platelets. Serum levels of valproic acid may be monitored to check on medication compliance and potentially to determine dosage adequacy, although the established therapeutic window is for seizure control rather than bipolar disorder. Carbamazepine has also been widely used in the treatment of acute mania and prophylaxis of mood cycling. It requires baseline and periodic liver function tests, complete blood count with platelets, and serum drug level monitoring. Carbamazepine induces its own hepatic metabolism and the hepatic metabolism of other drugs metabolized by the cytochrome P450 system. The other anticonvulsant medications listed in the previous paragraph would best be reserved for use in cases that are refractory to adequate trials of FDA-approved medications or as adjuncts to the other medications if necessary. Because clonazepam is a benzodiazepine, its use in the treatment of bipolar disorder in correctional populations is not recommended, for all of the reasons previously stated.

Many of the next-generation antipsychotic agents previously discussed have now been studied and approved by the FDA for treatment of bipolar disorder, particularly in the acute phase, but some have also been approved for maintenance treatment. Appropriate precautions noted with respect to metabolic consequences of atypical antipsychotic use are as relevant when these medications are prescribed for bipolar disorder as when they are prescribed for a primary psychotic disorder. Rapidly dissolving preparations of aripiprazole, olanzapine, and risperidone may be particularly useful in ensuring medication ingestion and compliance, particularly because all other mood stabilizers with the exception of lithium (which is available as a liquid) are available only in tablet or capsule forms that are easy for inmates to cheek.

In some instances, disorders that may not be considered serious mental illness, such as certain personality disorders (borderline and antisocial), may nevertheless manifest symptoms amenable to psychopharmacological intervention. High degrees of impulsivity leading to aggression and potential violence may be appropriately treated with medications discussed for the treatment of bipolar disorder (Citrome 2008).

Other Psychotropic Medications

Benzodiazepines have a limited use for inclusion in correctional formularies, as previously noted. Sedative-hypnotics should not be prescribed, except perhaps for time-limited periods during an acute stressor. Symptoms of anxiety may be treated with antidepressant medications (particularly the SSRIs). Other nonaddicting medications, such as buspirone (BuSpar) and hydroxyzine (Vistaril), are also viable alternatives for the treatment of anxiety in correctional populations.

Sympathomimetics should be included on the formulary in juvenile facilities for the treatment of attention-deficit/hyperactivity disorder (ADHD), and access to these medications in adult facilities may be appropriate as long as they are prescribed in accordance with FDA-approved indications and dosages. If ADHD is suspected in an adult, securing documentation of outside treatment or corroboration of symptoms through a second-opinion consultation is recommended. If treatment is indicated, a trial of atomoxetine (Strattera), a newer medication approved for use in adults as well as children with ADHD, should be considered before an off-formulary request for a sympathomimetic is undertaken. Atomoxetine is not a controlled substance and may therefore be a viable alternative to sympathomimetics in adult (as well as juvenile) correctional facilities. Ready availability of sympathomimetics on the formulary of adult facilities is strongly discouraged, given the challenges related to addictive potential and security concerns. However, an off-formulary mechanism to access sympathomimetics, combined with appropriately controlled and objectively measured clinical response to treatment, may be appropriate in adult facilities.

CONCLUSION

Psychotropic medications are a necessary component of correctional mental health care. Correctional facilities are mandated to provide treatment for serious mental illnesses. Failing to do so constitutes a violation of the U.S. Constitution's Eighth Amendment, which prohibits cruel and unusual punishment. In general, psychotropic medication use in correctional settings should follow the same standard of care as that found in other community settings. Nevertheless, some unique factors need to be considered when practicing in correctional settings. Among these factors are securing informed consent in an environment that is inherently coercive; balancing an inmate's right to refuse medication with legitimate correctional interests of maintaining order in the institution and preventing harm to other inmates and staff; and understanding correctional medication administration processes. Factors requiring special consideration in correctional facilities include the very high prevalence rate of substance use disorders occurring in correctional populations, which dictates that formularies limit or exclude medications that have high abuse potential, and the environmental and other conditions (work details) that may exacerbate the already increased risk of malignant heat-related conditions occurring in persons taking some psychotropic medications.

Formulary considerations should be based on the facility's population characteristics as well as the duration and conditions of confinement. In facilities containing inmates with serious mental illnesses, psychotropic medication formularies must contain both classes of antipsychotic medications (conventional and next-generation), antidepressants, and mood-stabilizing medications. Prescribing practices are becoming increasingly standardized in the psychiatric community with the issuance of expert consensus medication guidelines and treatment algorithms. Correctional facilities may wish to consider adoption and implementation of these practices in that they demonstrate adherence to the community standard of care; evidence-based, medically accepted and defensible treatment rationales; uniformity in the provision of treatment; and improved clinical outcomes.

SUMMARY POINTS

Persons with serious mental illness are entitled to

- Treatment for their condition when confined in correctional facilities.

- Access to and appropriate utilization of psychotropic medication for the treatment of serious mental illness.

- Informed consent and the right to refuse treatment under specified circumstances.

Prescribers in a correctional environment should

- Be familiar with the correctional facility's medication administration procedures, because they may impact medication choice, frequency of dosing, timing of laboratory studies, and inmate medication compliance.

- Recognize environmental risks (e.g., heat-related problems) associated with psychotropic medication, and educate inmates and medical and security administrative staff on these issues.

- Limit the use of benzodiazepines because of the development of dependence, high abuse potential, and security issues regarding illegitimate use of these drugs in a population with a high prevalence of substance use.

- Consider implementation of expert consensus, evidence-based treatment guidelines or medication algorithms for the treatment of certain psychiatric disorders.

- Develop a mechanism to access consultation if psychotropic medications are being prescribed above recommended dosing guidelines or for indications not formally approved by the U.S. Food and Drug Administration.

Correctional administration should

- Include representative medications from the following classes of medication: antipsychotic medications (both conventional and next generation), antidepressant medications, and mood-stabilizing medications.

- Provide access to other types of psychotropic medication on a case-by-case basis to ensure that inmates are not denied appropriate treatment of serious mental health needs.

REFERENCES

American Diabetes Association, American Psychiatric Association, American Association of Clinical Endocrinologists, et al: Consensus Development Conference on Antipsychotic Drugs and Obesity and Diabetes. Diabetes Care 27:596–601, 2004

American Psychiatric Association: Psychiatric Services in Jails and Prisons, 2nd Edition. Washington, DC, American Psychiatric Association, 2000

Bezchlibnyk-Butler KZ, Jeffries JJ (eds): Clinical Handbook of Psychotropic Drugs. Seattle, WA, Hogrefe & Huber, 2009

Burns KA: Jail diversion and correctional psychotropic medication formularies, in Management and Administration of Correctional Health Care. Edited by Moore J. Kingston, NJ, Civic Research Institute, 2003

Citrome LL: Psychopharmacology and electroconvulsive therapy, in Textbook of Violence Assessment and Management. Edited by Simon RI, Tardiff K. Washington, DC, American Psychiatric Publishing, 2008, pp 301–323

Cohen F: The Mentally Disordered Inmate and the Law. Kingston, NJ, Civic Research Institute, 1998

Kashner TM, Rush AJ, Crismon ML, et al: An empirical analysis of cost outcomes of the Texas Medication Algorithm Project. Psychiatr Serv 57:648–659, 2006

Meyer JM: Antipsychotic safety and efficacy concerns. J Clin Psychiatry 68 (suppl 14):20–26, 2007

Munetz M, Benjamin S: How to examine patients using the Abnormal Involuntary Movement Scale. Hosp Community Psychiatry 39:1172–1177, 1988

Pinals DA, Buckley PF: Novel antipsychotic agents and their implications for forensic psychiatry. J Am Acad Psychiatry Law 27:7–22, 1999

Ruiz v Estelle, 503 F.Supp. 1265 (S.D. Tex. 1980)

Rush AJ, Crismon ML, Kashner TM, et al: Texas Medication Algorithm Project, phase 3 (TMAP-3): rationale and study design. J Clin Psychiatry 64:357–369, 2003

Washington v Harper, 494 U.S. 210 (1990)

CHAPTER 13

Creating Wellness Through Collaborative Mental Health Interventions

Shama B. Chaiken, Ph.D.

Catherine Prudhomme, Ph.D.

People who have a mental illness are overrepresented in the corrections population compared with in the general population (Beck and Maruschak 2001). About 16% of individuals in the U.S. corrections population require treatment for a mental illness (Ditton 1999), compared with approximately 5% of people who have never been incarcerated (Kessler et al. 1998). In five states, the corrections population treated with psychotropic medication for mental illness approaches or exceeds 20%. Four states have reported that more than 25% of the incarcerated population receive mental health treatment. Compared with same-gender individuals without mental illness, men with mental illness are four times more likely to be incarcerated, and women with mental illness are eight times more likely to be incarcerated (Teplin et al. 2004).

In several states, federal courts have mandated the treatment of severe mental illness in incarcerated populations. Severe (or serious) mental illness is generally defined to include psychotic disorders, major depressive disorder, bipolar disorder, and other conditions that cause significant disability or dysfunction. Psychotropic medications that treat biological sources of mental illness may be effective for individuals who are compliant with the treatment; however, data indicate that incarcerated individuals are reluctant to participate in mental health treatment systems that depend solely on the use of medication (Beck and Maruschak 2001). Adjunct therapies are often necessary for individuals to increase insight, develop or maintain medication compliance, learn new skills and alternative behaviors, and identify triggers for worsening symptoms. In this chapter, we review evidence-based methods that are appropriate for application during incarceration and community reentry and for reduction of symptoms of mental illness that impair functioning. We also discuss mental health treatment that is focused on improving the quality of life for people who require treatment for mental illness. Although reduction of recidivism is not regularly identified as the main focus of mental health treatment in correctional facilities, it is an important outcome to consider in identifying effective treatment for inmates with mental illness.

In the case of *Estelle v. Gamble* (1976), the U.S. Supreme Court held that prisons cannot be "deliberately indifferent" to the serious medical needs of inmates. Since this important ruling, states with proactive legislatures, and others under prescriptive court order, have provided basic mental health treatment programs for incarcerated individuals. Approximately 70% of correctional facilities housing state prison inmates screen individuals for mental health problems at intake, 65% conduct psychiatric assessments, and 51% provide 24-hour mental health care (Beck and Maruschak 2001). Legal and ethical requirements for treatment of inmates with mental illness are established through community standards, federal court mandates, and professional associations. In this chapter, we provide an update regarding mental health interventions and describe an evolution of focus from quantity of care to quality of care. We discuss best practices for correctional mental health intervention and for assisting incarcerated individuals to successfully reenter the community. Throughout this chapter, we highlight evidence of the effectiveness of multiple-agency partnerships and blended service models.

MENTAL HEALTH INTERVENTIONS IN CORRECTIONAL SETTINGS

Overview

The types of mental health treatment in correctional settings generally parallel those available in the community. Levels of care include crisis intervention, hospitalization, "day treatment" programs, "outpatient" programs, and walk-in clinics. The availability of pharmacological treatment is widely accepted as an element critical to the success of any correctional mental health treatment program. The adequacy of correctional mental health programs has historically been measured by the *quantity* of care provided. Empirical research on *quality* of care and consensus about specific treatment outcomes that should be measured are lacking. A 2004 U.S. Department of Justice report (Hills et al. 2004) on effective prison mental health services included "guidelines to expand and improve treatment" and contained little research regarding specific therapeutic modalities except treatment with psychotropic medications.

Although increasing attention is focused on the development of specific standards of quality mental health care, most treatment methods have not been tested with incarcerated populations. The Substance Abuse and Mental Health Services Administration (SAMHSA) created a National Registry of Evidence-based Programs and Practices (see http://www.nrepp.samhsa.gov). The National GAINS Co-Occurring Disorders and Justice Center, which is part of SAMHSA (see http://gainscenter.samhsa.gov/html/ebps/default.asp), lists evidence-based practices for mental health treatment, some of which are discussed in this chapter. However, most of the recommended treatment methods focus on transition to the community. The only approaches that are recommended by this group for use during incarceration include "illness management and recovery," "integrated treatment for co-occurring mental health and substance abuse disorders," and "treatment of trauma-related symptoms." Determination regarding application of approaches supported by federal agencies requires close examination of the specific population studied and the specific outcome measures. In a meta-analysis of research on evidence-based practices in corrections, Blank et al. (2004) noted that differences in research methods resulted in a lack of clarity about which practices are truly effective.

Efforts have been made to adapt mental health interventions for use in correctional settings, with varying fidelity to proven practices (Osher and Steadman 2007). Treatment methods that have been found effective for mental health treatment of inmates include cognitive-behavioral therapy, dialectical behavior therapy, behavioral reinforcement programs, integrated dual diagnosis treatment, forensic assertive community treatment, trauma-informed approaches, and telepsychiatry. We discuss these methods in this chapter, as well as the benefits of the wellness and recovery model, which is supported by research, emerging community standards, and federal court mandate, and can be implemented in conjunction with other evidence-based approaches. In addition, treatment using the therapeutic community model has been applied in many corrections and reentry settings and is recommended for a subset of the incarcerated population.

Best Practices and Standards for Correctional Mental Health Treatment

Sources for information about best practices in correctional mental health are increasing in number and quality. The Criminal Justice/Mental Health Consensus Project, coordinated by the Council of State Governments (2002), provides a compilation of issues, research, and resources related to mental health treatment in the criminal justice continuum. The American Correctional Association is an accreditation agency that serves all disciplines within correctional settings and provides practitioners with guidelines for best-practice standards of care based on empirical data (American Correctional Association 2009). Similar standards have been developed by the National Commission on Correctional Health Care (NCCHC), which was established in the early 1980s in response to a correctional health care system that was poorly organized and inadequate. Initial guidelines developed by NCCHC recommended improvement in the quantity and efficiency of health care services, including mental health treatment. Recent changes have highlighted the quality of services provided to inmates, with a focus on multidisciplinary treatment. In addition to the original goals of reducing symptoms and improving individual functioning, guidelines are provided for proactive programs focused on individuals with a few specific diagnoses, such as schizophrenia. Along with detailed standards based on best-practice models of mental health treatment, the organization offers assistance in meeting those standards (National Commission on Correctional Health Care 2008).

As part of court negotiation processes in several states, standards are emerging in corrections for confidentiality of inmate–patient communications, treatment of specialized populations within the group of inmates who require treatment for mental illness, suicide prevention, and parole planning. Improvement of treatment in California's administrative segregation units and reception centers was required as a result of *Coleman v. Wilson* (1995). Court cases in other states have ordered similar improvements in the standard of care for incarcerated individuals with mental illness. In Florida, the *Osterback v. Moore* (2001) case alleged inhumane treatment of inmates confined to close management units, which are designed for individuals who have heightened security needs. Court proceedings in Florida and in the California *Madrid v. Gomez* (1998) case required the exclusion of inmates with chronic and severe mental illness from units in which sensory deprivation contributed to exacerbation of symptoms.

MENTAL HEALTH INTERVENTION MODELS
Wellness and Recovery Model

Mental health interventions in prisons have primarily targeted symptom reduction. Medication compliance, insight development, and behavior change are the most common objectives of treatment. Some federal court cases regarding the adequacy of treatment for inmates with severe mental illness in state hospitals have required a shift from a traditional medical symptom management model to a broader focus on wellness and recovery. *Wellness* is defined as "an active process through which people become aware of, and make choices towards, a more successful existence" (National Wellness Institute 2009). Wellness is the process through which a person in recovery is empowered to make purposeful choices that lead to a more satisfying and healthy lifestyle. It includes physical, emotional, intellectual, social, environmental, occupational, leisure, and spiritual dimensions, and incorporates disease prevention and health promotion approaches. A wellness lifestyle leads to positive outcomes that can be measured in terms of improved health status, greater productivity, enhanced social relationships, and participation in purposeful activity—all of which provide meaningful opportunities for healing, personal growth, and an improved quality of life (Swarbrick 1997, 2006). The concept of *recovery* requires a shift in focus from symptom relief and involves treatment focused on the development of meaning and purpose in life.

Efficacy of the wellness and recovery model is measured differently from that of other evidence-based programs, because the treatment involves a paradigm shift from symptom reduction to other indicators of wellness (Copeland 2002). Outcome measures include the individual's ability to recognize his or her own early warning signs or symptoms of deteriorating mental health, ability to identify specific skills and tools to cope with these symptoms, and ability to incorporate tools for staying well into a daily routine. This model is effective in reducing the severity of relapse and the disabling effects of mental illness, and in preventing rehospitalization (Mueser et al. 2002). Tools commonly employed in this model include a crisis plan, in which individuals identify the interventions that they prefer during periods of crisis, and people who will be most likely to help them return to a state of wellness (Copeland 2002).

Empirical research on outcomes of mental health treatment indicates that the quality of the therapeutic relationship is a leading predictor of effectiveness (Cruz and Pincus 2002). A growing body of literature supports the use of wellness and recovery models for mental health treatment and indicates that this approach is successful because it motivates the person who has mental illness by allowing him or her to set personally meaningful goals for treatment (Jacobson and Greenley 2001). Specific therapies demonstrate improved outcomes for individuals with certain diagnoses (e.g., cognitive-behavioral treatment for panic disorder); however, the relationship with the therapist remains an important variable impacting success of treatment. Unlike patients in the community, incarcerated individuals do not generally choose their mental health clinician, so the clinician's responsibility to tailor the therapy to the needs of the specific person is critical.

In medical models of mental health treatment, the trained clinician assesses mental health symptoms, develops a diagnosis, and develops a treatment plan with input from the patient. The implication of treatment based on the medical model is that the clinician knows what is best for the patient. This model, which is commonly used in correctional settings, is not particularly helpful in overcoming barriers to therapeutic rapport. In the wellness and recovery model, each individual is considered the expert in his or her own experience, and the clinician encourages the pursuit of options related to the achievement of personal aspirations. The treatment may or may not be focused on reduction of mood or psychotic symptoms, based on the interests of the person receiving mental health services. Implementation of interventions based on wellness and recovery concepts in the corrections environment requires a shift from traditional systems of mental health services delivery. Improvement in treatment compliance, satisfaction with the therapeutic relationship, and reduction of symptoms are noted as benefits of using a wellness and recovery approach to treatment.

In some mental health treatment programs, both staff members and individuals who receive treatment each develop a personalized wellness and recovery action plan. These plans focus on identification of signs of wellness. After describing what he or she is like when well, each individual develops "tools" that are useful for staying well and relieving symptoms. Choices for tools include peer and family interaction, relaxation and guided imagery, journaling, medications, psychotherapy, exercise, affirmations, and music. Triggers (e.g., use of alcohol and other drugs, ingesting too much caffeine, sleeping too little or too much, and interacting with certain people) are also identified. Each individual develops a maintenance plan, including things to do every day to maintain wellness and triggers that can be avoided. The individual identifies early warning signs of serious and dangerous symptoms, as well as an action plan for intervention. Crisis planning includes instructions for things that are helpful when symptoms become severe and things that can worsen the situation. Table 13–1 demonstrates the difference between a routine visit progress note that reflects a medical model approach and one that reflects a wellness and recovery approach.

Federal courts have supported the wellness and recovery model as a treatment standard. In May 2006, the federal government ordered changes in mental health treatment standards, in a court case naming the state of California and Metropolitan State Hospital as defendants (*United States of America v. State of California* 2006). The court ordered a shift in philosophy toward a recovery model of mental health care and specified numerous changes, including individual participation in the development of treatment plans, the use of positive behavioral support systems, and strength-based rehabilitation strategies.

Rehabilitation Model

Some states, especially those faced with severe prison overcrowding, have implemented rehabilitation programs designed to reduce recidivism. These programs focus on academic classes, vocational training, substance abuse prevention, and a set of core curricula related to reduction of criminal behaviors. California, Vermont, and Rhode Island have enacted legislation with goals of increasing public safety and reducing recidivism by improving the chances of success for individuals returning from prison. Individuals with severe mental illness may have difficulty participating in traditional rehabilitation programs because of psychotic and mood symptoms that lead to problems with attention, concentration, or logical thinking. In some cases, mental illness is manifested by behavior that is incompatible with a classroom setting. For individuals with severe mental illness who are returning to their communities after incarceration, effective rehabilitation programming, at minimum, needs to incorporate continuity of mental health care and address any connection between the individual's mental illness and his or her criminal behavior. People who are significantly disabled by mental illness may require assistance with application for disability benefits, supportive housing, and assistance with obtaining food and other basic needs.

Research has shown that being effectively employed can be an important part of mental health treatment (Illinois Department of Human Services 2007). Supported employment programs help with interviews, benefits planning, routines and schedules, work relationships, managing and learning from job loss, and finding the best job fit. Research has not

TABLE 13–1. Medical model versus wellness and recovery model: routine progress note

	Medical model note	Wellness and recovery model note
Subjective	Inmate patient reports reduction of auditory hallucinations. Reports feeling bothered by mild dry mouth, and wants medication reduced. States that he is upset that he has not heard from his mother, but denies thinking about suicide. Discussed ways to cope with feeling abandoned, including writing letters to other family members and increased social interaction. Responded defensively when questioned about poor hygiene. Discussed upcoming transition to parole.	Mr. J has identified that he feels well because the voices he hears in his head do not keep him from reading and enjoying watching television. Describes dry mouth, which is a trigger for stopping medication. An additional trigger for increased suicide risk is when he is feeling abandoned. Currently has not heard from his mother but has been following plan to write letters to other family members and to play chess with his cell mate. Reports that understanding the early warning sign of feeling abandoned and then implementing the wellness plan has been helpful. Discussed adding self-care and hygiene to wellness plan, but Mr. J does not see this as a problem. Began to generate a new wellness plan with triggers and interventions relevant to parole.
Objective	Presents mildly disheveled with clothing wrinkled and shirt untucked. Hygiene remains poor. Good eye contact. Speech is slow but clear and goal directed with occasional response to internal stimuli. Insight fair. Judgment impaired.	Speaks clearly and slowly, with good eye contact. Content is mostly focused on wellness plan. Occasionally speaks to voices that an observer cannot hear, but does not appear distressed by this.

TABLE 13–1. Medical model versus wellness and recovery model: routine progress note *(continued)*

	Medical model note	Wellness and recovery model note
Assessment	Schizoaffective disorder, depressed, in partial remission on medication. Positive and negative symptoms remain present but stable. No acute distress. No evidence of increased risk of suicide or violence.	Ability to identify early warning signs and use wellness plan interventions is improving. Recognizes that psychotic and mood symptoms are present, but reports that maintenance and early warning interventions are working to prevent increased risk of suicide or violence.
Plan	Return to session in 1 week. Continue to monitor symptoms. Refer for medication evaluation to determine whether symptoms can be better controlled on medication. Continue to discuss parole plans.	Mr. J will continue to monitor symptoms and report back in 1 week. Wellness plan includes medication compliance and requesting adjustment of medication to reduce side effects. He is working on his wellness plan for parole and identifying ways that the plan needs to be modified for the different environment.
Education	Reinforced continued need for medication compliance and improvement of hygiene.	Provided education about why medication causes dry mouth.

yet explored whether supported employment is equally effective for people with mental illness who are returning from a period of incarceration.

IMPLEMENTATION OF MENTAL HEALTH INTERVENTIONS

Role of Clinicians

Clinicians who provide mental health treatment in the correctional setting are required to balance competing responsibilities to maintain the safety and security of the institution and to avoid a dual relationship with the individual receiving treatment. Mental health staff members regularly make difficult ethical choices about when to report misconduct, whether to advocate for inmate rights, and how to respond to interactions between individuals working in and incarcerated in the correctional setting. Some clinicians adapt to the correctional environment by providing only the most basic elements of mental health care, whereas others violate boundaries by becoming overinvolved in the lives of the individuals who receive treatment. Differences of opinion about appropriate roles for clinicians can cause significant conflict that ultimately impacts the provision of mental health care. Supervisors and managers can alleviate some problematic situations by communicating clear decisions and expectations about the quality of interventions in the correctional setting, guidance regarding boundary issues that are specific to working in corrections, and direction regarding maintaining the confidentiality of communications with inmate patients.

Screening and Identification of Inmates With Mental Disorders

Correctional standards require that all inmates be screened for mental health symptoms and be provided with appropriate levels of mental health care based on their individual needs. Systems should be in place for mental health assessment at the time of arrival and transfer, and upon request from any inmate, staff member, or inmate's family member. Effective screening and assessment of mental health problems have reduced management problems, improved care, and reduced liability of correctional institutions (Maue 2001). Correctional mental health programs usually employ an interdisciplinary treatment team whose members work together to assess inmates' need for mental health care, make decisions about the appropriate level of care, and determine appropriate treatment interventions. Regularly scheduled treatment team meetings allow correctional staff psychiatrists, psychologists, social workers, counselors, primary care physicians, nurses, psychiatric technicians, recreational therapists, educational instructors, vocational instructors, substance abuse treatment providers, and custody personnel to collaborate regarding the needs of each incarcerated individual. Participation of the largest variety of interdisciplinary staff in the correctional setting is useful to gather collateral data regarding inmates' current symptoms and self-reported mental health history.

Confidentiality and Informed Consent

Mental health clinicians are generally well trained in community standards related to privileged communication between a patient and psychotherapist. However, in many situations, clinicians have difficulty following legal and ethical principles of confidentiality that were developed for noncorrectional settings. Custody staff are exposed to traditionally confidential mental health information when they participate in interdisciplinary treatment team meetings, provide security during medication distribution, and escort individuals to their mental health appointments. Although preferred treatment settings prevent the overhearing of clinical sessions by custody staff and provide visual privacy from other inmates, the facilities for this type of treatment environment are not always available. In addition, all staff members in correctional settings are expected to disclose information necessary to protect the safety and security of an institution, such as communication from an inmate about escape plans, possession of contraband, acute intoxication, or drug trafficking, but these types of disclosures would not be allowed according to community standards. Disclosure of information revealed during mental health treatment interventions can impact the length of time an individual remains incarcerated and the security level in which the individual is housed. Documentation in health records may also be accessible during parole reviews, as well as for decisions related to specialized programs for offenders with mental disorders and sexually violent predators upon parole. Disclosure, and even routine documentation, can therefore create an ethically challenging dual relationship between clinician and patient.

Legal standards for parameters of confidentiality of inmate–patient communications indicate that unless criteria for mandatory or permissible disclosure are met, information shared during a clinical encounter is confidential and may not be divulged outside of the treatment team. When disclosure is necessary, only limited and relevant information necessary to meet legal mandates or prevent harm should be disclosed, and only to individuals who have a need to know. Correctional staff who overhear inmate–patient communications to a mental health clinician are also required to maintain confidentiality about the communication. Clinicians may not use the inmate disciplinary system to report the thoughts, feelings, or fantasies of individuals who receive mental health care unless specific criteria for disclosure are met. Clinicians in corrections are more likely than those in the community to be informed by a patient about past crimes; in most cases, they are required to maintain the confidentiality of this information. Use of alcohol and other drugs in the correctional setting is a particularly difficult topic because intoxicated inmates can pose a significant risk to the safety and security of an institution. However, mental health clinicians need to be able to hear about alcohol and drug use in the correctional setting without disclosing the information, so they can provide treatment for co-occurring disorders. Acute intoxication may be reported only when necessary to prevent harm and when other options, such as providing a medical setting for treatment of the individual, are not available or will not reduce the potential danger. When information obtained by a clinician is disclosed outside of the treatment team, the clinician is responsible for addressing the impact on the therapeutic rapport, and the treatment team should consider whether assignment of a different clinician is indicated.

Consultation with experienced clinical and legal staff is recommended when a clinician has any doubt about how to weigh the potential risks and benefits of disclosure. For example, when a clinician obtained information during a clinical session that contraband cell phones were available to inmates in a specific housing unit, the clinician had to consider ethical issues related to confidentiality, the risks related to inmates having access to unlimited communication with individuals outside of prison, and the concern about access to the Internet and other public domains. One option in this situation was to disclose the information in a general statement to custody staff without identifying the source of the information. Incarcerated individuals must be informed of the limits of confidentiality before they engage in mental health treatment; a form for documenting this disclosure should be included in a standardized confidentiality policy.

Table 13–2 provides criteria for mandatory and permissible disclosure of information established through federal court negotiation in California adult prisons.

Mental Health Levels of Care

Levels of care provided in the correctional setting may differ from those in the community because all programs in corrections are necessarily "residential." The term *outpatient* in corrections is commonly used to describe programs for individuals who do not require care with 24-hour

TABLE 13–2. Mandatory and permissible disclosure of inmate patient communication during mental health treatment

Mandatory disclosure

- The inmate patient presents a clear risk to a reasonably identifiable victim or victims, and disclosure is necessary to discharge the clinician's duty to protect.

- Legal and ethical criteria from community standards are met, requiring a report of child or elder abuse.

- The inmate patient presents a danger to self or to the person or property of another, and disclosure is necessary to prevent the danger. Concerns include the following:

  — Possession of a weapon

  — Acute intoxication

  — Information about drug trafficking

- The inmate has plans for escape or internal disorder such as a riot.

- The clinician observes sexual misconduct or is informed of plans for sexual misconduct.

Permissible disclosure

- The inmate is at risk for suicide, and nonclinical staff are engaged to provide suicide observation or other duties required to protect the inmate.

- The inmate is prescribed specific psychotropic medications that may cause side effects or interfere with the ability to follow directions or participate in correctional programs.

- The inmate is noncompliant with medications, and custody staff need to be alert for behavioral indicators of decompensation.

- Transfer to a different treatment setting or higher level of care is required.

nursing support. In some settings, individuals with chronic symptoms due to psychotic illness, who are unlikely to ever return to the general correctional housing environment, are separated from those who have a better prognosis for significant symptom remission. Individuals who become gravely disabled or those who are a danger to themselves or others require treatment in acute inpatient programs with 24-hour nursing care. Some individuals do not require acute care but cannot be safely treated in the outpatient setting because of severe psychotic symptoms, intensive need for assistance with activities of daily living, or severe mood disorders that impact judgment. These individuals require longer-term intermediate inpatient care and may require frequent short-term acute inpatient admissions.

Some individuals can be housed with the rest of the prison population while receiving mental health care using a basic case management model. Individual therapy at least every 90 days and group therapy as clinically indicated are established treatment standards for individuals at this case management level of care. Individuals with psychotic or mood symptoms may be appropriate for this level of care, but they should be referred to a higher level of care if the symptoms cause more than mild impairment in communication, social interactions, daily living skills, or ability to participate in regular prison programs. Individuals who have symptoms that cause moderate functional impairment often require housing that is separate from the rest of the prison population. These individuals should be offered frequent individual psychotherapy and a daily schedule of activities, including group therapy.

Three common approaches to providing correctional mental health interventions include group therapy, individual therapy, and a therapeutic community. Each approach is summarized below.

Group Therapy

Group therapy in the correctional setting serves several different purposes (see Table 13–3). One purpose is to provide information and build life skills. Another is to provide opportunities for recreation and development of appropriate social interaction. These two types of groups require very little self-disclosure and are tolerated well by the corrections population. In the community, group therapy is usually for the purpose of peer support and for development of insight through shared experience. Group therapy based on the premise that individuals can safely process emotionally charged topics, express personal vulnerability, and/or disclose their criminal history should be handled with caution in the correctional setting because inmates can potentially harm each other by inappropriately exposing sensitive information. Although this type of group therapy can and should be offered in the correctional setting, it requires careful selection of participants, candid discussion of risks and benefits of participation, and follow-up with individual participants to detect misuse of information disclosed during group therapy.

Designing therapeutic group treatment for inmates requires attention to the unique correctional culture. Issues of safety and confidentiality must be addressed in general policy and with group therapy participants. Group therapy can be harmful to participants unless rules and consequences for breaking the rules are clarified from the outset. For example, in some group therapy sessions, use of profanity is allowed, and

TABLE 13–3.   Types of group therapy in the correctional setting

Information and skill building	Peer support and insight development
Advanced education	12-step meetings
Anger management	Adjustment issues
Assertiveness vs. aggression	Coping with a life term
Basic neurology, the human brain	Domestic violence reduction
Cause and effect of substance abuse	Empathy
Cognitive and memory rehabilitation	Family issues
Communication skills	Grief and bereavement
Cultural differences	Parole preparation
General education	Reduction of impulsivity
Human sexuality	Sexual predators
Life span development	Specific mental disorder focus
Medication education	Spiritual growth
Occupational therapy	Substance abuse prevention
Parenting	Survivors of physical abuse and neglect
Problem solving	Survivors of sexual abuse
Relaxation	Victimization, cycle of violence
Social skills	
Recreational groups	**Process groups**
Art (drawing, painting, creative arts)	Open discussion facilitated by the clinician; this type of group is patient led, and topics may vary from session to session
Book club	
Current events	
Drama	
Exercise, yoga, physical games	
Meditation	
Movie discussion	
Music appreciation	
Origami	
Recreational games	

in others, similar language would lead to disciplinary action. Having clear documented rules about how inappropriate behavior and conflict between participants will be handled is especially important in the correctional setting (Chaiken et al. 2005).

Physical safety during group sessions can be improved through group room design and early intervention when conflicts arise. Group facilitators should always have closest access to the room's exit and a means to summon correctional staff. In most settings, both an alarm system and close custody presence are implemented. In high-security settings, participants may be held in individual locked cells during treatment. When conflict begins to arise between participants, the group facilitator must quickly decide if the interaction can be used in a therapeutic context or if the behavior needs to be extinguished. Facilitators who work with patients who have a history of violent behavior should be trained to summon help quickly if attempts to diffuse the situation are unsuccessful. Even in group situations that employ individual treatment cells for patients, conflict between participants can quickly lead to assaultive behavior, such as spitting or throwing urine, or to self-injurious behavior (Chaiken et al. 2005).

Individual Psychotherapy and the Person-Centered Approach

Individual meetings with a mental health clinician are an established part of the standard of care for treatment of severe mental illness. Many patients in correctional settings have experienced few relationships with people who are consistent, honest, direct, and caring. Patients in jail or prison often perceive mental health staff as part of the bureaucracy of the correctional setting. The first task of the therapist is to differentiate himself or herself from custody staff, correctional counselors, legal consultants, and other medical personnel. The use of a person-centered approach is key to the development of therapeutic rapport, but such an approach can be challenging in the correctional setting due to the emphasis on uniformity and compliance with a prescribed set of rules and expectations. Systems of incarceration remove options for expression of individual differences that exist in the outside community. Uniform clothing creates the illusion of homogeneity. Standardized building structure and unvarying routine add to the monotony of incarceration. The role of mental health clinicians differs from that of most other correctional staff in that quality treatment requires recognizing the strengths and challenges of each individual person.

The person-centered approach recognizes that under adverse conditions, individuals do not fulfill their own potential for growth. The model maintains that the following three core conditions are necessary to provide a climate conducive to growth and therapeutic change:

1. Unconditional positive regard
2. Empathic understanding
3. Congruence (authentic, genuine presentation of the clinician)

Clinicians who react to these concepts with reflexive distaste are often solidly invested in maintaining a retributive justice system (as opposed to a rehabilitative justice system) that acts only as a punishment and deterrent of criminal behavior. Provision of compassionate mental health treatment is generally incompatible with this attitude, and ethical principles require that these clinicians reassess their motivations for working in correctional mental health.

Maintaining "unconditional" positive regard and empathic understanding can at times be difficult for even the most compassionate clinician, because doing so is overtly discouraged by conditions in the correctional setting. Because the treatment population can be dangerous and the clinical setting can be used for secondary gain, many mental health clinicians establish a guarded and skeptical attitude. To conduct accurate assessment and provide appropriate treatment, clinicians need to understand the crimes committed by incarcerated individuals and be aware that particularly heinous crimes may trigger countertransference reactions. Clinicians are generally concerned about the perception that they may be inappropriately involved or "overfamiliar" with inmates, and therefore may avoid necessary advocacy roles to avoid disapproval from other corrections staff. However, maintenance of safety and security can be accomplished and even improved by clinicians who display confidence in the ability of each individual to achieve meaningful treatment goals.

The mental health clinician who is congruent does not present an aloof professional façade and is able to connect to the inmate in an empathic manner and to show respect for the individual's opinions and experience. Correctional clinicians are careful to avoid disclosure of any personal information and generally to uphold boundaries that are more rigid than in community practice. However, personable interaction does not require disclosure of private information, and correctional clinicians have a responsibility to overcome numerous situational barriers in an effort to gain the confidence of the individuals they treat. Motivational interviewing (Miller and Rollnick 2002; Swanson et al. 1999) is a nonjudgmental, nonconfrontational, and nonadversarial evidence-based approach, which is consistent with the person-centered approach. Training in motivational interviewing allows the clinician to recognize each individual's readiness for change and to address discrepancies between how a person wants his or her life to be compared with the current reality. Originally developed for substance abuse treatment, this method has been expanded for use in motivating more general behavior change.

Cultural issues play an important role in the development of clinical rapport. Inmates who are newly incarcerated are adjusting to the correctional culture and may be unsure of the roles of different staff. Issues related to age, race, ethnicity, language, gang affiliation, commitment offense, length of term, educational level, socioeconomic status, religion, political associations, and other values and beliefs related to group affiliation should be addressed as they relate to clinical rapport. Clinicians can help the development of the therapeutic relationship by asking incarcerated individuals whom they would choose as a clinician, if they had the choice, and about reasons that they might not trust that the therapist will act in their best interests.

Clinical Case 13–1

I was escorted to the treatment room, and the doctor asked the officer to stand outside. That was the first difference. Most of the doctors just let the corrections officer sit in the doorway or leave the door open. She asked my permission to discuss personal issues and told me the difference between things that could be kept confidential and things that she would have to report to custody. She said that she saw I was talking to others in my head and asked if I like to do that. She asked me if I had the choice, who I would choose as my therapist. When I said I would like a black male therapist, we talked about problems in my relationships with women and white people. She explained that we would not be friends, because friends share information about their lives with each other, and that she would not be sharing that type of information with me, because the therapy time is about me and my needs, about setting my goals and helping me reach them. I told her I was not going to take medication because it makes me less creative. She said that it's important for me to be creative and that we would figure out together whether medication was a good or bad idea. She came to my cell and looked at my artwork. I don't know if I can trust her. I told her I don't think she really cares about me and that she's getting paid to talk to me. I think if I tell her too much, they will force me to take medication. She said that it was a good idea to take time before deciding whether to trust someone and that we would talk again next week. I still don't like white people, and the voices say she's evil.

Only after the development of adequate clinical rapport can treatment of trauma-related symptoms occur. The National GAINS Center (see http://gainscenter.samhsa.gov) indicates that trauma, especially when untreated, can have severe negative impacts on a person's physical and emotional well-being. Trauma has been linked to hallucinations and delusions, depression, suicidal tendencies, chronic anxiety, hostility, interpersonal sensitivity (i.e., poor social skills), somatization (i.e., chronic fatigue syndrome), eating disorders, and dissociation.

Therapeutic Community Treatment

Therapeutic community treatment (National Institute on Drug Abuse 2002) is used successfully with incarcerated individuals who tend to value peer influence over advice from those in positions of power, including treatment providers. Originally used as a treatment specifically for substance abuse disorders, the perspective of therapeutic community treatment has expanded to include difficult behaviors in all aspects of life. Participants learn through interaction with peers in a community setting, designed to promote wellness, how to change dysfunctional behaviors and acquire positive life skills. In addition to focusing on behavior change and physical health, the treatment addresses critical aspects of wellness, including spirituality, life skills, and the improvement of emotional and psychological states. Because this modality requires goal-directed thinking and is facilitated by the participants, it is not recommended for individuals who have psychotic symptoms that impact communication or organization.

Delaware was one of the first states to implement the therapeutic community model in the treatment of cocaine-dependent prisoners. The KEY/CREST program commenced in July 1988 at the Multi-Purpose Criminal Justice Facility in Wilmington, Delaware, and included 20 individuals with lengthy criminal histories and long-term drug dependence. These individuals were separated from the general prison population, and a therapeutic community was established inside the correctional facility. Later, some inmates were also involved in a work-release therapeutic community. At 18-month follow-up, those individuals who had been involved in both an in-prison therapeutic community and a work-release therapeutic community were significantly less likely to have been rearrested than individuals in the control group (23% vs. 44%). They were also much less likely to have a relapse to drug use, as measured by self-report and urinalysis (53% vs. 84%) (Martin et al. 1999). On the basis of the success of the KEY/CREST program, Delaware obtained additional funding and now has 550 in-prison treatment beds, 530 community-residential beds, and aftercare services for another 400 patients (Hooper 2003).

In prison and jail mental health programs in which patients can safely gather with staff in groups, therapeutic community–type meetings help create a setting where patients have input into program guidelines, rules, and procedures. Regularly scheduled therapeutic community meetings also work to facilitate conflict resolution, teach social skills and leadership, and help patients learn self-advocacy and prosocial behavior. Mental health and custody supervisors should intermittently be present at therapeutic community meetings to validate and resolve reasonable concerns of the patients. Keeping an official agenda and recording minutes are helpful to document issues, discussion, and decisions made (Chaiken et al. 2005).

An impressive, evidence-based therapeutic community is the Delancey Street Foundation. Delancey Street functions at no cost to taxpayers or the client by engaging participants in vocational training in profitable industry. Numerous participants in the Delancey Street program have a criminal history or are diverted from incarceration. The Delancey Street Web site includes references to outcome studies and indicates that

> Delancey Street has been viewed and reviewed by a wide variety of people. Dr. Karl Menninger (the founder of the Menninger Clinic and often considered the grandfather of the American mental health movement at its height) conducted a long-term study on Delancey Street graduates that demonstrated a phenomenal success rate of 98%. He summarized his findings with the statement, "Delancey Street is an incredible mixture of hard practicality and idealism. It is the best and most successful rehabilitation program I have studied in the world." Studies have been performed by the California State Board of Corrections, and by independent evaluators who have used success indicators such as arrest, recidivism of drug use, risk behaviors, social and emotional well being indicators such as perceived self-worth, education achievement indicators, among others. All the studies demonstrated success among [Delancey Street Foundation] participants. (Delancey Street Foundation 2007)

This model has been expanded to several states and is beginning to be applied in other countries. Core principles of the model have been implemented in the jail setting, and research indicates success in reduction of recidivism. Although the Delancey Street Foundation programs do not accept individuals who take psychotropic medications or have severe mental illness, the model could potentially be expanded to include services for people who have well-controlled mental health symptoms.

SELECT TREATMENT MODALITIES FOR THE INCARCERATED POPULATION

Cognitive-Behavioral Therapy

The focus of cognitive-behavioral therapy (CBT) is on the interaction of the three domains of human behavior: thought, emotion, and behavior. Simply put, because thinking affects behavior, by modifying thoughts, long-term behavioral changes can be effected. CBT, which can be delivered by trained practitioners in either group or individual settings, is a mainstay of treatment in various correctional settings because it is useful in targeting problem behaviors and maladaptive patterns of thinking. This form of therapy has been used by the Florida and Illinois Departments of Corrections, among others.

In the correctional setting, clinicians may use CBT to target antisocial, socially maladaptive patterns of thinking or behavior. It can also be used to treat disorders that may have less of an association with criminality or disruption of the milieu (e.g., panic disorder or obsessive-compulsive disorder). This approach is both practical and effective because CBT models have shown positive short-term effects for the treatment of violent offenders and inmates with severe personality disorders, even psychopathy (Serin 1996). Several treatment models that use CBT have been developed for the corrections population, including moral reconation therapy (Little 2006), a nationally recognized evidence-based approach for reducing recidivism (National Registry of Evidence-based Programs and Practices; see http://www.nrepp.samhsa.gov), and Thinking for a Change, a curriculum endorsed by the National Institute of Corrections. CBT, in combination with social skills training, has also been shown to be an effective treatment for sexual offenders. In several studies, the treatment groups showed reduced anxiety, improved self-esteem (Seto and Barbaree 1995), and lower levels of sexual reoffending when compared with controls (Hanson et al. 2002; Schwartz and Cellini 1995, 1999). However, more long-term evaluations and follow-up are needed to evaluate the efficacy of these methods in treating individuals who are diagnosed with severe mental illness.

Dialectical Behavior Therapy

Dialectical behavior therapy (DBT) is a cognitive-behavioral approach to treatment that includes perspectives akin to Eastern philosophy (Linehan 2003). Rather than "curing" upsetting symptoms, participants in DBT are encouraged to accept and manage difficulties through shifts in perspective that note the impermanence of upsetting emotions. DBT has been effectively used to treat serious problem behaviors (e.g., self-injurious behavior, violence toward others). This form of therapy has particularly targeted inmates with borderline personality disorder, who constitute a significant minority of the jail and prison population (Chaiken et al. 2005).

Participants are encouraged to work through difficulties, at times using relaxation techniques to reduce the impact of stressful emotional states. Rather than expecting that difficulties will disappear over time, individuals in DBT treatment are taught to expect and manage problems as they arise. DBT has been implemented successfully in both federal and state prisons (Trestman and Bergins 2004), and data indicate that it is a good modality for treatment of disruptive and aggressive behaviors. Additional details regarding DBT treatment can be found in Chapter 8, "Managing the Disruptive or Aggressive Inmate."

Behavioral Incentive Programs

Behavioral incentive programs and token economies have long been used to help mental health patients change maladaptive behaviors. Inmates are given opportunities to earn privileges by exhibiting appropriate behaviors and participating in beneficial activities designated by their treatment teams. These types of programs are employed at various correctional facilities around the country, including the Tamms Correctional Center in Illinois and two prisons in the California Department of Corrections and Rehabilitation. This type of intervention is appropriate for individuals with severe mental illness who may respond less well to modalities that require insight and internal motivation.

In the corrections environment, behavioral incentive programs should avoid providing incentives that cause patients to malinger mental illness so they can be included in the program. In the California Department of Corrections, a reinforcement system was created for the supermaximum security mental health program. Staff first identified all of the privileges (as opposed to constitutional rights) allowed inmates housed in this security level. Privileges included possession of property not necessary for legal purposes; use of radios and televisions; access to canteen and packages; use of small group yards; and out-of-cell time to clean the unit (which also allows conversation with other staff and inmates). In behavioral incentive programs in mental health units, all these privileges are initially restricted and can be earned only through appropriate behavior and participation in treatment activities designated in the treatment plan. Medication compliance is not required for acquisition of privileges. Unless a patient meets criteria for involuntary medication, the patient's behavior is a more ethical and legal measure of his or her progress in treatment. Patients receive an orientation handbook explaining the details of behavioral incentive programs, and the mental health staff help lower-functioning patients understand the criteria required to earn privileges (Chaiken et al. 2005).

Other Treatment Approaches

Integrated dual diagnosis treatment is critical because more than 70% of incarcerated males and females have a co-occurring substance abuse disorder (Beck and Maruschak 2001; Teplin and Abram 1991). Motivational interviewing (Swanson et al. 1999) is a commonly used evidence-based practice for substance abuse treatment, and preliminary evidence indicates that it is useful for psychiatric and dually diagnosed patients. For details regarding substance abuse treatment for inmates with mental illness, see Chapter 7, "Evaluating and Treating Substance Use Disorders."

Assertive community treatment (ACT) and *forensic assertive community treatment* (FACT) are evidence-based approaches to providing "wraparound"-type services for people with severe mental illness (Bond et al. 2001; Dixon 2000). The ACT model was developed in New York in the 1960s as an approach to treating individuals with chronic mental illness who are difficult to serve in traditional settings. In this model, a multidisciplinary team is proactive rather than reactive in assisting with housing and other support services and maintaining continuity of care across agencies. The FACT model has been used in Texas to address the needs of individuals with mental illness who frequently enter and exit the corrections system. This program focuses on goals such as reducing recidivism and homelessness, diversion from correctional to mental health treatment settings (e.g., hospital admission instead of incarceration), providing treatment in the least restrictive environment, and ensuring timely access to disability benefits. FACT is a high-cost, high-intensity intervention, and research on outcomes is in early stages (Weisman et al. 2004).

Trauma-informed approaches are supported by SAMHSA. The SAMHSA Web site lists specific methods for treating trauma survivors and indicates that

> when a human service program takes the step to become trauma-informed, every part of its organization, management, and service delivery system is assessed and potentially modified to include a basic understanding of how trauma impacts the life of an individual seeking service. Trauma-informed organizations, programs, and services are based on an understanding of the vulnerabilities or triggers of trauma survivors that traditional service delivery approaches may exacerbate, so that these services and programs can be more supportive and avoid re-traumatization.
>
> Trauma-specific interventions are designed specifically to address the consequences of trauma in the individual and to facilitate healing. Treatment programs generally recognize the survivor's need to be respected, informed, connected, and hopeful regarding their own recovery; the interrelation between trauma and symptoms of trauma (e.g., substance abuse, eating disorders, depression, anxiety, etc.); and the need to work in a collaborative way with survivors (and also with family and friends of the survivor) and with other human services agencies in a manner that will empower survivors. (National Mental Health Information Center 2009)

Telepsychiatry (the use of videoconferencing techniques for the provision of health-related services) has been growing in popularity in recent years, due in part to limited access to health care. This technique is particularly useful in rural counties, where limited numbers of health care professionals provide treatment to individuals over wide geographic areas. Correctional systems have started to recognize the benefits of using technology to provide health-related services, especially mental health services, to individuals who are incarcerated. A number of benefits accompany the use of videoconferencing for psychological or psychiatric consultation, including reduction in the need to transport inmates, improved overall cost, and improved access to mental health care. Ax et al. (2007) found that incarcerated individuals who used telepsychiatry did not report a difference between in-person versus videoconferenced mental health treatment sessions. Morgan et al. (2008) reported that satisfaction with telepsychiatric services depended on diagnosis, with persons with psychotic disorders reporting higher levels of satisfaction than those with affective disorders. Although use of the technology is minimal at this point, it holds some promise for the provision of services to individuals in situations where adequate care is difficult to access.

PARTICIPATION IN CORRECTIONAL PROGRAMS

Individuals with mental illness have a right to access prison programs available to other inmates, including work, education, vocational training, religious services, and rehabilitative programming. This concept can conflict with the systemic responsibility to maintain the safety of individuals who, because of mental illness, may be more vulnerable when they interact with the rest of the corrections population. Separation of individuals who receive treatment for mental illness can contribute to dangerous stigmatization of the population; however, it may be appropriate to separate individuals with chronic severe forms of mental illness from those who require treatment for mental illness but who have a better prognosis for remission from symptoms. Lack of access to beneficial activities can worsen symptoms of mental illness. Careful decision making is therefore needed to determine how each system, and each treatment team, can best provide for needs of each inmate patient to participate in the maximum amount of available activities at the facility, in the least restrictive environment.

SPECIALIZED TREATMENT GROUPS IN CORRECTIONS

Reception Centers and Parole Violators

Court decisions in the California *Valdivia v. Davis* (2002) case determined that individuals cannot be returned to a correctional system from parole solely on the basis of failure to comply with mental health care recommendations. However, many individuals who receive treatment for mental illness while incarcerated do not receive the same consistency of care in the community. Mental illness may be a contributing factor to the commission of new crimes or to the violation of requirements of parole. Individuals who quickly move between correctional settings and the community require unique interventions to facilitate assessment, treatment, and continuity of mental health care. Mental health clinicians should play a role in resolving barriers to successful community integration, including need for Social Security and other identification cards, benefits or financial planning, family systems needs, housing and transportation needs, social support systems, and linkage to community mental health services.

Administrative Segregation Units

Another group requiring unique services within the correctional setting includes individuals who are placed into administrative segregation units. Placement into segregation is a significant risk factor for suicide, both for individuals previously identified as requiring mental health treatment and for those who do not present with severe mental illness (Thienhaus and Piasecki 2007). Mental health clinicians need to be trained to be persistent in developing therapeutic rapport with those individuals housed in segregation who may have experienced recent trauma or may be facing new consequences. Decisions about placement into segregation should include consideration of an individual's mental illness, and clinicians need to be aware of the impact of recent stressors and environmental conditions in segregation so they can provide adequate treatment. The creation of treatment space in segregation, where confidential communication can occur, is critical.

COORDINATED CLINICAL DECISION MAKING

Correctional systems often involve numerous facilities that provide treatment of mental illness within a large bureaucracy that includes disparate custody and clinical cultures. Consultation about complicated clinical decisions should therefore not be limited to the local level. Case conferences can be helpful to discuss treatment plans for specific individuals, especially those who require difficult clinical decisions and/or communication between providers at different locations. Case conferences for large statewide systems should include senior-level clinicians familiar with different treatment options within the entire system; all providers involved with the case; and, when necessary, custody staff responsible for classification, transport, and housing. Communication between providers, especially about inmate patients who present with a complicated or unclear array of symptoms, cannot be accomplished solely through written documentation. Continuity of care and effective treatment planning can be improved by establishing systems for verbal communication between providers.

MENTAL HEALTH INTERVENTIONS LINKING CORRECTIONAL AND COMMUNITY SETTINGS

Multiple-Agency Collaboration

The Criminal Justice/Mental Health Consensus Project, coordinated by the Council of State Governments (2002), states that

> people with mental illness who have become involved (or are at risk of becoming involved) with the criminal justice system frequently have multiple needs that can be addressed only through the collaborative efforts of several agencies working within the constraints of diverse systems. The failure of these systems to connect effectively endangers lives, wastes money, and threatens public safety—frustrating crime victims, consumers, family members, and communities in general.

Ideally, communication between agencies should begin well before individuals are released from prison. Multiple-system partnerships that offer an array of services based in both the prison and the community can better provide for the ongoing monitoring of service delivery and can follow the released or paroling person into the community. Nowhere is multiagency cooperation more important than for those individuals challenged with serious psychiatric conditions who are expected to subsist outside of the structure of prison. Individuals with serious mental disorders often experience the task of rebuilding a life "on the outside" as even more daunting than the years spent waiting for release from prison.

Clinical Case 13–2

Mr. W, age 39, was due to be paroled in 1 week, after serving nearly 20 years for armed robbery. Ninety days prior to his parole date, he met with a social worker, who completed a needs assessment for him as part of a transitional service for inmates with mental illness. He wasn't too concerned that the social worker had been unable to make contact with his sister. He figured that he would call an old friend to see if he could stay with him for a while. He was thinking about not taking his medications when he got out. They didn't help much with the voices anyway. He was able to live on the streets before he got locked up, so he figured he could make it now without too much trouble. But he was beginning to feel that people were planning to trip him up so he couldn't leave.

Rehabilitative programs that attempt multiagency collaboration must manage in the complex and often conflicting world of prison, parole, state, and county mental health systems. Several common themes have emerged in the design of the growing number of programs that provide effective multiagency partnership. Successful programs have as their cornerstone ongoing communication between service providers that have distinctly different services but that require collaboration to benefit participants. Services that are provided over an extended period of time, with a gradual reduction in supervision, are showing improved outcomes for recipients. Several programs offer personal assistance to participants in the form of case managers who provide individual guidance across programs. At times, that personal connection is the key to successful rehabilitation for persons who are challenged with both mental illness and a history of incarceration.

Individualized Needs Assessment

Efforts to assist individuals who are returning to their communities from prison have evolved to include detailed assessment of individual needs, a process that includes the use of multiple assessment tools and the development of a needs hierarchy. Complex assessments have highlighted the need for habilitation—the acquisition of skills that were never developed—not only for individuals who struggle with mental illness, but also for those whose early circumstances and life choices failed to offer them the opportunities to learn basic, life-sustaining skills.

The Correctional Offender Management Profiling for Alternative Sanctions is a validated and reliable measure that defines risk and needs factors for individuals preparing for parole and guides criminal justice practitioners regarding placement and other management decisions (Brennan et al. 2009). Another assessment tool used to guide the provision of services can be found in the field of developmental disabilities. The Supports Intensity Scale (Thompson et al. 2004) provides detailed information about the type of support needed by consumers. It relies heavily on family input, an element that is often missing in corrections at the state level but one that could enhance rehabilitative efforts for individuals who may not be able to provide accurate accounts of their own histories. The support systems highlighted as a consequence of this assessment tool can serve as models for services provided to people with mental illness who are transitioning from correctional settings to their communities.

Job-Based Initiatives and Supportive Employment

Several state correctional systems have developed programs with supportive employment as a fundamental component of preparation for reentry into the community. Typically, participants receive training for positions that are likely to exist outside prison. The most successful supportive employment programs include outreach to potential employers in the community. Many of the programs that focus on the employment prospects of incarcerated individuals are not specifically designed for participants with serious mental illness. An open forum sponsored by the National GAINS Center (Osher et al. 2002) concluded that data indicate that supportive employment is effective among persons with mental illness, but that the research has not yet demonstrated an impact on criminal justice outcomes.

CONCLUSION

Effective treatment of individuals with mental illness in U.S. correctional facilities depends on a shift in perspective and practice toward quality care. The shift has already begun, due in part to court requirements that have targeted insufficient and indifferent practices. A number of correctional institutions are beginning to recognize that beyond adequate treatment, quality treatment is essential if true rehabilitation of incarcerated individuals is to be achieved. Standards are emerging that address the importance of focusing on a whole-person model of recovery, with collaboration between entities responsible for mental health treatment, substance abuse prevention, education and vocational training, and family systems support.

Success in treating individuals with mental illness is possible only with complex solutions at both personal and societal levels. Improved treatment designs require collaboration among complex systems within corrections and within the communities to which incarcerated individuals will eventually return. Numerous models of interagency collaboration are emerging at the community level, with multiple systems involved in clinical decision making. Mentorship programs, diversion strategies, and person-centered approaches are expanding and improving the treatment of individuals with severe mental illness. The measurement of treatment success and recidivism reduction requires a new focus on each individual's ability to reach personalized life goals. Research designs that incorporate these concepts are needed to guide future program development.

SUMMARY POINTS

- Court decisions indicate that incarcerated individuals have a right to quality mental health treatment in the correctional setting.

- Quality mental health treatment requires collaboration between consumers of mental health care; family members; providers; and federal, state, and local agencies.

- Correctional settings meet legal and ethical standards of care by integrating traditional mental health treatment approaches with person-centered approaches focused on wellness, recovery, and rehabilitation.

- Select evidence-based models of treatment may be used in the correctional setting, whereas others require modification for use with the incarcerated population.

- Incarcerated individuals require treatment interventions tailored to meet the needs of specialized populations, especially as these individuals reenter their communities from correctional settings.

- Treatment planning extends beyond the reduction of symptoms to include spiritual, social, educational, vocational, and reentry needs of the population.

- Research that measures each individual's ability to reach personalized life goals is needed to guide future program development.

REFERENCES

American Correctional Association: Standards & accreditation. 2009. Available at: http://www.aca.org/standards. Accessed April 8, 2009.

Ax RK, Fagan TJ, Magaletta PR, et al: Innovations in correctional assessment and treatment. Crim Justice Behav 34:893–904, 2007

Beck AJ, Maruschak LM: Mental health treatment in state prisons, 2000. Washington, DC, U.S. Department of Justice, Office of Justice Programs, Bureau of Justice Statistics, 2001

Blank A, Pogorzelski W, Maschi T: Can we determine what works? A meta-analysis of research methods used to evaluate behavioral health interventions in criminal justice settings. Paper presented at the annual meeting of the American Society of Criminology, Nashville, TN, November 2004

Bond GR, Drake RE, Mueser KT, et al: Assertive community treatment: critical ingredients and impact on patients. Disease Management and Health Outcomes 9:141–159, 2001

Brennan T, Dieterich W, Ehret B: Evaluating the predictive validity of the COMPAS risk and needs assessment system. Crim Justice Behav 36:21–40, 2009

Chaiken SB, Thompson CR, Shoemaker W: Mental health interventions in correctional settings, in Handbook of Correctional Mental Health. Edited by Scott CL, Gerbasi JB. Washington, DC, American Psychiatric Publishing, 2005, pp 122–127

Coleman v Wilson, 912 F.Supp. 1282 (1995)

Copeland ME: Wellness Recovery Action Plan. West Dummerston, VT, Peach Press, 2002

Council of State Governments: Criminal Justice/Mental Health Consensus Project, 2002. Available at: http://consensusproject.org/downloads/Entire_report.pdf. Accessed April 8, 2009.

Cruz M, Pincus HA: Research on the influence that communication in psychiatric encounters has on treatment. Psychiatr Serv 53:1253–1265, 2002

Delancey Street Foundation: Frequently asked questions. 2007. Available at: http://www.delanceystreetfoundation.org/faq.php. Accessed April 8, 2009.

Ditton PM: Mental health treatment of inmates and probationers. Washington, DC, U.S. Department of Justice, Office of Justice Programs, Bureau of Justice Statistics, 1999

Dixon L: Assertive community treatment: twenty-five years of gold. Psychiatr Serv 51:759–765, 2000

Estelle v Gamble, 429 U.S. 97 (1976)

Hanson RK, Gordon A, Harris AJ, et al: First report of the collaborative outcome data project on the effectiveness of psychological treatment for sex offenders. Sex Abuse 14:169–197, 2002

Hills H, Siegfried C, Ickowitz A: Effective Prison Mental Health Services: Guidelines to Expand and Improve Treatment: 2004 Edition. Washington, DC, U.S. Dept of Justice, National Institute of Corrections, 2004. Available at: http://www.nicic.org/pubs/2004/018604.pdf. Accessed Accessed April 8, 2009.

Hooper R: Something works: therapeutic communities in the treatment of substance abuse, in Correctional Psychology: Practice, Programming, and Administration. Edited by Schwartz B. Kingston, NJ, Civic Research Institute, 2003, pp 12/1–12/17

Illinois Department of Human Services: Evidence-based practices: state-of-the-art strategies to help recover from mental illnesses. 2007. Available at: http://www.dhs.state.il.us/OneNetLibrary/27897/documents/Brochures/4657.pdf. Accessed April 8, 2009.

Jacobson N, Greenley D: What is recovery? A conceptual model and explication. Psychiatr Serv 52:482–485, 2001

Kessler RC, Berglund EE, Walters PJ, et al: A methodology for estimating the 12-month prevalence of serious mental illness, in Mental Health, United States 1999. Edited by Manderscheid RW, Henderson MJ. Washington, DC, U.S. Government Printing Office, 1998

Linehan MM: Cognitive-Behavioral Treatment of Borderline Personality Disorder. New York, Guilford, 2003

Little GL: Review of one- to three-year recidivism of felony offenders treated with MRT in prison settings. Cognitive-Behavioral Treatment Review 15:1–3, 2006

Madrid v Gomez, 150 F.3d 1030 (9th Cir. 1998)

Martin S, Butzin C, Saum C, et al: Three year outcomes of therapeutic community treatment for drug-involved offenders in Delaware: from prison to work release to aftercare. Prison J 79:294–320, 1999

Maue FR: An overview of correctional mental health issues. Corrections Today 63:5, 8, 2001

Miller WR, Rollnick S: Motivational Interviewing: Preparing People for Change. New York, Guilford, 2002

Morgan RD, Patrick AR, Magaletta PR: Does the use of telemental health alter the treatment experience? Inmates' perceptions of telemental health vs. face-to-face treatment modalities. J Consult Clin Psychol 76:158–162, 2008

Mueser KT, Corrigan PW, Hilton DW, et al: Illness management and recovery: a review of the research. Psychiatr Serv 53:1272–1284, 2002

National Commission on Correctional Health Care: NCCHC's 2008 mental health standards and accreditation program. Available at: http://www.ncchc.org/resources/2008_standards/mentalhealth.html. Accessed April 8, 2009.

National Institute on Drug Abuse: Research report series: therapeutic community (NIH Publ No 02-4877). Washington, DC, National Institute on Drug Abuse, 2002

National Mental Health Information Center: Trauma-informed care. Rockville, MD, Substance Abuse & Mental Health Services Administration, 2009. Available at: http://mentalhealth.samhsa.gov/nctic/trauma.asp. Accessed April 10, 2009.

National Wellness Institute: Defining wellness. 2009. Available at: http://www.nationalwellness.org/index.php?id_tier=2&id_c=26. Accessed April 8, 2009.

Osher FC, Steadman HJ: Adapting evidence-based practices for persons with mental illness involved in the criminal justice system. Psychiatr Serv 38:1472–1478, 2007

Osterback v Moore 2000 U.S. 7846, 121 S.Ct. 587 (2001). Available at: http://www.hrw.org/reports/2003/usa1003/Florida_Osterback_PlaintiffsResponse.pdf. Accessed April 8, 2009.

Schwartz BK, Cellini HR: Female sex offenders, in The Sex Offender: Corrections, Treatment, and Legal Developments. Edited by Schwartz BK, Cellini HR. Kingston, NJ, Civic Research Institute, 1995, pp 5/1–5/22

Schwartz BK, Cellini HR: Sex offender recidivism and risk factors in the involuntary commitment process, in The Sex Offender: Theoretical Advances, Treating Special Populations and Legal Developments. Edited by Schwartz BK. Kingston, NJ, Civic Research Institute, 1999, pp 8/1–8/22

Serin R: Violent recidivism in criminal psychopaths. Law Hum Behav 20:207–217, 1996

Seto MC, Barbaree HE: The role of alcohol in sexual aggression. Clin Psychol Rev 15:545–566, 1995

Swanson AJ, Pantalon MV, Cohen KR: Motivational interviewing and treatment adherence among psychiatric and dually diagnosed patients. J Nerv Ment Dis 187:633–635, 1999

Swarbrick M: A wellness model for clients. Mental Health Special Interest Section Quarterly 20:1–4, 1997

Swarbrick M: A wellness approach. Psychiatr Rehabil J 29:311–314, 2006

Teplin LA, Abram KM: Co-occurring disorders among mentally ill jail detainees: implications for public policy. Am Psychol 46:1036–1045, 1991

Teplin LA, Abram KM, McClelland GM: Prevalence of psychiatric disorders among incarcerated women: pretrial jail detainees. Arch Gen Psychiatry 53:730–737, 2004

Thienhaus OJ, Piasecki M (eds): Correctional Psychiatry: Practice Guidelines and Strategies. Kingston, NJ, Civic Research Institute, 2007

Thompson JR, Bryant BR, Campbell EM, et al: Supports Intensity Scale. Washington, DC, American Association on Mental Retardation, 2004

Trestman RL, Bergins LG: The development and implementation of dialectical behavior therapy in forensic settings. International Journal of Forensic Mental Health 3:93–103, 2004

United States of America v State of California (May 2006). Available at: http://www.usdoj.gov/crt/split/documents/metro-napa_hosp_compl_5-2-06.pdf. Accessed April 8, 2009.

Valdivia v Davis, 206 F.Supp. 2d 1068 (E.D. 2002)

Weisman RL, Lamberti JS, Price N: Integrating criminal justice, community healthcare, and support services for adults with severe mental disorders. Psychiatr Q 75:71–85, 2004

CHAPTER 14

Monitoring a Correctional Mental Health System

Jeffrey L. Metzner, M.D.

Class-action litigation has been instrumental in jail and prison reform over the past three decades. Correctional mental health systems have significantly benefited from such litigation related to increased resources and mandated implementation of basic policies and procedures necessary for a sound system. This type of litigation has frequently resulted in jails and prisons becoming more humane and safer for both prisoners and correctional staff (Metzner 2002).

Newly initiated consent decrees related to class-action litigation involving correctional mental health services have virtually become nonexistent following the passage of the Prison Litigation Reform Act of 1995 (PLRA), which was actually passed during 1996 (Belbot 2004; Boston 2004; Schlanger 2003), although private settlement agreements and/or memoranda of agreements have essentially emerged as replacements for the consent decree process. These agreements typically lack judicial enforcement other than the reinstatement of the pertinent civil proceedings. The monitoring processes in these types of agreements are generally quite similar to those previously used in consent decrees.

In this chapter, I describe the monitoring process involved in class-action litigation concerning correctional mental health systems that has resulted in remedial plans being either court ordered or agreed upon via a private settlement agreement, pre-PLRA consent decree, or some other mechanism (e.g., a memorandum of agreement) between the parties. Perspectives from both the monitor's viewpoint and that of the correctional institution (i.e., the defendant) are briefly referenced to help prepare the institutional staff to succeed in the implementation of remedial plans.

MONITOR SELECTION

Class-action litigation in correctional facilities can be conceptualized as having the following three phases (Metzner 2002):

1. Liability phase (legally determining whether or not constitutional deficiencies exist)
2. Remedial phase (developing a remedy to constitutional deficiencies found)
3. Implementation phase (implementing the remedial plan)

Selecting a monitor or monitors is a crucial step in the process for many reasons, which I summarize in this section. A monitor is usually selected during either the remedial or the implementation phase. The decisions that need to be made in this selection process are summarized in Table 14–1.

Monitor selection models include the following:

1. *The monitor has not previously been involved in the litigation process concerning the named correctional mental health system.* The main advantage of this model is the apparent neutrality of the selected monitor, who presumably has been approved by both parties. The disadvantage is that the monitor will not be familiar with the history of the case, although review of relevant documents and discussions with the attorneys can quickly mitigate this potential disadvantage. In some respects, this initial lack of familiarity can be an advantage because the monitor will often be able to present a fresh and less biased perspective of relevant issues that may have become particularly difficult to resolve between the involved parties due to tension generated by the adversarial process. Thus, this model is attractive when the process leading up to the settlement has been acrimonious.
2. *The monitor has previously been involved in the litigation process.* Frequently, the monitor was working with the defendants but had also established credibility with the plaintiffs. The advantage of this model is that the monitor has a working knowledge of the correctional mental health system with established relationships that will facilitate the monitoring process and, hopefully, the implementation of the remedial plan.

TABLE 14–1. Selection and monitoring issues

Is more than one monitor needed?

Should the monitor have been involved in an earlier phase of the litigation process?

What are the responsibilities and authority of the monitor?

What is the frequency of the on-site monitoring, and over what period of time?

What outcome measures are to be monitored? How are they to be measured (objectively or subjectively; through chart review, inmate interviews, or staff interviews; etc.)?

What are the format and frequency of the monitoring reports?

3. *The monitoring is carried out by a joint monitoring team consisting of a monitor selected by the plaintiffs and a monitor selected by the defendants.* Such a monitoring team needs to be willing to work together, with their mission being the monitoring of the remedial plan in contrast to advocating from either the plaintiffs' or defendants' perspectives. Often, especially when the settlement process has been collaborative, these monitors will have served as expert witnesses for the respective parties.

The selection of one monitor versus two or more monitors is generally based on the size of the system to be monitored and cost considerations, although other factors such as the specifics of the remedial plan are often considered. For example, a psychiatrist is often needed because of medication issues that cannot be adequately assessed by a psychologist or psychiatric social worker.

Monitor selection is a crucial component of the implementation phase for many reasons. Most remedial plans include elements that will eventually require 1) interpretations regarding the meaning of the requirements and 2) clinical assessments concerning compliance, both of which are significantly influenced by and/or determined by the monitor. The monitor has an essential role in setting the tone of the implementation phase, with the tone established having a significant impact on both staff morale and the success of this phase. Also, as the monitoring process proceeds, the monitor commonly provides useful consultations (independent of the monitoring process) relevant to the correctional mental health system that are unlikely to occur in a productive manner if the monitoring process is not working well. The monitor should always carefully label recommendations as either consultative (and thus optional) or mandatory elements of the settlement agreement or consent decree.

The obvious reason for selecting a monitor during the remedial phase is to assist in developing the remedial plan. The major advantage of involving the monitor at this stage is that the monitoring instrument and/or monitoring process will likely be more apparent to the parties prior to beginning the implementation phase, because the actual monitoring process is likely to be discussed more accurately with the monitor's earlier involvement. However, commonly, the parties have not selected or involved a monitor at this stage because both sides want to develop the remedial plan based on their extensive history with the litigation leading up to the plan.

Complaints about monitors, which may be accurate or reflect poor implementation of the remedial plan and subsequent displaced anger or inappropriate projection of blame, include the following: 1) the monitor creates "moving targets"—that is, by changing the outcome measures relevant to the remedial plan (in some cases unilaterally and even arbitrarily), the monitor changes the goal lines; 2) the monitor is unclear about outcome measures; 3) the monitor does not want to give up a cash cow (i.e., the monitoring job); 4) the monitor is plaintiff (or defense) oriented; and 5) the monitor makes conclusions based on inadequate data. A well-drafted agreement and proper selection of a monitor can prevent these complaints from being made in the first place or defend the monitoring process when the complaints are untrue.

REMEDIAL PLAN

Although the particular elements of a remedial plan will vary based on the factors specific to the litigation and the size and type of the correctional facility (e.g., small jail, large jail, large prison, entire prison system), the basic structures of many correctional mental health care system remedial plans are quite similar and are usually related to well-accepted national standards and guidelines (American Psychiatric Association 2000; Council of State Governments 2002; National Commission on Correctional Health Care 2008a, 2008b) and well-known court decisions (*Coleman v. Wilson* 1995; *Madrid v. Gomez* 1995; *Ruiz v. Estelle* 1980). These guidelines, standards, and court decisions essentially provide the details to the "access" concept described by Cohen (2008). Cohen specified three elements required to establish a constitutionally adequate correctional mental health system: 1) adequate physical resources (treatment program space and supplies), 2) adequate human resources (numbers of properly trained and/or experienced mental health staff who will identify and/or provide treatment to inmates with serious mental illness), and 3) adequate access for inmates to these physical and human resources within a reasonable period of time.

TABLE 14–2. Policies and procedures

1. Mission and goals
2. Administrative structure
3. Staffing (job descriptions, credentials, privileging, caseload ratios when appropriate)
4. Reliable and valid methods for identifying inmates with mental illnesses (i.e., receiving screening, intake mental health screening, mental health evaluations, referral process)
5. Treatment programs available (which should include level of mental health care, such as outpatient treatment, crisis stabilization units, intermediate care housing units, and access to inpatient psychiatric hospitalization)
6. Special issues related to mental health services provided to inmates in locked-down housing units such as disciplinary segregation (e.g., mental health screening upon admission, regular mental health rounds, exclusion from such housing when clinically appropriate)
7. Involuntary treatments for mental health purposes (e.g., restraints, medication, psychiatric hospitalization)
8. Other medicolegal issues (e.g., obtaining informed consent)
9. Limits of confidentiality during assessment and treatment sessions, with relevant exceptions described
10. Quality improvement process
11. Suicide prevention program
12. Cross-training of correctional staff concerning mental health issues and of mental health staff regarding correctional and security issues
13. Research guidelines (Metzner 1997)

Source. Adapted from Metzner 1997.

Policies and procedures form the framework for implementation of a remedial plan. A *policy* is a facility's official position on a particular issue related to an organization's purpose. A *procedure* describes in detail how the policy is carried out (National Commission on Correctional Health Care 2008a). These correctional mental health policies and procedures, which should be reviewed on an annual basis and revised as needed, should cover at least the areas summarized in Table 14–2 (Metzner 1997).

MONITORING PROCESS

An initial, major focus of monitoring is to review these policies and procedures for adequacy of content and process. Both the writing of the policies and procedures by the administrators of the correctional mental health program and the review for adequacy by the monitor are laborious tasks, which typically require at least several rewrites. However, this process is very important, because during the implementation phase, the monitoring will essentially focus on the adequacy of implementation of these policies and procedures. In addition, the quality improvement program, which has become an essential element of most remedial plans, will in large part be based on these policies and procedures, with many of the indicators being defined by them. Quality improvement is a crucial management tool that helps assess and improve system issues relevant to the correctional mental health system, which should also help to determine the state of compliance with the remedial plan.

Little has been written about the evaluation and/or monitoring process from the perspective of a clinician monitor or clinical consultant. Metzner (2002; Metzner and Dubovsky 1986), Elliott (1997), and Wills (2007) emphasized the importance of a structured systematic approach that includes 1) relevant pre–site visit document reviews and 2) on-site visits that involve interviews with inmates and correctional, mental health, and medical staffs; inspection of physical plant resources (e.g., office space, treatment/programming space, all types of housing units, including general population and segregation units, and infirmaries); and an assessment of the quality improvement process.

Monitoring generally requires review of the following essential areas:

1. The condition and adequacy of the physical plant (e.g., program and office space) of the correctional facility, especially in the context of the average inmate population
2. The adequacy of allocations and credentials of the mental health staff
3. Access to mental health care
4. The clinical appropriateness and quality of the mental health care provided
5. Medication management practices
6. Suicide prevention program
7. The quality improvement process
8. Interface between custody and mental health staffs

Pre–Site Visit Information

The remedial plan provides the structure for the monitoring process. The monitor's job is to report whether or not the settlement agreement is being implemented and the data upon which such conclusions are based. As much as possible, monitors should rely on objective information to support their conclusions about compliance. To the extent possible, the monitor should receive information relevant to the remedial plan several weeks prior to scheduled site visits. The information obtained will help to identify both strengths and weaknesses of the mental health system. The process of obtaining the information will often provide important data concerning the mental health program from a systems perspective (e.g., whether the information was difficult to obtain in a timely manner despite reasonable requests, and if so, why). Based on the answers to these process issues, important information concerning the correctional mental health system's quality improvement process and management information system will become apparent, both of which are essential elements of an adequate correctional mental health system.

The on-site assessment will often be shorter in duration and more efficiently performed if the pre–site visit information is reviewed in advance, assuming the obtained information is accurate. Obtaining this information in electronic form will also facilitate the timely production of the site visit report because of the ease of managing the electronic data for report-writing purposes. Pre–site visit information requests will vary based on the stage of the litigation process, issues specific to the litigation (e.g., the requirements of the remedial plan), the current level of compliance, and other relevant factors.

Table 14–3 summarizes a typical pre–site visit information request that should result in obtaining very helpful information relevant to the site assessment process. This list is very comprehensive and includes the kinds of data that will enable the institution's leaders and the monitor to demonstrate adherence (or failures to adhere) to the requirements of the settlement agreement and implementation plan. Pre–site visit information should be obtained prior to each site visit, although the information requested will vary based on prior site visits and the specifics of the remedial plan. The monitor should select only those items that are relevant and essential to monitoring the particular remedial plan, to prevent the institution from spending unnecessary time in responding to the request.

When requesting pre–site visit information, the monitor should advise correctional facility staff that if any of the requests are very burdensome to produce, they should contact the monitor before proceeding with the specific request. Although this information often provides very useful

TABLE 14–3.   Pre–site visit information

Overview

1. Mental health system's organizational chart, listing each position, name of person filling position, and his or her credentials (e.g., degrees, licenses).

2. Written program description of current mental health system, highlighting notable successes, problems, and challenges. This summary should report on any mission changes at the institution or major population changes, as well as any obstacles (e.g., lockdowns, space limitations) to provision of mental health treatment or compliance with policies and procedures.

3. Any internal or external reviews (e.g., accreditation survey reports) relevant to mental health system.

Census

4. Total number of inmates in institution(s) and number of inmates by custody level (e.g., maximum security, medium security) and legal status (e.g., pretrial, sentence serving).

5. Annual number of admissions to and discharges from the institution.

6. Total number of inmates on mental health caseload on a given day, enumerated by level of care and/or treatment program (e.g., outpatient, residential treatment housing, infirmary, inpatient).

7. Total number of inmates in locked-down units, such as administrative (and all other forms of) segregation; number and percentage of these inmates who are on mental health caseload; and average and median lengths of stay in these units.

Mental health caseloads

8. Average daily census in mental health treatment units (e.g., intermediate care, infirmary) on a monthly basis during past 6 months.

9. Monthly average (stated as percentage) of total population of inmates who received mental health treatment (i.e., average mental health caseload).

10. Total number of inmates who have been prescribed psychotropic medications.

11. Average and median lengths of stay in infirmary (or equivalent unit) for inmates admitted for mental health purposes.

TABLE 14–3. Pre–site visit information *(continued)*

Staffing

12. Staffing information, including a list of all authorized (i.e., funded) mental health positions by program or area (e.g., reception/ receiving area, administrative segregation, general population). For each position, indicate person's name, professional degree, start date, and percentage of full-time equivalent if not full-time. If position is vacant, provide date position became vacant. For any staff on extended leave, indicate date that leave began. Information pertinent to the use of contract clinicians should be provided.

13. Percentage of mental health clinical staff who have state licensure in their respective disciplines.

14. If clinicians are not licensed, a description of any supervision provided.

15. Number of patients on each clinician's and psychiatrist's caseload.

16. Staffing information regarding pharmacy, laboratory, medical records department, and nonpsychiatric nursing staff, which should be provided due to their significant impact on the mental health care delivery system.

Reception/receiving center

17. Protocol for mental health screens/assessments/evaluations for new commitments (assuming the institution maintains a new arrival function).

18. Number of persons admitted through reception/receiving center annually and average number of intakes per day.

19. Statistical information pertinent to the reception/receiving center screening of inmates:

    a. Number of persons screened on a daily, weekly, or monthly basis for the past 6 months

    b. Percentage of inmates who have positive screens from a mental health perspective

    c. Percentage of inmates with positive screens who enter the continuum of mental health services

    d. Percentage of all newly admitted inmates who enter the continuum of mental health services

TABLE 14–3. Pre–site visit information *(continued)*

Quality improvement

20. Quality improvement (formerly called "quality assurance") documents (e.g., reports, reviews, minutes) pertinent to the mental health system that were generated since previous monitoring visit.

21. Description of relevant inmate management information system(s) and copies of reports regularly generated from the system(s) that are used for mental health system review and planning.

Medication issues

22. Copy of drug formulary or changes in formulary since previous monitoring visit, and description of process for maintaining and changing formulary.

23. Documentation of any medication errors reported, and results of any summary and classification of errors in the pharmacy or related committee examining these reports.

24. List of any inmates who received psychotropic medications on an involuntary basis.

25. Description of procedure used to identify inmates taking psychiatric medications who move within the institution and to provide them medication without significant interruption.

26. Description of procedure used to identify and manage inmates taking psychiatric medications who are nonadherent with medications.

27. Audits (quality improvement reports) relevant to continuity of medication for newly admitted inmates and inmates who have changed housing units within the institution, medication expirations and renewal of orders, and medication nonadherence issues.

28. Information relevant to timing of "pill call" (i.e., the medication administration process) and length of pill-call lines.

Access to care

29. Description of the procedures for collecting, triaging, assigning, responding to, and recording mental health referrals.

30. Data concerning response time frames for routine, urgent, and emergency mental health referrals.

31. Number of inmates transferred to higher levels of mental health care, such as crisis bed units (with 24-hour nursing care) or inpatient psychiatric units, and length of time from referral to actual transfer to such units.

32. Number of inmates with three or more transfers to mental health units with 24-hour nursing care during previous 6 months.

TABLE 14–3. Pre–site visit information *(continued)*

Suicides and suicide prevention

33. Names of any inmates who committed suicide or made serious attempts, including copy of psychological autopsy and/or serious incident review, if performed.

34. Training requirements for custody staff relevant to suicide prevention and other mental health issues.

35. Percentage of custody officers currently working who have completed the required suicide training.

36. Minutes of the suicide prevention committee meetings.

37. Data relevant to suicide attempts.

Custody reports

38. Serious incident reports pertinent to mental health, including information relevant to use of force involving inmates with mental illness.

39. Grievances relating to mental health care.

40. Copies of any disciplinary write-ups for inmates involving self-injurious behavior.

Discharge planning

41. Information relevant to discharge planning:

    a. Process that identifies inmates in need of discharge planning

    b. Elements of the discharge planning process (e.g., entitlement benefits, linkages for mental health treatment, provision of discharge medications, housing referrals)

    c. Proof of practice regarding the above elements

---

information about the management information system and other system issues, it is often not a good use of time for the institution to commit many hours of work to produce data that are not easily obtainable for pre–site visit information purposes only. Whenever possible, the information provided to the monitor should be routinely used by the facility's leaders to manage the mental health program. Part of the monitor's consultative and educational mission may be to teach the facility how to monitor itself, thereby hastening the day when the expensive external monitoring process can end.

Review and initial analysis of the pre–site visit information will greatly assist the monitor in 1) formulating areas of inquiry to be explored during the site visit and 2) structuring the monitoring visit. Even under the best of circumstances, the requested site information imposes a significant time commitment on many of the monitored institutional mental health staff; the monitor should recognize the staff for their efforts in a positive manner.

On-Site Assessment

The on-site assessment, especially at the beginning of the monitoring process, is very stressful for most of the staff involved, especially the clinical and administrative leadership. The staff's response is often dependent on the dynamics and events leading to the monitoring process. In other words, the correctional and mental health staff are often initially defensive when faced with monitoring of the mental health system. No one likes being told that his or her work is inadequate or deficient, and the litigation is commonly a result of resource issues. The monitor needs to take a nonblaming, positive approach to the monitoring process.

The staff's response to the monitoring process can be demonstrated by their treatment of the monitor's arrival at the institution. At the one extreme, the staff may make it difficult for the monitor to actually get into the institution. The monitor would do well not to react in a narcissistic manner but instead to take the situation in stride, remain respectful, and proceed with obtaining entrance via the pertinent chain of command. At the other extreme, by providing a reserved parking space or offering simple refreshments for the monitor, the institution signals a lack of defensiveness and indicates the potential for a more collegial relationship between the monitor and the correctional mental health system.

Most monitoring visits begin with an opening session attended by the institution's leadership, such as wardens or jail directors, deputy wardens, correctional captains, and key clinical or administrative health care staff, obviously including the mental health program leadership. As the monitoring process becomes less of an unknown, these opening meetings become shorter in duration, more focused, and more useful in facilitating the monitoring process.

To start the actual "hands-on" portion of the on-site review process, the monitor should ask to meet with key clinical and administrative staff to question them about specific elements of the remedial plan. At this time, the monitor can also seek clarification of information provided in the pre–site visit information process.

One effective way to implement a settlement agreement is to create a series of specific corrective action plans (CAPs) to remedy those elements of the implementation plan that have not yet been successfully developed or implemented. Excluding the first monitoring visit, a status report for each written CAP should be provided by the facility to the monitor as part of the pre–site visit information package. The monitor should review the current status of the CAP with the relevant staff and obtain pertinent information through interviews with staff and inmates, reviews of records and quality improvement studies, and other relevant sources.

Unfortunately, obtaining accurate and relevant information from staff is not always a straightforward process. Questions must be worded clearly, and data sources must be checked (at least on a random basis) for accuracy. Although inaccurate information might result from an intentional desire to mislead, it is far more likely due to a misunderstanding of what the monitor wants to know.

For various reasons, mental health and custody staff do not always provide complete, relevant, or accurate answers to questions asked by the monitor. The monitor usually discovers such inaccuracies or omissions either by adhering to a sound methodological assessment approach or perhaps by accident. Credibility issues are then raised, and the often unwelcome result is an increase in documentation requirements of the staff for monitoring purposes. The staff usually realize fairly quickly that the question is *how long* it will take the monitor to obtain essential information, not *whether* the information will be obtained by the monitor. Basically, the less cooperative the staff are, the longer the site visit will take. Related to this issue, in addition to asking very specific questions, the monitor should emphasize during the assessment process that any other relevant information regarding implementation of the remedial plan not specifically requested by the monitor should be provided. For example, the monitor should ask, "Is there anything else about the mental health system that I have not asked about but should know?"

The monitor should be aware that line staff often exaggerate the problems within the correctional mental health system because they lack familiarity with the actual data and/or feel overwhelmed by job duties and/or job dissatisfaction. Collateral information needs to be obtained to check the accuracy of information provided by line or administrative staff.

If the monitor is reasonable and has the opportunity to develop a working relationship with the monitored staff, credibility issues on both sides will be minimal and the monitoring process should help the system improve and meet the remedial plan requirements. Obstacles that impede development of a good working relationship include the following:

1. Interference by the attorneys on either side that creates an adversarial relationship between the monitor and the correctional and/or mental health staff; for example, not allowing the line staff to talk with the monitor without the defendants' attorney present is not helpful to the monitoring process.

2. Instructions to the mental health staff from administrative staff to not volunteer information and/or to talk to the monitor only in the presence of supervisory staff.
3. A monitor who uses the information obtained from staff in a manner that causes the staff to experience actual or perceived subsequent retaliation.

After obtaining pertinent information from the staff as described above, the monitor needs to confirm the accuracy of the information and/or obtain additional information for reasons previously summarized. Potential sources of information for this process are summarized in Table 14–4. The length of the site visit is often a limiting factor in obtaining information from some of these sources.

TABLE 14–4. Sources of primary and/or collateral information

Line mental health care staff

Nursing, medical, medical records, and pharmacy staffs

Correctional staff (administrators, supervising correctional officers, and line correctional officers)

Inmates (predominantly, but not exclusively, mental health care caseload inmates)

Review of health care and custody records, including a variety of relevant logbooks

Review of quality improvement studies, other audits relevant to the mental health system, and pertinent committee minutes (e.g., suicide prevention committee, mental health quality improvement committee)

Attendance at mental health team meetings, such as treatment planning meetings, shift briefings, or routine morning meetings

Observation of treatment activities such as group therapy sessions and community meetings

Observation of custody classification committee procedures and custody disciplinary hearings, especially involving inmates with mental illness

In general, the monitor should meet with line mental health staff, including all available clinicians and clerical staff, without supervisory staff present. Meeting with these staff in the middle of the site visit enables the monitor to confirm the accuracy of information already obtained and to elicit relevant information that the monitor can verify during the remainder of the site assessment. This meeting should not become a "gripe session" regarding specific disagreements between staff and their supervisors; instead, it should be limited to broad and systemic issues. The staff should be told that the information they provide is not confidential and that the monitor can judge how it will be used, although a monitor rarely discloses the specific source of information except through use of the generic term *staff*. Supervisors are not present at this meeting because they may inhibit free discussion with the monitor by the line staff. Requests by staff for individual interviews with the monitor are discouraged for various reasons, which include time limitations. Providing preliminary feedback to the staff regarding implementation of the remedial plan is helpful for establishing a better working relationship with them.

Interviews with inmates with mental illness are also very useful in assessing compliance issues with the remedial plan. An effective mechanism is the use of group interviews, for which the inmate participants are selected from a caseload list provided by the staff. The monitor might select a skewed sample to include a larger number of inmates with serious mental illnesses; however, the monitor should make clear that this process is not intended to represent a random sample of inmates or to generate prevalence estimates. The number of groups of inmates interviewed will depend on the size of the institution. In large facilities, the monitor should interview inmates from different yards or housing units in an attempt to have a more representative sample. In special housing units for inmates with mental illnesses, interviews in a community meeting setting can be very helpful and efficient in obtaining relevant information.

After clearly explaining the purpose of the process to the inmates, the monitor should ask questions that focus on issues regarding access to care, medication continuity, quality of treatment, interactions with mental health and custody staffs, and other issues relevant to the remedial plan. The records of a sample of these inmates should be reviewed to confirm the accuracy of problems identified during the interview process.

In a locked-down setting, such as an administrative segregation unit, the monitor can observe (or "perform") mental health rounds to obtain information pertinent to the remedial plan. A limited number of individual interviews (not at the cell front) may also be useful, for both locked-down inmates and general population inmates. However, due to time limitations, some form of screening process should be developed to increase the chances that these interviews will be useful to the monitoring process. The screening process may include suggestions from the plaintiff's attorneys, mental health staff, and/or correctional officers, or may be based on the monitor's triage process during observation of mental health rounds, general interactions with inmates (e.g., while walking in the yards), or review of incident reports or logbooks (e.g., repeat admission to the infirmary for mental health purposes).

Information obtained from custody staff is also useful and can be obtained in a variety of ways, including group interviews and informal interactions with custody staff during the site visit. Observation of custody interactions with inmates and mental health staff is also informative. Such observations often reveal that problems in the working relationship between custody staff and mental health staff are not just one-sided (i.e., both staffs contribute to the problem).

Sustained compliance with the remedial plan is almost always associated with implementation of an adequate quality improvement process. In the early stages of the monitoring process, the correctional system essentially uses (often unknowingly) the monitoring process as a quality improvement process. Under these circumstances, the monitoring is initially structured to perform audits that should have been performed by the institution's mental health system. As a result, in a short period of time, a monitor commonly obtains information about the mental health system that was not apparent to the system. Although the monitoring will eventually assist the correctional system in developing its own internal quality improvement system, this process is easier said than done for many reasons, including staff turnover, inadequate management information systems, and inexperience with the quality improvement process. As the system's own quality improvement process becomes adequate, as confirmed by the monitoring process, compliance with the remedial plan will likely follow close behind, assuming that needed resources as specified in the remedial plan have been obtained.

THE MONITORING REPORT

The format of the report, which varies for many reasons, should be negotiated with, or at least announced to, the parties before the first report is issued. The format should be structured according to the remedial plan, to facilitate tracking of the degree of compliance with the plan. A helpful suggestion is to summarize 1) the administrative staff's description of the current status of various remedial plan elements; 2) the data obtained by the monitor from other sources of information, as previously summarized; and 3) the monitor's assessment of the current progress toward compliance of the specific remedial plan element. Prior to or during the early stages of the monitoring process, the parties should agree on definitions and guidelines regarding terms such as *noncompliance, partial compliance, compliance,* and *sustained compliance* used in the context of the remedial plan elements.

Unfortunately, reports are commonly provided to the parties in an untimely manner, for various reasons. For example, if a report is not distributed until 6 months after the site visit, and if the monitoring assessments occur every 6 months, the correctional facility will not have the benefit of reviewing the previous report in a thoughtful manner prior to the subsequent site visit. Such problems can be mitigated via exit interviews at the end of a site visit. However, exit interviews can also be problematic, because 1) the monitor has not had adequate time to synthesize the site visit assessment and 2) the correctional mental health staff may not adequately understand the findings summarized during the exit interview due to fatigue, anxiety, or other reasons.

SUMMARY POINTS

- Correctional mental health systems have significantly benefited from being monitored because of increased resources and mandated implementation of basic policies and procedures related to the monitoring process.

- Selecting a monitor or monitors is a crucial step due to the important role of the monitor(s) in the assessment process.

- The access concept provides a framework for the remedial plan, and relevant policies and procedures help to structure the monitoring process.

- Obtaining relevant pre–site visit information is an essential component of the monitoring process.

- Obtaining information from multiple sources during the on-site assessment is essential to accurately assess the degree of implementation of the remedial plan.

- Reports should be structured to correspond to the elements of the remedial plan and produced in a timely manner.

REFERENCES

American Psychiatric Association: Psychiatric Services in Jails and Prisons: A Task Force Report of the American Psychiatric Association, 2nd Edition. Washington, DC, American Psychiatric Association, 2000

Belbot B: Report on the Prison Litigation Reform Act: what have the courts decided so far? Prison J 84:290–316, 2004

Boston J: The Prison Litigation Reform Act. 2004. Available at: http://www.wnylc.net/pb/docs/plra2cir04.pdf. Accessed April 10, 2009.

Cohen F: The Mentally Disordered Inmate and the Law, 2nd Edition. Kingston, NJ, Civic Research Institute, 2008

Coleman v Wilson, 912 F.Supp. 1282 (E.D. Cal. 1995)

Council of State Governments: Criminal Justice/Mental Health Consensus Project. New York, Council of State Governments, 2002

Elliott RL: Evaluating the quality of correctional mental health services: an approach to surveying a correctional mental health system. Behav Sci Law 15:427–438, 1997

Madrid v Gomez, 889 F.Supp. 1146 (N.D. Cal. 1995)

Metzner JL: An introduction to correctional psychiatry, part I. J Am Acad Psychiatry Law 25:375–381, 1997

Metzner JL: Class action litigation in correctional psychiatry. J Am Acad Psychiatry Law 30:19–29, 2002

Metzner JL, Dubovsky SL: The role of the psychiatrist in evaluating a prison mental health system in litigation. Bull Am Acad Psychiatry Law 14:89–93, 1986

National Commission on Correctional Health Care: Standards for Health Services in Jails. Chicago, National Commission on Correctional Health Care, 2008a

National Commission on Correctional Health Care: Standards for Health Services in Prisons. Chicago, National Commission on Correctional Health Care, 2008b

Prison Litigation Reform Act of 1995, Pub. L. No. 104-134, H.R. 3019, 104th Cong. (1996)

Ruiz v Estelle, 503 F.Supp. 1265 (S.D. Texas 1980)

Schlanger M: Inmate litigation: results of a national survey. National Institute of Corrections Large Jail Network Exchange, July 2003, pp 1–12

Wills CD: PRAMS: a systematic method for evaluating penal institutions under litigation. J Am Acad Psychiatry Law 35:103–108, 2007

CHAPTER 15

Clinically Oriented Reentry Planning

Henry A. Dlugacz, M.S.W., J.D.

Erik Roskes, M.D.

> *Insanity: doing the same thing over and over again and expecting different results.*
>
> Albert Einstein

Historically, correctional health care was conceptualized as being conducted in a host environment, with its mission subordinate to the primary mission of confinement. Over time, this limited vision and understanding of correctional health care has grown to encompass public health concepts, including smoking cessation, tuberculosis case finding, screening for HIV, and approaches to treating addiction. Recently, at least one of the original pioneers in the field has begun to promote the idea that the provision of health care to such a large group of multiproblem patients in a congregate setting is a public health mission of equal importance to the confinement role of corrections, particularly in light of the significantly reduced number of public hospitals (King 2005).

We assert that a similar evolution is taking place with regard to correctional mental health care. Correctional mental health services initially were developed primarily as a means of suicide prevention and secondarily as a crisis intervention program, often in response to court-imposed mandates (see Chapter 14, "Monitoring a Correctional Mental Health System"). Over the past several decades, in the context of deinstitutionalization, the public mental health system has deteriorated to the point that for many persons with mental illness, the correctional system has become the primary provider of assessment and care (President's New Freedom Commission on Mental Health 2003). Thus, just as with public health and preventive medicine, the case identification and mental health treatment missions of jails and prisons have become far more salient. In this context, reentry planning[1] for mentally ill inmates has begun to evolve from a best practice toward a standard of care (Metzner 2007).

Clinically oriented reentry planning requires critical assessment of the mental health service delivery model typically found within correctional institutions. This assessment may include an expanded definition of *mission* as well as revisions to specific organizational, staffing, technological, and assessment aspects of a correctional mental health program. In contrast to crisis-oriented mental health care within a correctional setting, clinically oriented reentry planning is, by definition, community based in orientation and proactive in nature. As a result, its outlook in terms of assessment techniques and foci, as well as its measures of success, should extend into the community (see Chapter 2, "Criminal Justice System and Offenders Placed in an Outpatient Setting"). Whatever outcome measure is employed, some degree of integration of correctional care with the public mental health system is required. The nature and extent of this integration are highly dependent on jurisdiction.

Correctional systems vary significantly in their size, location, and service delivery models. In addition, correctional systems differ in their detention role, with widely varying average incarceration lengths and predictability. Furthermore, inmates' circumstances vary according to their illness, their connection with mental health treatment while incarcerated, and their ability to function in the community (Metzner 2007). In the following sections, we review a variety of promising approaches to clinically oriented reentry planning. However, we do not suggest that all

---

[1]The term *reentry planning* is typically used in correctional settings when describing the process of preparing inmates for returning to their communities. It is roughly analogous to the *discharge planning* process used in a hospital setting. Sowers and Rohland (2004) suggested replacing the term *discharge planning* with *transition planning* because they believe it better captures the concept of continuing care. Each of these terms has specific strengths vis-à-vis the movement of individuals between systems of care; for clarity's sake, we use the term *reentry planning* except where one of the other terms is preferable for specific reasons.

jurisdictions apply all of these approaches. Rather, our aim is to describe the characteristics shared by successful programs and discuss innovative approaches that can inform clinically sound reentry planning. Jurisdictions interested in improving the transition of inmates or detainees with mental illness need to adapt these approaches to the specific needs and capabilities of their specific systems of care.

The approaches outlined in this chapter focus primarily on addressing the needs of the inmate or detainee whose presentation is primarily that of a serious mental illness. Reentry poses particular risks for this population, including recidivism, hospitalization, and morbidity. Within 18 months of release, two-thirds of all seriously mentally ill inmates are rearrested and one-half are hospitalized (Feder 1991; Hartwell 2003, 2008). Of great concern, a recent study from Washington State found that inmates were almost 13 times more likely to die within the first 2 weeks of release than were other people with similar demographics (Binswanger et al. 2007a, 2007b).

Except for how the release date is determined, the clinical elements of the reentry planning process from a short-term correctional setting are *conceptually* similar to discharge planning in a hospital or other community setting. Indeed, ensuring continuity of care for patients with low socioeconomic status and minority patients leaving psychiatric hospitals proves likewise a significant challenge. The details of the reentry planning process will vary with the type and mission of the correctional agency (Adair 2007). For longer-term incarcerations, the stress of reentry may, in fact, be greater and more complex than it is from a hospital setting (Draine et al. 2005). Most community-based discharge planning occurs when individuals are released from higher to lower levels of care; in these instances, the treating clinicians can be expected to "speak the same language." In contrast, coordinating correctional institution–based and community-based care may demand the input and coordination of custody staff, correctional mental health staff, parole officers, and community-based clinicians, all of whom may have quite distinct views as to the nature and goals of treatment. Draine et al. (2005) noted that "community reintegration is more complicated than would be suggested by a list of psychiatric needs and criminogenic risk factors, or by the model used in planning for patients leaving a psychiatric hospital" (p. 691).

We acknowledge that many inmates and detainees have both a mental illness and interpersonal and social characteristics that may complicate reentry planning. Recent research suggests that inmates with mental disorders may have risk factors for reoffense that are disproportionately higher than those of the overall criminal justice population (Skeem et al. 2008). To the extent that a mentally ill inmate leaving jail or prison has risk factors for recidivism, such as substance use, procriminal attitudes, or criminogenic companions (Andrews and Bonta 2003; Bonta 2002), the reentry issues may closely resemble those of inmates without serious mental illness. Even where such risk factors are prominent, the existence of a serious mental illness will require reentry planners to address acute symptoms and the social context before an offender can be expected to avail himself or herself of transition strategies aimed at reducing recidivism. To the extent that symptom levels, social needs, and risk factors are independent and may vary temporally, an individualized assessment must be made to decide in what order and in what way they will be addressed. Reentry planning efforts must account for the interaction of symptom levels, social needs, and risk factors. Much scholarship indicates that mental illness per se is only a modest predictor of recidivism (Bonta et al. 1998; Skeem et al. 2008). However, a recent large-scale study of inmates serving sentences in the Texas prison system found that those with major psychiatric disorders—defined as major depressive disorder, bipolar disorders, schizophrenia, and nonschizophrenic psychotic disorders—had much greater risks of multiple incarcerations over the 6-year study period (Baillargeon et al. 2008). Also, a singular focus on recidivism per se may be overly simplistic because probationers and parolees with mental illness fail supervision disproportionately, often due to technical violations (Skeem et al. 2008). Although empirical study is required to enhance understanding of the relationship between mental illness and risk for incarceration, this group clearly requires focused, clinically based reentry planning as part of a comprehensive strategy to address this concern. In addition, related but independent public health, public safety, and fiscal rationales exist for providing clinically oriented reentry planning to people with serious mental illness (Dlugacz et al. 2007).

In this chapter, we discuss the theoretical underpinnings driving correctional systems to engage or not engage in clinically oriented reentry planning programs. We also review the evolving clinical and legal standards that apply to correctional systems vis-à-vis transitional care of inmates and detainees with mental illness. We then outline current approaches to reentry planning, identifying the characteristics of successful models. Finally, we put forth our recommendations as to how these clinical, ethical, and legal requirements may be met.

THEORETICAL UNDERPINNING OF CLINICALLY ORIENTED REENTRY PLANNING

Confidence in society's ability to effect positive change in the correctional population has ebbed and flowed over the years, reflecting variations in political, religious, and psychological theories in vogue at the time. As stated by the prominent federal judge Jack B. Weinstein, there has been a "rise and fall of the belief in rehabilitation—that many of those who commit crimes can be, with appropriate attention and intervention, brought back into society as productive, valued members" (Weinstein and Wimmer, in press). In 1974, Robert Martinson published a very influential paper titled "What Works? Questions and Answers About Prison Reform." Although it was an oversimplification of Martinson's work, the answer was widely understood to be "nothing works," with the implication that engaging in rehabilitative efforts is a waste of time and resources. The thinking embodied in this view contributed to a profound lack of attention to individual rehabilitation in correctional settings in the ensuing years. In contrast to the Canadian approach to reentry, which emphasizes rehabilitation focused on empirically substantiated cognitive restructuring techniques, the focus on reentry planning in the United States has eschewed efforts to treat individual offenders, focusing instead primarily on sociological analysis.

This mistrust of the concept of rehabilitation characterized in recent U.S. approaches to this issue became enshrined in the federal sentencing guidelines (U.S. Sentencing Commission 2008). These guidelines were upheld by the Supreme Court in *Mistretta v. United States* (1989), although more recent Supreme Court cases have held that the guidelines were advisory rather than mandatory (*Gall v. United States* 2007; *United States v. Booker* 2005). The guidelines, with their formulaic approach to sentencing, discarded rehabilitation as an important factor in deriving sentences. In fact, the U.S. Senate report to the act establishing the guidelines stated the view that the previous system was "based largely on an outmoded rehabilitation model" (S. Rep. No. 98-225 at 38 [1984]; cited in Weinstein and Wimmer, in press). Furthermore, the guidelines made departure from prescribed sentences on the basis of the mental illness of the defendant difficult but not impossible. The policy statement accompanying the guidelines articulated the position that mental conditions are not "ordinarily relevant" when determining a sentence (Perlin and Gould 1995). Consistent with cognitive, motivational, and recovery approaches, we suggest that reentry work with inmates with mental disabilities be individually based, with a reliance on positive rather than negative reinforcements (Petersilia 2004). Also, reentry planning must emphasize patient strengths and the mobilization of support systems. A number of specific clinical interventions and perspectives are relevant to this endeavor. The late, respected corrections professional John Conrad said that correctional institutions need to be "lawful, safe, industrious, and hopeful" (Beto 1992). The approaches we discuss tend to engender hope, in our view an essential albeit difficult to quantify ingredient to constructive change.

Unfortunately, the overarching resistance to considering rehabilitation as one of the primary goals of corrections has sometimes pervaded even the mind-set of those charged with treating patients in this setting. This is clear when one considers the constitutional rationale for requiring treatment in corrections: it is the Eighth Amendment's prohibition against cruel and unusual punishment, and not an ethical or clinical imperative to help people get better, that animates many treatment requirements (*Estelle v. Gamble* 1976). This mind-set contributes to the isolation that providers of care in corrections experience and reinforces the disconnection of care and inadequate attention to clinically oriented reentry planning in correctional settings.

EVOLVING STANDARDS OF CARE

Statistical Background

Each year, an estimated 650,000 adults are released from prisons and 7 million are released from local jails (Council of State Governments 2002). A very large number of these individuals have mental illness, as highlighted in Chapter 5, "Conducting Mental Health Assessments in Correctional Settings." Estimates indicate that between 15% and 50% of incarcerated individuals have mental health needs during their incarceration (Ditton 1999; James and Glaze 2006). A large proportion of incarcerated individuals with mental illness have comorbid addictions. Individuals with mental illness account for a disproportionately large percentage of intakes and releases from correctional settings. Approximately 97% of the vast number of people detained or incarcerated return to live in the community at some point (Council of State Governments 2002; Dlugacz et al. 2007; Travis and Waul 2004), making effective reentry planning, particularly for those with serious mental illness, a meaningful goal of the public psychiatry system.

Clinical Bases of Reentry Planning

The importance of planning for prisoners to reenter society is becoming increasingly well accepted. Professional standards governing the provision of care in the wider community emphasize continuity of care as patients transition across systems of care and among services (Joint Commission 2008). For example, NPSG.08.02.01 of the 2009 National Patient Safety Goals Behavioral Health Care Program (Joint Commission 2008) states in part that

> [w]hen a [patient] is referred to or transferred from one [organization] to another, the complete and reconciled list of medications is communicated to the next provider of service, and the communication is documented. Alternatively, when a [patient] leaves the [organization]'s care to go directly to his or her home, the complete and reconciled list of medications is provided to the [patient]'s known primary care provider, the original referring provider, or a known next provider of service. (p. 10)

Given the importance of medication continuity and the difficulty encountered by patients in many communities in accessing timely psychiatric care upon release from incarceration, we suggest that jurisdictions provide those leaving correctional facilities who have been taking psychotropic medications with a reasonable supply of medications and/or prescriptions, as well as patient education consistent with the aftercare plan for ongoing treatment. Individual clinical circumstances vary, as does access to community-based treatment. In specific instances, the decision as to how long a supply of medication to provide should be subject to the clinical judgment of the psychiatrist, informed by knowledge concerning the capacity of community treatment providers. Professional organizations focused more specifically on correctional health care have, over time, become unanimous that some form of postrelease planning is an essential component of adequate treatment. The National Commission on Correctional Health Care (NCCHC; 2008) standards mandate that discharge planning be "provided for inmates with serious health needs whose release is imminent." This language is consistent with a prior version of the NCCHC standards. Mental health–focused commentary provided additional guidance to the unchanged earlier standards (NCCHC 2003):

> The mental health considerations for this [M-E-13] standard focus on a need for a seamless system of care between the correctional environment and the community. The intent of this standard is that facility clinicians ensure patients' health needs are met during transition to a community provider. Successful return to the community, particularly for patients with mental health or substance abuse problems, depends on effective discharge planning and linkage to community providers, including funding sources where possible. (NCCHC 2003, pp. 90–91)

The American Psychiatric Association (APA; 2000b) has also promulgated standards on psychiatric services in jails and prisons. The APA standards note that "timely and effective discharge planning is essential to continuity of care and an integral part of adequate mental health treatment" (p. 18). The American Public Health Association's (2003) standards governing health care in correctional institutions require transition planning: Standard III states that "there must be a plan for continuity of care, whether a prisoner is transferred to another correctional system or facility or returned to the community" (p. 39).

Medical ethical standards relevant to the psychiatrist practicing in the correctional setting further reinforce the importance of transition planning. In what could be seen as an ethical take on the legal prohibition on the abandonment of a patient by his or her physician, the American Medical Association's (1990) ethical guidelines provide that

> the patient has the right to continuity of health care. The physician has an obligation to cooperate in the coordination of medically indicated care with other health care providers treating the patient. The physician may not discontinue treatment of a patient as long as further treatment is medically indicated, without giving the patient reasonable assistance and sufficient opportunity to make alternative arrangements for care.

An individual psychiatrist working in a correctional institution cannot meet this standard acting alone. The system would have to support the physician's ability to effectuate this ethical standard, raising complex ethical questions for all physicians working in correctional health and mental health care, particularly for those in leadership positions.

Although the standards discussed above lack specific guidance as to the intensity or nature of reentry planning, contemporary professional standards, taken as a whole, require correctional systems to, in some fashion, attend proactively and systematically to the needs of inmates and detainees leaving their systems.

Complicating this picture is a gap between what the U.S. Constitution requires as a matter of constitutional law and what ethical principles, public health constructs, accreditation bodies, and perhaps state or local laws require. As far back as 1979, in a case involving conditions of pretrial detention (*Bell v. Wolfish* 1979), the U.S. Supreme Court held that professional standards are not dispositive but are only advisory in determining the minimum constitutional standard. The fact that a certain level of care is generally required by professional standards does not necessarily mean that it is constitutionally mandated (*Estelle v. Gamble* 1976). Also complicating an assessment of the prevailing standard of care is what we perceive as a chasm between prevailing notions in health care that transition planning is critical and should be universally practiced in some form and the current reality that many jurisdictions do little or nothing to make this occur. For example, a Bureau of Justice Statistics survey (Beck and Maruschak 2001) conducted in 2001 found that only 51% of jurisdictions responding indicated that they provided released inmates with any assistance in connecting with community services. The extent of the assistance ranged from the provision of lists of providers to comprehensive case management. Furthermore, it is not uncommon for "model" reentry programs to specifically disqualify from participation those with mental illness (Byrne and Taxman 2004; Dlugacz et al. 2007).

A 2002 study of correctional facilities in New Jersey found that release planning occurred in less than half of that state's county jails (Wolff et al. 2002). Programs for reentry specifically targeting inmates with mental illness remain uncommon, especially when such services are not part of a program designed to service inmates with co-occurring substance abuse (Peters et al. 2004).

This empirical reality should be compared with the impression one might gain from involvement with such pioneering organizations as the Council of State Governments (CSG) Justice Center (2008) and the Urban Institute's Reentry Policy Council (Solomon et al. 2006), where the importance of reentry planning for inmates with mental illness has been promoted in a scholarly, cross-disciplinary manner for the past decade. Such a comparison reveals that much has been done to raise awareness among policymakers and corrections professionals that reentry planning is sound policy on the fiscal, public safety, and public health levels, but that substantial work remains to be done before comprehensive, clinically oriented reentry planning can truly be considered an ongoing national practice.

Legal Bases for Reentry Planning

As in other areas of correctional health care, a complex and mutually reinforcing interaction exists between professional standards and legal requirements. The U.S. Supreme Court, in *Estelle* (1976), held that the Eighth Amendment's prohibition of cruel and unusual punishment required correctional institutions to avoid deliberate indifference to an inmate's serious medical need. *DeShaney v. Winnebago Department of Social Services* (1989) established the principle that jurisdictions are required to provide services only to individuals in the custody of the jurisdiction; therefore, an inmate's right to this minimal level of health care generally terminates immediately following release from custody (Cohen 2008; Perlin and Dlugacz 2008).

Some groundbreaking cases have begun to erode this bright line, however gradually and minimally, either by extending the constitutional right to adequate health care slightly beyond the prison's walls or by finding successful legal theories based on state laws not restricted by the minimal federal standard laid out in *Estelle* (1976). As an example of the former approach, the U.S. Court of Appeals for the Ninth Circuit, in *Wakefield v. Thompson* (1999), held that the Constitution required that a released prisoner who had been prescribed psychotropic medications while incarcerated be given a supply of that medication sufficient to allow him or her time to seek medical advice and possible treatment continuation. The only required action was the provision of a supply of medication adequate for the transition period, but the case is a landmark in that it introduced the principle that prisoners' constitutional right to health care, in carefully defined circumstances, could be briefly extended beyond the time of release. As stated in *Wakefield* (1999),

> As the cases themselves recognize, it is clear that while a prisoner is actually incarcerated the state restricts completely his ability to secure medical care "on his own behalf." For that reason, the Court has held, the state must provide prisoners with the medical care they need during the period of their incarceration....It is a matter of common sense, however, that a prisoner's ability to secure medication "on his own behalf" *is not necessarily restored the instant he walks through the prison gates and into the civilian world* [emphasis added]. Although many patients must take their medication one or more times a day, it may take a number of days, or possibly even weeks, for a recently released prisoner to find a doctor, schedule an examination, obtain a diagnosis, and have a prescription filled [footnote omitted]. Accordingly, the period of time during which prisoners are unable to secure medication "on their own behalf" may extend beyond the period of actual incarceration. Under the reasoning of Estelle and DeShaney, the state's responsibility to provide a temporary supply of medication to prisoners in such cases extends beyond that period as well.

Several subsequent cases have followed *Wakefield* (1999). In *Lugo v. Senkowski et al.* (2000), a New York federal district court applied the reasoning of *Wakefield* to a situation involving an inmate who had surgery to remove kidney stones. This surgery occurred shortly prior to his release on parole, and the inmate was told that within weeks he would require surgery to remove a metal stent that had been placed in his kidney. The court held that

> the state has a duty to provide medical services for an outgoing prisoner who is receiving continuing treatment at the time of release for the period of time reasonably necessary for him to obtain treatment on his own behalf....A parolee just having been released after a stay in prison is often in no position to immediately find the alternative medical attention that he needs.

In *Griffith v. Hofmann et al.* (2006), an inmate who received a diagnosis of manic-depressive disorder claimed that because he had no health insurance, he was not immediately able to obtain needed medication upon his release. In response to a defense motion to dismiss the case, the court held that the inmate should be allowed to argue that the failure to provide him with medication upon his release violated his constitutional rights. Also, in *Jacobs v. Ramirez et al.* (2005), the U.S. Court of Appeals for the Second Circuit found that a parolee had a potentially cognizable claim sufficient to withstand a motion to dismiss against a parole officer whom Jacobs claimed violated his civil rights by, among other things, paroling him to his mother's unsafe and unsanitary residence and denying his request to move to a homeless shelter. Following the reasoning of *Wakefield* (1999), the court accepted the idea that a parolee, although not strictly in state custody, nonetheless is not fully free to fend for himself or herself.

One landmark case, decided entirely on state law grounds and involving reentry planning for detainees with mental illness, greatly exceeded *Wakefield*'s (1999) constitutionally based requirements. The stipulation of settlement in *Brad H. v. City of New York* (2000) requires a comprehensive, multiagency, multidisciplinary approach to the provision of reentry planning to the large numbers of inmates with mental illness released from New York City's correctional system (commonly referred to as Rikers Island). Provisions are made for community referrals; medication continuity, including medicine and prescriptions; and assistance in applying for benefits, supportive housing, and transportation after release. The settlement also requires specific agencies to provide case management and linkage services for detainees released at court. Broadly speaking, the theory of the case extended the state statutory rights of inmates and detainees with mental illness to discharge planning similar to that enjoyed by patients receiving psychiatric services in the community or in psychiatric hospitals.

Programmatically, the *Brad H.* (2000) stipulation is noteworthy for its comprehensive approach to reentry planning and for its efforts to account for the often precipitous release of a predominantly detainee population in a large urban jail. With regard to legal standards, it is exceptional for its innovative reliance on state law. This latter feature, however, limits its applicability to other jurisdictions, except those states that have analogous state laws and a judiciary willing to interpret those laws to cover incarcerated individuals with mental illness.

Some federal class-action litigations challenging the constitutionality of the correctional mental health care provided within state prison systems have included some attention to reentry planning as an aspect of the resultant consent decrees. Examples include *Dunn v. Voinovich* (1995) in Ohio, *D.M. v. Terhune* (1999) in New Jersey, and *Coleman v. Schwarzenegger* (1995) in California.

Relevant federal legislation also attempts to deal with the issue of reentry planning. The Mentally Ill Offender Treatment and Crime Reduction

Reauthorization and Improvement Act of 2008 was recently reauthorized. It provides funding of $50 million per year for the next 5 years. Among other goals, it directs the U.S. attorney general to give priority to grant applications that promote effective strategies to identify and treat offenders with mental illness.

In our view, there is a confluence of events in the evolving litigations and statutes discussed in this section, the clinical and ethical guidelines reviewed above, and the growing expert consensus surrounding the need for reentry planning. Although reentry planning programs are important for these reasons, they may also bring fiscal, public safety, and public health benefits to jurisdictions choosing to implement them (see, e.g., Dlugacz et al. 2007; Ridgely et al. 2007; Ventura et al. 1998). As such, we suggest that reentry planning for offenders with serious mental illness is an important undertaking beyond what may be legally required or, in fact, aside from what impact it may or may not have on violent offending in the population.

DEVELOPMENT AND IMPLEMENTATION OF CLINICALLY ORIENTED REENTRY PLANNING SERVICES

From a pure symptom-management perspective, the correctional mental health staff may develop an up-to-date understanding of the patient that is superior to that of any previous community-based providers. In such instances, clinical information critical for successful aftercare should flow from the institution to the community. In this respect, it might be said that the correctional mental health staff become the primary caregivers, passing the care of the patient on to community providers on the patient's release. This may be especially so for individuals serving long prison sentences, individuals incarcerated during a first episode, or individuals who have never cooperated with community-based treatment but who willingly accept treatment while incarcerated. This is less true with regard to an assessment of social adaptation, where even a thorough understanding of an individual's functioning within the highly structured and unique correctional environment may be of limited utility in predicting his or her coping style and level of functioning in the community. A central thesis of this section is that staff assigned to develop reentry plans must have a biopsychosocial orientation and that attention to the social context of the individual patient is as important as attention to the biological diagnosis.

Clinically oriented reentry planning, therefore, requires a sophisticated integration of biopsychosocial data culled from the patient, from collateral sources of information in the community where the offender lived prior to incarceration, and from current correctional treatment providers. How practicable this data gathering is in a particular setting depends on the length of stay, on levels of cooperation of the patient and of collateral information sources, and on institutional resources. In addition, crafting a plan likely to succeed requires matching the individual patient's needs, as defined by the totality of the available data, to a program or set of services designed to meet those needs. Assessment of reentry needs for this population should focus on the six major areas listed in Table 15–1.

Meeting the patient's clinical needs, addressing patient motivation for treatment and services, devising clinically sound approaches to identified barriers to an individual patient's successful reentry, and working to reduce risks associated with criminal justice involvement require more than diagnosing the patient's mental illness and managing its symptoms. Clinical staff must attend specifically to the psychosocial and environmental problems faced by the patient during incarceration and/or after release, with the goal of identifying and bolstering strengths and mobilizing and enhancing the existing support system. In some cases, however, individuals with serious mental illness have untreated or unremitted symptoms that constituted the primary factor leading to their incarceration.

Clinical Case 15–1

Mr. A is a 27-year-old man charged with loitering, resisting arrest, and disturbing the peace. The police were called to a subway station, where Mr. A was found talking excitedly on the pay phone. He refused to leave the area, and bystanders reported that he had been at the phone for the past half-hour or more. He reportedly was swinging his fist at anyone who came close to him to use the telephone. Police reported that they felt they had to arrest Mr. A because he had not engaged in behavior of sufficient dangerousness to be hospitalized involuntarily under state law. After he was detained by police, a check of phone records indicated that nobody was on the other end of the line. A review of the "datalink" indicated that Mr. A was a current assertive community treatment patient, was a recipient of Supplemental Security Income and Medicaid benefits, and was living with his parents as recently as 4 days prior to the arrest.

Far more common in our experience are individuals who, although mentally ill, are also homeless, poor, or socially disconnected and for whom these latter problems are the immediate causative factor(s) related to the arrest and incarceration. Failure to address these additional

TABLE 15–1.   Six major assessment areas to evaluate reentry needs

1. Clinical needs (major medical and psychiatric diagnoses, including substance abuse)

2. Social support and connectedness (family, significant others, peer counseling, spiritual support, etc.)

3. Housing needs

4. Financial needs (including employment and benefits from social programs)

5. Motivation

6. Risk factors associated with failed reentry

problems may interfere with a patient's successful reentry, even in the face of complete symptom remission. Although challenging, addressing these needs is as essential to a successful reentry plan as are correct diagnosis and treatment interventions. In fact, the Housing First approach argues that meeting housing needs may not even require addressing symptomatic needs first (Tsemberis and Eisenberg 2000). Addressing these other needs may be particularly important for those released on parole or under other forms of supervised release, where the failure to attend scheduled treatment sessions or meetings with parole officers can be in and of itself a violation of parole, leading to reincarceration. Inasmuch as unmet basic needs—such as housing (Roskes and Osher 2006), financial support (Social Security Administration 2009), and access to medical insurance—relate to failures to comply with release conditions, the jurisdiction has not adequately enabled the correctional system to plan for such individuals' releases.

The individual's level of functioning, as captured on Axis V (American Psychiatric Association 2000a), is also important to consider. Many people function quite differently in a correctional setting than they do in the community. Although some respond positively to the predictability and structure of incarceration, many others decompensate as a result of the rigid and sometimes harsh nature of the correctional setting. Some inmates are able to avoid the destructive use of substances while incarcerated, whereas others continue to risk lengthier incarcerations by seeking illegal drugs or inappropriately using psychiatric treatment to obtain medications that they intend to abuse. An individual's ability to meet daily needs may be difficult to assess in the correctional setting, where housing, meals, medical care, and sometimes employment are provided or may even be forced. Often, inmates without any legitimate employment history in the community responsibly perform menial tasks for pennies per hour while incarcerated. Interestingly, at least one study found that men with mental illness showed higher success rates than did other men in a prison work release program (Way et al. 2007). Similarly, educational opportunities have been shown to improve postrelease outcomes (Harer 1994).

Some clinicians attempting to use the Global Assessment of Functioning (GAF) scale score to inform treatment planning find it to be of limited usefulness in a correctional setting. A principal limitation has been that at the lower levels of functioning, the GAF scale may be more sensitive to the acuity of symptoms than to psychological, social, or occupational functioning (Dixon 2004). With the incarcerated patient divorced from the realities of day-to-day life in the community, clinicians assessing a patient's GAF may find assigning ratings both difficult and arbitrary in a setting that, no matter how deforming and abnormal, provides most of life's necessities.

As an alternative, the Kennedy Axis V (Kennedy 2003) provides a comprehensive approach to generating what is described as a "K-axis." Rather than attempting to condense functioning into one number, this scale uses the following seven subscales designed to maintain a level of detail that permits a more comprehensive assessment of functioning:

- Psychological Impairment
- Social Skills
- Violence
- Activities of Daily Living—Occupational Skills
- Substance Abuse
- Medical Impairment
- Ancillary Impairment

The fact that each subscale requires individual attention and its own rating forces the clinician to assess each of these important areas, better accounting for a variety of psychosocial issues and less severe symptoms at the higher end of the rating continuum (Dixon 2004). This approach requires interdisciplinary collaboration and, to the extent that information is available and reasonably accessible, an understanding of functioning outside the highly structured correctional environment. Examining an inmate's functioning in this manner should lead to a more focused assessment of the areas required for sound, clinically oriented reentry planning.

Figure 15–1 depicts our view of the interrelationship of symptoms and functioning. This model can be considered in two directions: in-

creased symptoms and poorer social functioning can be mutually reinforcing, but conversely, reduced symptoms and improved social function
can also be mutually reinforcing. Thus, for some individuals, symptom
resolution may produce improved social function. For example, resolving a serious depression may assist an individual in achieving and maintaining employment. However, in other cases, focusing on enhancing
social function may ameliorate a patient's symptoms. One well-known example of this is the Housing First approach to assisting individuals who
are mentally ill and homeless (Greenwood et al. 2005). Giving attention to
specific issues that are often of importance to offenders returning to the
community, such as benefits and housing, may increase their overall engagement in the reentry plan, thus leading to reduced symptomatology
over time (Draine and Herman, in press).

An individual's psychosocial functioning may be viewed quite differently during confinement compared with in the community (Rotter et al.
2005). The observations of custody and of clinical staff are significant and
should not be overlooked in this regard. Because of these differences, we
suggest that a critical aspect of assessment of functional levels requires
contact with collateral sources of information concerning the patient's
functioning in the community, which may be quite distinct from that observed within the jail or prison.

In our view, a proper and complete assessment of the transitional needs
of inmates requires an interdisciplinary and integrated approach that includes the active participation of the patient, custody staff, and, when
possible, the family and community provider. Staff involved in developing reentry plans for inmates or detainees with serious mental illness
must consider each individual's biological, psychological, social, cultural,
and spiritual background, and attempt to integrate data and support
from community sources into reentry efforts. As noted by Draine et al.
(2005), successful reentry "depends upon the individual's willingness
and ability to act in accordance with specific social norms as well as the
community's willingness and capacity to support the individual's prosocial efforts" (p. 691). For these reasons, the reentry planning function
should not be organizationally isolated from clinical practice internally or
separate from community resources. To the contrary, these tasks should be
merged to the greatest degree practicable. For most systems, regular interdisciplinary treatment planning meetings, which should already be a
routine part of mental health care for inmates with special needs, are the
natural forum in which such integration can occur. These meetings
should always strive for the active participation of the offender.

Frequently, given the nature of correctional systems and of the health
care delivery systems within them, adequate care requires the collabora-

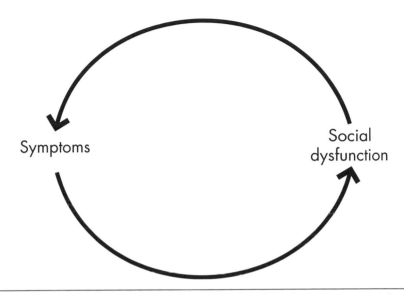

FIGURE 15–1. Model showing interrelationship of symptoms and functioning.

tion of agencies outside the jail or prison. For this reason, the establishment of a reentry planning delivery model requires efforts to create buy-in among critical stakeholders. Typically, this group includes policymakers, funders, consumers, law enforcement personnel, treatment and housing providers, agencies managing financial and medical benefits, and advocates. The CSG's Criminal Justice/Mental Health Consensus Project is perhaps the quintessential embodiment of this approach; the report and ongoing work stemming from it have included input of and consensus across a wide range of disciplines and agencies. The CSG Consensus Project approach to program creation mirrors at the macro level the cross-agency communication and problem solving that any successful program needs to achieve and sustain at the micro level.

Broner et al. (2001) described a typical progression in which, at early phases of such a process, seemingly insurmountable problems are first identified. These problems include funding, staff training, complex treatment issues, benefits applications, and confidentiality requirements thought to impede the required information sharing. Over time, solutions can be developed. These solutions may include changing current operating procedure or altering agency rules and regulations or even local or state statutes (Lamon et al. 2002; National GAINS Center 1999a, 1999b). A primary rule of successful collaboration involves an appreciation that just because an agency has functioned one way in the past does not justify its continuing to do so in the future. All assumptions must be open for exploration. On a clinical level, preparation for release demands that patients be assisted when moving toward this type of self-examination—a critical question regarding past behavior being, "How did that work out for you?" On the organizational level, correctional and treatment systems should be no less willing to engage in this type of critical self-exploration.

For inmates with longer periods of incarceration, especially those with predictable release dates, a global approach to the reentry process can be applied. For those inmates or detainees with shorter incarcerations, the best approach might be to attempt to identify and intervene in the one or two key factors having the greatest salience to a given individual. For all inmates leaving correctional settings, the central questions are these:

• What is (are) the greatest obstacle(s) to this patient's making it safely from the point of release from the jail or prison to an adequate living and treatment situation?
• What strengths and supports can this person call on or mobilize to increase the likelihood of overcoming the specific obstacle(s)? This is entirely consistent with the wellness and recovery model (see Chapter 13, "Creating Wellness Through Collaborative Mental Health Interventions").

EXAMPLES OF PROMISING APPROACHES WITH RELEVANCE TO REENTRY PLANNING PROGRAMS

Brief Motivational Interviewing

Brief motivational interviewing (BMI) is a scientifically tested approach to counseling that has demonstrated effectiveness in assisting patients who are confronting a variety of physical and psychological illnesses (Rubak et al. 2005). BMI is an evidence-based practice that has been shown to improve a person's ability to examine himself or herself, contemplate change, talk about change, and ultimately change behaviors. It has been shown to be successful in numerous rigorous studies and has been applied with success to a variety of areas, including substance abuse. This therapeutic approach can be adapted to the engagement of patients in a variety of settings and with a variety of problems, including incarcerated individuals with mental illness. Any reentry plan, no matter how well crafted, is only as useful as its implementation. Assessing a patient's motivation for treatment and improving that motivation to the extent possible can help to increase the likelihood that the patient will engage in treatment after release.

Regarding the application of BMI to substance use disorders, BMI might be expected to have a positive effect on postrelease violent behavior in three-fourths of the offender population with mental illness, given the association between substance use and violence (Skeem and Louden 2006; Steadman et al. 1998). Motivational techniques have also been found to be promising in promoting treatment adherence among people with schizophrenia (Zygmunt et al. 2002). As such, the application of BMI to reentry efforts could be viewed as reinforcing medication adherence, a protective factor (Haddock and Lewis 2005).

Rollnick and Miller (1995) defined *motivational interviewing* as "a directive, client-centered counseling style for eliciting behavior change by helping clients to explore and resolve ambivalence" (p. 325). Therapists using this technique often begin with an exploration of the client's readiness for change (Prochaska et al. 1992). People generally do not change entrenched behaviors overnight or progress in a linear progression to a healthier lifestyle. Rather, they undergo various stages, as described in Table 15–2; incarcerated individuals tend to cluster in the earlier stages.

The role of a clinician focusing on reentry planning with incarcerated individuals is often to assist them in moving toward considering ways to change their lives, consistent with the tasks of precontemplation and contemplation. Understanding a patient's stage is critical to the task of clinically oriented reentry planning. A typical strategy in motivational interviewing with early-stage patients includes reviewing with the patient a typical day as a means for developing rapport and avoiding an inordinate emphasis on problems (Miller and Rollnick 2002). People are then encouraged to look back in an effort to examine what life was like prior to the onset of their current difficulties. This approach is designed to engender hope by reminding the person of his or her strengths. Next, the clinician may focus on reviewing what is good and what is less good about the activity explored. Inherent in this exploration is a nonjudgmental stance and an acknowledgment that all behaviors can reflect some attempt, no matter how maladaptive or seemingly self-destructive, to deal with life's challenges (Luhrmann 2008; Rotter et al. 2005). This notion should be familiar to the correctional psychiatrist who has considered the overdetermined nature of many so-called manipulative behaviors encountered in the correctional population.

TABLE 15–2. Stages of change and role of professional staff

Stage	Where is the patient?	Staff role(s)
Precontemplation	Not considering change Denies existence of problem or attributes problem to external factors outside of his or her control	Generating motivation to consider change (e.g., motivational interviewing)
Contemplation	Considering changes Weighing pros and cons of changes	Generating motivation to consider change (e.g., motivational interviewing)
Preparation	Testing possible changes	Helping patients learn from experience (e.g., cognitive-behavioral approaches)
Action	Making commitment and carrying it through	Supportive approaches Solidifying patient's learning from experience Peer support
Maintenance	Incorporating changes into all aspects of life	Supportive approaches Peer support Relapse prevention
Relapse	Demoralized Starting over (usually at preparation or action stage)	Supportive approaches Helping patient learn from experience Peer support

Source. Adapted from Prochaska et al. 1992.

Clinical Case 15–2

Ms. B is a 22-year-old woman incarcerated for the third time on charges of drug possession and solicitation. She was diagnosed on admission with opiate and cocaine dependence and depression. On admission, she reported that she was not an addict and had no intention of stopping her drug use. At this point, she could be considered a "precontemplation" patient.

After being treated for 4 months with fluoxetine and regular therapy visits, she began engaging in a conversation with her therapist about the use of drugs as a "numbing" strategy to help her forget about her prior traumatic experiences, beginning in childhood. Discussion of the drug use helped her realize how much damage the drug use had done to her physically, emotionally, and socially—she was recently diagnosed with hepatitis C, continues to struggle with depression and anxiety, and is homeless and disconnected from any support system. She began to consider entering drug rehabilitation programs tied to supportive housing and therapeutic opportunities. Ms. B would be considered now to be in the contemplation stage of readiness for change.

In a model such as this, the clinical goal in treatment planning for successful transition to the community is to assist the person in moving along the change spectrum toward a position in which he or she is motivated to change his or her life. The length and predictability of the incarceration will be the primary nonclinical factors in determining how far the treatment can progress. Even brief incarcerations in jails or truncated stays in state prisons secondary to parole violations can provide fertile ground for this type of exploration. Incarceration has obvious and well-documented destructive effects on people with mental illness; however, it can also produce a constructive sense of crisis and reevaluation, which, aided by possible forced remission of substance abuse, can be harnessed by the use of BMI.

In our experience, genuine motivation for change animated by the crisis of arrest and incarceration does not automatically translate into follow-through with reentry plans upon release. The individual is more likely to evince strong motivation for change while incarcerated, where the choices are limited and the pain of separation from loved ones is most acute. Once released, however, an offender is faced with a myriad of choices. Many of these choices involve decisions about engaging in potentially perilous behaviors, such as using illegal substances, abusing alcohol, or associating with people engaged in criminal activity, all of which increase risk in a number of areas such as violence, criminal recidivism, and psychiatric decompensation. Recently released individuals may make entirely rational, albeit psychiatrically risky, decisions based on the fact that proposed reentry plans simply do not meet their needs. These decisions are particularly likely when concrete and critical foundational issues such as housing and benefits are not addressed (Draine and Herman, in press).

Although ultimately a released inmate with mental illness must take personal responsibility for his or her treatment, our contention is that a primary focus of reentry efforts should be a preparation for continuation of treatment upon release. Explorations of BMI's applicability to the criminal justice system have tended to focus on individuals released on probation, but the possibility for the use of BMI within institutions has also been explored (Miller 1999). Further enhancing its potential in corrections is the possibility of training staff with a wide range of skill sets in its use. With its focus on the service provider as a facilitator for the exploration of motivation by the patient, BMI is consistent with modern notions of strength-based recovery that eschew the traditional symptom-oriented medical model. This technique has been shown to produce lasting effects that can be accomplished in relatively brief periods of time. Like other evidence-based clinical interventions, such as cognitive-behavioral therapy, BMI can positively influence future behavior and choices. Thus, it is a cost-effective, easily applied approach in a correctional setting, with potentially significant benefits.

Critical Time Intervention

Originally developed as a method for enhancing linkages for people in homeless shelters and hospitals (Draine and Herman 2007), critical time intervention (CTI) has been demonstrably effective in moving homeless individuals into housing (Herman et al. 2007). Greenberg and Rosenheck (2008) investigated the rates and correlates of homelessness in the adult male jail population. They found that recent homelessness was 7.5 to 11.3 times more common in this population than in the general population, concluding that "[h]omelessness and incarceration appear to increase the risk of each other, and these factors seem to be mediated by mental illness and substance abuse..." (p. 170). Therefore, it seems reasonable to view incarcerated people with mental illness and homeless people with mental illness as belonging to analogous populations.

CTI is designed as a 9-month, staged intervention consisting of three phrases: transition to community, try-out, and transfer of care. During the transition phase, a treatment plan is formulated by the client and case manager. The focus is on areas considered critical to stable functioning in the community, such as medication, money, and housing; crisis management; substance abuse problems; and family interventions (Herman et al. 2007). Linkage to community resources is the fundamental task at this stage. The support systems developed as a result of the first phase are tested during the try-out stage, at which time required adjustments are made. Observations and interventions are made in vivo. The emphasis during this phase is on filling gaps found in the preexisting plan. Longer-term plans are then created so that ongoing supports can be put in place for the final phase, transfer of care (New York Presbyterian Hospital and Columbia University 2009).

Recent scholarship has explored CTI's potential use in improving the continuity of care for people with mental illness released from jails or prisons (New York Presbyterian Hospital and Columbia University 2009). The first stage would ideally be provided during the incarceration, and the later stages would be implemented following release. The creation of linkages prior to release is crucial. The primary emphasis is on improving problem-solving skills through the use of motivational coaching and advocacy with service agencies in the community. As such, CTI is fully compatible with BMI techniques, which can be seen as one part of this more broad-based approach. Draine and Herman (2007) have reported on CTI's potential use with the criminal justice population and suggested that although relevant, the model would have to be modified for use with this population.

Sensitizing Providers to the Effects of Correctional Incarceration on Treatment and Risk Management (SPECTRM)

Even promising approaches to treatment and reentry planning for people with severe mental illness will require adaptation by the clinician to the criminal justice population. Some posit that this is the result of inherent characteristics of incarcerated people. In a best-practice approach called Sensitizing Providers to the Effects of Correctional Incarceration on Treatment Risk Management (SPECTRM), Rotter et al. (2005) described a set of presentation styles and skills acquired by many inmates that are adaptive in prison but that are often misinterpreted by clinicians as pathological symptoms. Some of these culturally bound attitudes include mistrust, intimidation, and minding one's own business. Rotter et al. (2005) described these collectively as *prisonization*.

Because mental health care providers often lack knowledge and training about these traits, they may interpret them clinically as signs of resistance, lack of interest in treatment, personality pathology, or even acute symptoms of a mental illness such as paranoia. These missed cues can reduce empathy between the provider and the patient, interfere with the formation of a therapeutic alliance, and present difficulties for the inmate specifically upon reentry, when suddenly the inmate is faced with a new and distinct set of expectations regarding socially appropriate behavior and the need for openness and self-exploration in a therapeutic setting. Direct discussions of these differences are suggested, as is the taking of an incarceration history. Rotter et al. (2005) described a training program for staff providing treatment to individuals released from prison so that the staff could approach these behaviors in a nonjudgmental, neutral manner. Similarly, this clash of cultural expectations can be discussed frankly with inmates prior to release so that they can anticipate this critical transition.

CSG Assessment Tool

The CSG Reentry Policy Council has published an interactive assessment tool that embodies the comprehensive approach advocated in this chapter (Council of State Governments Justice Center 2008). This assessment tool is useful in breaking down each crucial area, with a focus based on time frame. The areas of focus suggested are physical health, substance abuse, mental health, family relationships, housing, employment and education, financial status, and recidivism risk. Specific tasks are outlined for the prerelease and immediate postrelease periods, as well as for the midterm and long-term postincarceration periods.

Risk–Need–Responsivity

Pioneered in Canada (Andrews et al. 1990), risk–need–responsivity (RNR) is an approach to offender risk assessment and rehabilitation grounded in the cognitive social learning theory of criminality (Bonta and Andrews 2007). This approach to recidivism reduction has three core principles. First, the assessment of *risk* involves the prediction of criminal behavior, specifically identifying those offenders at highest risk for reoffending (see the seven major risk factors for recidivism, listed in Table 15–3); these individuals will be the group for whom this treatment approach is focused, as suggested by research demonstrating that providing treatment to low-risk offenders may actually increase the failure rate for high-risk offenders (Lowenkamp and Latessa 2004). Some correctional systems may congregate large numbers of inmates with significant risk factors, and thus the majority may fall into the high-risk category. Further, it may be that other interventions and treatment settings may be effective for those assessed as lower risk; further study is required of this important question. We believe that it would be unfortunate indeed if, reminiscent of Martinson's (1974) work, we were too quick to conclude in the modern era that "nothing works" for the subpopulation of offenders who are at the lower end in terms of risk of the very high risk group. The second principle, *need*, places an emphasis on matching treatment to crimino-genic needs—that is, those factors that tend to produce criminal behaviors. The third principle, *responsivity*, advocates using cognitive-behavioral treatment tailored to the individual's strengths, abilities, moti-vation, and learning style (Bonta and Andrews 2007)—this aspect of the RNR approach bears some similarities to the BMI approach, described earlier.

In the RNR schema, a major mental disorder is considered a non-criminogenic or minor need (Bonta and Andrews 2007). However, the extraordinarily high prevalence of substance use disorders among in-mates with mental illness renders this population as a whole at higher risk of recidivism (Steadman et al. 1998). Existing RNR research also makes clear that the best results obtain from treatment provided in the commu-nity rather than in correctional settings.

This approach to recidivism reduction has many important implica-tions for reentry planning for individuals with serious mental disorders. Many of the major risk factors revolve around the primary foci of reentry planning, which are social factors and support systems. We have also noted the destructive cycle between acute symptoms and social functioning that can occur. Thus, we conclude that stabilization of serious mental illness is likely a necessary prerequisite for successful engagement in the cognitive-behavioral treatment approach promoted by RNR (Bonta and Andrews 2007).

Forensic Assertive Community Treatment

Assertive community treatment (ACT) is an approach that provides com-prehensive services to individuals with severe mental illness in the com-munities where they live. Pioneered by Stein and Test (1980), the model includes the basic precepts of low client:staff ratios, services that are not time limited, and cross-training among team members to engender a full team approach. ACT has been extensively studied and is frequently found to reduce hospitalization, to increase time spent in stable housing, and to increase satisfaction with treatment and quality of life (Essock et al. 2006).

Although applying this basic model to the treatment of populations following release from corrections may have seemed logical, studies did not show evidence that treatment with the unmodified ACT model pro-duced any meaningful reductions in recidivism among the offending population (Lamberti et al. 2004). As a result, modifications have been developed that augment ACT teams by adding members with experience with the criminal justice system, such as probation officers and peers with

---

TABLE 15–3.   Seven major risk factors for recidivism

Antisocial personality pattern

Procriminal attitudes

Social supports for crime

Substance abuse

Family and/or marital relationships

School and/or work (poor performance and low levels of
   satisfaction)

Lack of involvement in prosocial recreational activities

Source.   Bonta and Andrews 2007.

---

criminal histories. This approach is called forensic assertive community treatment (FACT). As often occurs with promising approaches, the use of FACT in the field has outpaced the empirical study of its effectiveness (Lamberti et al. 2004; Morrissey and Meyer 2005). Although studies regarding its effectiveness show the need for more investigation, FACT is a promising and emerging model in this area (Lamberti et al. 2004). To the extent that FACT teams are located in or near the communities to which offenders with mental disorders will be returning and within reasonable proximity of the location of their incarceration, having FACT teams following clients during or at least near the end of their incarceration may assist in the transition to community treatment. In this way, FACT could facilitate two basic tenets of this chapter: 1) the need for greater integration of correction and community treatment and 2) the notion that a primary focus of correctional mental health treatment must be the preparation of the individual to use services upon release.

RECOMMENDATIONS

In addition to planning for follow-up treatment for mental illness, the comprehensive assessment of postrelease needs during an incarceration demands a sophisticated understanding of the patient's functioning prior to incarceration as well as his or her response to prior treatment in the community so that the proper level and type of service(s) can be accessed upon release. This goal will be achieved to differing degrees depending on individual and systemic variables. This assessment requires specific emphasis on an interdisciplinary assessment of psychosocial and environmental problems captured by Axis IV as well as on functional levels as assessed by Axis V or similar rating systems (American Psychiatric Association 2000a; Kennedy 2003). Additionally, no reentry plan is of any utility if the patient does not follow through with it upon release. Approaches such as motivational interviewing techniques and other forms of gauging and increasing the patient's readiness for change are often required, further changing the focus of correctional treatment toward nonemergent treatment and treatment planning.

Intervening in a cycle of social dysfunction, symptom exacerbation, and arrest is an ambitious goal. A jurisdiction wishing to begin the process of tackling this issue must consider and critically evaluate its correctional mental health program with regard to the following:

- Mission and vision
- Assessment tools and protocols
- Staffing, in terms of both staffing levels and staff skill sets
- Service delivery model, including consideration of what entity or mix of entities is to provide health, mental health, and reentry planning services and the ability of these providers to integrate their work with that of community-based providers
- Technology

The inclusion of a clinically oriented approach to reentry has implications regarding the way mental health care is structured, necessary staffing competencies, and the integration of correctional care with community care. Even the core functions of existing correctional mental health services, such as stabilization of active psychosis or other crises and amelioration of acute suicide risk, can be accomplished more effectively when a clinician communicates with community treatment providers, family members, or other sources of collateral information regarding a patient. Two obvious examples are understanding a patient's triggers for suicidal behavior and knowledge of the efficaciousness of particular medications for a given person. The effectiveness of interventions of this nature is judged contemporaneously, and in most cases treatment plans can be revised on the basis of observable behaviors and reactions. For example, adherence to a medication regimen can be monitored weekly with data provided by the pharmacy; similarly, the efficacy of a prescribed medication in the abatement of the acute symptoms of psychosis can be assessed regularly by the psychiatrist during clinical encounters, which include self-report by the patient and the contemporaneous observations of the physician as well as other health care and custody staff.

In contrast, the efficacy of a reentry plan is only known following release. In the absence of systematically tracked outcome measures, only those failures represented by a reincarceration in the same facility will come to the attention of the treatment team. Reincarcerations in other systems will not become evident, and, more importantly, successful reentry plans will be unknown to the correctional staff who created them, absent some form of feedback from community settings and providers. Therefore, a jurisdiction desiring to systematically improve its reentry planning on the basis of empirical observation must not only create linkages with community services but also develop internal mechanisms through its continuous quality improvement plan for 1) identifying returning inmates for whom reentry plans were developed and 2) critically examining what revisions might be made to the current plan. Examining prior reentry plans to determine what worked and what did not can help teams to avoid repeating mistakes.

Creating outcome measures consistent with the program's mission is also important. This task requires an examination of how reentry planning for individuals with mental disorders relates to reentry programs for the system's overall population and what reentry services are available for those with overlapping needs, such as medical problems or substance abuse. A thorough examination of the program's goals is also required. Is "success" measured only in terms of recidivism reduction, and if so, is reduction in violent recidivism the only acceptable outcome measure? Are reentry plans that lead to decreased hospitalization rates or lengths of stay acceptable measures of success for this population? Is there a role for tracking percentage of appointments kept after release? Would fiscal efficiencies resulting from improved acceptance rates for Supplemental Security Income or other federally funded benefits programs be considered sufficient for local jurisdictions? Is there a place for more subjective measures, such as increased client satisfaction and connection with services or improved integration with families upon release? The process of developing and using meaningful outcome measures may lead to improvements over time at both the individual inmate level and the system level.

These concepts have far-reaching implications in a number of seemingly disparate areas. For example, staff morale is negatively affected when their only feedback is in the form of treatment failures, which promotes a destructive sense of learned helplessness. Likewise, a lack of feedback regarding the outcome of reentry planning efforts increases the counterproductive sense of isolation frequently encountered by institutional treatment providers. In contrast, becoming aware of inmates who made successful transitions to the community with the aid of sound reentry planning and improved communication with community clinicians who are providing postrelease treatment can improve a sense of purpose and pride in clinicians working on reentry planning.

Technology is becoming increasingly pervasive in most areas of professional life; this is true as well for mental health care and reentry planning, where the ability to communicate with outside providers and family members is an integral part of the job. Dedicated phones with voice mail, individual e-mail accounts that are secure and checked regularly, functioning fax machines, and dedicated hotlines are all essential tools of the trade for professionals involved in reentry planning. In addition, the development of computerized or Web-based databases can assist staff in the preparation of clinically appropriate and achievable reentry plans for their patients.

No reentry plan will result in improved outcomes if that plan is not discussed with the inmate. In the world of corrections, where space is at a premium, sufficient allocations of office space in which to conduct reentry planning cannot be taken for granted. Visual and auditory privacy is essential to primary reentry planning functions, such as individual sessions, group sessions, telephone interviews with the Social Security Administration or other agencies, or meetings with community treatment providers to aid in transition. Also essential in large correctional institutions is the availability of escort officers to transport inmates to meetings with staff providing reentry planning services. Finally, central to this type of assessment and targeted intervention is an understanding of the person's motivation for change; psychological, social, and/or spiritual supports; triggers or high-risk situations; and past community functioning.

In our view, preparing incarcerated inmates and detainees for release requires as much integration of services as possible. This has many implications for the service delivery model used to provide reentry planning. In many jurisdictions, correctional providers are highly disconnected from community treatment providers, frustrating efforts toward interagency collaboration. Correctional systems are complex organizations that use various models for providing care, custody, and control. Some are privatized entirely, whereas others rely on a mixture of public and private providers. In some systems, health care may be privatized, whereas mental health care is a public function. Similarly, mental health care may be delivered by public employees, but contracts may be let specifically for reentry planning services. We suggest that, where possible, systems specifically consider the need for integrated, comprehensive reentry planning when developing their service delivery and funding model. In some settings, inviting community providers to conduct "inreach" programs to engage inmates nearing their release may be a successful model (Roskes et al. 2001), because those providers can target specific patient populations and identify the appropriate community services to meet their patients' needs. In other settings it may be more efficient to develop specialized discharge planning services within their overall correctional mental health operation (*Brad H. v. City of New York* 2000). Another approach is the forensic transition team model, in which specialized reentry planners work neither in the correctional setting nor in the community, but instead as "boundary spanners" (Hartwell 2008).

Despite the significant variation inherent in different correctional systems, successful reentry programs appear to share certain characteristics, in spite of their superficial differences. King (2005), in a presentation about reentry programs in general rather than those specifically directed at individuals with mental disabilities, identified these characteristics as follows:

- The mission or vision of the correctional agency explicitly includes preparation of inmates for successful reentry as a priority, both in words and in actions.
- Leaders of both the correctional and the health care enterprises manifest consistent support for reentry preparation programs and their continuous enhancement.
- The reentry initiatives are based on a holistic perspective inclusive of social, economic, cultural, environmental, physical, and mental health factors likely to affect each individual's prospects for successful reentry.
- The current approaches to reentry were achieved through sustained efforts and investments over periods of 5 to 10 years.
- As reentry initiatives have grown behind the walls, program staff members have acquired a reservoir of knowledge of and collaborative relationships with pertinent people and agencies in the communities and counties to which the majority of released persons are likely to return.
- Costs and staffing of the reentry initiatives, including transitional health care planning, are integral components of the correctional agency and health program operating budgets.
- The programs start the reentry planning process with assessment at the time of initial incarceration. Planning, education, and preparation are intensified in the last three to six months before release.
- These model programs emphasize the salient role of individual accountability by each inmate in preparing to overcome the many problems and obstacles to success he or she will encounter when returning home.
- Concentrating soon-to-be-released persons and reentry preparation resources in facilities geographically proximate to where former inmates will return is seen as especially beneficial.

CONCLUSION

Correctional systems need to engage in clinically oriented reentry planning for the large number of inmates and detainees with mental illness.

The details of these programs will undoubtedly vary depending on the nature of the correctional entity, the population served, and the individual needs of each patient. Correctional institutions cannot be responsible for this effort alone; other relevant participants include the community treatment providers, benefits agencies, housing providers, and policymakers. We have outlined a series of recommendations that jurisdictions may use in an effort to engage in this important work.

SUMMARY POINTS

- Reentry planning for inmates with mental illness is becoming a core function of correctional mental health. It is at minimum a best practice, appears to be required by ethical guidelines, and is evolving into a standard of care.
- Clinically oriented reentry planning requires integration of reentry concerns into ongoing treatment planning.
- Despite the above two summary points, comprehensive reentry programs for inmates with mental illness remain surprisingly uncommon.
- The extent and nature of reentry planning will be influenced not only by correctional factors such as size, location, and mission, but also by individual patient characteristics.
- Although mental illness per se may be only a modest risk factor for recidivism, a large-scale study found that inmates with major psychiatric disorders had a substantially increased risk of multiple incarcerations.
- Clinically oriented reentry planning for inmates with serious mental illness is critical because 1) a public health imperative exists for improving continuity of care, 2) abatement of psychiatric symptoms can be a necessary step in programming that targets criminal behavior, 3) symptoms and environmental risk factors interact in complex ways within this heterogeneous population, and 4) people with inadequately treated mental illnesses are at elevated risk for destructive interactions with law enforcement and the criminal justice system even when not committing crimes.
- Because reentry planning must account for community-based functioning, communication with collateral sources of information should be encouraged.
- Assessment of psychosocial and environmental problems (Axis IV) and global assessment of functioning (Axis V) are particularly important in planning for reentry, because these factors are often involved causally in the person's current incarceration.

- Promising clinical approaches, such as the use of the Kennedy Axis V, motivational interviewing techniques, critical time intervention, and the SPECTRM (Sensitizing Providers to the Effects of Correctional Incarceration on Treatment Risk Management) training program, should be considered and adapted to specific systems' requirements. All of these approaches are consistent with the recovery model.

- Jurisdictions considering the implementation of a reentry program should convene key stakeholders' meetings, at which all assumptions concerning the function of various stakeholders should be subject to reexamination.

REFERENCES

Adair CE: Postdischarge follow-up: research and practice disconnect (editorial). Psychiatr Serv 58:1521, 2007

American Medical Association: E-10.01 Fundamental elements of the physician-patient relationship. Chicago, American Medical Association, 1990. Available at: http://www.ama-assn.org. Accessed April 12, 2009.

American Psychiatric Association: Diagnostic and Statistical Manual of Mental Disorders, 4th Edition, Text Revision. Washington, DC, American Psychiatric Association, 2000a

American Psychiatric Association: Psychiatric Services in Jails and Prisons: A Task Force Report of the American Psychiatric Association, 2nd Edition. Washington, DC, American Psychiatric Association, 2000b

American Public Health Association: Standards for Health Services in Correctional Institutions. Washington, DC, American Public Health Association, 2003

Andrews DA, Bonta J: The Psychology of Criminal Conduct, 3rd Edition. Cincinnati, OH, Anderson, 2003

Andrews DA, Bonta J, Hoge RD: Classification for effective rehabilitation: rediscovering psychology. Crim Justice Behav 17:19–52, 1990

Baillargeon J, Binswanger IA, Penn JV, et al: Psychiatric disorders and repeat incarcerations: the revolving prison door. Am J Psychiatry 166:103–109, 2008

Beck A, Maruschak LM: Mental health treatment in state prisons, 2000 (Rep No NCJ 188215). Washington, DC, U.S. Department of Justice, Office of Justice Programs, Bureau of Justice Statistics, 2001

Bell v Wolfish, 441 U.S. 520 (1979)

Beto GJ: Prison administration and the Eighth Amendment. Texas Probation, Summer 1992. Cited in: Dlugacz H, Broner N, Lamon S: Implementing reentry: establishing a continuum of care of adult jail and prison releasees with mental illness, in Correctional Psychiatry: Practice Guidelines and Strategies. Edited by Thienhaus OJ, Piasecki M. Kingston, NJ, Civic Research Institute, 2007, pp 12-2–12-30

Binswanger IA, Stern MF, Deyo RA, et al: Correction to "Release from prison: a high risk of death for former inmates." N Engl J Med 356:536, 2007a

Binswanger IA, Stern MF, Deyo RA, et al: Release from prison: a high risk of death for former inmates. N Engl J Med 356:157–165, 2007b

Bonta J: Offender risk assessment: guidelines for selection and use. Crim Justice Behav 29:355–379, 2002

Bonta J, Andrews DA: Risk-need-responsivity model for offender assessment and rehabilitation. Ottawa, ON, Public Safety Canada, 2007. Available at: http://www.publicsafety.gc.ca/res/cor/rep/risk_need_200706-eng.aspx. Accessed April 12, 2009.

Bonta J, Law M, Hanson K: The prediction of criminal and violent recidivism among mentally disordered offenders: a meta-analysis. Psychol Bull 123:123–142, 1998

Brad H v City of New York, 712 N.Y.S.2d 336 (S. Ct. 2000), 716 N.Y.S.2d 852 (App. Div. 2000)

Broner N, Franczak M, Dye C, et al: Knowledge transfer, policymaking and community empowerment: a consensus model approach for providing public mental health and substance abuse services. Psychiatr Q 72:79–102, 2001

Byrne JM, Taxman FS: Targeting for reentry: inclusion/exclusion criteria across eight model programs. Fed Probat 68:53–61, 2004

Cohen F: The Mentally Disordered Inmate and the Law, 2nd Edition. Kingston, NJ, Civic Research Institute, 2008

Coleman v Schwarzenegger, 912 F.Supp. 1282 (E.D. Cal. 1995)

Council of State Governments: Criminal Justice/Mental Health Consensus Project. New York, Council of State Governments, 2002. Available at: http://consensusproject.org/downloads/Entire_report.pdf. Accessed April 12, 2009.

Council of State Governments Justice Center: CSG Justice Center releases innovative Web-based tool to help state and local officials improve prisoner/inmate reentry. New York, Council of State Governments Justice Center, August 5, 2008. Available at: http://www.reentrypolicy.org/announcements/assessments_tool. Accessed April 12, 2009.

DeShaney v Winnebago Department of Social Services, 429 U.S. 189 (1989)

Ditton PM: Mental health and treatment of inmates and probationers (NCJ 174463). Washington, DC, U.S. Department of Justice, Office of Justice Programs, Bureau of Justice Statistics, 1999

Dixon S: Book reviews: Mastering the Kennedy Axis V: A New Psychiatric Assessment of Patient Functioning, and Fundamentals of Psychiatric Treatment Planning, 2nd Edition. Psychiatr Serv 55:196–197, 2004

Dlugacz H, Broner N, Lamon S: Implementing reentry: establishing a continuum of care of adult jail and prison releasees with mental illness, in Correctional Psychiatry: Practice Guidelines and Strategies. Edited by Thienhaus OJ, Piasecki M. Kingston, NJ, Civic Research Institute, 2007, pp 12-2–12-30

DM v Terhune, 67 F.Supp.2d 401 (D. N.J. 1999)

Draine J, Herman DB: Critical time intervention for reentry from prison for persons with mental illness. Psychiatr Serv 58:1577–1581, 2007

Draine J, Herman D: Critical times and critical issues in reentry for people with mental illness: CTI as an intervention for prison and jail reentry, in Reentry Planning for Offenders With Mental Disorders: Policy and Practice. Edited by Dlugacz H. Kingston, NJ, Civic Research Institute (in press)

Draine J, Wolff N, Jacoby JE, et al: Understanding community re-entry of former prisoners with mental illness: a conceptual model to guide new research. Behav Sci Law 23:689–707, 2005

Dunn v Voinovich, C1-93-0166 S.D. Ohio (1995)

Essock SM, Mueser KT, Drake RE, et al: Comparison of ACT and standard case management for delivering integrated treatment for co-occurring disorders. Psychiatr Serv 57:185–196, 2006

Estelle v Gamble, 429 U.S. 97 (1976)

Feder L: A comparison of the community adjustment of mentally ill offenders with those from the general population. Law Hum Behav 15:477–493, 1991

Gall v United States, 128 S. Ct. 586 (2007)

Greenberg GA, Rosenheck RA: Incarceration, homelessness, and mental health: a national study. Psychiatr Serv 59:170–177, 2008

Greenwood RM, Schaefer-McDaniel NJ, Winkel G, et al: Decreasing psychiatric symptoms by increasing choice in services for adults with histories of homelessness. Am J Community Psychol 36:223–238, 2005

Griffith v Hofmann et al, 2006 WL 2585074 (D. Vt. 2006)

Haddock G, Lewis S: Psychological interventions in early psychosis. Schizophr Bull 3:697–704, 2005

Harer MD: Recidivism among federal prisoners released in 1987. August 4, 1994. Available at: http://www.bop.gov/news/research_projects/published_reports/recidivism/oreprrecid87.pdf. Accessed April 12, 2009.

Hartwell S: Short-term outcomes for offenders with mental illness released from incarceration. Int J Offender Ther Comp Criminol 47:145–158, 2003

Hartwell S: Community reintegration of persons with SMI post incarceration. Center for Mental Health Services Research Brief 5, May 2008. Available at: http://www.umassmed.edu/uploadedFiles/Brief37Reintergration.pdf. Accessed April 12, 2009.

Herman D, Conover S, Felix A, et al: Critical time intervention: an empirically supported model for preventing homelessness in high risk groups. J Prim Prev 28:295–312, 2007

Jacobs v Ramirez et al, 400 F.3d 105 (2d Cir. 2005)

James DJ, Glaze LE: Mental health problems of prison and jail inmates (NCJ 213600). Washington, DC, U.S. Department of Justice, Bureau of Justice Statistics, 2006

Joint Commission: 2009 National Patient Safety Goals Behavioral Health Care Program. June 13, 2008. Available at: http://www.jointcommission.org/PatientSafety/NationalPatientSafetyGoals/09_bhc_npsgs.htm. Accessed April 12, 2009.

Kennedy JA: Mastering the Kennedy Axis V: A New Psychiatric Assessment of Patient Functioning. Washington, DC, American Psychiatric Association, 2003

King L: Correctional medicine and community reentry: the meaning of it all. Paper presented at the National Conference on Correctional Health Care, Denver, CO, October 2005

Lamberti JS, Weisman R, Faden DI: Forensic assertive community treatment: preventing incarceration of adults with severe mental illness. Psychiatr Serv 55:1285–1293, 2004

Lamon SS, Cohen NL, Broner N: New York City's system of criminal justice mental health services, in Serving Mentally Ill Offenders and Their Victims: Challenges and Opportunities for Social Workers and Other Mental Health Professionals. Edited by Landsberg G, Rock M, Berg L, et al. New York, Springer, 2002, pp 144–156

Lowenkamp CT, Latessa EJ: Understanding the Risk Principle: How and Why Correctional Interventions Can Harm Low-Risk Offenders. Washington, DC, National Institute of Corrections, 2004

Lugo v Senkowski et al, 14 F.Supp. 2s 11 (N.D. N.Y. 2000)

Luhrmann TM: "The streets will drive you crazy": why homeless psychotic women in the institutional circuit in the United States often say no to offers of help. Am J Psychiatry 165:15–20, 2008

Martinson R: What works? Questions and answers about prison reform. Public Interest 35:22–54, 1974

Mentally Ill Offender Treatment and Crime Reduction Reauthorization and Improvement Act of 2008, S. 2304

Metzner JL: Evolving issues in correctional psychiatry. Psychiatric Times 24, September 1, 2007. Available at: http://www.psychiatrictimes.com/display/article/10168/54766?pageNumber=2. Accessed April 12, 2009.

Miller W: Pros and cons: reflections on motivational interviewing in correctional settings. Motivational Interviewing Newsletter: Updates, Education and Training 6:2–3, 1999

Miller WR, Rollnick S: Motivational Interviewing: Preparing People for Change. New York, Guilford, 2002

Mistretta v United States, 488 U.S. 361 (1989)

Morrissey J, Meyer P: Extending ACT to criminal justice settings: applications, evidence, and options. Paper presented at the Evidence-Based Practice for Justice-Involved Individuals: Assertive Community Treatment Expert Panel Meeting, Bethesda, MD, February 18, 2005. Available at: http://gains-center.samhsa.gov/text/ebp/Papers/ExtendingACTPaper.asp. Accessed April 12, 2009.

National Commission on Correctional Health Care: Correctional Mental Health Care: Standards and Guidelines for Delivering Services, 2nd Edition. Chicago, National Commission on Correctional Health Care, 2003

National Commission on Correctional Health Care: Standards for Mental Health Care in Correctional Facilities. Chicago, National Commission on Correctional Health Care, 2008

National GAINS Center: Maintaining Medicaid Benefits for Jail Detainees With Co-occurring Mental Health and Substance Use Disorders. Delmar, NY, National GAINS Center, 1999a

National GAINS Center: Using Management Information Systems to Locate People With Serious Mental Illness and Co-occurring Substance Use Disorders in the Criminal Justice System. Delmar, NY, National GAINS Center, 1999b

New York Presbyterian Hospital and Columbia University: The Critical Time Intervention Training Manual. New York. Available at: http://www.hrsa.gov/homeless/main_pages/lcw/materials/transition/7ctimanual.pdf. Accessed April 12, 2009.

Perlin ML, Dlugacz HA: Mental Health Issues in Jails and Prisons: Cases and Materials. Durham, NC, Carolina Academic Press, 2008

Perlin ML, Gould KK: Rashomon and the criminal law: mental disability and the federal sentencing guidelines. American Journal of Criminal Law 22:431–460, 1995

Peters RH, LeVasseur ME, Chandler RK: Correctional treatment for co-occurring disorders: results of a national survey. Behav Sci Law 22:563–584, 2004

Petersilia J: What works in prisoner reentry? Reviewing and questioning the evidence. Fed Probat 68:4–9, 2004

President's New Freedom Commission on Mental Health: Achieving the promise: transforming mental health care in America (Publ No SMA 03-3832). Rockville, MD, Department of Health and Human Services, President's New Freedom Commission on Mental Health, 2003

Prochaska JO, DiClemente CC, Norcross JC: In search of how people change. Am Psychol 47:1102–1114, 1992

Ridgely MS, Engberg J, Greenberg MD, et al: Justice, treatment, and cost: an evaluation of the fiscal impact of Allegheny County Mental Health Court. Santa Monica, CA, RAND Corporation, 2007. Available at: http://www.rand.org/pubs/technical_reports/TR439. Accessed April 12, 2009.

Rollnick S, Miller WR: What is motivational interviewing? Behav Cogn Psychother 23:325–334, 1995

Roskes E, Osher F: Jails and prisons, in Clinical Guide to the Treatment of the Mentally Ill Homeless Person. Edited by Gillig PM, McQuistion HL. Washington, DC, American Psychiatric Association, 2006, pp 131–140

Roskes E, Craig R, Strangman A: A prerelease program for mentally ill inmates. Psychiatr Serv 52:108, 2001

Rotter M, McQuistion HL, Broner N, et al: The impact of the "incarceration culture" on reentry for adults with mental illness: a training and group treatment model. Psychiatr Serv 56:265–267, 2005

Rubak S, Sandbaek A, Lauritzen T, et al: Motivational interviewing: a systematic review and meta-analysis. Br J Gen Pract 55:305–312, 2005

Skeem J, Louden JE: Toward evidence-based practice for probationers and parolees mandated to mental health treatment. Psychiatr Serv 57:333–342, 2006

Skeem J, Nicholson E, Kregg C: Understanding barriers to re-entry for parolees with mental disorder. March 2008. Available at: https://webfiles.uci.edu/skeem/Downloads_files/barrierstoreentry.pptx.pdf. Accessed June 8, 2009

Social Security Administration: Understanding Supplemental Security Income: SSI Spotlight on Prerelease Procedure, 2009 Edition. Washington, DC, Social Security Administration, 2009. Available at: http://www.ssa.gov/ssi/spotlights/spot-prerelease.htm. Accessed February 14, 2009.

Solomon AL, Visher C, La Vigne NG, et al: Understanding the challenges of prisoner reentry: research findings from the Urban Institute's prisoner reentry portfolio. Washington, DC, Urban Institute, 2006. Available at: http://www.urban.org/publications/411289.html. Accessed April 12, 2009.

Sowers WE, Rohland B: American Association of Community Psychiatrists' principles for managing transitions in behavioral health services. Psychiatr Serv 55:1271–1275, 2004

Steadman HJ, Mulvey EP, Monahan J, et al: Violence by people discharged from acute psychiatric inpatient facilities and by others in the same neighborhoods. Arch Gen Psychiatry 55:393–401, 1998

Stein LI, Test MA: Alternative to mental hospital treatment, I: conceptual model, treatment program, and clinical evaluation. Arch Gen Psychiatry 37:392–397, 1980

Travis J, Waul M: Prisoners Once Removed: The Children and Families of Prisoners. Washington, DC, Urban Institute, 2004

Tsemberis S, Eisenberg RF: Pathways to housing: supported housing for street-dwelling homeless individuals with psychiatric disabilities. Psychiatr Serv 51:487–493, 2000

United States v Booker, 543 U.S. 220 (2005)

U.S. Sentencing Commission: Federal Sentencing Guidelines, 2008. Available at: http://www.ussc.gov/guidelin.htm. Accessed June 12, 2009.

Ventura L, Cassel C, Jacoby J, et al: Case management and recidivism of mentally ill persons released from jail. Psychiatr Serv 49:1330–1337, 1998

Wakefield v Thompson, 177 F.3d 1160 (9th Cir. 1999)

Way BB, Abreu D, Ramirez-Romero D, et al: Mental health service recipients and prison work release: how do the mentally ill fare compared to other inmates in prison work release programs? J Forensic Sci 52:965–966, 2007

Weinstein WB, Wimmer C: Sentencing in the United States, in Reentry Planning for Offenders With Mental Disorders: Policy and Practice. Edited by Dlugacz H. Kingston, NJ, Civic Research Institute (in press)

Wolff N, Plemmons D, Veysey B, et al: Release planning for those with mental illness compared with those who have other chronic illnesses. Psychiatr Serv 53:1469–1471, 2002

Zygmunt A, Olfson M, Boyer CA, et al: Interventions to improve medication adherence in schizophrenia. Am J Psychiatry 159:1653–1664, 2002

PART III

Special Inmate Populations

CHAPTER 16

Supermax Units and Death Row

James L. Knoll IV, M.D.

Gary E. Beven, M.D.

In an idyllic world, a psychiatrist would have little work in either a super-maximum security (supermax) setting or death row because few inmates with mental illness would be present in those settings. These prison structures, however, are currently a permanent part of the correctional landscape, and psychiatrists must be prepared to engage in effective evaluations and treatment of the offenders with mental disorders who reside in them. In this chapter, we present an overview of supermax confinement; the inherent difficulties faced by inmates housed in these settings; and the potentially deleterious psychological effects of prolonged isolation, especially for offenders with mental illness. We discuss common barriers to rendering adequate mental health treatment in administrative segregation. We provide guidelines for the effective screening, monitoring, and treatment of segregated inmates so that both community standards of care and constitutional requirements are met. Finally, we review the psychiatric and legal aspects of evaluation and treatment of death row inmates.

Readers may be surprised by how little is understood about supermax and death row units from either a correctional or a psychiatric perspective (Pizarro and Narag 2008). At least part of the confusion may be attributed to the significant variability in the terms used by different prisons to describe supermax confinement. For example, one entire prison may be called a supermax prison, whereas another, medium-security facility may have a single unit that is run as a supermax facility. In addition, these housing units may be called a variety of names, including supermax custody units, special management units, secure housing units, intensive management units, and special control units (Arrigo and Bullock 2008; Haney 2003). The National Institute of Corrections has defined a supermax prison as a "free-standing facility, or a distinct unit within a facility that provides for the management and secure control of inmates who have been officially designated as exhibiting violent or seriously disruptive behavior while incarcerated" (National Institute of Corrections 1997). Most of these units have similar distinctive features, allowing for some collective categorization and analysis. In this chapter, we use the terms *supermax unit* and *supermax confinement* to refer to the most isolative, incapacitating, and restrictive of penal settings.

The provision of mental health care in supermax units presents a difficult challenge. Psychiatrists may be required to evaluate and treat offenders with serious behavior disorders who are housed in these facilities for extended periods. These settings may be stressful for both inmates and staff. Significant barriers to providing adequate care can stand in the way of the mental health clinician's mission, and ensuring the provision of clinically necessary treatment may be at odds with institutional security requirements (Eshem et al. 2001). Furthermore, supermax units and death row are often the target of legal scrutiny and extensive litigation. Such litigation involves the basic constitutional right to adequate mental health care, as well as the related legal right to avoid penal conditions so harsh that they "cause" mental illness or exacerbate an existing condition (Cohen 1988, 2008).

SUPERMAX CONFINEMENT

Prison administrative staff use supermax confinement as a management tool for the control of prisoners who are deemed disruptive, dangerous, or predatory, or who otherwise violate institutional rules of conduct. Supermax units are considered to be the most isolative, incapacitating, and restrictive of penal settings (Holton 2003; Riveland 1999). Built specifically to house the most dangerous offenders, supermax units provide an extreme form of administrative segregation. Unique characteristics of these facilities include prolonged lengths of stay, an architectural design that relies on diminished human contact, greatly diminished environmental stimulation, and austere privilege restrictions. More modern supermax facilities have been described as "high-tech," mechanized, impersonal facilities that are subject to continual "hardening" in terms of security and surveillance (Rhodes 2007). Special correctional security teams may be equipped with stun technology, "stun shields," and other methods for effectuating cell extractions or quelling disturbances. Because of the combination of isolation, privilege restriction, and a lowered level of tolerance for disruptive behavior, high levels of patience and submission are demanded of inmates. Although considerable variability exists across prisons in the use, operation, and management of supermax units, some elements of supermax confinement are fairly consistent across facilities (see Table 16–1).

The professed rationale for the supermax unit is to segregate the "most dangerous" inmates to protect prison staff and other inmates, while attempting to exert a deterrent effect on other would-be violent offenders. In essence, this confinement is a form of "double incarceration," in which the inmate is isolated from the general prison population. Supermax confinement is ostensibly reserved for those inmates who have demonstrated extreme violence and/or are considered uncontrollable in a less restrictive setting. While the lay perception may be that this is a homogeneous group of the "worst of the worst," the reality is quite different. Some inmates may be sent to a supermax facility as a result of questionable administrative decision making. Others may be there for either protective or preventive reasons, and up to 30% meet criteria for serious mental illnesses (Cloyes et al. 2006). Because of a lack of uniform reporting, few studies have addressed the composition of inmates in supermax units. Lovell et al. (2000) suggested that this population is heterogeneous and that in addition to those inmates who truly pose a serious risk of dangerous or disruptive behavior, these units may include inmates who require protective custody, have difficulty coping in the general population of the prison, have committed disciplinary infractions, have a mental illness, or prefer isolation or simply want their own cell.

No matter its duration, life in a supermax unit is a hardship. The restrictions placed on inmates in such settings are many, and although incarceration itself is difficult, the contrast between life in the general population and life in supermax segregation is striking. In our experience, a jaunt through a typical correctional institution's general population often reveals a great deal of relatively normal activity, such as a baseball game in the recreation yard, inmates returning from work in the prison industry building, and religious celebration in the chapel. One may encounter a gymnasium with inmates playing basketball, a busy dining hall, and a visiting area filled with offenders and their families and children. Supermax

TABLE 16–1.   Supermax confinement conditions

Small cell (approximately 7×10 feet)

Diminished environmental stimulation

Restriction to cell for 22–23 hours per day

Meals restricted to cell

Treatment encounters or programs restricted to cell

No physical contact

Exercise alone in a small, secure area

Noncontact visitation

No work

No religious programs

No, or restricted, access to TV, radio, and phone

Restricted commissary list

Restricted list of personal items in cell

Source.   Adapted from Beven 2005, pp. 209–228.

units, in contrast, are generally devoid of such activities, and living conditions are often unpleasant. The restrictions placed on offenders in these settings are burdensome, and virtually every aspect of an inmate's life is adversely affected. A walk through any supermax unit will likely reveal prisoners sleeping, reading, drawing, pacing, praying, staring out the cell door, and otherwise engaged in solitary activity. The unit may be nearly silent or, alternatively, deafening due to a chorus of pounding, racial epithets, insults, accusations, and profanity, all of which may suggest that unceasing boredom and anger have taken their toll.

The Supermax Debate

The U.S. penitentiary in Marion, Illinois, which opened in 1963, is typically cited as the country's first official supermax unit (Christianson 2004). This facility's severe approach to inmate discipline influenced the development and proliferation of secure housing units (SHUs) in U.S. state prisons over the next 40 years (Arrigo and Bullock 2008). Despite the lack of evidence supporting their efficacy, supermax settings have held enormous appeal for corrections administrators. The number of such facilities in the country has increased to approximately 60 (Briggs et al. 2003). In 2000, over 40,000 individuals were confined in such facilities in the United States (Camp and Camp 2001). Due to the continual growth of the U.S. prison population over the past decade, this number has likely risen. Presently, intense debate is ongoing in corrections over this extreme form of human control and surveillance, and it is slowly gaining momentum as a human rights issue (Human Rights Watch 1997, 2000).

Some have alleged that supermax prisons are inhumane, nonrehabilitative, and psychologically injurious, especially for offenders with mental illness (Grassian and Friedman 1986; Haney and Lynch 1997; Kupers 1999). Consequently, these facilities have triggered controversy and considerable litigation, the most basic of which challenges the confinement of inmates with a history of mental illness in these facilities (Harrington 1997; Metzner 2002a). Another concern centers on the problems, in terms of psychological well-being and ability to improve interpersonal skills, that result from such a high degree of isolation. Most ethical and humanitarian objections to the use of supermax confinement concern the psychological effects of social or sensory deprivation and of hostile conditions (Arrigo and Bullock 2008). Regarding such hostile conditions, some authors have noted that supermax units may be prone to cultivating an environment characterized by physical and verbal abuse by staff, and in which a "wartime" mentality characterizes inmate–staff relationships (Arrigo and Bullock 2008; Rhodes 2007).

Put simply, those who support supermax confinement view it as a "necessary evil" and an indispensable corrections tool, whereas opponents view it as inhumane and unconstitutional (Mears and Castro 2006). Proponents maintain that inmates confined in supermax units are very unlikely to be dissuaded from future violence and are likely to pose a danger to staff and inmates in less restrictive settings. Proponents also claim that punitive isolation serves an invaluable purpose in corrections that could not be achieved by any other means, given current correctional resource limitations. For example, the Colorado State Penitentiary, which houses "the most violent and disruptive offenders" in the state, claims to be an "austere environment" designed to "provide enough time to allow for significant behavior changes in inmate behavior" (Atherton 2001, pp. 100, 101).

Conversely, others have voiced serious concerns about supermax confinement, referring to it as "custodial overkill...liable to enhance rather than reduce the violence potential of inmates" (Toch 2001, p. 376). The controversy over whether supermax units successfully serve as a deterrent to crimes committed by inmates in less restrictive settings remains unresolved from a research perspective (Pizarro and Stenius 2004). No empirical evidence has supported the notion that supermax conditions are effective in deterring violence and maintaining order in the general population. Only one study has addressed this issue directly, finding that the opening of a supermax facility did not significantly reduce levels of inmate-on-inmate violence (Briggs et al. 2003). Table 16–2 gives a list of commonly cited issues on both sides of the supermax debate.

Supermax Case Law Review

As early as 1890, the U.S. Supreme Court considered the potential adverse effects of solitary confinement on inmates' mental health. In the case of *In re Medley*, the Court noted that some inmates in solitary confinement "became violently insane; others still, committed suicide; while those who stood the ordeal were not generally reformed, and in most cases did not recover sufficient mental activity to be of any subsequent service to the community" (*In re Medley* 1890). Most contemporary supermax litigation involves claims of Eighth and Fourteenth Amendment violations. Challenges to the Eighth Amendment, which prohibits cruel and unusual punishment, have typically focused on the following three claims:

1. Isolation leading to mental health deterioration
2. Excessive use of force (e.g., cell extractions)
3. Excessively harsh conditions of isolative confinement

The extreme conditions of social and environmental isolation have resulted in litigation targeting supermax prisons over the past several decades. In *Sandin v. Conner* (1995), the U.S. Supreme Court held that short-term solitary confinement did not violate due process. However, *indefinite* confinement in supermax conditions was found to be a severe deprivation of liberty in *Koch v. Lewis* (2001). Despite an awareness of the potential harm caused by supermax facilities, most courts have held that placement of mentally and physically healthy inmates in supermax settings does not violate the Eighth Amendment. The courts have traditionally given substantial deference to correctional administrators in terms of the use and procedures of supermax confinement. Challenges to supermax procedure invariably confront the U.S. Supreme Court's decision in *Turner v. Safley* (1987), which instructed trial judges to give deference to prison administrators' overriding objectives of institutional safety and security. Therefore, unless the isolated population consists of youth or those with a diagnosed mental condition, the courts are simply not receptive to legal challenges.

In cases involving notorious conditions of solitary confinement, such as *Madrid v. Gomez* (1995) and *Jones'El v. Berge* (2001), experts described an informal "syndrome" experienced by inmates confined to highly restrictive conditions for long periods (Ferrier 2004). Some of the symptoms of this secure housing unit syndrome (SHU syndrome) are believed

TABLE 16–2. The supermax debate

Intended goals	Unintended negative impacts
Increase prison safety, efficiency	Damages inmate–staff relations
Improve order and control of inmates	Reduces resources for other prison efforts
Reduce influence of gangs	Exacerbates mental illness
Punish violent or disruptive inmates	Increases potential for abuse of inmates
Improve living conditions for inmates in general population	Impedes inmate reintegration
	Decreases inmates' physical health

Source. Mears and Watson 2006.

to be pervasive anxiety, hypersensitivity to external stimuli, perceptual distortions, impulsivity, aggressive fantasy, and suicidal ideation. Both *Madrid* and *Jones'El* also dealt with mental health issues specific to punitive isolation. In *Madrid*, the Court described conditions of punitive isolation at the Pelican Bay SHU as residing "on the edge of what is humanely tolerable." In addition, mental health services in the SHU were found to be markedly deficient. In *Jones'El*, Wisconsin's Supermax Correctional Institution was found to have deficient mental health services, particularly in the areas of adequate numbers of mental health staff and methods for screening for mental illness. The courts have been criticized for attempting to ease tensions around the supermax debate by denouncing such conditions for inmates with mental illness but finding them constitutional for "healthy" inmates (Haney 2003).

Psychological Effects of Supermax Confinement

Prolonged Isolation and Confinement in Analogue Environments

Prolonged isolation and confinement of any kind may cause psychological deterioration, and a subclinical syndrome of psychological decrement appears to be common to humans in such circumstances. Indeed, the deleterious consequences of long-term isolation and confinement have been identified in disparate populations, including Russian cosmonauts (Kanas 2000; Kozerenko et al. 2000), Antarctic researchers (Palinkas et al. 2000), and incarcerated felons (Toch 2001).

Russian psychologists have documented that cosmonauts participating in long-duration space missions have experienced psychological distress, especially those aboard early space stations, including the Salyut stations and Mir (Kanas and Manzey 2008). These early space stations were small, and contact with the ground was generally limited to sporadic radio contact with the Russian mission control center. Anecdotal reports of subclinical symptoms similar to SHU syndrome were described by crew members. This long-duration spaceflight syndrome, called "asthenia," included symptoms of fatigue, weakness, irritability, tension, dysphoria, emotional lability, withdrawal, territorial behavior, sleep and appetite disturbance, and attention and memory deficits (Kanas and Manzey 2008). Asthenia has been defined by Russian psychologists as a "nervous or mental weakness manifesting itself in tiredness…and quick loss of strength, low sensation threshold, extremely unstable moods, and sleep disturbance" (Petrovsky and Yaroshevsky 1987, p. 28). This condition appears to be one of cumulative mental fatigue that develops over time and appears in mild form after 1–2 months in space, but increases in intensity after 4 months. American astronaut Jerry Linenger, who spent nearly 5 months aboard Mir in 1997, later reported, "I was astounded at how much I had underestimated the strain of living cut off from the world in an unworldly environment. The isolation was extreme in every way" (Linenger 2000, p. 152). Indeed, because of these earlier adverse experiences aboard Russian space stations, psychological countermeasures provided to astronauts aboard the International Space Station are comprehensive, including weekly private family video conferences and biweekly private psychological conferences (Beven et al. 2008; Sipes and Vanderark 2005). Because of the risk that prolonged isolation and confinement pose for astronauts, one of the hurdles to a potential 36-month mission to Mars is the ability of NASA (National Aeronautics and Space Administration) to successfully provide psychological countermeasures and monitor astronauts' ability to tolerate the extreme isolation and related psychological stress that such a voyage would entail (Arehart-Treichel 2002).

A similar negative psychological syndrome, called "winter-over syndrome," has been described by those who have experienced the harsh and isolated environment of the Antarctic winter. Antarctic explorers and researchers have documented progressively worsening depression, hostility, sleep disturbance, cognitive functioning, and paranoia (Rothblum 1990). Symptoms of winter-over syndrome were first documented by Dr. Frederick Cook, the polar explorer who served as physician aboard the Belgica on the first Belgian Antarctic expedition of 1898–1899. This was the first expedition to spend an entire year in the Antarctic and to overwinter within the Antarctic Circle, and for most of the time, the ship was locked in the frozen Bellingshausen Sea. Cook (1900/1998) painstakingly documented symptoms among the crew that included dejection, loneliness, boredom, hopelessness, lethargy, and insomnia. Many years later, similar findings were reported by the U.S. Navy Medical Neuropsychiatric Research Unit, which noted a high incidence of sleep disturbance, depression, anxiety, aggression, and somatic complaints, as well as a progressive impoverishment of social relationships as the winter progressed (Gunderson 1963; Gunderson and Nelson 1963). The similarity of symptoms common to asthenia, winter-over syndrome, and SHU syndrome is uncanny and speaks to a common psychological and physiological response to prolonged human isolation and confinement.

Prolonged Segregation Confinement

Although some offenders may remain entirely unscathed by segregation, long-term segregation confinement is potentially psychologically detrimental (Metzner 2003; National Commission on Correctional Health Care 2003; Toch 2001). Supermax units have been observed to produce or enhance feelings of resentment, rage, and psychological deterioration (Korn 1988). Even for inmates with no previous history of a psychiatric disorder, prolonged solitary confinement may lead to a decrement in functioning and the insidious development of psychological deterioration (Grassian 1983; Grassian and Friedman 1986; Haney and Lynch 1997). Indicators of behavioral decline may include the following:

1. Restlessness and agitation
2. Concentration and memory impairment
3. Irritability, anger, and frustration intolerance
4. Apathy, social withdrawal, and dysphoria
5. Mood and affective lability
6. Generalized anxiety and panic attacks
7. Irrational suspicion and paranoia

For obvious ethical and humanitarian reasons, performing methodologically sound research in this area is quite difficult. As a result, existing data are limited and may be subject to methodological criticisms. The following are findings of early research:

- Approximately 20% of Washington State supermaximum unit (SMU) residents met criteria for serious mental illness (Cloyes et al. 2006).
- Washington State SMU residents with serious mental illness had an average Brief Psychiatric Rating Scale score in the marked to severe range (on measures of suspiciousness, hostility, anxiety, and depression) (Cloyes et al. 2006).

- Inmates in disciplinary segregation measured with the Brief Symptom Inventory had significantly more feelings of rage, anger, inferiority, and social withdrawal than did general population inmates (Miller and Young 1997).
- The SMU environment produced extreme social isolation, decreased inmate stimulation, and sensory distortion (Rhodes 2005).
- Inmates in solitary confinement appeared to have distorted personal boundaries and extreme dependency on staff (Haney 2003).
- Inmates subjectively related that solitary confinement either "broke" them (produced psychological decompensation) or produced a hardened, recalcitrant sense of rage (Rhodes 2002).

Based on these findings, the conclusion is that inmates in supermax settings demonstrate at least moderate levels of psychosocial impairment. The degree of negative psychological impact caused by prolonged segregation has been correlated with several factors, including the duration of segregation, the extent of isolation, the degree of environmental stimulation deprivation, and the inmate's premorbid psychological fitness (Grassian and Friedman 1986; Haney and Lynch 1997). Factors with more subtle influence on the psychological impact of segregation include the inmate's perception of the justness underlying the decision to implement the segregation, expectations regarding the inmate's ability to earn release, the length of the inmate's prison sentence, and the inmate's ability to use rationalization as a defense mechanism. This defense may allow the inmate to discover something uniquely positive about the segregation experience, such as freedom from fear of sexual assault in the general population or the time to immerse oneself in religious study.

Many offenders already labor under strongly ingrained feelings of societal persecution (Hyatt-Williams 1998). We have observed that some inmates seem to function with relatively fixed feelings of mistreatment and frustration at what they misperceive as "intentional" harm, or "purposeful" and unnecessary withholding of privileges. In long-term isolation, inmates may experience increasing levels of distress and develop more paranoid cognitions, such as distrusting all authority, or unfounded beliefs that they are being singled out for especially punitive treatment. The previously discussed negative psychological effects of isolation in supermax confinement are often insidious and may not be expressed directly by the prisoner.

Over time, a mental health clinician making regular rounds on a supermax unit may begin to notice a previously "normal" inmate pacing restlessly; becoming unaware of the date or the time spent in isolation; refusing family visitation and correspondence; declining meals; failing to regularly shower, clean the cell, or exercise; revealing sudden and irrational fits of anger or accusation; ignoring entreaties of therapeutic interaction; sleeping throughout the day and remaining awake during the night; mumbling or speaking to himself or herself; and refusing medical or psychiatric evaluation. In our experience, inmates without preexisting mental illness who develop signs of psychological decline in punitive segregation typically improve when they are released and/or returned to a general population living environment. As a side note, the effects of supermax settings on staff who work in them are not presently known.

Suicide in Solitary Confinement

Correctional authorities have long theorized that punitive isolation is associated with an increased risk of suicide (American Psychiatric Association 2000; "Prison Suicide Increase" 2007). In a study of the 132 suicides in the New York State prison system between 1993 and 2003 (Way et al. 2007), 32 (24%) were found to have taken place while the inmate was housed in a special disciplinary unit, or SHU. When the authors examined the timing of these 32 suicides, they found that inmates spent a median of 63 days in solitary housing before committing suicide. Therefore, the first 2 months of SHU placement may constitute a high-risk period during which extra attention is warranted. The aggregate median sentence being served in the SHU for the 32 inmates who committed suicide was 298.5 days. The vast majority of the 32 inmates who committed suicide in the SHU had been there for a fairly short time (i.e., less than 2 months). However, 5 of the 32 were unusual in that they had been in the SHU for more than 1 year, leading the authors to wonder about individual "triggers" for these inmates. Ultimately, the most desirable supermax suicide prevention effort would involve administrative and process measures (see "Disciplinary Hearings" section, later in chapter) for effective identification, diversion, or removal of vulnerable inmates. Single-cell disciplinary housing typically occurs without close observation or attentive mental health presence. Enhanced observation of inmates in special housing has been recommended, particularly in light of findings that most inmates who commit suicide in solitary housing do so within the first 2 months of placement there (Way et al. 2007).

If one conceives of punitive segregation as a rather severe form of social exclusion, the "escape theory" of suicide may help explain why some inmates are at increased risk of suicide and self-harm in supermax units. Research findings in nonincarcerated populations have suggested that social exclusion has been found to increase feelings of meaninglessness and to decrease self-awareness and the ability to self-regulate behavior (Baumeister et al. 2005; Twenge et al. 2005). Baumeister (1990) speculated that when the drive to avoid negative affect, meaning, and self-awareness becomes strong enough, an individual has a significantly increased risk of suicide and/or self-destructive behaviors. This theory has been called the *escape theory* of suicide to denote the suicidal individual's motivation to escape from aversive self-awareness. Escape theory may have relevance to the psychology of suicidal inmates, particularly where the inescapable structure and discipline of a supermax unit reduce their ability to avoid aversive affect and self-awareness. According to escape theory, when the individual is unable to avoid negative affect and aversive self-awareness, a process of "cognitive deconstruction" occurs in which there is a rejection of meaning, increased irrationality, and disinhibition. Suicide then becomes an acceptable option in the effort to escape from painful affects and nihilistic cognitions. Escape theory is consistent with previously observed research findings in correctional suicide. For example, strong feelings of hopelessness (whereby an inmate no longer perceives meaning or purpose in life) and suicidal behavior are significantly correlated in prison suicides (Ivanoff and Jang 1991). In addition, poorer coping skills and more severe affective symptoms have been observed in inmates who harm themselves than in inmates who do not (Pen et al. 2003).

Serious Mental Illness in Supermax Units and Barriers to Treatment

Offenders with a history of psychiatric illness are often placed in supermax units because of behavior that is related to their mental disorder (National Commission on Correctional Health Care 2001). Inmates with serious mental illnesses that cause behavior problems are prone to placement in supermax units when they demonstrate difficulties following rigid prison rules, or when their symptoms lead to continual episodes of disruptiveness, intrusiveness, or outbursts of anger. Inmates in this category may include those with mental retardation, borderline personality disorder, mania, organic mental disorders, or impulse control disorders. Prolonged isolation produces a more damaging effect on inmates previously diagnosed as being mentally ill, and this group of offenders is more commonly harmed by the experience (Metzner 2002b). The stress of long-term segregation may exacerbate preexisting symptoms of mental illness or cause remitted symptoms to reemerge. The situation is often compounded by the loss of previously effective multidisciplinary treatment in general population and the subsequent inadequacy of mental health care in many administrative segregation facilities.

Inmates who deteriorate psychiatrically while in administrative segregation can become enmeshed in a futile cycle in which behavioral dyscontrol is interpreted by custody staff as intentional disobedience or disruptiveness (Holton 2003). Such an interpretation results in further administrative intervention and prolonged segregation, in some cases with even greater austerity. This scenario may produce a downward spiral of psychiatric decompensation, behavioral instability, and increasingly self-defeating, yet reflexively administered, punitive sanctions that persist indefinitely or until a tragedy ends the cycle.

Security and safety are the cardinal interests of segregation unit custody staff; these issues supersede all others. Consequently, mental health clinicians assigned to work within an administrative segregation facility often have a discouraging task. Some segregation unit custody staff may assign mental health issues low priority. Within this setting, even highly dedicated and capable mental health clinicians can experience a disquieting sense that their efforts to intercede on behalf of segregated inmates are discounted or, worse, meaningless. An awareness of common obstructions to providing adequate care is necessary to overcome them and also avoid feelings of apathy.

Barriers to the provision of mental health care in administrative segregation generally fall into two categories (Metzner 2003). The first category involves *philosophical impediments* arising from the conviction that segregated offenders manifesting behavior problems should be addressed with orthodox correctional methods, principally additional disciplinary and control measures. This approach, based on correctional tradition and training, is effective with inmates whose disruptiveness emanates from volitional actions unrelated to symptoms of mental illness. However, inmates with mental illness often respond poorly to greater restrictions. Subsequent therapeutic intervention by mental health clinicians, including advocacy to divert disruptive offenders with mental illness from administrative segregation into a treatment setting, may be met with derision by custody staff. An awkward scenario may then ensue, in which correctional mental health clinicians feel trapped between a professional duty to an inmate with a mental disorder and an allegiance to fellow institutional staff who are responsible for ensuring the clinician's safety. A by-product of this circumstance is a potential overreliance on the diagnosis of malingering, even in the face of significant behavioral disturbance and self-injury (Bonner 2001). The diagnosis of malingering may also arise insidiously as "burned-out" clinicians become desensitized by incessant exposure to abusive and indignant offenders; repeatedly observe disturbing scenes of psychological deterioration (e.g., fecal smearing); have their therapeutic efforts continually thwarted; and meet with the concomitant indifference, or perhaps even callousness, of some supermax unit custody staff.

The second category of barriers to mental health treatment in administrative segregation involves *resource limitations*. Examples include mental health staff shortages; lack of office space for private interviews and counseling; the absence of secure mental health group program facilities; segregation cells that afford inadequate observation, communication, and ventilation; the unavailability of maximum security residential care facilities; insufficient custody staff to escort inmates to treatment; and insufficient availability of acute psychiatric hospitalization. In the face of such physical and human resource inadequacies, only abbreviated and often substandard mental health care may be rendered, even if a clinician works in a segregation facility where collegiality and compassion are evident. If a mixture of indifference and resource limitations is present, a culture of neglect nearly invariably arises. Table 16–3 presents a summary of characteristics common to supermax facilities that provide substandard mental health care.

TABLE 16–3. Characteristics of supermax units with inadequate mental health care

---

Inmates experience long-term segregation confinement.

Mental health diversion efforts are absent or discounted.

Inmates with serious mental illness are overrepresented.

An adversarial relationship or poor boundaries exist between mental health staff and custody staff.

Cursory mental health screening and monitoring are available.

Inmates with mental illness are disciplined for disruptive behavior regardless of etiology.

Cells have poor lighting, poor ventilation, and inadequate observation.

Interviews of inmates occur without privacy or confidentiality.

Units often have vacant mental health staff positions and large clinician caseloads.

Psychotherapy and group programs are unavailable.

Self-injurious and suicidal inmates are regularly labeled as malingerers.

Psychiatric medication is the sole therapeutic modality for most inmates.

Maximum security residential care is unavailable.

Psychiatric hospitalization is severely limited or unattainable.

Source.   Adapted from Beven 2005, pp. 209–228.

Treatment in Supermax

Screening and Diversion

Although formal policies may differ, for inmates with mental illness who are being considered by correctional staff for supermax confinement, intervention should be initiated soon after the disciplinary ticket is given but before sanctions are considered by the institutional disciplinary committee. Following a disruptive or aggressive action by an offender with mental illness, the recommended action is for mental health clinicians to assist custody staff in determining if symptoms of mental illness influenced the inmate's behavior and if the offender has adequate understanding of the disciplinary proceedings (Metzner 2003; National Commission on Correctional Health Care 2001). This is crucial if the prisoner is known to be seriously and chronically mentally ill.

Inquiry by correctional mental health staff into an inmate's behavioral instability should include the offender's diagnosis, medication compliance, recently observed symptoms, and possible precipitating or mitigating factors. If the inmate's conduct is related to symptoms of mental illness, treatment rather than discipline is needed, and diversion into a secure correctional mental health unit may avert further psychiatric deterioration in an administrative segregation facility (Kupers 1999). For example, in the case of an agitated inmate with paranoid schizophrenia who attacks another inmate without provocation, further inquiry may uncover poor antipsychotic medication compliance, the development of persecutory delusions, and recent discharge from a residential treatment unit into an outpatient setting. Despite the serious nature of the infraction, correctional mental health clinicians advocating for diversion to a secure residential treatment unit make a wise judgment that addresses both institutional security concerns and the inmate's treatment needs.

Unfortunately, the majority of disciplinary circumstances are not as clear as this example. In some cases, disruptive or violent acts may be in response to common emotions, including anger, greed, and fear, regardless of mental illness. In these cases, mental health staff involvement in adjudication and punitive sanction determination may be less helpful. An offender with well-controlled bipolar disorder who sexually assaults another inmate provides an example. If subsequent investigation indicates the offense was unrelated to active symptoms of the inmate's mental illness, placement into administrative segregation is likely to be unavoidable. Nevertheless, the necessary monitoring and ongoing treatment requirements of the segregated offender should become the primary focus of correctional mental health staff.

Disciplinary Hearings

Disciplinary hearings are intrafacility hearings to determine the consequences of disciplinary infractions by inmates. They are typically conducted by a senior correctional officer in the presence of another correctional staff member and the inmate. Punishment for disciplinary infractions may involve a "sentence" of anywhere from 2 weeks in a disciplinary segregation unit to reclassification followed by months to years in a supermax unit. Disciplinary hearings have very serious consequences for offenders with mental illness. These inmates are more likely to be charged with rule violations than inmates without mental illness (James and Glaze 2006), and therefore have an increased rate of disciplinary infractions and placement in punitive segregation (Lovell et al. 2000; Toch and Adams 1986). In some cases, accumulated punitive segregation time extends the mentally ill offender's sentence beyond his or her maximum sentence date. The inmate with mental illness who is charged with a disciplinary infraction may or may not be entitled to mental health consultation or expert testimony.

In practice, the criteria and procedures for placing inmates in administrative segregation vary considerably. A formal disciplinary or classification hearing may or may not be required, depending on the facility's policies. Prison administrators may make such decisions based on factual data or merely the perception that the inmate is a danger. Some facilities use this reasoning to place gang members in a supermax unit, even if the inmate has not been found to have engaged in any disciplinary infractions. Other facilities may have elaborate supermax placement procedures. For example, the Ohio Department of Corrections requires a "factual basis" for eligibility (*Wilkinson v. Austin* 2005). In *Wolff v. McDonnell* (1974), the U.S. Supreme Court held that although prisoners are entitled to some due process protections in prison disciplinary proceedings, they are not entitled to "the full panoply of rights due a defendant" in a criminal prosecution.

The subject of mental health testimony at inmate disciplinary hearings has been largely neglected until fairly recently. Lack of mental health clinician consultation and expert testimony at disciplinary hearings is often the final turn of the key for the inmate who has violated prison rules due to his or her mental illness. Even if the inmate is not hindered by disorganized thought and speech, a lack of insight and awareness of the legal implications of his or her behavior may preclude the inmate's ability to testify rationally or effectively at a hearing (Buckley et al. 2004). In a nationwide survey, considerable diversity was found across states regarding the role of mental health staff in disciplinary hearings (Krelstein 2002).

Although most states had policies on the issue, no clear consensus existed on whether mental health staff should offer "ultimate opinions" regarding inmates' competency or sanity in the disciplinary process. Complicating matters further are concerns about dual agency problems, mental health staff shortages, and the creation of conflict between mental health staff and correctional staff (Metzner 2002b). Many of these issues were addressed in *Powell v. Coughlin* (1991), where the Second Circuit Court of Appeals addressed mental health representation at inmate disciplinary hearings.

The *Powell* decision raised some concern that the court's deference to prison administrators' interests might lead to a neglect of the rights of inmates with mental illness (Dvoskin et al. 1995). Despite these concerns, private settlement agreements have suggested that the courts will, in fact, attend to the rights of mentally ill inmates at disciplinary hearings. For example, in *Anderson v. Coughlin* (1987), both parties entered into a private settlement that was approved by the U.S. District Court for the Northern District of New York. In *Anderson,* a workable agreement was reached regarding mental health expert testimony at disciplinary hearings, which resulted in amendments to the New York Department of Corrections' SHU regulations. The amendments included 1) specific criteria to be used by hearing officers in determining when an inmate's mental state or intellectual capacity is at issue during a hearing, 2) adjournment of the hearing when the hearing officer believes the inmate is unfit to proceed, and 3) specific criteria that alert hearing officers to inquire about the inmate's mental state and intellectual capacity. In addition, the agreement outlined the issues that mental health clinicians should address in their expert testimony:

1. The extent to which the inmate's current mental health status affects his or her fitness to proceed with the hearing
2. The extent to which the inmate's mental status at the time of the incident did or did not affect his or her responsibility for the offense
3. The extent to which the inmate's current mental health status or clinical history makes him or her suitable or unsuitable for SHU placement

The Anderson agreement specified that mental health staff who testify must be trained to do so. The New York Office of Mental Health (2006), in consultation with Central New York Psychiatric Center, has developed a reasonably sophisticated but workable process and a testimony checklist for mental health staff to follow. An example of items contained in the checklist is given in Table 16–4. Mental health staff do not give opinions on the ultimate issues. For example, when testifying about responsibility, they are instructed to give their "clinical opinions" on "the extent to which the inmate's mental status at the time of the incident does or does not affect his responsibility for the offense." Similarly, regarding sentence duration, they are instructed to give their clinical opinions on suitability for SHU, as well as "the extent to which the inmate's current mental health status or clinical history should be considered in determining the duration of the sentence to SHU." Only mental health professionals not involved in the inmate's treatment serve as representatives at the disciplinary hearings, which satisfies the National Commission on Correctional Health Care recommendation that "the services of outside providers or someone on the institution's staff who is not involved in a therapeutic relationship with the inmate should be obtained" for such proceedings (National Commission on Correctional Health Care 2003, Standard J-I-03, cited in American Psychiatric Association 2000, p. 20).

Supermax Transfers

Transgressions of a very serious nature, such as rape or attempted escape, may trigger a recommendation that the offender be transferred to a supermax unit. At present, best practice indicates that inmates with serious mental illness, or with a psychological disposition to behavioral decay under severe stress, should be precluded from transfer to such facilities unless adequate mental health resources are available (Metzner 2002b). Inmates vulnerable to deterioration in supermax include those with any serious mental illness; mental retardation; cognitive disorders such as dementia; a history of self-injury or mutilation; severe personality disorders (e.g., borderline personality disorder); or a related record of functional impairment due to depression, suicidality, or brief psychosis (Metzner 2003). Prudent record review, a clinical interview, and documentation of any exclusionary factors should occur prior to approval for transfer of an inmate to a supermaximum security institution, and also upon reception at the secure facility. Prisoners who pass through conscientious screening methods but behaviorally deteriorate later due to the stress of supermaximum security confinement should be transferred to a segregation facility with fewer restrictions or greater access to mental health treatment.

Mental Health Treatment in Supermax

As noted above, every effort should be made to reduce the chances that inmates with serious mental illness, extreme psychological vulnerability, or intellectual disabilities will be housed in segregation, especially for long periods of time. Nevertheless, some of these inmates undoubtedly will be placed in segregation, and other inmates without such disabilities

TABLE 16–4. Testimony checklist for mental health at disciplinary hearings

Treatment history (hospitalizations, intermediate care program residence, suicide watches, etc.)

Last clinical contact with inmate and clinical status

Diagnoses, service level, housing/program location

Behaviors associated with diagnosis

Medications (current and at time of disciplinary infraction)

Compliance with medications and effects of noncompliance

Side effects of medications

Past history of SHU time and ability to cope

Clinical opinions on

　Fitness to proceed

　Responsibility for offense

　Suitability for SHU

　Duration of SHU sentence

Note. This list does not represent the full New York State Office of Mental Health testimony checklist.
SHU=secure housing unit.

Source. Office of Mental Health 2006

may experience psychological or emotional crises while housed there. Mentally ill inmates and those in psychological crisis who are housed in administrative segregation require a full range of multidisciplinary care to treat active symptoms, maintain psychiatric stability, and prevent deterioration (American Psychiatric Association 2000). Professional treatment guidelines for major mental illness such as schizophrenia, bipolar disorder, and major depressive disorder cannot be neglected because of incarceration (American Psychiatric Association 2002). Regardless of a prisoner's security needs or prior behavior, the standard of care for the treatment of mental illness should be followed. Although this task is difficult in any supermax setting, comprehensive mental health care must be offered if mentally ill inmates are consigned to long-term segregation. This care should include evaluation, monitoring, psychotherapy, psychiatric medication, crisis care, secure residential treatment unit care including group programs, and acute psychiatric hospitalization. Table 16–5 includes a list of characteristics of supermax units providing effective mental health care.

TABLE 16–5. Characteristics of supermax units with effective mental health care

Inmates with serious mental illness are diverted into a secure treatment setting.

Acutely mentally ill inmates are rarely in supermax units.

Inmates are frequently monitored by mental health staff.

Collaborative professional relationship exists between mental health staff and custody staff.

Disruptive inmates with mental illness are addressed by mental health staff and are not routinely disciplined.

Mental health interviews and counseling occur in a private setting.

Individual psychotherapy and group programs are available in an appropriately secure setting.

Crisis intervention occurs promptly and without reflexive assumption of malingering.

Multidisciplinary team provides care and actively engages the inmate to meet behavioral goals.

Psychiatric care considers segregated offender's unique needs.

Psychiatric hospitalization is readily available when needed.

Inmates stabilized via hospitalization are not transferred directly back into segregation but are placed into an appropriately secure residential treatment unit.

Maximum security residential treatment unit placement is available, which affords a balance of security and treatment needs.

Source. Adapted from Beven 2005, pp. 209–228.

Monitoring Inmates in Supermax

Correctional mental health staff should monitor all inmates in long-term segregation confinement, but particular attention should be given to offenders with mental illness (American Psychiatric Association 2000). At a minimum, mental health staff should make weekly cell-front visits to mentally ill inmates for informal inquiry and observation for signs of decline (Metzner 1997). During these "house calls," the staff can judge cell cleanliness and the inmate's attire, attitude, attention, energy level, interaction with others, and general sense of well being—preferably within the context of a consultative relationship with corrections officers assigned to the unit. The findings gleaned can be communicated to other members of the treatment team, including the treating psychiatrist. If inmates not previously identified as being mentally ill reveal indications of distress, they should be referred for more comprehensive evaluation.

Although cell-front interviews can be meaningful and necessary, such contact is insufficient for the initial comprehensive evaluation or individual psychotherapy. All therapeutic contact beyond simple monitoring should occur in private, where confidentiality can be maintained. Ideally, this may take place in a nearby mental health office or interview area designated for such a purpose. Security concerns are undeniably important but can be appropriately addressed by active collaboration with the supermax security chief.

Clinical Case 16–1

Mr. D, a young man without any known history of mental illness, was placed into punitive segregation after he stabbed another inmate. The assault was the result of a dispute between rival prison gangs. Mr. D had been chosen by his gang leader to commit the offense and bear the subsequent disciplinary consequences, which he did with apparent stoicism. Mr. D was seen weekly at cell-front by the mental health clinician assigned the task of monitoring inmates in segregation. Initially rather brash, Mr. D consistently denied any problems and often sarcastically told the mental health clinician to "leave me alone....I'm no nut case." The conversation between the two usually consisted of informal, relatively friendly banter.

After 6 months of segregation, Mr. D's hygiene noticeably worsened, and he began to look deconditioned, having gained 15 pounds. Ordinarily well groomed and quite lean, Mr. D now rarely showered and had stopped exercising. His cell became dirty, and Mr. D's demeanor changed as well, turning sullen and unfriendly. As the weeks passed, he began pacing restlessly in his cell and started to ignore the mental health clinician entirely. Segregation unit corrections officers reported that Mr. D was "no problem," although they too noticed that he was becoming increasingly withdrawn. Growing concerned, the mental health clinician arranged for a private interview in a nearby office, with a corrections officer nearby. Initially hesitant to speak, the young inmate admitted to feeling depressed and anxious, as well as sleeping only 3–4 hours each night. He found it very difficult to concentrate and felt that "I might be going crazy." Mr. D was referred for psychiatric evaluation, leading to a diagnosis of major depressive disorder. Treatment with an antidepressant medication combined with individual psychotherapy rapidly produced a positive outcome.

The Supermax Unit Mental Health Team

The combination of cell-front visitation, psychotherapy, and consultation with security staff should occur as a collaboration between a psychiatrist and other correctional mental health providers working closely as a team with the custody staff, especially in the case of segregated inmates with serious mental illness (Metzner 1997). Treatment team members may include social workers, psychology staff, activity therapists, and representatives from custody and administration. This multidisciplinary model of care requires treatment team meetings between the segregated inmate, correctional mental health clinicians, and other correctional staff involved in his or her care, usually at 30- to 90-day intervals. During these encounters, active participation by the offender should be solicited and management of the inmate's mental illness addressed. Behavioral improvement may be augmented if the prisoner is advised that the treatment team will recommend eventual administrative segregation release if the inmate's disordered behavior ceases.

In high-profile cases involving behavioral instability and extreme violence, senior administrative staff, such as a deputy warden, should be encouraged to attend a treatment team meeting to affirm behavioral expectations leading to supermax release and to be made aware of the mental health department's role. Such involvement preferably should occur in a venue that preserves confidentiality by focusing on important custodial concerns without discussion of personal information or psychiatric treatment. A balanced effort, achieved through multidisciplinary teamwork, provides for the greatest chance of treatment success and the prevention of philosophical rifts between mental health and custody personnel.

Psychiatric Treatment in Supermax

The psychiatrist should play an active role in the monitoring, evaluation, and treatment of inmates in supermax units. Isolation may exacerbate or produce distress that requires a treatment response using psychotropic medication (Burns 2003). All psychiatrists—including those who use telemedicine equipment to furnish care and do not have the opportunity to witness the correctional environment directly—must have a comprehensive awareness of both patient care risks and custodial concerns.

Characteristics of segregation facilities may cause treatment problems. The medication-administering nurse may be unable to see clearly into an inmate's cell to properly determine if an inmate is "cheeking" (i.e., not swallowing) medication. This scenario may raise concerns about certain inmates hoarding medication for an overdose or planning to sell to other inmates. Some mentally ill offenders with poor insight or concern about side effects may refuse all medication, rendering treatment efforts useless. During summer months, segregation cells may be stifling, leading to an increased risk of hyperthermia.

A psychiatrist's treatment response to the idiosyncrasies of segregation will be distinct for each prison and each patient, but may entail prescribing medication in liquid form, using medications with a lower potential for lethality in overdose, educating nursing and corrections staff on the risk of hyperthermia, relying on medication serum levels to assist with determination of compliance, and resolutely focusing on patient education and medication compliance issues. Correctional psychiatrists who treat segregated inmates should also be vigilant against the use of polypharmacy, especially where several psychiatrists provide care based on a coverage rotation, making continuity of care difficult to achieve. If several classes of psychiatric medications are being prescribed at increasing or maximal dosages, one must consider the possibility of environmentally caused deterioration or treatment resistance, and the need for inmate transfer to a secure intermediate care unit. The illicit diversion of medication to other segregated inmates or medication-seeking behavior in an offender with a history of drug addiction should also be considered.

Psychiatrists who treat inmates in supermax confinement also require considerable patience. Strict security requirements slow the pace of work, and segregated offenders often require longer interviews due to adverse environmental circumstances and a greater need for therapeutic contact. A psychiatrist who normally examines 15–20 inmates per day in a general population venue may see only half as many patients in administrative segregation. This should not be considered a reflection of professional inadequacy, but rather a genuine need for clinical deliberateness within the constraints of a maximum security context.

Occasionally, segregation custody staff who work with the most disruptive and aggressive offenders may inadvertently influence the correctional psychiatrist to view such inmates in a negative light. Countertransference may also play a role in such cases and in a worst-case scenario can lead to compromised professionalism. The outcome may include ignoring signs of an inmate's emotional distress or failing to implement available modes of treatment, including hospitalization, when clinically indicated. Such a scenario may occur when the segregated offender is incarcerated for a heinous crime or if the prisoner has seriously injured a fellow staff member. Psychiatrists who choose to work in supermax settings should remain mindful of their role as physicians and be willing to make unpopular decisions to ensure patient safety and provide effective care despite their own negative personal feelings or the pointed opinion of others.

Crisis Intervention and Malingering

Effective crisis intervention services are greatly needed in supermax, because inmates periodically engage in destructive or bizarre behaviors related to mental illness or merely to extreme loneliness and antipathy (Bonner 2001). Such behaviors include fecal smearing, head banging, self-inflicted lacerations, destruction of personal property, fire setting, and suicidal statements. Although this behavior may represent an inmate's effort to feign mental illness, correctional mental health clinicians are strongly advised to consciously avoid making a reflexive diagnosis of manipulation or malingering. The stress of prolonged segregation can cause offenders with mental illness to engage in unusual acts of self-harm, such as swallowing foreign objects or consuming excrement. Inmates without a history of mental illness may become seriously depressed and consider suicide as a means to escape continued isolation. Additionally, a desperate inmate who strives to maintain some control over his or her austere environment may destroy what few personal belongings he or she has—making a bad situation even worse.

Offenders who engage in acts of self-injury or irrational aggression deserve prompt crisis intervention regardless of the underlying motives (National Commission on Correctional Health Care 2001). The clinical response may include suicide watch procedures, seclusion, therapeutic restraint, emergency medication, and careful multidisciplinary evaluation. Inmates with serious mental illness may ultimately require a more intensive level of care elsewhere. Inmates with severe personality disorders may benefit from more frequent, structured therapeutic contact. Prisoners who clearly do not have mental illness, but orchestrate labor-intensive mental health crises, should be evaluated, counseled, and referred to appropriate administrative staff for complaint resolution. Irrespective of the final conclusion, correctional mental health clinicians must use careful judgment and caution. The risk of error can be very high, with suicide one potential result if signs of genuine distress are discounted, and explosive violence another possible outcome if release to a less secure facility occurs without adequate forethought.

Psychiatric Hospitalization

Despite the mental health treatment team's best efforts, segregated inmates may precipitously deteriorate or harm themselves so severely that transfer to a secure psychiatric hospital becomes necessary. The venue of hospital-level care varies across correctional systems but commonly involves transfer to a designated prison hospital facility or a forensic unit of a state hospital. Psychiatric hospitalization, or any other clinically necessary medical intervention, must not be disallowed solely because of security concerns or an inmate's segregation status (American Psychiatric Association 2000; National Commission on Correctional Health Care 1997). If clinical indications for hospitalization arise, such as a near-lethal suicide attempt or the development of florid psychosis, transfer should be expedited. It is incumbent upon the hospital facility to ensure adequate security while also providing patient care.

Following hospitalization, diversion into a secure residential treatment unit setting should occur. Immediate return to segregation risks negating the clinical gains achieved during hospitalization, especially if ongoing treatment requirements cannot be met or if the effects of isolation trigger exacerbation of the newly stabilized illness. This scenario often results in an expensive and futile cycle of deterioration, hospitalization, stabilization, segregation, deterioration, and rehospitalization (National Commission on Correctional Health Care 2001). Effective care after hospitalization increases the likelihood of behavioral improvement and diminishes the risk of further misconduct (Haddad 1999; Lovell et. al. 2001).

Secure Residential Treatment

Factors giving rise to psychiatric instability in supermax confinement may be negated if maximum security residential care is made available (Eshem et al. 2001). The development of a secure residential treatment facility, designed exclusively for the provision of mental health treatment to violent and disruptive mentally ill offenders, can pay great dividends, including a decrease in inmate aggression and subsequent disciplinary response (Condelli et al. 1994; Rayford and Trestman 2002).

Inmates with serious and persistent mental illness who would otherwise be transferred to administrative segregation and disrupt customary unit activities can in many cases be diverted to a secure mental health unit following serious misconduct. In this manner, both institutional security needs and individual psychiatric treatment requirements may be addressed without the perception that the transgression of prison rules has provoked no disciplinary response. Segregated offenders suspected of malingered psychosis may undergo psychiatric evaluation in a secure setting without there being a risk of potentially ignoring genuine symptoms. Inmates in supermax facilities who develop active suicidal ideation or otherwise behaviorally decline can be properly evaluated and afforded care without security measures having to be spared. Segregated inmates with mental illness may be discharged from an acute care facility to a secure residential program for ongoing treatment so that progress attained during hospitalization is not imperiled. Finally, prisoners thought to be entirely beyond hope, including those who engage in continual acts of irrational aggression, rebellion, and self-injury, may receive intensive evaluation and care in a setting that provides a chance of psychosocial rehabilitation and behavioral improvement when all previous correctional interventions have failed. A maximum security residential treatment unit may have the greatest results with this group of offenders, and the behavioral reformation of an intractably disturbed and unmanageable inmate previously "buried" in punitive segregation may appear miraculous.

Clinical Case 16–2

Following his assault of a corrections officer, Mr. J had been in supermax confinement for over 3 years. Having borderline intellectual intelligence, a seizure disorder, serious impulse control problems, and illiteracy, he was thought to be hopelessly disruptive. Over the course of his segregation, Mr. J developed a repertoire of increasingly maladaptive behaviors, including smearing and throwing feces, spitting on corrections officers, exposing himself to female staff, threatening others and himself, destroying prison property, flooding his cell, head banging, swallowing foreign objects, and self-mutilation. Increasingly restrictive privileges, isolation from other inmates, and frequent custody staff intervention failed to improve Mr. J's conduct. The intermittent use of restraint and suicide watch precautions, with subsequent release back into segregation, appeared to reinforce his self-injurious behavior.

Mr. J was admitted to a maximum security residential treatment unit, and a multidisciplinary treatment plan was developed with input from mental health, unit management, and custody staff. Mr. J began 15 hours per week of therapeutic group programs. Psychiatric evaluation prompted use of a mood-stabilizing anticonvulsant for enhanced impulse control. A recreation program was begun under the supervision of an activity therapist, who implemented a structured exercise regimen, and a reading tutor was assigned. Psychotherapy was initiated, with the principal goals being improved impulse control and frustration tolerance. All therapeutic modalities occurred in a secure setting under the direct observation of corrections officers with specialized mental health training.

Over the course of 6 months, Mr. J's behavior substantially improved. A mental health professional, present at all security-level review hearings, reported the progress to custody and administrative staff. Following a 6-month period entirely free of prison rule infractions or conduct reports, Mr. J was released to the prison general population after nearly 4 years of segregation confinement, a feat considered by many to be a "miracle."

The successful implementation of a maximum security residential treatment unit depends on adequate human and physical resources (Haddad 1999; Metzner 1998). The following resources are often necessary: activity therapy staff for therapeutic group and recreational programs; psychiatric nurses; psychology staff; social workers; psychiatrists; and unit management staff sensitive to the needs of mentally ill offenders. Supplementary mental health training for correctional officers assigned to work in a maximum security residential treatment unit is of critical importance. Such officers should have a genuine interest in correctional mental health issues and have a demonstrated history of compassion, flexibility, and professionalism. Custody staff without additional training who may be randomly assigned to the mental health unit and/ or not accustomed to working with inmates with mental illness may inadvertently undermine the mental health treatment team's best therapeutic efforts.

The secure mental health unit should also provide adequate private office space for clerical work and treatment records; cells that afford adequate observation, communication, and ventilation; indoor and outdoor recreation facilities; and secure group program space, such as adjacent holding cells linked in a semicircle. Although maximum security residential treatment units are initially costly, the start-up expenses may be balanced over time by a decreased risk of litigation, reduced need for psychiatric hospital care, and less need for emergency medical care following self-inflicted injury. Morale also improves, because most corrections officers are freed to work with offenders who are not mentally ill and correctional mental health staff can focus on the mission of providing treatment in a setting that greatly enhances the prospect of therapeutic success.

The Future of Supermax Confinement

The use of supermax confinement is likely to continue due to the tradition of judicial deference to prison administration, as well as the powerful symbolic meaning behind supermax facilities. Supermax confinement can be said to serve as a symbol of the state's posture of being "tough" on crime and "prevailing" over it with consequences that appear to ensure order and safety. A nationwide survey found a consensus among state prison wardens that supermax prisons "serve to increase system-wide safety, order, and control," and that "they are successful in achieving these goals" (Mears and Castro 2006, p. 420). These views, however, cannot be attributed to data-driven conclusions, because research on the effectiveness of supermax prisons is generally lacking (Mears 2008; Pizarro and Narag 2008).

The use of supermax confinement will continue to require the presence of competent mental health staff to ensure that appropriate treatment is available to offenders with mental illness. Mental health and human rights advocates may, over time, be successful in making recommendations and proposals for reducing the psychological harm caused by supermax confinement. For example, one proposal for reformation has suggested that corrections begin to view prolonged isolation in the same way that mental health views the use of seclusion and restraints—that is, it should be used only for control, not punishment, and only for certain, time-limited circumstances (Cohen 2006). Other recommendations for the reform of supermax confinement are listed in Table 16–6.

DEATH ROW

Absent the wait for an impending execution, inmates' conditions on death row are not substantially different from those of supermax confinement. Prisoners on death row are confined to small cells for up to 23 hours per day (Hudson 2000). The cells are often small, and their livability varies with the resources available. Psychiatric research on death row–related issues is not well developed; this is unfortunate because forensic and treating psychiatrists could benefit from more guidance in this ethically complex environment.

Ethical Dilemmas

Diverse opinions exist about the ethical permissibility of psychiatrists' participation in death penalty cases. In a survey of 290 forensic psychiatrists (Leong et al. 2000), only 8.5% believed that it was never acceptable to evaluate a condemned prisoner. About half believed that an inmate who is incompetent to be executed should be treated to restore competence. Most respondents supported a role for psychiatric evaluations of death row inmates, but they were divided on whether incompetent death row inmates should be treated if treatment would result in the inmates' competence to be executed.

The constitutionality of the death penalty was generally upheld by the Supreme Court in *Gregg v. Georgia* (1976), and its application to specific offender groups has been considered over the past several decades. For example, in *Ford v. Wainwright* (1986), the U.S. Supreme Court ruled that the Eighth Amendment prohibits the execution of a prisoner who is insane. In *Ford*, the Court gave little guidance on a standard for competence to be executed, other than an arguably vague "test" involving whether the prisoner is aware of the impending execution and the reason for it. After lower courts struggled with this application, the U.S. Supreme Court

TABLE 16–6. Recommendations for reform of supermax confinement

Careful screening, monitoring, and removal of inmates with serious mental illness, or any inmate who is psychologically vulnerable

Immediate removal of decompensated inmates

Privacy when inmates meet with mental health staff

Humane conditions—modifying harsh conditions of confinement

Providing meaningful activities and programming

Sufficient space for exercise and recreation

Access to visitor or family contact

Step-down programming

Strict time limits

Prohibition of any form of staff abuse of inmates

Adequate training and supervision for all staff

More well-designed supermax research on the effects, costs and benefits, and needs

Improved classification and hearing procedures used to place inmates in isolation

Source.   Arrigo and Bullock 2008; Cohen 2006; Haney 2003; Mears 2008; Mears and Watson 2006.

remained reluctant to establish a rule governing all competence-to-be-executed determinations in *Panetti v. Quarterman* (2007). However, the Court clarified that "a prisoner's awareness of the State's rationale for an execution is not the same as a rational understanding of it." Thus, a mentally ill death row inmate's simple, concrete awareness of a state's reason for execution may nevertheless be inadequate where the inmate has a "delusion that the stated reason is a sham." In *State v. Perry* (1992), the Louisiana Supreme Court ultimately held that the state may not forcibly medicate a defendant found incompetent to be executed. The court, however, did leave open the possibility for the state to reinstate the defendant's execution should he become competent to be executed without the use of medication.

The U.S. Supreme Court has addressed the death penalty in other select populations, such as individuals with developmental disabilities and youthful offenders. In *Atkins v. Virginia* (2002), the Court held that executing a criminal with mental retardation was cruel and unusual punishment prohibited by the Eighth Amendment. The Court cited "evolving standards of decency" and the fact that a significant number of states had

concluded that "death is not a suitable punishment for a mentally retarded criminal." This conclusion would appear to be supported by the
social science research finding that juries were less likely to view mentally
retarded and mentally ill offenders as "death worthy" (Boots et al. 2003).

Regarding youthful offenders, the constitutionality of the death penalty was initially upheld for juveniles age 16 years and older (*Stanford v.
Kentucky* 1989) but prohibited for offenders age 15 years and younger
(*Thompson v. Oklahoma* 1988). More recently, the U.S. Supreme Court
overturned these decisions in *Roper v. Simmons* (2005), which challenged
the constitutionality of capital punishment for persons who were under
age 18 at the time they committed murder. The challenge was based on
Eighth Amendment protections against cruel and unusual punishment.
The Court invoked the "evolving standards of decency" test, and cited a
body of sociological and scientific research suggesting that juveniles lack
the brain maturity and decision-making abilities of adults (E. Scott and
Grisso 1997; Sowell et al. 2001). In addition, the majority cited the abol-
ishment of juvenile capital punishment in 30 states as evidence of an evolving consensus, as well as the notion that age 18 is often where the law
draws the line between minority age and adulthood.

The American Academy of Psychiatry and the Law (2001) has called
for a moratorium on capital punishment "at least until death penalty
jurisdictions implement policies and procedures that: A) Ensure that
death penalty cases are administered fairly and impartially in accordance
with basic due process; and B) Prevent the execution of mentally disabled persons and people who were under the age of 18 at the time of
their offenses." The American Medical Association's Council on Ethical
and Judicial Affairs has taken the unequivocal position that any physician's direct participation in an execution is unethical. Under any circumstances, treatment of death row inmates demands that the psychiatrist
function in a highly complex ethical arena (Matthews and Wendler
2006).

Distinguishing Treatment From Evaluation

In navigating the complex death row terrain, psychiatrists must first
make a clear distinction between providing treatment to inmates on
death row and performing a forensic evaluation of a death row inmate
for the courts. The American Medical Association's Council on Ethical
and Judicial Affairs (1995) concluded that evaluating an inmate's competence to be executed is permissible given that the physician is acting as
an advocate of the justice system and not as part of the process of punishment. Burns (2007), however, recommended that a treating psychiatrist
never offer a forensic opinion on a patient's competence to be executed.

When an inmate has been found incompetent to be executed, two important questions typically arise (C. Scott 2006): 1) Should the psychiatrist initiate psychotropic medication or continue to treat with medications when this may result in a restoration of competence to be executed? 2) Can the inmate who refuses medication be involuntarily medicated to restore competence to be executed? Professional ethical guidelines will often be helpful in answering the first question. As a foundational guideline, the American Medical Association has clearly stated that psychiatrists should never treat an inmate for the purpose of restoring competence to be executed. Treatment expressly for the purpose of restoring competence to be executed is ethically suspect, because the psychiatrist could be seen as closely linked to facilitating the state's interest in executing the inmate (Matthews and Wendler 2006). Table 16–7 provides a list of ethical guidelines for treating death row inmates.

The question of how to approach the psychiatric treatment of an incompetent death row inmate can be guided by the traditional medical ethic of *primum non nocere* (Latin for "first, do no harm"). Thus, the psychiatrist's objective may be focused on treating solely to reduce pain and suffering caused by a serious mental illness. Once some individualized degree of rational mental capacity has been restored, the patient may make his or her own decision about receiving further treatment. In this way, the question of whether treatment is ultimately beneficial or harmful is left to the patient (Bonnie 1990). Should an inmate decide that treatment is not desired, the psychiatrist may then refrain from treatment based on both ethical grounds and the patient's informed decision. Ultimately, commutation of the death sentence for inmates who are incompetent to be executed may be the best resolution for psychiatrists tasked with the treatment of death row inmates (Matthews and Wendler 2006).

Another important consideration for psychiatrists is whether they can remain objective while treating or evaluating death row inmates. In particular, the moral burden is likely to "fall most heavily on those who hold the greatest moral doubts about the death penalty" (Bonnie 1990, p. 18). Indeed, some research evidence suggests that a moral opposition to the death penalty is associated with a reluctance to participate in evaluations of competence to be executed (Deitchman et al. 1991). The persistence and resilience of the death penalty in the United States may be explained by acknowledging its strong emotional variables, which ultimately undergird all so-called rational debate (Bandes 2008). Because such emotional variables cannot be ignored, psychiatrists should acknowledge their own emotional responses to working on death row and consider how their responses may affect treatment or evaluation decisions.

TABLE 16–7.   Treating death row inmates: ethical guidelines

Primum non nocere—first, do no harm.

Do not treat for the purpose of restoring competence to be executed.

Treat all death row inmates undergoing extreme suffering as a result of a psychiatric disorder.

If an inmate's rational mental capacity has been restored, allow the inmate to make a decision about receiving further treatment.

Arrange for reevaluations of competence to be performed by an independent, nontreating psychiatrist.

Obtain consultation in difficult cases.

Source. American Medical Association's Council on Ethical and Judicial Affairs 1992; Bonnie 1990; Scott 2006.

Psychiatric Disorders in Death Row Inmates

The potential for condemned inmates living on death row to develop mental and emotional distress has long been recognized by the courts. In *California v. Anderson* (1972), the California Supreme Court held that "the cruelty of capital punishment lies not only in the execution itself... but also in the dehumanizing effects of the lengthy imprisonment prior to execution." Taking a more descriptive approach, a Massachusetts court stated that

> a condemned man knows...the time and manner of his death....He must wait for a specific death, not merely death in the abstract....Having to face an inevitable death, any man, whatever his convictions, is torn asunder from head to toe. (*District Attorney for Suffolk District v. Watson* 1980)

Attention has been focused on how the length of time the condemned inmate spends on death row appears to be associated with worsening mental suffering. In *Furman v. Georgia* (1972), the U.S. Supreme Court noted that "mental pain is an inseparable part" of the death sentence, and that a pending execution "exacts a frightful toll during the inevitable long wait." *Lackey v. Texas* (1995) dealt with this issue directly, with the Court finding that extended death row stays have the potential to cause "the gratuitous infliction of suffering." Subsequent to this case, a "Lackey claim" has come to represent a claim of an Eighth Amendment violation due to an unreasonably long delay on death row while going through the appeals process (*Lackey v. Scott* 1995).

In 2005, the average time that a condemned inmate spent on death row in the United States was 12 years 3 months (Snell 2006). In some cases, extended stays on death row have been associated with psychiatric decompensation ("Mental Suffering Under Sentence of Death" 1972). Prisoners on death row have been found to demonstrate aberrant behavior and paranoia (Bluestone and McGahee 1962). Some have referred to a "death row phenomenon" or "death row syndrome" characterized by mental and physical deterioration (Hudson 2000), although this purported syndrome has not yet been adequately studied. One study called attention to the "destruction of spirit, undermining of sanity, and mental trauma" ("Mental Suffering Under Sentence of Death" 1972). The phenomenon is believed to be related to the environmental and emotional conditions of life on death row, the length of time spent on death row, and the stress of awaiting one's own execution (Hudson 2000). Other factors, such as sensory deprivation, harassment, and social isolation, may also play a role (Cunningham and Vigen 2002).

Treating psychiatrists may encounter death row inmates experiencing overwhelming fear, helplessness, recurrent depression, and self-mutilation (Blank 2006; Cunningham and Vigen 2002; "Mental Suffering Under Sentence of Death" 1972). Like other supermax conditions, the conditions of confinement on death row may also aggravate existing mental disorders (Cunningham and Vigen 2002). Well-designed studies of psychiatric disorders on death row are lacking. However, death row inmates have invariably been convicted of some type of murder. In a study of 95 persons with severe mental illness (not on death row) who had been convicted of murder, almost three-quarters were found to have a mood disorder (Matejkowski et al. 2008). Some early studies, such as that by Lewis et al. (1986), have suggested that death row inmates may have an increased likelihood of having experienced closed head injuries, although the Lewis et al. study has been criticized as having methodological shortcomings. Death row inmates may be intellectually impaired and often have developmental histories of trauma and substance abuse (Cunningham and Vigen 2002). Treating psychiatrists should also be aware that the suicide rate of male death row inmates was found to be approximately five times higher than the rate among men in the community (Lester and Tartaro 2002). Most research indicates that the majority of death row inmates do not exhibit violence in prison, even after they were released to more open institutional settings (Cunningham and Vigen 2002).

Another phenomenon not uncommonly seen on death row is an inmate who voluntarily waives appeals in an effort to hasten the execution. The motivations of these so-called volunteers may be rooted in depression, resentment, or simple demoralization. On the other hand, some may choose to waive their appeals to avoid the long delay before the inevitable. Between 1976 and 2003, of those executed in the United States,

10% were volunteers (Blank 2006). Whether the death row phenomenon represents a legitimate mental disorder or simply the demoralization of a "morbid existential distress" is not yet clear (Schwartz 2005). When a treating psychiatrist notices this behavior in a death row inmate, it may signal the need for an independent consultation or evaluation of the inmate's competence to be executed. One of us (Knoll) helped evaluate the competence to be executed of a death row volunteer who had been brutally beaten by his death row peers during routine movement of death row inmates, because they feared that the volunteer's actions would hasten their own executions.

CONCLUSION

Despite the many disadvantages associated with providing mental health services to inmates in supermax confinement, such efforts are indispensable and have the potential to be professionally gratifying. Prior to confinement in the most restrictive and isolative part of the correctional system, mentally ill inmates in supermax settings have repeatedly been declared a failure and written off by family, the educational system, the public mental health system, the private health care sector, the juvenile justice system, and, finally, the adult criminal justice system.

Mental health providers who work in supermax units should take solace that their work is vitally important because they are often the last hope for inmates caught in a downward spiral of psychiatric illness and criminality. To attain any level of treatment success in this challenging setting can be very rewarding. All correctional mental health clinicians who dedicate time and effort to this underserved population should be rightfully proud of their accomplishments.

Mental health staff choosing to work on death row function in an ethically, morally, and emotionally complex environment. Careful attention to ethical guidelines and clear separation between treatment and forensic evaluative roles are critical. Ultimately, conscientious use of consultation and/or supervision with colleagues is both prudent and likely to help resolve the many ethical and moral dilemmas encountered.

SUMMARY POINTS

- Supermax units are designed to provide the highest level of security precautions.
- Supermax confinement is a form of prolonged solitary confinement with severe privilege restrictions.

- Prolonged supermax confinement is potentially psychologically harmful and has significant potential for exacerbating mental illness.
- Offenders with mental illness are often placed in supermax units due to behavior caused by mental illness.
- Significant barriers exist to providing adequate mental health treatment to segregated offenders.
- Inmates whose unruly conduct is caused by mental illness should receive psychiatric treatment and not be placed in supermax facilities.
- All inmates in supermax confinement should be monitored for signs of mental deterioration.
- Offenders with mental illness in supermax should be afforded multidisciplinary treatment via a team approach.
- Supermax inmates who engage in self-injurious behavior require comprehensive evaluation without reflexive presumption of malingering.
- Offenders with serious mental illness in supermax confinement should be afforded secure psychiatric hospitalization based on clinical need alone.
- After psychiatric hospitalization, inmates should not be placed back into supermax confinement unless adequate mental health treatment is available.
- Maximum security residential treatment is a valuable resource in the care and management of inmates with mental illness presenting a security risk.
- Treatment of death row inmates demands that psychiatrists function in a highly complex ethical arena.
- Treatment and forensic evaluative roles on death row must be clearly distinguished.
- A treating psychiatrist should never offer a forensic opinion on a patient's competence to be executed.
- Psychiatrists should never treat an inmate for the purpose of restoring competence to be executed.
- Inmates living on death row are vulnerable to mental and emotional distress.
- Confinement on death row may aggravate preexisting mental disorders.
- The suicide rate of male death row inmates is five times higher than in the community.

REFERENCES

American Academy of Psychiatry and the Law: Death penalty. 2001. Available at: http://www.aapl.org/positions.htm. Accessed April 15, 2009.

American Medical Association's Council on Ethical and Judicial Affairs: Physician Participation in Capital Punishment (adopted as CEJA opinion 2.06). Chicago, American Medical Association, 1992

American Medical Association's Council on Ethical and Judicial Affairs: Physician participation in capital punishment: evaluations of prisoner competence to be executed: treatment to restore competence to be executed (CEJA Report 6-A-95). House of Delegates Proceedings of 144th annual meeting, June 18–22, 1995

American Psychiatric Association: Psychiatric Services in Jails and Prisons: A Task Force Report of the American Psychiatric Association, 2nd Edition. Washington, DC, American Psychiatric Association, 2000

American Psychiatric Association: Practice Guidelines for the Treatment of Psychiatric Disorders: Compendium 2002. Washington, DC, American Psychiatric Association, 2002

Anderson v Coughlin, N.D. N.Y. (1987)

Arehart-Treichel J: NASA addresses mental health of Mars-mission members. Psychiatr News, February 2002, p 5

Arrigo BA, Bullock JL: The psychological effects of solitary confinement on prisoners in supermax units: reviewing what we know and recommending what should change. Int J Offender Ther Comp Criminol 52:622–640, 2008

Atherton E: Incapacitation with a purpose. Corrections 63:100–103, 2001

Atkins v Virginia, 536 U.S. 304 (2002)

Bandes S: The heart has its reasons: examining the strange persistence of the American death penalty. Studies in Law, Politics and Society 42:3–51, 2008

Baumeister R: Suicide as escape from self. Psychol Rev 97:90–113, 1990

Baumeister R, DeWall C, Ciarocco N, et al: Social exclusion impairs self-regulation. J Pers Soc Psychol 88:589–604, 2005

Beven G: Offenders with mental illnesses in maximum and supermaximum security settings, in Handbook of Correctional Mental Health. Edited by Scott CL, Gerbasi JB. Washington, DC, American Psychiatric Publishing, 2005, pp 209–228

Beven G, Holland A, Sipes W: Psychological support for U.S. astronauts on the International Space Station. Aviat Space Environ Med 79:1124, 2008

Blank S: Killing time: the process of waiving appeal: the Michael Ross death penalty cases. Journal of Law and Social Policy 14:735–749, 2006

Bluestone H, McGahee C: Reaction to extreme stress: impending death by execution. Am J Psychol 119:393–396, 1962

Bonner R: Rethinking suicide prevention and manipulative behavior in corrections. Jail Suicide/Mental Health Update 10:7–8, 2001

Bonnie R: Healing-killing conflicts: medical ethics and the death penalty. Hastings Center Report, May/June 1990

Boots D, Cochran J, Heide K: Capital punishment preferences for special offender populations. J Crim Justice 31:553–565, 2003

Briggs C, Sundt J, Castellano T: The effect of supermaximum security prisons on aggregate levels of institutional violence. Criminology 41:1341–1378, 2003

Buckley PF, Hrouda DR, Friedman L, et al: Insight and its relationship to violent behavior in patients with schizophrenia. Am J Psychiatry 161:1712–1714, 2004

Burns KA: Jail diversion and correctional psychotropic medication formularies, in Management and Administration of Correctional Health Care. Edited by Moore J. Kingston, NJ, Civic Research Institute, 2003, pp 13-1–13-13

Burns K: The red zone: boundaries of clinical vs. forensic work in correctional settings, in Correctional Psychiatry: Practice Guidelines and Strategies. Edited by Thienhaus O, Piasecki M. Kingston, NJ, Civic Research Institute, 2007

California v Anderson, 493 P.2d 880 (Cal. 1972)

Camp C, Camp G: Corrections Yearbook 2001: Adult Systems. Middletown, CT, Criminal Justice Institute, 2001

Christianson S: Notorious Prisons: An Inside Look at the World's Most Feared Institutions. Guilford, CT, Lyons Press, 2004

Cloyes K, Lovell D, Allen D, et al: Assessment of psychosocial impairment in a supermaximum security unit sample. Crim Justice Behav 33:760–781, 2006

Cohen F: Legal Issues and the Mentally Disordered Prisoner. Washington, DC, National Institute of Corrections, 1988

Cohen F: Isolation in penal settings: the isolation-restraint paradigm. Washington University Journal of Law and Policy 22:295–324, 2006

Cohen F: The Mentally Disordered Inmate and the Law, Volumes I and II, 2nd Edition. Kingston, NJ, Civic Research Institute, 2008

Condelli WS, Dvoskin JA, Holanchock H: Intermediate care programs for inmates with psychiatric disorders. Bull Am Acad Psychiatry Law 22:63–70, 1994

Cook F: Through the First Antarctic Night—Centennial Edition. Pittsburgh, PA, Polar Publishing, Frederick A Cook Society, 1998. (Original work published 1900)

Cunningham M, Vigen M: Death row inmate characteristics, adjustment, and confinement: a critical review of the literature. Behav Sci Law 20:191–210, 2002

Deitchman M, Kennedy W, Beckham J: Self-selection factors in the participation of mental health professionals in competency for execution evaluations. Law Hum Behav 15:287–299, 1991

District Attorney for Suffolk District v Watson, 411 N.E. 2d 1274 (Mass. 1980)

Dvoskin JA, Petrila J, Stark-Riemer S: Powell v. Coughlin and the application of the professional judgment rule to prison mental health. Mental and Physical Disability Law Reporter 19:108–114, 1995

Eshem S, Hasan A, Beven G: New treatment modality in a maximum security prison: administrative control unit for the seriously mentally ill. Correctional Mental Health Report 2:90–92, 2001

Ferrier RM: An atypical and significant hardship: the supermax confinement of death row prisoners based purely on status—a plea for procedural due process. Ariz Law Rev 46:291–315, 2004

Ford v Wainwright, 477 U.S. 399 (1986)

Furman v Georgia, 408 U.S. 238, 288 (1972)

Grassian S: Psychopathological effects of solitary confinement. Am J Psychiatry 140:1450–1454, 1983

Grassian S, Friedman N: Effects of sensory deprivation in psychiatric seclusion and solitary confinement. Int J Law Psychiatry 8:49–65, 1986

Gregg v Georgia, 428 U.S. 153, 188 (1976)

Gunderson E: Emotional symptoms in extremely isolated groups. Arch Gen Psychiatry 9:362–368, 1963

Gunderson E, Nelson P: Adaptation of small groups to extreme environments. Aerosp Med 34:1111–1115, 1963

Haddad J: Treatment for inmates with serious mental illness who require specialized placement but not psychiatric hospitalization. Correctional Mental Health Report 1:49–62, 1999

Haney C: Mental health issues in long-term solitary and "supermax" confinement. Crime Delinq 49:124–156, 2003

Haney C, Lynch M: Regulating prisons of the future: a psychological analysis of supermax and solitary confinement. Rev Law Soc Change 23:477–570, 1997

Harrington SPM: Caging the crazy: "supermax" confinement under attack. Humanist 57:14–20, 1997

Holton SMB: Managing and treating mentally disordered offenders in jails and prisons, in Correctional Mental Health Handbook. Edited by Fagan TJ, Ax RK. Thousand Oaks, CA, Sage, 2003, pp 101–122

Hudson P: Does the death row phenomenon violate a prisoner's rights under international law? European Journal of International Law 11:833–856, 2000

Human Rights Watch: Cold storage: super-maximum security confinement in Indiana. 1997. Available at: http://www.hrw.org/legacyreports/1997/usind. Accessed April 15, 2009.

Human Rights Watch: Out of sight: super-maximum security confinement in the United States. February 2000. Available at: http://www.hrw.org/legacyreports/2000/supermax. Accessed April 15, 2009.

Hyatt-Williams A: Cruelty, Violence and Murder: Understanding the Criminal Mind. Northvale, NJ, Jason Aronson, 1998

In re Medley, 134 U.S. 160 (1890)

Ivanoff A, Jang S: The role of hopelessness and social desirability in predicting suicidal behavior: a study of prison inmates. J Consult Clin Psychol 59:394–399, 1991

James DJ, Glaze LE: Mental health problems of prison and jail inmates (NCJ 213600). Washington, DC, U.S. Department of Justice, Bureau of Justice Statistics, 2006

Jones'El v Berge, 164 F.Supp. 2d 1096, 1101–1102 (W.D. Wis. 2001)

Kanas N: Asthenia: does it exist? (abstract) Aviat Space Environ Med 71:271, 2000

Kanas N, Manzey D: Space Psychology and Psychiatry. El Segundo, CA, Microcosm Press, 2008

Koch v Lewis, 216 F.Supp. 2d 994 (D. Ariz. 2001)

Korn R: The effects of confinement in the high security unit at Lexington. Soc Justice 15:8–20, 1988

Kozerenko OP, Kozlovskaya IB, Grigoriev AI: Psychological support in long-term space flights (abstract). Aviat Space Environ Med 71:349, 2000

Krelstein M: The role of mental health in the inmate disciplinary process: a national survey. J Am Acad Psychiatry Law 30:488–496, 2002

Kupers T: Prison Madness: The Mental Health Crisis Behind Bars and What We Must Do About It. San Francisco, CA, Jossey-Bass, 1999

Lackey v Scott, 885 F.Supp. 958 (W.D. Tex. 1995)

Lackey v Texas, 514 U.S. 1045, 1422 (1995)

Leong G, Silva J, Weinstock R, et al: Survey of forensic psychiatrists on evaluation and treatment of prisoners on death row. J Am Acad Psychiatry Law 28:427–432, 2000

Lester D, Tartaro C: Suicide on death row. J Forensic Sci 47:1108–1111, 2002

Lewis D, Pincus J, Feldman M, et al: Psychiatric, neurological and psychoeducational characteristics of 15 death row inmates in the United States. Am J Psychiatry 143:838–845, 1986

Linenger J: Off the Planet: Surviving Five Perilous Months Aboard the Space Station Mir. New York, McGraw-Hill Professional, 2000

Lovell D, Cloyes K, Allen D, et al: Who lives in super maximum custody? A Washington State study. Fed Probat 64:33–43, 2000

Lovell D, Allen D, Johnson C, et al: Evaluating the effectiveness of residential treatment for prisoners with mental illness. Crim Justice Behav 28:83–104, 2001

Madrid v Gomez, 889 F.Supp. 1146 (N.D. Cal. 1995)

Matejkowski J, Cullen S, Solomon P: Characteristics of persons with severe mental illness who have been incarcerated for murder. J Am Acad Psychiatry Law 36:74–86, 2008

Matthews D, Wendler S: Ethical issues in the evaluation and treatment of death row inmates. Curr Opin Psychiatry 19:518–521, 2006

Mears D: An assessment of supermax prisons using an evaluation research framework. Prison J 88:43–68, 2008

Mears D, Castro J: Wardens' views on the wisdom of supermax prisons. Crime Delinq 52:398–431, 2006

Mears D, Watson J: Towards a fair and balanced assessment of supermax prisons. Justice Quarterly 23:232–270, 2006

Mental suffering under sentence of death: a cruel and unusual punishment. Iowa Law Rev 57:814–833, 1972

Metzner JL: An introduction to correctional psychiatry, part II. J Am Acad Psychiatry Law 25:571–579, 1997

Metzner JL: An introduction to correctional psychiatry, part III. J Am Acad Psychiatry Law 26:107–114, 1998

Metzner JL: Class action litigation in correctional psychiatry. J Am Acad Psychiatry Law 30:19–29, 2002a

Metzner J: Commentary: the role of mental health in the inmate disciplinary process. J Am Acad Psychiatry Law 30:497–499, 2002b

Metzner JL: Trends in correctional mental health care, in Management and Administration of Correctional Health Care. Edited by Moore J. Kingston, NJ, Civic Research Institute, 2003, pp 12-2–12-18

Miller H, Young G: Prison segregation: administrative detention remedy or mental health problem? Crim Behav Ment Health 7:85–94, 1997

National Commission on Correctional Health Care: Standards for Health Services in Prisons. Chicago, National Commission on Correctional Health Care, 1997

National Commission on Correctional Health Care: Correctional Health Care: Guidelines for the Management of an Adequate Delivery System. Chicago, National Commission on Correctional Health Care, 2001

National Commission on Correctional Health Care: Correctional Mental Health Care: Standards and Guidelines for Delivering Services. Chicago, National Commission on Correctional Health Care, 2003

National Institute of Corrections: Supermax housing: a survey of current practice. Special Issues in Corrections, March 1997. Available at: http://www.nicic.org/pubs/1997/013722.pdf. Accessed April 15, 2009.

Office of Mental Health: Confidential tier III testimony checklist (outpatient), in Outpatient Operations Policy & Procedure Manual. Albany, New York State Office of Mental Health, June 2006

Palinkas LA, Gunderson EKE, Holland AW, et al: Predictors of behavior and performance in extreme environments: the Antarctic space analogue program. Aviat Space Environ Med 71:619–625, 2000

Panetti v Quarterman, 551 U.S. 930 (2007)

Pen J, Esposito C, Schaeffer L, et al: Suicide attempts and self-mutilative behavior in a juvenile correctional facility. J Am Acad Child Adolesc Psychiatry 42:762–769, 2003

Petrovsky AV, Yaroshevsky MG: A Concise Psychological Dictionary. Moscow, Progress Publishers, 1987

Pizarro J, Narag R: Supermax prisons: what we know, what we do not know, and where we are going. Prison J 88:23–42, 2008

Pizarro J, Stenius V: Supermax prisons: their rise, current practices, and effect on inmates. Prison J 84:248–264, 2004

Powell v Coughlin, 953 F.2d 744, 750 (2d Cir. 1991)

Prison suicide increase: isolation the culprit. Correctional Mental Health Report 8(6):87, 2007

Rayford BS, Trestman RL: The intensive mental health unit in Connecticut's Department of Correction: a model treatment program. The Psychiatric Times 19(suppl):2–3, 2002

Rhodes L: Psychopathy and the face of control in supermax. Ethnography 3:442–466, 2002

Rhodes L: Pathological effects of the supermaximum prison. Am J Public Health 95:1692–1695, 2005

Rhodes L: Supermax as a technology of punishment. Soc Res (New York) 74:547–566, 2007

Riveland C: Supermax Prisons: Overview and General Considerations. Washington, DC, National Institute of Corrections, 1999

Roper v Simmons, 543 U.S. 551 (2005)

Rothblum E: Psychological factors in the Antarctic. J Psychol 124:253–273, 1990

Sandin v Conner, 515 U.S. 472, 486 (1995)

Schwartz H: Death row syndrome and demoralization: psychiatric means to social policy ends. J Am Acad Psychiatry Law 33:153–155, 2005

Scott C: Psychiatry and the death penalty. Psychiatr Clin North Am 29:791–804, 2006

Scott E, Grisso T: The evolution of adolescence: a developmental perspective on juvenile justice reform. J Crim Law Criminol 88:137–189, 1997

Sipes W, Vanderark S: Operational behavioral health and performance resources for International Space Station crews and families. Aviat Space Environ Med 76(suppl):B36–B41, 2005

Snell TL: Capital punishment, 2005 (NCJ 215083). Washington, DC, U.S. Department of Justice, Bureau of Justice Statistics, December 2006

Sowell E, Thompson P, Tessner K, et al: Mapping continued brain growth and gray matter density reduction in dorsal frontal cortex: inverse relationships during postadolescent brain maturation. J Neurosci 15:8819–8829, 2001

Stanford v Kentucky, 492 U.S. 361 (1989)

State v Perry, 608 So.2d 594 (La. 1992)

Thompson v Oklahoma, 487 U.S. 815 (1988)

Toch H: The future of supermax confinement. Prison J 81:376–388, 2001

Toch H, Adams K: Pathology and disruptiveness among prison inmates. Journal of Research in Crime and Delinquency 23:7–21, 1986

Turner v Safley, 482 U.S. 78 (1987)

Twenge J, Catanese K, Baumeister R: Social exclusion and the deconstructed state: time perception, meaninglessness, lethargy, lack of emotion, and self-awareness. J Pers Soc Psychol 85:409–423, 2005

Way B, Sawyer D, Barboza S, et al: Inmate suicide and time spent in special disciplinary housing in New York State prison. Psychiatr Serv 58:558–560, 2007

Wilkinson v Austin, 545 U.S. 209 (2005)

Wolff v McDonnell, 418 U.S. 539, 556 (1974)

CHAPTER 17

Female Offenders in Correctional Settings

Catherine F. Lewis, M.D.

$\mathbf{A}$t the end of 2007, more than 2.2 million people were incarcerated in prisons or jails in the United States. Even though women represent the majority of the general population (51.6%), the overwhelming majority of these inmates were male (82.3%) (Greenfeld and Snell 1999; West and Sabol 2008). It is not surprising, then, that existing policy, treatment, and programming within correctional systems have been derived predominantly from research and experience with male offenders (Lewis 2006).

The rate of incarceration for women rose more rapidly than that for men from 2000 to 2006 (3.2% vs. 2.7%), and women are being arrested for more serious offenses than in the past (West and Sabol 2008). Felony arrests for women increased substantially during the years associated with the "war on drugs"—specifically, 10% of incarcerated women were arrested on a drug-related offense in 1980; this number skyrocketed to 33% by 2000 (Beck and Stephen 1999). As a result of these trends, increased numbers of women with substance use disorders and drug charges are in state jails and prisons.

Women and men differ in both their likelihood to offend and their patterns of offending. A significant if not the major risk factor for overall crime is male gender; men are arrested more often than women for every offense other than prostitution, running away, and embezzlement. The difference in offense patterns is particularly striking for violent crimes, in which men are perpetrators in 85% of cases; women account for one in 20 assaults, one in 10 aggravated assaults and murders, and one in 50 sexual assaults (Greenfeld and Snell 1999). Women are more likely than men to have opposite-gender accomplices and to victimize people they know; in two-thirds of homicides committed by women, the victim is an intimate or relative, whereas in three-quarters of homicides committed by men, the victim is an acquaintance or stranger (Fox and Zavitz 2004; Greenfeld and Snell 1999).

When women do offend, they are likely to commit nonviolent offenses such as prostitution, drug possession, and larceny (Lewis 2006). Perhaps because of the less violent nature of their offenses, the majority of women with criminal justice involvement in the United States are in supervised placements in the community (Beck and Stephen 1999). The differences in criminal behavior prevalence and patterns of offending between the sexes beg the question, "Who are the women who end up incarcerated?" In this chapter, I explore that question while outlining treatment strategies for female offenders.

Incarcerated women are a socioeconomically disadvantaged, vulnerable group with substantial physical and mental health needs. They have often experienced breakdown of their family units, as well as social isolation and economic hardship. Although slightly more than half of incarcerated women are high school graduates, they are less likely than their male counterparts to be employed at the time of their arrest and are more likely to have income of less than $600 per month or to be on welfare (Greenfeld and Snell 1999). Before incarceration, women more commonly live at or below the poverty level, despite being responsible for single-family households (Glaze and Maruschak 2008; Greenfeld and Snell 1999).

Most female state prisoners are minorities (33% white, 48% black, 15% Hispanic) in the reproductive age group and have never been married (Greenfeld and Snell 1999). The majority (70%) of these women have minor children; the average number of minor children per female inmate in state prison is 2.4 (Brooks 1993). Immediately before incarceration, women were more likely than men to live with their children, be a primary caretaker for their children, or be the head of a household. Currently, in the United States, more than 65,000 children have mothers who are incarcerated. The rate of incarceration of mothers has risen more than 120% since 1991, while that of fathers has risen only 77% (Glaze and Maruschak 2008). Clearly, parenthood is a major issue to be considered in caring for incarcerated women.

A past history of abuse or victimization, particularly in childhood, is more common for women than men in the correctional system. Childhood victimization, especially sexual abuse, is associated with psychiatric morbidity in adulthood, including major depression, suicide attempts, substance dependence, increased risky behavior, posttraumatic stress disorder (PTSD), and other anxiety disorders (Brodsky et al. 2001). Childhood victimization may be specifically associated with female criminality. One prevailing theory suggests that female criminality is based on the need to survive abuse and poverty, coupled with substance dependence (Steffensmeier and Allen 1996). Trauma history, substance dependence, limited socioeconomic resources, and externalizing behavior together result in "spiraling marginality" marked by a decline in functioning. Despite difficulties with past trauma, addiction, and mental and physical health problems, most women entering the correctional system do not have medical insurance at the time of their arrest (Henderson 1998; Smith 1993). Treatment has been sparse and often has had limited effect on behavior.

Research on incarcerated women has been a neglected area (Singer et al. 1995) for several reasons, including that women are a minority of all offenders, accounting for less violent crime, and perhaps that women tend to be given a lower priority for access to services and for research (Rasche 1974). The recent surge in arrests of women has caused clinicians, policymakers, and researchers to examine the treatment needs of female offenders more closely. A consensus is emerging that incarcerated women have treatment needs that differ from those of incarcerated men or nonincarcerated women. Research on treatment of incarcerated women is in its infancy. In this chapter, I discuss issues of specific relevance to incarcerated women and implications for mental health treatment in the correctional system.

EPIDEMIOLOGY OF PSYCHIATRIC DISORDERS IN INCARCERATED WOMEN

Existing research on incarcerated women suggests that women arriving in the correctional system are far more likely to have psychiatric disorders than their male counterparts (DiCataldo et al. 1995; Maden et al. 1994; Teplin et al. 1996). An estimated one-third to two-thirds of women entering correctional facilities require mental health treatment (American Correctional Association 1990; Guy et al. 1985; Singer et al. 1995; Teplin et al. 1997), and about one-fifth arrive at correctional facilities with a history of taking psychotropic medication (Beck 1993). Women use more psychiatric services than men while incarcerated (Maden et al.

1994; Steadman et al. 1991) and are extremely likely to have comorbid substance-related diagnoses and Axis I or Axis II psychopathology (Jordan et al. 1996; Lewis 2006; Singer et al. 1995; Warren et al. 2002b).

In a study of 1,272 female jail detainees, Teplin et al. (1996) used the Diagnostic Interview Schedule for DSM-III-R (DIS; Robins et al. 1981, 1988) to assess psychopathology. The study assessed 6-month and lifetime prevalence of a variety of psychiatric disorders, including PTSD, antisocial personality disorder (ASPD), schizophrenia, mania, panic disorder, generalized anxiety disorder, major depression, and drug or alcohol abuse/dependence. A comparison of Teplin et al.'s results with the results of three other studies, including the National Comorbidity Survey (Kessler et al. 1994, 1995), is given in Table 17–1. In the Teplin et al. sample, a high percentage of women (80%) met criteria for a lifetime psychiatric disorder, and the majority (70%) had psychiatric symptoms at the time of incarceration. The most common diagnoses included drug abuse/ dependence, alcohol abuse/dependence, and PTSD.

Jordan et al. (1996) studied newly convicted female felons in North Carolina, using the Composite International Diagnostic Interview (Robins et al. 1981, 1988) supplemented with the DIS for assessment of ASPD. The study assessed disorders including major depression, ASPD, borderline personality disorder (BPD), drug or alcohol abuse/dependence, and dysthymia. The study also assessed exposure to extreme traumatic events via a survey instrument used in a past national study of the prevalence of rape (Resnick et al. 1993), and reported a prevalence of PTSD based on inmate report of symptoms. The results of this study appear in Table 17–1. Jordan et al. (1996) found a high prevalence of psychopathology in the sample, with highest lifetime prevalence for drug and alcohol abuse/ dependence, PTSD, major depressive disorder, and ASPD. Six-month prevalence of BPD was also high (data not shown in Table 17–1).

Lewis (2006) examined a sample of 136 sentenced female felons in Connecticut, using the Semi-Structured Assessment for the Genetics of Alcoholism (Bucholz et al. 1994). Unlike the earlier studies by Jordan et al. (1996) and Teplin et al. (1996), Lewis's study differentiated drug and alcohol abuse from dependence and reported lifetime prevalence for dependence for a variety of drugs. As shown in Table 17–1, Lewis (2006) found high lifetime prevalence of alcohol and drug dependence, major depressive disorder, PTSD, and ASPD. The most common drugs of dependence were cocaine (49%) and heroin (35.7%). More than half of the women were dependent on more than one substance and had comorbid Axis I and Axis II psychopathology. The prevalence of ASPD, although higher than that for newly incarcerated female felons reported by Teplin et al. (1996), is consistent with other recent studies of female felons (Zlotnick 1997).

TABLE 17–1. Lifetime prevalence of psychiatric diagnoses in female offenders (in percentages)

Disorder	Teplin et al. 1996[a] (N=1,272)	Jordan et al. 1996[b] (N=805)	Lewis 2006[c] (N=136)	National Comorbidity Survey (Kessler et al. 1994, 1995)[d]
Schizophrenia	1.4	—	2.4	0.8
Mania	2.4	—	4.1	1.7
Major depressive disorder	16.9	13.0	36.2	21.3
Dysthymia	9.6	7.1	4.6	8.0
Substance abuse/dependence	70.2	—	65.4	—
Alcohol abuse	32.3	38.0	22.3	6.4
Alcohol dependence	—	—	43.8	8.2
Drug abuse	63.6	44.2	14.0	3.5
Drug dependence	—	—	56.6	5.9
Panic disorder	1.6	5.8	3.8	5.0
Generalized anxiety disorder	2.5	2.7	5.4	6.6
Posttraumatic stress disorder	33.5	30.0	40.8	10.4
Antisocial personality disorder	13.8	11.9	32.3	1.2

Note. — = not reported.
[a]Newly admitted female felons.
[b]Female jail detainees.
[c]Female felons serving sentence.
[d]National sample of women in community (N>9,000).

These three studies, drawn from three different populations and using different assessment instruments and methods of recruitment, suggest that psychopathology among female incarcerated offenders is high regardless of whether they are in jail, are new arrivals to prison, or are in the midst of their prison terms. Lifetime prevalence of drug abuse/dependence, alcohol abuse/dependence, PTSD, ASPD, and major depression is significantly elevated in female inmates. The high prevalence of comorbidity among incarcerated women suggests that psychiatric treatment may be challenging. The difference in prevalence of psychiatric psychopathology from the women in the National Comorbidity Survey (Kessler et al. 1994, 1995, 1997) indicates that approaches to the treatment of psychiatric disorders in incarcerated women may need to differ from approaches to psychiatric disorders in women in the general population.

PSYCHIATRIC DISORDERS AND BEHAVIORS IN CORRECTIONAL SETTINGS

Substance Abuse and Dependence

Epidemiology

Prevalence of substance dependence is extraordinarily high in female offenders (Jordan et al. 1996; Kessler et al. 1994, 1995, 1997; Lewis 2006; Teplin et al. 1996). Although the prevalence rate of substance dependence for women in the community is far below that for men, the difference begins to erode in the correctional population. Figure 17–1 highlights the prevalence rates of substance dependence in community and incarcerated samples of men and women.

In the National Comorbidity Survey, a large community-based sample, only 8.2% of women had alcohol dependence, but between one-third and one-half of the incarcerated female population was alcohol dependent; similarly, although only 5.9% of women in the community were drug dependent, a majority of incarcerated women had a diagnosis of drug dependence (Jordan et al. 1996; Lewis 2006; Teplin et al. 1996). In Lewis's (2006) study, which used strict criteria for identifying substance dependence versus abuse, the prevalence of alcohol dependence among incarcerated women approached that of incarcerated men (43.8% vs. 51.1%), and the prevalence of drug use by incarcerated women exceeded that by incarcerated men (56.6% vs. 32.4%). These numbers are striking and suggest that with respect to prevalence and severity of substance dependence, incarcerated women may be a group quite distinct from women and even men in the community.

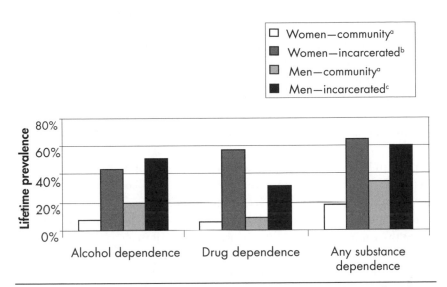

FIGURE 17–1. Gender difference in substance dependence disorders.

[a]Kessler et al. 1997; [b]Lewis 2006; [c]Teplin et al. 1996.

Alcohol. Alcohol dependence has significant implications for the health of female inmates. Women who are dependent on alcohol are likely to develop physical sequelae sooner than men (Ashley et al. 1977; Schuckit et al. 1995). These sequelae include cirrhosis, hypertension, obesity, anemia, fatty liver, and malnutrition. Some sequelae (e.g., cervical cancer, HIV), although not directly caused by alcohol use, are likely related to lifestyle issues (e.g., comorbid substance abuse, including nicotine; promiscuity). Alcohol use increases the likelihood of fetal alcohol syndrome, domestic violence, and marital dissolution, negative sequelae that affect future generations (Anda et al. 1988; Greenfeld 1998). Alcohol dependence also worsens the prognosis for women with other psychiatric disorders, including major depression (Drake et al. 1996; Hesselbrock et al. 1985; Kranzler et al. 1996). Women with alcohol dependence are more likely than men to develop dependence on other substances and to have comorbid non-substance-related psychiatric disorders (Kessler et al. 1997; Regier et al. 1990). These women tend to attribute difficulties to drug use rather than to alcohol use, which renders treatment difficult (Weisner and Schmidt 1992). Finally, alcohol use has been linked to recidivism and reincarceration, violent behavior including suicide and homicide, poverty, and unemployment (Greenfeld 1998).

Drugs. Women differ from men in their patterns of addiction to illegal drugs. They most commonly are introduced to substance use by men

(Daly 1994; Lex 1995), and their partners are likely to use drugs. Whereas men use drugs for hedonistic reasons, women tend to use drugs for escapist reasons, such as numbing and comfort (Amaro 1995). Female drug abusers have more positive family history for alcohol and drug use than do men and have often experienced abuse and neglect (Finkelstein et al. 1997). They also experience "telescoping" with alcohol and drug use, a phenomenon in which significant symptoms occur over a shorter period of time than in men (Blume 1990; Finkelstein et al. 1997; Nespor 1990).

Women who are incarcerated are more likely than their male counterparts to have used drugs in the months preceding their incarceration. Sixty percent of women entering the correctional system used drugs in the month before arrest, half used daily, and 40% were using at the time of their offense (Greenfeld and Snell 1999). Female inmates are more likely than male inmates to be intravenous drug users (Hammett et al. 1999), to have partners who are intravenous drug users (Schilling et al. 1994), and to smoke rather than snort cocaine (Grella 1996; Wilsnack et al. 1997). Intravenous drug use is linked to physical illness, including hepatitis C and HIV, and psychiatric disorders, including alcohol dependence, major depression, and ASPD (Dinwiddie et al. 1992; Rounsaville et al. 1982).

Drug-addicted women are more likely than drug-addicted men to experience socioeconomic hardship and to prostitute to get money for drugs (Guyon et al. 1999). Addiction is closely linked to criminality in both men and women and is associated with a more serious criminal record, an earlier age at onset of criminality, and more HIV risk behaviors (Guyon et al. 1999). A higher percentage of female arrestees versus male arrestees use "hard" drugs (heroin, cocaine) and have at least one other mental health disorder (Wellisch et al. 1994). Possibly, the emphasis on drug-related offenses by the criminal justice system is actually pushing psychiatrically impaired women into the correctional system (Chesney-Lind 1998).

Treatment Issues

Given the higher likelihood of addiction with psychiatric illness, socioeconomic hardship, and history of trauma among incarcerated women versus men, women would likely benefit from treatment structured for their specific needs. Use of drugs and alcohol by women is generally less socially acceptable than use by men; this can lead to reluctance to identify addictive problems, punitive or negative attitudes toward the female substance abuser, and treatment that fails to address addiction. Treatment may fail because it focuses on mental health issues and excludes the issue of substance dependence (e.g., when a woman identifies herself as only a trauma survivor rather than an addict who has been traumatized) (Chasnoff 1989). Women are more likely than men to seek treatment when having problems with addiction, but they are less likely to receive addiction-specific treatment; most of the time they get treatment for other mental health–related issues (Green-Hennessy 2002; Weisner and Schmidt 1992). The failure to adequately address substance dependence is associated with relapse, decreased treatment compliance, and poorer overall treatment outcomes.

Cognitive-behavioral therapy and interpersonal therapy have been found more effective than other types of therapy in the treatment of addiction in female offenders. Several studies offer evidence of the value of cognitive-behavioral therapy in incarcerated populations. Peters et al. (1997) studied 435 female and 1,220 male detainees in a Florida jail who underwent a 6-week substance abuse program. Compared with men, women had significantly more extensive drug use, psychiatric histories, and trauma histories, as well as more past suicide attempts. Peters et al. reported that 12-step programs, with their emphasis on personal accountability and abstinence, were potentially damaging to traumatized women, who experienced the groups as demoralizing and overwhelming. They recommended the use of cognitive-behavioral interventions aimed at enhancing self-esteem and social functioning.

In a study of 1,326 male and 318 female federal prisoners who volunteered for a 12-month residential program, Langan and Pelissier (2001) concurred with previous authors' assessment that addicted incarcerated women's needs were not getting met by traditionally male programs (Miller 1984; Wellisch et al. 1993). Like Peters et al. (1997), Langan and Pelissier (2001) observed that compared with men, women used harder drugs; used drugs more often; and had more educational, family, mental health, and physical problems. Langan and Pelissier stressed the need to focus on well-being rather than self-control in treating addicted women, to prevent regression and worsening of anxiety and depression during treatment. They also noted that harmful effects of alcohol should be less of a focus than recovery from trauma and empowerment for incarcerated women. Specifically, women with substance use disorders are likely to remain in negative relationships with their partners even as they try to stay abstinent (Anglin et al. 1987; Steffensmeier and Allen 1996). Treatment must therefore address interpersonal issues and issues related to reenacting past traumatic experience. Emphasis should be placed on strengthening competencies rather than emphasizing deficits (Langan and Pelissier 2001).

Cognitive-behavioral interventions at the group level offer the potential for streamlined treatment in correctional settings. In a study of male and female detainees at the Baltimore City Jail, Peyrot et al. (1994) found that a cognitive-behavioral intervention emphasizing concepts such as consequential thinking, anger management, and stress management led to better outcomes than traditional substance abuse education programs. The outcome measures involved information retained by the participants rather than long-term assessments of sobriety.

Contingency management, a therapy often paired with traditional cognitive-behavioral therapy, has been proven effective in HIV-positive, antisocial, and drug-addicted community populations (Higgins et al. 1991; Messina et al. 2003) but has had limited application in correctional settings. Further research is needed on integrated cognitive-behavioral and contingency-based treatment in secure settings.

The treatment of substance-dependent incarcerated women requires the recognition of acute medical and psychiatric issues. Detoxification should be provided when necessary, preferably in a special unit. Because of the medical sequelae of alcohol and drug dependence, women should undergo careful physical examination and testing when appropriate. Sociocultural and psychopathological issues are of critical importance to addicted incarcerated women. General clinical considerations include recognition of and sensitivity to trauma-related issues and depressive symptoms, and recognition of the importance of interpersonal relationships to sobriety for women. Treatment matching should occur (Farabee et al. 1999) such that women with the most serious dependence are placed in the most intensive treatment settings (e.g., hospital, therapeutic community) and women with less serious dependence are placed in less intensive settings. This approach is rarely taken in correctional settings, where addiction is often viewed as a yes-no phenomenon and the gradation of addictive disorders is not recognized (Farabee et al. 1999).

The therapeutic community may be the most effective mode of treatment for incarcerated women with severe addiction (De Leon 1995; Farabee et al. 1999). Therapeutic communities assist inmates with the social learning process. Once the inmate has completed the program, follow-up treatment and transition to aftercare are critical. During incarceration, motivational interviewing can be used with inmates; in other populations, motivational interviewing has been found to be more effective when more individual sessions occur during the beginning of treatment and when the success of previous program graduates is demonstrated (De Leon 1995; Miller 1984). Once an inmate has completed treatment in the therapeutic community and is released to the community or transferred to another prison unit, he or she should have continuity of care to minimize the risk of treatment dropout (Prendergast et al. 1996; Singer et al. 1995).

Treatment of underlying depressive illness is particularly important in addicted incarcerated women. This treatment has been shown to decrease relapse risk and compromise from depressive symptoms in non-incarcerated populations (Greenfield et al. 1998; Mason et al. 1996). Psychopharmacological treatment for symptoms of major depression should not be withheld because of a recent history of drug abuse or dependence. Care must be taken, however, to avoid creating iatrogenic drug dependence (e.g., benzodiazapines), given the comorbid history of addiction, and to avoid prescribing multiple medications at subtherapeutic levels. Promising work on psychopharmacological interventions to diminish craving in community samples (Kranzler et al. 1996) should be extended to prerelease incarcerated women, who would then be followed longitudinally.

Clinical Case 17–1

Ms. M, a 28-year-old mother of two, was incarcerated for armed robbery and possession of heroin and crack cocaine. Shortly after booking Ms. M, correctional officers called mental health services because she was agitated and appeared "hyper." When assessed, she said she had been drinking a quart of vodka a day and using intravenous heroin and cocaine daily up to the time of her arrest. She also said she has bipolar affective disorder but had stopped taking her medication about 10 days earlier. Ms. M recognized that she needed mental health treatment but expressed that she did not want any medication metabolized by her liver because she has hepatitis C. This was, in fact, the reason why she had stopped taking the medication previously prescribed to her. She expressed having no desire to harm herself or others but conceded that she has felt that she is "thinking too fast" and has been feeling very nervous.

This case illustrates the complexity of presentation of polysubstance-dependent women in correctional settings. The following are important considerations when treating women such as the one in the clinical example:

- Conduct a physical examination, including vital signs, to assess for signs of withdrawal. Even if no signs are present at the time of booking, the woman should be monitored for withdrawal and placed on a detoxification protocol for alcohol and heroin.
- Obtain relevant laboratory work. A liver function panel can be drawn to assess the woman's degree of liver impairment. A pregnancy test as well as HIV and hepatitis B and C testing should also be performed.

- Provide education about the risks and benefits of medication, including the possibility of using medication not metabolized by the liver or using hepatically metabolized medication at lower doses.
- Consider admission to a detoxification unit, where the woman's mental health needs, as well as her impending withdrawal, could be addressed.

Personality Disorders and Psychopathy

Epidemiology

Personality disorders are prevalent among female inmates, and comorbidity between Axis I and Axis II disorders is high. In a study of 261 female felons, Warren et al. (2002a) found, using the Structured Clinical Interview for DSM-IV Axis II Personality Disorders (SCID-II; First et al. 1997), 200 women who screened positive for Cluster B personality pathology (e.g., antisocial, borderline, histrionic, or narcissistic personality traits). The most common personality disorder was ASPD (43%), followed by paranoid personality disorder (27%) and BPD (24%). Warren et al. suggested that paranoid personality disorder may be overdiagnosed in correctional populations, because women responding affirmatively to questions targeting paranoid symptoms may, in fact, be accurately reporting reasonable feelings and experiences, given their traumatic and dangerous environments. Most women in the sample evidenced more than one personality disorder. For example, 43% of the women with ASPD also met criteria for BPD, and there was high co-occurrence between ASPD and Cluster A disorders (e.g., schizoid 54%, schizotypal 56%). An earlier study of male and female offenders (Coid 1992) found a similarly high degree of comorbidity between ASPD and BPD and a high number of mean personality disorders per offender (3.6). Coid suggested that given the high comorbidity of personality disorder diagnoses in inmates, personality pathology should be viewed as a recurring pattern of covariant traits versus a single unified diagnosis.

Despite the high comorbidity between ASPD and BPD, women with ASPD appear to have distinct characteristics. For example, Zlotnick (1999) found a strong association between poor anger modulation and ASPD, even after controlling for BPD and PTSD. This elevated state of arousal was not associated with past childhood abuse, contrary to previous reports of association of abuse with ASPD (Windle et al. 1995). Additionally, self-mutilation was not associated with ASPD in the absence of BPD.

Treatment Issues

Female inmates with severe personality pathology who attempt to harm themselves pose a unique challenge to the correctional system. *Parasui-*

cidal behavior, defined as self-harm whose intent is not death but improvement in one's emotional state (e.g., through cutting or burning), is a common problem in correctional settings for women. The Intensive Healing Program was developed by the Canadian Correctional System specifically to address parasuicidal behavior among female inmates (Roth and Presse 2003). The program uses Linehan et al.'s (1999) model for dialectical behavior therapy (DBT). The fundamental concepts associated with DBT are described in Chapter 13, "Creating Wellness Through Collaborative Mental Health Interventions."

DBT has been shown to be effective in reducing parasuicidal behavior in patients in noncorrectional populations (Alper and Peterson 2001; Linehan et al. 1999). The therapeutic environment is critical to treatment; women are housed in a specified unit where adaptive behaviors are reinforced and crisis management is readily available. Components of the program include a therapeutic community, individual counseling, group activities (e.g., anger management; DBT; relapse prevention; psychoeducation on violence, parenting, empathy), and educational and vocational training. Primary therapists are based on the inmate's housing unit, and therapeutic protocol exists to handle parasuicidal behavior. Examples of the protocol include giving no additional psychoactive medications after a parasuicidal act, making verbal contracts not to engage in self-harm, and conducting behavioral chain analysis of the incident of self-harm. Evaluation of this program with a control group has not yet been reported.

Anger management is another problem often seen in female inmates with personality disorders, particularly those with Cluster B pathology. Warren et al. (2002a) noted that the combination of narcissistic psychopathology and paranoid psychopathology seen in Cluster A disorders (e.g., paranoid, schizoid, schizotypal) may be particularly associated with violent behavior both before and during incarceration, whereas ASPD is associated with violence during incarceration. Interventions targeting anger management benefit women with affect dysregulation (Zlotnick 1999). A constant tension exists between the need for institutional sanctions and psychiatric interventions. The optimal treatment consists of collaborative efforts with custody and mental health staff. Such collaboration sets reasonable limits while ensuring physical safety and treatment of comorbid psychopathology (e.g., addiction, major depression).

ASPD has a prevalence of only 1% in women in the community, but that prevalence rises to 12% among alcoholic women (Blume 1990). It is therefore not surprising that the prevalence of ASPD is greatly elevated among female offenders, a majority of whom are substance dependent. The importance of this elevation is, at times, eclipsed by a common belief that male offenders of all types (e.g., jail, prisons, mid-sentence felons) are much more likely to have ASPD, female offenders with a history of trauma may not have ASPD, or trauma in and of itself causes ASPD. Recent studies of mid-sentence female felons, perhaps the most serious female offenders, have found a prevalence of ASPD ranging from 31% to 43% (Lewis 2006; Warren et al. 2002a; Zlotnick 1999). These data approach those of male correctional samples and cannot be ignored. ASPD is an important, prevalent diagnosis with specific implications for treatment efficacy in the correctional system. Individuals with ASPD are difficult to treat and have worse prognoses than those without. ASPD is associated with earlier onset; more severe and rapidly progressive substance dependence; polysubstance dependence; attempted or completed suicide; and poorer outcomes from treatment. Existing literature suggests that individuals with ASPD benefit more from developing coping skills than from participating in interactional treatment (Bucholz et al. 1994; Hesselbrock et al. 1988; Lewis 2006).

A related and important issue is identification of individuals with psychopathy in female correctional populations. Psychopathy is among the most robust indicators of treatment failure and recidivism among forensic populations (Hare et al. 2000; Warren et al. 2002a). Although the most commonly used measures of psychopathy are normed on men, scores consistent with psychopathy are also associated with recidivism and institutional infractions in female correctional populations. Initial work suggested that the prevalence of psychopathy was low (i.e., less than 10%) among female inmates (Hare et al. 2000; Warren et al. 2002b), but more recent studies of female felons show prevalence rates that approach those for males (15%–25%) (Warren et al. 2002a). These results suggest that a minority but significant group of female offenders may be treatment resistant and disruptive to treatment programs. This group should be identified and offered specialized programming to avoid group contagion.

Clinical Case 17–2

Ms. R, a 23-year-old single woman serving a 6-year sentence for prostitution and drug possession with the intent to distribute, was referred to mental health services by correctional officers, who reported she had been scratching herself with her fingernails until her arms and legs bled. The woman was well known to mental health staff and had been on the inpatient unit at least six times. When questioned about her symptoms, Ms. R reported feeling "empty, like a shell," "very, very sad like I wished I was gone," and "alone." She reported feeling "relaxed" and "free" when she hurts herself. She reported a history of severe childhood sexual abuse beginning at age 4. Although she said she would not mind if she died, she adamantly denied thoughts or intent to kill herself. She had a history of two suicide attempts before incarceration (by drug overdose) and one attempt (labeled a gesture by some staff members) where she placed a sheet around her neck and tied it to her bed, and then lay on her cell floor. Correctional staff felt that she was not safe in her own cell and needed mental health intervention. Mental health staff and correctional staff described her as "manipulative."

This case illustrates the nuances of dealing with a patient who self-mutilates, has a history of suicide attempts, and yet denies suicidal intent or thoughts. A challenge of a case such as this is to provide a safe environment for the patient without repeatedly hospitalizing her in the inpatient unit for brief periods in a "revolving door" scenario. Interventions that may be considered include the following:

- Transfer to a housing unit for inmates with mental illness who are not ill enough to require inpatient hospitalization. The unit would optimally have a variety of groups that could address issues such as anger management, surviving trauma, achieving abstinence from substances, and avoiding revictimization.
- Referral to a psychiatrist to consider medication to assist with depressive symptoms, impulsivity, affective lability, and anxiety.
- Enrollment in treatment involving manualized therapy such as DBT to assist in the management and treatment of symptoms related to trauma and the urge to self-harm.

Trauma and Posttraumatic Stress Disorder

Epidemiology

Incarcerated women are likely to have experienced physical abuse, sexual abuse, and exploitation before arriving at correctional facilities (Lewis 2003, 2005, 2006; Zlotnick 1997). PTSD is the most common diagnosis other than substance abuse in multiple studies involving incarcerated women (Hutton et al. 2001; Jordan et al. 1996; Lewis 2003, 2006; Teplin et al. 1996). In a study of 805 convicted felons, Jordan et al. (1996) found that 30% of the women had been exposed to trauma severe enough to cause symptoms of PTSD. In a similar study of 85 randomly selected incarcerated women, Zlotnick (1997) noted that 78%–85% of the participants had experienced at least one traumatic event and that this percentage was higher than for women in the general population (69%)

(Lake 1993; Resnick et al. 1993). Zlotnick (1997) also found high prevalence of current PTSD (48.2%) and lifetime PTSD (20%). Hutton et al. (2001) interviewed 177 female prisoners and found a 33% lifetime prevalence of PTSD and a 15% prevalence of current PTSD. Lewis (2003, 2006) found a similar prevalence of lifetime PTSD in a sample of 136 female felons but a higher prevalence of lifetime PTSD (72%) in a sample of 81 HIV-positive inmates (Lewis 2005). These findings suggest that HIV-positive incarcerated women may be a group at particular risk for PTSD.

What is clear from the existing literature is that traumatic experiences are common among incarcerated women and that the prevalence of PTSD among incarcerated women is two to three times that of women in the general population (Kessler et al. 1995). PTSD and trauma history are especially important to assess because they are associated with suicidal ideation and attempts (Brodsky et al. 2001; Kotler et al. 2001; Lewis 2006), HIV high-risk behavior (Kimmerling and Goldsmith 2000; Logan and Leukefeld 2000), and substance abuse (Brady et al. 1994; Brown et al. 1998).

The traumas experienced by incarcerated women are diverse and repetitive and occur early in their lives. A Bureau of Justice Statistics survey of 38,978 women in prison found that 43% had been assaulted, 34% had been physically abused, and 34% had been sexually abused before their incarceration. Of the women reporting sexual abuse, 56% had had a completed rape (Snell and Morton 1994). In a survey of 1,720 women, the American Correctional Association (1990) found that 53% of incarcerated women had experienced physical abuse and 36% had experienced sexual abuse. Of those sexually abused, one-third had been abused between ages 5 and 14 years. Other authors, using more detailed question strategies, found higher prevalences of abuse in female inmates and noted the severity of the abuse experienced. Bloom et al. (1994) found that 29% of female inmates interviewed had been physically abused by a parent, 31% had experienced childhood sexual abuse, 60% had been physically abused as an adult, and 23% had been sexually abused as an adult. In another study of female inmates, Browne et al. (1999) reported high prevalence rates of childhood physical abuse (70%), childhood sexual abuse (59%), and physical abuse in adulthood by an intimate (75%). These prevalence rates are far higher than those reported for the general population for childhood sexual abuse (Finkelhor 1994) or physical abuse (Tjaden and Thoennes 1992). Also, women are more likely to develop PTSD than men exposed to similar trauma, and early-onset abuse is associated with more severe later psychopathology (Kessler et al. 1995).

The interrelationships of PTSD and other psychiatric disorders, including addiction, are complex, and substantial comorbidity exists (Bremner et al. 1992; Kessler et al. 1994; van der Kolk et al. 1996). PTSD has been associated with higher preference for "hard" drugs, such as heroin and cocaine (Najavits et al. 1996). PTSD is also associated with development of other psychiatric disorders, including BPD, major depressive disorder, and substance abuse (Shalev et al. 1998; Zlotnick 1997). Symptoms of PTSD worsen during early abstinence (Brady et al. 1994), and PTSD worsens comorbid psychiatric conditions (Shalev et al. 1998). Childhood trauma is associated with a variety of psychiatric symptoms, including dissociation, somatization, affect dysregulation, and persistent hyperarousal (van der Kolk et al. 1996).

Treatment Issues

PTSD is often underdetected by medical and mental health treatment providers (Grossman et al. 1997). A critical first step in the treatment of PTSD in female offenders is recognition of the disorder. Evaluation of past trauma history and ongoing symptoms should be considered for inclusion in mental health screening for newly incarcerated inmates. Screening questionnaires for trauma (e.g., Najavits et al. 1998a) can be used in initial assessments when available. The treatment of PTSD ideally would address issues related to low self-esteem, physical and sexual abuse, depression, anxiety, self-abuse, and addiction (Gil-Rivas et al. 1996; Najavits et al. 1996).

Research on therapy for incarcerated women with PTSD is limited. Najavits et al. (1998b) and Zlotnick et al. (2003) evaluated a cognitive-behavioral intervention, Seeking Safety, through a pilot study of 17 incarcerated women with PTSD and addiction who were in a residential unit. The treatment was manual based and addressed cognitive, behavioral, and interpersonal aspects of treatment over eight sessions each. Seeking Safety combines educational intervention, cognitive-behavioral therapy for addiction, and treatment for PTSD (Herman 1992). The program goals are abstinence and personal safety. Women participating in the program had a decrease in PTSD symptoms that was maintained at 3 months and decreased substance abuse at 6 weeks postrelease. Their likelihood of relapse with substances after 6 weeks, however, remained high. Given the prevalence of addiction among incarcerated women and the comorbidity of addiction with PTSD, continued development of services addressing victimization and drug abuse is critical (Austin et al. 1992; Henderson 1998; Prendergast and Wellisch 1995).

The importance of cognitive strategies for trauma treatment is underscored by the limited efficacy of psychoeducational interventions for symptom management. Pomeroy et al. (1998) studied 13 incarcerated women who underwent a psychoeducational group intervention that focused on topics including low self-esteem, victimization, depression, symptoms of PTSD, and basic life skills. Participants met three times a week for 90 minutes over 5 weeks. At the end of the study, the participants self-reported greater improvement in symptoms of anxiety and depression than in symptoms of stress and trauma.

Bradley and Follingstad (2003) compared a small sample of incarcerated women who participated in DBT and writing assignments with a matched sample of women who had treatment as usual (i.e., supportive therapy and psychopharmacological interventions where appropriate). DBT focused on skills training related to self-esteem, management of trauma, anxiety and depressive symptoms, and development of trust and self-control. Participating inmates self-reported reduction in PTSD as well as mood and interpersonal symptoms.

The relationship between PTSD and substance dependence is a complex and important one. Substance-abusing women are often victimized through exposure to risky situations, and women who have experienced victimization are often substance dependent (Lewis 2003, 2006; Najavits et al. 1998b). Some evidence indicates that substance-dependent women often have experienced trauma that predates substance abuse (Lewis 2006). These data are confounded by the presence of childhood conduct disorder, which has been linked to trauma and addiction (Lewis 2006; Warren et al. 2002b). Further study is needed about the trajectory of symptoms among female offenders, with particular attention to early-onset childhood conduct disorder as a mediator of symptom development (e.g., PTSD, substance dependence) and severity. Regardless of the relationship, comorbidity of PTSD and addiction is important and has important clinical consequences for incarcerated women, including in the areas of prognostic outcome, service utilization, life problems such as loss of child custody, and suicide attempts (Najavits et al. 1998b).

The implications of these trials are not clear because of their small sample sizes and the absence of control groups. The treatment of PTSD in incarcerated women remains a largely unexplored field. Nonetheless, preliminary results suggest that an integrated approach, including psychoeducational, interpersonal, and cognitive-behavioral interventions, might be of benefit. Psychopharmacological interventions can also be used to treat depressive or anxiety symptoms related to underlying traumatic experience.

Suicide

Epidemiology

Suicide among incarcerated women is an important but understudied topic. Data from the general population suggest that compared with men, women are more likely to attempt but less likely to complete suicide (Moscicki 1994). Incarcerated women have multiple risk factors for suicidal behavior, including mood disorders, high total numbers of psychiatric disorders, comorbid Axis I and II disorders (Hawton et al. 2003; Kessler et al. 1999), drug and alcohol dependence (Hesselbrock et al. 1988; Roy 2003; Schuckit 1986), and childhood trauma (Canetto and Lester 1995; Kingree et al. 1999). Additional risk factors for suicide attempts include low social support and socioeconomic status (Murphy and Robins 1967) and younger age (Gomberg 1989).

Studies from the general U.S. population indicate that the rate of suicide for men (19.5 per 100,000) is about four times that of women (4.6 per 100,000) (Centers for Disease Control and Prevention 2008). The rate of suicide in prisons and jails is overall higher than in the general population for both men and women, but the gender difference is not as great. Specifically, women in prison have a rate of suicide of 10 per 100,000, whereas men have a rate of 14 per 100,000; women in jails have a rate of 32 per 100,000, whereas men have a rate of 50 per 100,000 (Mumola 2005). These results are striking, show the heightened risk of suicide for incarcerated women, and make sense given the high prevalence of substance dependence and ASPD in incarcerated women. Table 17–2 summarizes gender differences in suicide rates between men and women in the community, jails, and prisons.

TABLE 17–2. Gender difference in suicide rates

	Suicide rate (per 100,000)		
	Community[a]	Jail[b]	Prison[b]
Women	4.6	32.0	10.1
Men	19.5	50.0	14.0

[a]Centers for Disease Control and Prevention 2008.
[b]Mumola 2005.

TABLE 17–3.   Suicide history in sample of 136 female prisoners

Have you ever thought of suicide? ($n=94$)	69.4%
Reported that thoughts lasted for a full week	44.1%
Reported having had a plan	82.1%
Have you ever tried to kill yourself? ($n=71$)	52.0%

Source.   Lewis 2006.

The suicidal behavior seen in incarcerated women often predates incarceration and has lasted many years. In a study of 136 incarcerated female felons, Lewis (2006) found a high number of women with positive histories for suicidality when in the community. The majority of women (69.4%) had thought of suicide; of those who had thought of suicide, most (82.4%) had had a plan and had actually tried (52%) to take their lives. Of those who had attempted, close to half had tried to kill themselves multiple times. Tables 17–3 and 17–4 summarize findings on suicide thoughts and suicide attempts in a sample of female offenders.

What is salient in Lewis's (2006) study is the severity of attempts (e.g., proportion of women requiring medical treatment, hospitalization) and reported desire and intent to die. About one-third of the women had attempted suicide when using drugs and one-quarter when using alcohol. The most common methods of suicide attempts in this sample were cutting and overdose; hanging becomes more prevalent during actual incarceration. In this study, suicide attempts were associated with depressive symptoms, alcohol dependence, ASPD with childhood onset of severe symptoms, and PTSD. Further research is needed to assess patterns of suicide attempts and successful suicide attempts during incarceration.

Treatment Issues

The strong association among suicide attempts, severe substance dependence, affective illness, and/or past trauma is not surprising (Brodsky et al. 2001; Kingree et al. 1999). Treatment prevention strategies should include detailed screening for suicide, which requires assessment of trauma history, addiction severity, and ongoing affective symptoms. Depressive symptoms are closely associated with attempted and completed suicide (Roy 2003). Aggressive psychopharmacological treatment of these symptoms should occur even when recent substance abuse or dependence is present. Comorbidity heightens the risk of suicide (Hawton et al. 2003; Kessler et al. 1999; Roy 2003; Schuckit 1986). Multiple suicide attempts are themselves a risk factor for completed suicide; therefore, the argument that someone who has attempted and failed suicide is not serious

TABLE 17–4. Characteristics of 71 female prisoners with actual suicide attempt history

Required medical treatment	56.9%
Admitted to hospital	31.4%
Really wanted to die	84.3%
Sorry did not die	60.8%
Depressed at the time	94.1%
Using alcohol at the time	29.4%
Using drugs at the time	23.5%
Had severe intent to die	54.9%

Source. Lewis 2006.

about dying is erroneous (Roy 2003). Labeling multiple failed suicide attempts as "gestures," with the implication that they are not to be taken seriously or treated specifically, is inappropriate. Aggressive pharmacotherapy for depressive and traumatic symptoms in incarcerated women is an important component of suicide prevention. Aggressive treatment of withdrawal symptoms is also critical. Specialized housing units, such as group housing for inmates with suicidal ideation, have also shown potential benefit in correctional settings (Goss et al. 2002).

MEDICAL ISSUES IN CORRECTIONAL SETTINGS

General Medical Concerns

Incarcerated women often have physical illness, including sexually transmitted diseases, cervical dysplasia, obesity, hypertension, asthma, and hepatitis B or C (De Groot 2000; Lewis 2006; Onorato 2001). An initial physical examination accompanied by appropriate testing helps place psychiatric symptoms in context for effective treatment. Initial medical evaluation would optimally include a physical examination (including an obstetric-gynecological examination with pregnancy testing and assessment of hormonal levels where appropriate, Papanicolaou's test, HIV testing, testing for tuberculosis, testing for sexually transmitted diseases, and testing for hepatitis B and C); review of HIV risk factors; and mental health assessment, including assessment of trauma, depressive symptoms, and neurocognitive functioning. Other disorders, such as heart disease and osteoporosis, although less common in younger women, are likely to become more prevalent as the correctional population ages. Consideration should be given to medical issues with specific impact on psychiatric well-being in women (e.g., postpartum depression, perimenopausal depression, premenstrual dysphoric disorder). Effective and appropriate psychopharmacological intervention in the treatment of psychiatric symptoms is critical in optimizing psychiatric and physical health.

HIV and AIDS

Epidemiology

HIV is an important problem for the correctional system; currently close to 20,000 incarcerated people are HIV positive (Maruschak 2007). HIV seropositivity has a prevalence of 2.4% in incarcerated women, which is slightly higher than the 1.8% prevalence in incarcerated men but exponentially higher than the 0.15% prevalence for women in the general community (Maruschak 2001, 2007). The prevalence of HIV in incarcerated women has declined slightly since a peak in 1999, in part because of the rapidly growing population of female inmates without HIV and the overall decrease in HIV cases in women in the United States. During the 1990s, minority women were the group in which HIV infection rose most rapidly in the United States (De Groot 2000; Onorato 2001). In 1986, women represented 6.7% of all cases of HIV; by 1999, the percentage was 18% (Harris et al. 2003; Wish et al. 1990). This trend has leveled off; between 1999 and 2005, the prevalence of HIV fell 1% for incarcerated women and 0.4% for incarcerated men (Maruschak 2007).

Incarcerated women have a greater risk of HIV infection than their community peers because of high-risk lifestyles, which can include prostitution (Guyon et al. 1999), sexual abuse (Klein and Chao 1995), homelessness (Shlay et al. 1996), involvement with regular sexual partners who are at high risk for HIV (Berman and Brown 1990), and intravenous drug use (Guyon et al. 1999; Vlahov et al. 1991). HIV-positive incarcerated women are typically socioeconomically disadvantaged and lack basic necessities such as food, clothing, employment, housing, transportation, and health insurance (Lewis 2003; Sheu et al. 2002). Most HIV-positive incarcerated women are mothers who have never been married and are unemployed, having less than a high school education (Lewis 2003). Most are injection drug users (84%) (Brewer and Derrickson 1992; Farley et al. 2000), and about one-third of these injection drug users have engaged in prostitution. HIV-positive incarcerated women are likely to have experienced sexual abuse (67%) and to have a lifetime history of major depression (46%), ASPD (18%), PTSD (72%), alcohol dependence/abuse (81%), and drug dependence (95%) (Lewis 2003).

Treatment Issues

HIV-positive incarcerated women have complex medical and psychiatric pathology. Incarceration offers a unique opportunity to influence their lives through testing, counseling, and treatment of HIV and comorbid medical and psychiatric disorders. Women who are at risk for HIV infection or who are HIV positive are hard to reach in the community (Lubelczyk et al. 2002). Most women who are incarcerated are asymptomatic at the time they test positive for HIV, so their diagnosis may come as a surprise or shock (Farley et al. 2000). Pretest and posttest counseling are critical for inmates regardless of their serostatus. Medical issues are also important and can affect mental health. For example, women with HIV are more likely than non-HIV positive women to have hepatitis C and other sexually transmitted diseases (Onorato 2001). Consideration should be given early in treatment to the possibility that a woman is pregnant, to allow treatment with antiretrovirals to minimize transmission of HIV to the child.

Effective mental health treatment for HIV-positive incarcerated women should include HIV intervention (e.g., education about risky behaviors, education about illness, testing), treatment for addiction, and treatment for comorbid psychiatric conditions such as PTSD, major depression, and personality disorders. The high-risk behavior often seen in individuals with personality disorders has been linked to increased likelihood of transmission of HIV (Brooner et al. 1993; Jacobsberg et al. 1995). Programs designed to reduce risky behavior in incarcerated populations have been shown to be effective, and motivational interviewing for soon-to-be-released inmates has also shown potential efficacy (Lubelczyk et al. 2002). To increase social support among incarcerated women at high risk for HIV, el-Bassel et al. (1997) developed a cognitive-behavioral intervention that included support groups with former inmates, educational sessions, and cognitive-behavioral therapy to enhance coping and social support. Women who participated in the program were almost four times as likely to maintain safe sexual practices after release as were those women who only participated in an HIV information group (el-Bassel et al. 1997).

Continuity of care is an important concept in treating incarcerated women with HIV. Programs in which the same physician treats the HIV-positive inmate while in prison and after discharge to the community have been shown to increase treatment retention, decrease recidivism, and provide social support (Farley et al. 2000; Guyon et al. 1999). Because of the complexity of psychopathology, socioeconomic hardship, and medical issues of HIV-positive women, case management is an important intervention. Ideally, interventions would start for women jailed even for minor offenses, because these women exhibit high-risk behaviors yet are likely to return to the community relatively quickly (McClelland et al. 2002). Ultimately, services for HIV-positive female inmates should integrate medical treatment, psychiatric treatment (including treatment for substance use, traumatic symptoms, and personality disorders), and psychosocial interventions (vocational counseling, obtaining entitlements), with as much continuity of care as is feasible.

Pregnancy

One in four women entering prison has been pregnant in the year before her incarceration (Fogel 1993; Safyer and Richmond 1995), and 6% are pregnant at the time of incarceration (Snell and Morton 1994). Incarcerated women are at high risk for late entry into prenatal care, sexually transmitted diseases, HIV, substance abuse (including nicotine), and interpersonal violence (Snell and Morton 1994). Fewer than half of existing correctional facilities have programs for prenatal care, special prenatal diets, light work duty for pregnant women, or policies regarding pregnant women's control or travel; fewer than one in five offers instruction in birthing (e.g., Lamaze) (Siefert and Pimlott 2001). A survey of wardens identified multiple institutional limitations in dealing with pregnant inmates, including inadequate programs to deal with the trauma of miscarriage, unavailability of maternity clothes, institutional requirements that inmates wear belly chains, no separate visiting area for newborns, and the necessity of placing minimum security pregnant inmates in maximum security facilities to receive adequate care (Siefert and Pimlott 2001).

Data on the outcomes of inmate pregnancies are conflicting. Early work suggested that pregnant inmates have more frequent complications, including anemia, urinary tract infections, and bleeding (Fogel 1993; Shelton and Gill 1989). Later studies have suggested that length of incarceration is linked to pregnancy outcome; specifically, women with short incarcerations are more likely to have complications, including low-birth-weight babies. Women with longer incarcerations have higher-birth-weight babies and fewer complications (e.g., stillbirths, low Apgar scores, anemia) than women on parole (Cordero et al. 1991; Elton 1985; Martin et al. 1997) or in methadone maintenance programs (Kyei-Aboagye et al. 2000). The better physical outcomes for pregnant women having longer incarcerations may be associated with decreased access to substances of abuse, decreased exposure to sexually transmitted disease (including streptococcus B), better access to food and shelter, and decreased exposure to domestic violence (Cordero et al. 1991; Elton 1985; Martin et al. 1997).

Little information is available about the mental health of incarcerated pregnant women or their babies. The prevalence of depression may be higher in pregnant inmates than in nonpregnant inmates (Fogel 1993). Nicotine abuse remains an issue in some prison settings for pregnant women, even when they are participating in prenatal care within the facility (Cordero et al. 1991); smoking cessation programs would benefit pregnant female inmates. Although the prison environment may offer a certain type of stability that, on paper, enhances pregnancy outcomes, many variables remain unexplored. The impact of familial separation and loss of privacy on long-term mother–child bonding has not been explored in a correctional population. Very few facilities exist where mothers can stay with their babies after birth, and visiting with newborns is often limited (Wooldredge and Masters 1993). The effect of this separation is not known.

Treatment Issues

Research on treatment of pregnant offenders has focused primarily on community-based interventions as alternatives to incarceration (Barkauskas et al. 2002; Siefert and Pimlott 2001). Barkauskas et al. (2002) described a community-based residential program in which women were provided with family planning, prenatal and postpartum services, rehabilitation for addiction, job training, health care from conception through the fourth month, on-site child care, lactation consultation, labor assistance, and infant rooming-in. Such programs, which have reportedly good outcomes, are limited by cost and complexity of administration. The central concepts of community programs are transferable to correctional facilities that house pregnant women. Specifically, programs in correctional facilities would benefit from having nurse-midwives to coordinate care, education on nutrition and spacing of pregnancies, prenatal care, treatment for substance abuse, smoking cessation, parenting, childbirth, and stress management (Barkauskas et al. 2002; Fogel 1993). The Federal Bureau of Prisons allows most infants to stay with their mothers for 3 months postpartum; most state facilities do not currently have this option.

Clinical Case 17–3

Ms. G, a 32-year-old pregnant mother of three, complains of hearing voices during booking for a trespassing charge. She has a history of chronic schizophrenia and is treated at a local community mental health center. She reports being 6 weeks pregnant and says she has stopped all her medications because she does not want to hurt the baby. She has had no prenatal visits. Ms. G reports being HIV positive, but has stopped all medication for her HIV. She expresses reluctance to take medication for HIV because she remembers her brother taking it and "dying anyway." The patient says her most recent medications included an atypical antipsychotic and a mood stabilizer that she was told could "hurt the baby's heart." She admits to using intravenous drugs up to the day of her arrest and says she does not practice safe sex consistently.

This case illustrates the complex needs of a pregnant inmate who will likely stay in the correctional system for just a short time. The central issue in this case is coordination of care for the patient in the community after her discharge from the correctional system. The following considerations are important when working with such an inmate:

- Test to confirm pregnancy, assess nutritional status, rule out teratogenic medication (e.g., valproic acid), and assess for sexually transmitted diseases including HIV.
- Monitor withdrawal symptoms and begin detoxification.
- Begin immediate assignment to a case manager within the facility to begin discharge planning.
- Provide brief consultation from an HIV counselor regarding safe sexual practices.
- Arrange a physician appointment to discuss the advisability of starting a regimen of medication for HIV and to prevent transmission of HIV to the fetus.
- Arrange a psychiatry appointment, which would include a frank discussion about 1) the risks and benefits of various pharmacological options to treat the psychotic disorder during pregnancy and 2) the risks and benefits of no psychopharmacological intervention.

If the inmate's stay is short, all of these interventions may not be feasible. In this instance, the case manager at the correctional facility can contact the case manager at the mental health center to coordinate follow-up and transition to the community.

MOTHERHOOD IN CORRECTIONAL SETTINGS

Most incarcerated women (70%–80%) are mothers; of these mothers, 8%–10% have children in foster care (Barry 1985; McGowan and Blumenthal 1976). Maternal grandmothers care for the majority of the children of incarcerated women (Beckerman 1994). Female inmates are generally concerned about their children's welfare, miss their children, and want to reunite with them (Thompson and Harm 1995). Although most incarcerated women value the maternal role, they are often confused about their legal rights and responsibilities in regard to their children (Beckerman 1994; McGowan and Blumenthal 1976). The children experience loneliness, fear, and embarrassment (Hale 1988). They have an increased risk for mental illness, learning disabilities, teen pregnancy, and PTSD (Moses 1995). When the mother is incarcerated, the children have a deeper drop in economic resources and are more likely to have a change in their primary caretaker, dislocation, and family dissolution than when a father is incarcerated (Brooks 1993). More than half of the children of incarcerated women never visit their mothers in prison because of difficulty scheduling visits, remote locations of prisons, and difficulties negotiating the complexities of the child welfare system (Hufft 1999). Although contact between the incarcerated mother and the caseworker for her children is critical, such contact is often strained and infrequent (McGowan and Blumenthal 1976). Incarcerated mothers experience difficulty getting and making phone calls at specified times; coordinating family court visits; and receiving, understanding, and responding to correspondence about their children.

Treatment Issues

Incarcerated mothers with children would benefit from the assistance of a dedicated legal educator and advocate to help negotiate the child welfare system (Beckerman 1994). Given the high number of incarcerated mothers, assigning a specific caseworker or caseworkers to interface with the advocate would likely be advantageous. Interventions aimed at enhancing parenting skills would also be beneficial. A fundamental focus of treatment should be addressing substance abuse and dependence, both of which interfere with parenting ability (Kemper and Rivara 1993). Psychoeducational interventions should focus on enhancing self-esteem, increasing empathy, assisting with developing effective strategies for discipline, decreasing risk factors for child abuse, understanding the maternal role, decreasing recidivism, and addressing addiction (Browne et al. 1999; Thompson and Harm 1995). Another approach is to provide interventions for both children and mothers. Such interventions can include supervised visitation or programming that emphasizes providing appropriate adult role models, helping parents and children develop structured goals they can meet, and enhancing communication between parent and child (Hairston 1991; Hufft 1999).

CONCLUSION

In this chapter, I have reviewed issues of particular relevance to the treatment of women in the correctional system. Relationships between past traumatic experiences, substance abuse and dependence, ASPD, and depressive symptoms have been emphasized. The complex psychopathology seen in incarcerated women heightens their psychiatric morbidity and mortality and increases the risk of recidivism. Incarcerated women are a challenging treatment population.

Clear gender-related differences are apparent in incarcerated populations. The typical female offender is a single, minority mother in her reproductive years with polysubstance use, physical or sexual abuse often dating to childhood, and socioeconomic disenfranchisement (Greenfeld and Snell 1999; Lewis 2006; Teplin et al. 1996). Most research used to develop treatment interventions for incarcerated women has been based on research on male offenders or women in clinical samples, and the applicability of these studies is not clear (Lewis 2006). An erroneous assumption is that a program that worked for women in the community can be applied without modification to incarcerated women merely on the basis of gender. Women who are incarcerated differ from women in the community; in some populations, incarcerated women are more similar to their male counterparts in prevalence of substance dependence, suicidality, and ASPD (Lewis 2006; Warren et al. 2002a; Zlotnick 1999). Studies of treatment for incarcerated women with mental illness are few in number and rarely contain control groups to assess efficacy (Najavits et al. 1998b; Prendergast and Wellisch 1995). Indeed, incarcerated women represent a unique population, which has just begun to be researched from an epidemiological and treatment efficacy perspective (Lewis 2006).

Future research should address delineating epidemiology of psychiatric illness further among incarcerated women; assessing efficacy of treatment interventions; and gaining knowledge about factors associated with treatment entry, retention, and completion. More studies on incarcerated women with dual diagnoses are needed, and further development of modalities to treat substance abuse/dependence within this population is critical. The inexorable rise in the number of women incarcerated in the United States underscores the timeliness and critical nature of this research agenda.

The burgeoning population of female inmates with complex psychopathology taxes an already stressed system. Health care budgets can be twice as high for female versus male correctional facilities, and facilities providing care for women with HIV are among the most expensive programs in the country (De Groot 2000). Although integrative treatment and holistic approaches are likely to benefit incarcerated women, funding for such programs is a serious limitation to program implementation. Correctional mental health services will need to expand to meet the increasing demands of this heterogeneous population (Marquart et al. 2001;

Morash et al. 1994); this expansion will almost certainly require additional funding and optimization of health service delivery. Incarceration represents a unique opportunity to access a hard-to-reach population with complex medical and psychiatric needs. Successful interventions enhancing medical and psychiatric well-being of female inmates are likely to benefit not only the inmates but also their families, partners, and communities (Hammett 2001).

SUMMARY POINTS

- Substance dependence is the most common psychiatric disorder among incarcerated women.
- Incarcerated women have a high prevalence of antisocial personality disorder.
- Incarcerated women have multiple risk factors for completed suicide; this risk approaches that for male inmates.
- Female inmates have more complex psychopathology and higher comorbidity than male inmates.
- Mental health treatment for incarcerated women should include the following:
  1. Integrated treatment for comorbid mental health and addictive disorders
  2. Use of the therapeutic community: "one-stop shopping" for treatment
  3. Recognition that the population is challenging and the work is difficult
  4. Psychopharmacological management of symptoms where appropriate
  5. Treatment matching for severity of disorder and therapeutic setting
  6. Coordination and close linkage to HIV services and other medical services
  7. Counseling regarding pregnancy, motherhood, and familial interactions
  8. Vocational/educational training
  9. Making the case manager the "quarterback" for coordinating services and transitions
  10. Use of interpersonal therapy and cognitive-behavioral therapy when appropriate

REFERENCES

Alper G, Peterson SJ: Dialectical behavior therapy for patients with borderline personality disorder. J Psychosoc Nurs Ment Health Serv 39:38–45, 2001

Amaro H: Love, sex, and power: considering women's realities in HIV prevention. Am Psychol 50:437–447, 1995

American Correctional Association: The Female Offender. Washington, DC, St Mary's Press, 1990

Anda RF, Williamson DF, Remington PL: Alcohol and fatal injuries among U.S. adults: findings from the NHANES I Epidemiologic Follow-up Study. JAMA 260:2529–2532, 1988

Anglin MD, Hser YI, Booth MW: Sex differences in addict careers, 4: treatment. Am J Drug Alcohol Abuse 13:253–280, 1987

Ashley MJ, Olin JS, Le Riche WH, et al: Morbidity in alcoholics: evidence for accelerated development of physical disease in women. Arch Intern Med 137:883–887, 1977

Austin J, Bloom B, Donahue T: Female Offenders in the Community: An Analysis of Innovative Strategies and Programs. Washington, DC, National Institute of Corrections, 1992

Barkauskas VH, Low LK, Pimlott S: Health outcomes of incarcerated pregnant women and their infants in a community-based program. J Midwifery Womens Health 47:371–379, 2002

Barry E: Children of prisoners: punishing the innocent. Youth Law News 6:12–17, 1985

Beck AJ: Survey of state prison inmates, 1991 (NCJ 145321). Washington, DC, U.S. Department of Justice, Office of Justice Programs, Bureau of Justice Statistics, March 1993

Beck AJ, Stephen JJ: Correctional populations in the United States, 1996 (NCJ 170013). Washington, DC, U.S. Department of Justice, Office of Justice Programs, Bureau of Justice Statistics, April 1999

Beckerman A: Mothers in prison: meeting the prerequisite conditions for permanency planning. Soc Work 39:9–14, 1994

Berman J, Brown D: AIDS knowledge and risky behavior by incarcerated females: IV and non-IV drug users. Sociol Soc Res 75:8–16, 1990

Bloom B, Chesney L, Owen B: Women in California Prisons: Hidden Victims of the War on Drugs. San Francisco, Center on Juvenile and Criminal Justice, 1994

Blume SB: Chemical dependency in women: important issues. Am J Drug Alcohol Abuse 16:297–307, 1990

Bradley RG, Follingstad DR: Group therapy for incarcerated women who experienced interpersonal violence: a pilot study. J Trauma Stress 16:337–340, 2003

Brady K, Killeen T, Saladain M, et al: Comorbid substance abuse and posttraumatic stress disorder: characteristics of women in treatment. Am J Addict 3:160–164, 1994

Bremner JD, Southwick S, Brett E, et al: Dissociation and posttraumatic stress disorder in Vietnam combat veterans. Am J Psychiatry 149:328–332, 1992

Brewer T, Derrickson J: AIDS in prison: a review of epidemiology and preventive policy. AIDS 6:623–628, 1992

Brodsky BS, Oquendo M, Ellis SP, et al: The relationship of childhood abuse to impulsivity and suicidal behavior in adults with major depression. Am J Psychiatry 158:1871–1877, 2001

Brooks MK: How Can I Help? Working With Children of Incarcerated Parents: Serving Special Children, Vol 1. New York, Osbourne Association, 1993

Brooner RK, Greenfield L, Schmidt CW, et al: Antisocial personality disorder and HIV infection among intravenous drug abusers. Am J Psychiatry 150:53–58, 1993

Brown PJ, Stout RL, Gannon-Rowley J: Substance use disorder–PTSD co-morbidity: patients' perceptions of symptom interplay and treatment issues. J Subst Abuse Treat 15:445–448, 1998

Browne A, Miller B, Maguin E: Prevalence and severity of lifetime physical and sexual victimization among incarcerated women. Int J Law Psychiatry 22:301–322, 1999

Bucholz KK, Cadoret R, Cloninger CR, et al: A new, semi-structured psychiatric interview for use in genetic linkage studies: a report on the reliability of the SSAGA. J Stud Alcohol 55:149–158, 1994

Canetto S, Lester D: Women and Suicidal Behavior. New York, Springer, 1995

Centers for Disease Control and Prevention: Welcome to WISQARS: Web-based Inquiry Statistics Query and Reporting System. April 1, 2008. Available at: http://www.cdc.gov/injury/Wisqars/index.html. Accessed April 18, 2009.

Chasnoff IJ: Drug use and women: establishing a standard of care. Ann N Y Acad Sci 562:208–210, 1989

Chesney-Lind M: Women in prison: from partial justice to vengeful equity. Corrections Today 60:66–73, 1998

Coid J: DSM-III diagnosis in criminal psychopaths: a way forward. Crim Behav Ment Health 2:78–94, 1992

Cordero L, Hines S, Shibley KA, et al: Duration of incarceration and perinatal outcome. Obstet Gynecol 78:641–645, 1991

Daly K: Gender, Crime and Punishment. New Haven, Yale University Press, 1994

De Groot AS: HIV infection among incarcerated women: an epidemic behind the walls. HIV Education Prison Project 3:1–4, 2000

De Leon G: Therapeutic communities for addictions: a theoretical framework. Int J Addict 30:1603–1645, 1995

DiCataldo F, Greer A, Profit WE: Screening prison inmates for mental disorder: an examination of the relationship between mental disorder and prison adjustment. Bull Am Acad Psychiatry Law 23:573–585, 1995

Dinwiddie SH, Reich T, Cloninger CR: Psychiatric comorbidity and suicidality among intravenous drug users. J Clin Psychiatry 53:364–369, 1992

Drake RE, Mueser KT, Clark RE, et al: The course, treatment, and outcome of substance disorder in persons with severe mental illness. Am J Orthopsychiatry 66:42–51, 1996

el-Bassel N, Ivanoff A, Schilling R, et al: Skills building and social support enhancement to reduce HIV risk in women in jail. Crim Justice Behav 24:205–223, 1997

Elton P: Outcome of pregnancy among prisoners. J Obstet Gynaecol 5:241–244, 1985

Farabee D, Prendergast M, Cartier J, et al: Barriers to implementing effective correctional drug treatment programs. Prison J 79:150–162, 1999

Farley JL, Mitty JA, Lally MA, et al: Comprehensive medical care among HIV-positive incarcerated women: the Rhode Island experience. J Womens Health Gend Based Med 9:51–56, 2000

Finkelhor D: The international epidemiology of child sexual abuse. Child Abuse Negl 18:409–417, 1994

Finkelstein N, Kennedy C, Thomas K, et al: Gender-Specific Substance Abuse Treatment. Washington, DC, National Women's Resource Center for the Prevention and Treatment of Alcohol, Tobacco and Other Drug Abuse and Mental Illness, 1997

First MB, Gibbon M, Spitzer RI, et al: Structured Clinical Interview for DSM-IV Axis II Personality Disorders (SCID-II). Washington, DC, American Psychiatric Press, 1997

Fogel CI: Pregnant inmates: risk factors and pregnancy outcomes. J Obstet Gynecol Neonatal Nurs 22:33–39, 1993

Fox JA, Zavitz MW: Homicide trends in the United States: 2002 update (NIJ 204885). Washington, DC, U.S. Department of Justice, Office of Justice Programs, Bureau of Justice Statistics, November 2004

Gil-Rivas V, Fiorentine R, Anglin MD: Sexual abuse, physical abuse, and posttraumatic stress disorder among women participating in outpatient drug abuse treatment. J Psychoactive Drugs 28:95–102, 1996

Glaze LE, Maruschak L: Bureau of Justice special report: parents in prison and their minor children (NCJ 222984). Washington, DC, U.S. Department of Justice, Office of Justice Programs, Bureau of Justice Statistics, August 2008

Gomberg ES: Suicide risk among women with alcohol problems. Am J Public Health 79:1363–1365, 1989

Goss JR, Peterson K, Smith LW, et al: Characteristics of suicide attempts in a large urban jail system with an established suicide prevention program. Psychiatr Serv 53:574–579, 2002

Greenfeld LA: Alcohol and crime: an analysis of national data on the prevalence of alcohol involvement in crime (NCJ 168632). Washington, DC, U.S. Department of Justice, Office of Justice Programs, Bureau of Justice Statistics, April 1998

Greenfeld LA, Snell TL: Bureau of Justice Statistics special report: women offenders (NCJ 175688). Washington, DC, U.S. Department of Justice, Office of Justice Programs, Bureau of Justice Statistics, December 1999

Greenfield SF, Weiss RD, Muenz LR, et al: The effect of depression on return to drinking: a prospective study. Arch Gen Psychiatry 55:259–265, 1998

Green-Hennessy S: Factors associated with receipt of behavioral health services among persons with substance dependence. Psychiatr Serv 53:1592–1598, 2002

Grella C: Background and overview of mental health and substance abuse treatment systems: meeting the needs of women who are pregnant and parenting. J Psychoactive Drugs 28:319–343, 1996

Grossman LS, Willer JK, Stovall JG, et al: Underdiagnosis of PTSD and substance use disorders in hospitalized female veterans. Psychiatr Serv 48:393–395, 1997

Guy E, Platt J, Zwerling I, et al: Mental health status of prisoners in an urban jail. Crim Justice Behav 12:29–53, 1985

Guyon L, Brochu S, Parent I, et al: At-risk behaviors with regard to HIV and addiction among women in prison. Women Health 29:49–66, 1999

Hairston C: Family ties during imprisonment: important to whom and for what? J Sociol Soc Welf 18:87–104, 1991

Hale DC: The impact of mothers' incarceration on the family system: research and recommendations. Marriage Fam Rev 12:143–154, 1988

Hammett TM: Making the case for health interventions in correctional facilities. J Urban Health 78:236–240, 2001

Hammett TM, Harmon P, Rhodes W: The burden of infectious disease among inmates and releasees from correctional facilities. Prepared for the National Commission on Correctional Health Care–National Institute of Justice, Chicago, June 1999

Hare RD, Clarke D, Grann M, et al: Psychopathology and the predictive validity of the PCL-R: an international perspective. Behav Sci Law 18:623–645, 2000

Harris RM, Sharps PW, Allen K, et al: The interrelationship between violence, HIV/AIDS, and drug use in incarcerated women. J Assoc Nurses AIDS Care 14:27–40, 2003

Hawton K, Houston K, Haw C, et al: Comorbidity of Axis I and Axis II disorders in patients who attempted suicide. Am J Psychiatry 160:1494–1500, 2003

Henderson DJ: Drug abuse and incarcerated women: a research review. J Subst Abuse Treat 15:579–587, 1998

Herman JL: Trauma and Recovery. New York, Basic Books, 1992

Hesselbrock MN, Meyer RE, Keener JJ: Psychopathology in hospitalized alcoholics. Arch Gen Psychiatry 42:1050–1055, 1985

Hesselbrock M, Hesselbrock V, Syzmanski K, et al: Suicide attempts and alcoholism. J Stud Alcohol 49:436–442, 1988

Higgins ST, Delaney DD, Budney AJ, et al: A behavioral approach to achieving initial cocaine abstinence. Am J Psychiatry 148:1218–1224, 1991

Hufft AG: Girl Scouts Beyond Bars: a unique opportunity for forensic psychiatric nursing. J Psychosoc Nurs Ment Health Serv 37:45–51, 1999

Hutton HE, Treisman GJ, Hunt WR, et al: HIV risk behaviors and their relationship to posttraumatic stress disorder among women prisoners. Psychiatr Serv 52:508–513, 2001

Jacobsberg L, Frances A, Perry S: Axis II diagnoses among volunteers for HIV testing and counseling. Am J Psychiatry 152:1222–1224, 1995

Jordan BK, Schlenger WE, Fairbank JA, et al: Prevalence of psychiatric disorders among incarcerated women, II: convicted felons entering prison. Arch Gen Psychiatry 53:513–519, 1996

Kemper KJ, Rivara FP: Parents in jail. Pediatrics 92:261–264, 1993

Kessler RC, McGonagle KA, Zhao S, et al: Lifetime and twelve-month prevalence of DSM-III-R psychiatric disorders in the United States: results from the National Comorbidity Survey. Arch Gen Psychiatry 51:8–19, 1994

Kessler RC, Sonnega A, Bromet E, et al: Posttraumatic stress disorder in the National Comorbidity Survey. Arch Gen Psychiatry 52:1048–1060, 1995

Kessler RC, Crum RM, Warner LA, et al: Lifetime co-occurrence of DSM-III-R alcohol abuse and dependence with other psychiatric disorders in the National Comorbidity Survey. Arch Gen Psychiatry 54:313–321, 1997

Kessler RC, Borges G, Walters EE: Prevalence of and risk factors for lifetime suicide attempts in the National Comorbidity Survey. Arch Gen Psychiatry 56:617–626, 1999

Kimmerling R, Goldsmith R: Links between exposure to violence and HIV-infection: implications for substance abuse treatment. Alcohol Treat Q 18:61–70, 2000

Kingree JB, Thompson MP, Kaslow NJ: Risk factors for suicide attempts among low-income women with a history of alcohol problems. Addict Behav 24:583–587, 1999

Klein H, Chao BS: Sexual abuse during childhood and adolescence as predictors of HIV-related sexual risk during adulthood among female sexual partners of injection drug users. Violence Against Women 1:55–76, 1995

Kotler M, Iancu I, Efroni R, et al: Anger, impulsivity, social support, and suicide risk in patients with posttraumatic stress disorder. J Nerv Ment Dis 189:162–167, 2001

Kranzler HR, Del Boca FK, Rounsaville BJ: Comorbid psychiatric diagnosis predicts three-year outcomes in alcoholics: a posttreatment natural history study. J Stud Alcohol 57:619–626, 1996

Kyei-Aboagye K, Vragovic O, Chong D: Birth outcome in incarcerated, high-risk pregnant women. J Reprod Med 45:190–194, 2000

Lake ES: An exploration of the violent victim experiences of female offenders. Violence Vict 8:41–51, 1993

Langan NP, Pelissier BM: Gender differences among prisoners in drug treatment. J Subst Abuse 13:291–301, 2001

Lewis CF: Prevalence of psychiatric diagnoses in HIV positive incarcerated women. Paper presented at the annual meeting of the American Psychiatric Association, San Francisco, May 2003

Lewis CF: PTSD in HIV positive incarcerated women. J Am Acad Psychiatry Law 33:255–264, 2005

Lewis CF: Treating incarcerated women: gender matters. Psychiatr Clin North Am 29:773–789, 2006

Lex BW: Alcohol and other psychoactive substance dependence in women and men, in Gender and Psychopathology. Edited by Seeman MV. Washington, DC, American Psychiatric Press, 1995, pp 311–358

Linehan MM, Schmidt H 3rd, Dimeff LA, et al: Dialectical behavior therapy for patients with borderline personality disorder and drug-dependence. Am J Addict 8:279–292, 1999

Logan TK, Leukefeld C: Violence and HIV risk behavior among male and female crack users. J Drug Issues 30:261–282, 2000

Lubelczyk RA, Friedmann PD, Lemon SC, et al: HIV prevention services in correctional drug treatment programs: do they change risk behaviors? AIDS Educ Prev 14:117–125, 2002

Maden T, Swinton M, Gunn J: Psychiatric disorder in women serving a prison sentence. Br J Psychiatry 164:44–54, 1994

Marquart JW, Brewer VE, Simon P, et al: Lifestyle factors among female prisoners with histories of psychiatric treatment. J Crim Justice 29:319–328, 2001

Martin SL, Kim H, Kupper LL, et al: Is incarceration during pregnancy associated with infant birthweight? Am J Public Health 87:1526–1531, 1997

Maruschak LM: HIV in prisons and jails, 1999 (NCJ 196023). Washington, DC, U.S. Department of Justice, Office of Justice Programs, Bureau of Justice Statistics, July 2001

Maruschak LM: HIV in prisons, 2005 (NCJ 218915). Washington, DC, U.S. Department of Justice, Office of Justice Programs, Bureau of Justice Statistics, September 2007

Mason BJ, Kocsis JH, Ritvo EC, et al: A double-blind, placebo-controlled trial of desipramine for primary alcohol dependence stratified on the presence or absence of major depression. JAMA 275:761–767, 1996

McClelland GM, Teplin LA, Abram KM, et al: HIV and AIDS risk behaviors among female jail detainees: implications for public health policy. Am J Public Health 92:818–825, 2002

McGowan B, Blumenthal KL: Children of women prisoners: a forgotten minority, in The Female Offender. Edited by Crites L. Lexington, MA, DC Heath, 1976

Messina N, Farabee D, Rawson R: Treatment responsivity of cocaine-dependent patients with antisocial personality disorder to cognitive-behavioral and contingency management interventions. J Consult Clin Psychol 71:320–329, 2003

Miller RE: Nationwide profile of female inmate substance involvement. J Psychoactive Drugs 16:319–326, 1984

Morash M, Haarr R, Rucker L: A comparison of programming for women and men in U.S. prisons in the 1990s. Crime Delinq 40:197–221, 1994

Moscicki EK: Gender differences in completed and attempted suicides. Ann Epidemiol 4:152–158, 1994

Moses M: A synergistic solution for children of incarcerated parents. Corrections Today 57:124–126, 1995

Mumola CJ: Suicide and homicide in state prisons and local jails (NCJ 210036). Washington, DC, U.S. Department of Justice, Office of Justice Programs, Bureau of Justice Statistics, August 2005

Murphy GE, Robins E: Social factors in suicide. JAMA 199:303–308, 1967

Najavits LM, Weiss RD, Liese BS: Group cognitive-behavioral therapy for women with PTSD and substance use disorder. J Subst Abuse Treat 13:13–22, 1996

Najavits L, Weiss R, Reif S: The Addiction Severity Index as a screen for trauma and posttraumatic stress disorder. J Stud Alcohol 59:56–62, 1998a

Najavits LM, Weiss RD, Shaw SR, et al: "Seeking safety": outcome of a new cognitive-behavioral psychotherapy for women with posttraumatic stress disorder and substance dependence. J Trauma Stress 11:437–456, 1998b

Nespor K: Treatment needs of alcohol-dependent women. Int J Psychosom 37:50–52, 1990

Onorato M: HIV infection among incarcerated women. HIV and Hepatitis Education Prison Project 4:1–4, 2001. Available at: http://www.thebody.com/content/whatis/art12954.html. Accessed April 18, 2009.

Peters RH, Strozier AL, Murrin MR, et al: Treatment of substance-abusing jail inmates: examination of gender differences. J Subst Abuse Treat 14:339–349, 1997

Peyrot M, Yen S, Baldassano CA: Short-term substance abuse prevention in jail: a cognitive-behavioral approach. J Drug Educ 24:33–47, 1994

Pomeroy EC, Kiam R, Abel E: Meeting the mental health needs of incarcerated women. Health Soc Work 23:71–75, 1998

Prendergast M, Wellisch J: Assessment of and services for substance-abusing women offenders in community and correctional settings. Prison J 75:240–256, 1995

Prendergast M, Wellisch J, Wong M: Residential treatment for women parolees following prison-based drug treatment: treatment experiences, needs and services, outcomes. Prison J 76:253–274, 1996

Rasche C: The female offender as an object of criminological research. Crim Justice Behav 1:301–320, 1974

Regier DA, Farmer ME, Rae DS, et al: Comorbidity of mental disorders with alcohol and other drug abuse: results from the Epidemiologic Catchment Area (ECA) study. JAMA 264:2511–2518, 1990

Resnick HS, Kilpatrick DG, Dansky BS, et al: Prevalence of civilian trauma and posttraumatic stress disorder in a representative national sample of women. J Consult Clin Psychol 61:984–991, 1993

Robins LN, Helzer JE, Croughan J, et al: National Institute of Mental Health Diagnostic Interview Schedule: its history, characteristics, and validity. Arch Gen Psychiatry 38:381–389, 1981

Robins LN, Wing J, Wittchen HU, et al: The Composite International Diagnostic Interview: an epidemiologic instrument suitable for use in conjunction with different diagnostic systems and in different cultures. Arch Gen Psychiatry 45:1069–1077, 1988

Roth B, Presse L: Nursing interventions for parasuicidal behaviors in female offenders. J Psychosoc Nurs Ment Health Serv 41:20–29, 2003

Rounsaville BJ, Weissman MM, Kleber H, et al: Heterogeneity of psychiatric diagnosis in treated opiate addicts. Arch Gen Psychiatry 39:161–168, 1982

Roy A: Characteristics of drug addicts who attempt suicide. Psychiatry Res 121:99–103, 2003

Safyer SM, Richmond L: Pregnancy behind bars. Semin Perinatol 19:314–322, 1995

Schilling R, el-Bassel N, Ivanoff A, et al: Sexual risk behavior of incarcerated, drug-using women, 1992. Public Health Rep 109:539–547, 1994

Schuckit MA: Primary men alcoholics with histories of suicide attempts. J Stud Alcohol 47:78–81, 1986

Schuckit MA, Anthenelli RM, Bucholz KK, et al: The time course of development of alcohol-related problems in men and women. J Stud Alcohol 56:218–225, 1995

Shalev AY, Freedman S, Peri T, et al: Prospective study of posttraumatic stress disorder and depression following trauma. Am J Psychiatry 155:630–637, 1998

Shelton BJ, Gill DG: Childbearing in prison: a behavioral analysis. J Obstet Gynecol Neonatal Nurs 18:301–308, 1989

Sheu M, Hogan J, Allsworth J, et al: Continuity of medical care and risk of incarceration in HIV-positive and high-risk HIV-negative women. J Womens Health (Larchmt) 11:743–750, 2002

Shlay JC, Blackburn D, O'Keefe K, et al: Human immunodeficiency virus seroprevalence and risk assessment of a homeless population in Denver. Sex Transm Dis 23:304–311, 1996

Siefert K, Pimlott S: Improving pregnancy outcome during imprisonment: a model residential care program. Soc Work 46:125–134, 2001

Singer MI, Bussey J, Song LY, et al: The psychosocial issues of women serving time in jail. Soc Work 40:103–113, 1995

Smith BV: Special Issues of Women in the Criminal Justice System. Washington, DC, National Women's Law Center, 1993

Snell TL, Morton DC: Survey of state prison inmates 1991: women in prison (NCJ 145321). Washington, DC, U.S. Department of Justice, Office of Justice Programs, Bureau of Justice Statistics, March 1994

Steadman HJ, Holohean EJ Jr, Dvoskin J: Estimating mental health needs and service utilization among prison inmates. Bull Am Acad Psychiatry Law 19:297–307, 1991

Steffensmeier D, Allen E: Gender and crime: toward a gendered theory of female offending. Annu Rev Sociol 22:459–487, 1996

Teplin LA, Abram KM, McClelland GM: Prevalence of psychiatric disorders among incarcerated women, I: pretrial jail detainees. Arch Gen Psychiatry 53:505–512, 1996

Teplin LA, Abram KM, McClelland GM: Mentally disordered women in jail: who receives services? Am J Public Health 87:604–609, 1997

Thompson PJ, Harm NJ: Parent education for mothers in prison. Pediatr Nurs 21:552–555, 1995

Tjaden PG, Thoennes N: Predictors of legal intervention in child maltreatment cases. Child Abuse Negl 16:807–821, 1992

van der Kolk BA, Pelcovitz D, Roth S, et al: Dissociation, somatization, and affect dysregulation: the complexity of adaptation of trauma. Am J Psychiatry 153:83–93, 1996

Vlahov D, Brewer TF, Castro KG, et al: Prevalence of antibody to HIV-1 among entrants to U.S. correctional facilities. JAMA 265:1129–1132, 1991

Warren JI, Burnette M, South SC, et al: Personality disorders and violence among female prison inmates. J Am Acad Psychiatry Law 30:502–509, 2002a

Warren JI, Hurt S, Loper AB, et al: Psychiatric symptoms, history of victimization, and violent behavior among incarcerated female felons: an American perspective. Int J Law Psychiatry 25:129–149, 2002b

Weisner C, Schmidt L: Gender disparities in treatment for alcohol problems. JAMA 268:1872–1876, 1992

Wellisch J, Anglin MD, Prendergast ML: Treatment strategies for drug abusing women offenders, in Drug Treatment and Criminal Justice. Edited by Inciardi JA. Newbury Park, CA, Sage, 1993, pp 5–29

Wellisch J, Prendergast M, Anglin MD: Drug-abusing women offenders: results of a national survey (NCJ 149261). Washington, DC, U.S. Department of Justice, Office of Justice Programs, Bureau of Justice Statistics, 1994

West HC, Sabol WJ: Prisoners in 2007 (NCJ 224280). Washington, DC, U.S. Department of Justice, Office of Justice Programs, Bureau of Justice Statistics, December 2008

Wilsnack C, Vogeltanz NDI, Klassen AD, et al: Childhood sexual abuse and women's substance abuse: national survey findings. J Stud Alcohol 58:264–271, 1997

Windle M, Windle RC, Scheidt DM, et al: Physical and sexual abuse and associated mental disorders among alcoholic inpatients. Am J Psychiatry 152:1322–1328, 1995

Wish ED, O'Neil J, Baldau V: Lost opportunity to combat AIDS: drug abusers in the criminal justice system. NIDA Res Monogr 93:187–209, 1990

Wooldredge JD, Masters K: Confronting problems faced by pregnant inmates in state prisons. Crime Delinq 39:195–203, 1993

Zlotnick C: Posttraumatic stress disorder (PTSD), PTSD comorbidity, and childhood abuse among incarcerated women. J Nerv Ment Dis 185:761–763, 1997

Zlotnick C: Antisocial personality disorder, affect dysregulation and childhood abuse among incarcerated women. J Pers Disord 13:90–95, 1999

Zlotnick C, Najavits LM, Rohsenow DJ, et al: A cognitive-behavioral treatment for incarcerated women with substance abuse disorder and posttraumatic stress disorder: findings from a pilot study. J Subst Abuse Treat 25:99–105, 2003

CHAPTER 18

Individuals With Developmental Disabilities in Correctional Settings

Barbara E. McDermott, Ph.D.

The overall mission of the U.S. correctional system is multifaceted. Arguably, in addition to punishment and removal of the offender from society, one important component is rehabilitation. Training and habilitation programs may be useful in assisting facilities to maintain order and control (Hall 1992). Habilitation is particularly relevant with offenders with developmental disabilities. Although the research is controversial, most studies suggest that offenders with developmental delays commit less serious offenses yet serve more time in prison than offenders without such delays (MacEachron 1979; Petersilia 2000a). In 1975, Talent and Keldgord opined, "Less effort has been expended in the United States to rehabilitate the mentally retarded offender than any other group of offenders" (p. 39). Petersilia (2000a) noted that 25 years later this situation remained essentially unchanged.

In this chapter, I outline the progress that has been made in the identification and habilitation of individuals with developmental disabilities in the criminal justice system. I provide definitions, describe legal issues, present prevalence rates, and discuss the particular vulnerabilities that individuals with developmental delays present to the criminal justice system. Finally, I discuss screening, management, and habilitation in corrections arising directly from these vulnerabilities and describe model programs in several states. Included is an innovative program designed to keep offenders with developmental disabilities out of correctional facilities as well as model programs designed to meet the needs of such individuals while incarcerated.

DEFINITIONS

Federal law has provided a definition of the term *developmental disability*, which incorporates a spectrum of disorders. The Developmental Disabilities Assistance and Bill of Rights Act of 2000 (P.L. 106-402) outlines the legal standard required for an individual to be designated as having a developmental disorder and includes the following:

1. The disability is attributed to a mental or physical impairment or combination of the two.
2. The disability manifested before the age of 22.
3. The disability is likely to continue indefinitely.
4. The disability results in functional limitations in three or more of the following areas:

    a. Self-care
    b. Receptive or expressive language
    c. Mobility
    d. Self-direction
    e. Capacity for independent living
    f. Economic self-sufficiency

5. Individualized support is of a lifelong or extended duration and is individually planned.

Some states, such as California, have a more narrow definition of the term *developmental disability* (Petersilia 2000a). In 1977, California adopted the Lanterman Developmental Disabilities Services Act (2009), which delineates the state's responsibility to provide services to individuals with developmental disabilities. In Welfare and Institutions Code Section 4512(a) of the Lanterman Developmental Disabilities Services Act, *developmental disability* is defined as "a disability that originates before an individual attains age 18 years, continues, or can be expected to continue, indefinitely, and constitutes a substantial disability for that individual." Further, the definition includes mental retardation, cerebral palsy, epilepsy, and autism. This term shall also include disabling conditions found to be closely related to mental retardation or to require treatment similar to that required for individuals with mental retardation, but shall not include other handicapping conditions that are solely physical in nature.

According to the Centers for Disease Control and Prevention (1996), mental retardation is the most common developmental disability. For this reason, persons with mental retardation in the criminal justice system are the primary focus of this chapter. More recently, the term *mental retardation* has been changed to *intellectual disability*. Because sources vary in their use of terminology, both intellectual disability and mental retardation will be used interchangeably in this chapter.

The *Diagnostic and Statistical Manual of Mental Disorders*, 4th Edition, Text Revision (DSM-IV-TR) requires the following criteria for an individual to be diagnosed with mental retardation (American Psychiatric Association 2000):

1. Subaverage intellectual functioning (generally defined as an IQ of 70 or less)
2. Impairments in adaptive functioning
3. Onset before age 18

The severity of mental retardation is coded on the basis of the degree of intellectual impairment. The four DSM-IV-TR categories and their respective IQ ranges are as follows: *mild*, 50–55 up to 70; *moderate*, 35–40 up to 50–55; *severe*, 20–25 up to 35–40; and *profound*, below 20–25.

The American Association on Intellectual and Developmental Disabilities (AAIDD) (formerly the American Association on Mental Retardation [AAMR]) defines *intellectual disability* as "a disability characterized by significant limitations both in intellectual functioning and in adaptive behavior, which covers many everyday social and practical skills" (AAIDD 2009). The disability must originate before age 18 years. The AAIDD presents several issues to consider when evaluating an individual with intellectual disability:

1. Describing whether deficits exist in conceptual skills, social skills, or practical skills is necessary to develop an appropriate support plan.
2. The context of the individual's community environments, which are considered typical for his or her age, peers, and culture, must be considered when addressing limitations in current functioning.
3. Assessment must take into consideration cultural and linguistic diversity as well as differences in communication and sensory, motor, and behavioral factors.

4. It must be recognized that limitations and strengths coexist within an individual.
5. The life functioning of an individual with intellectual disability generally will improve with appropriate individualized support over a sustained period of time.

Table 18–1 summarizes the core aspects required for an individual to be considered developmentally disabled.

Some researchers have indicated that individuals with mental retardation are overrepresented within the criminal justice system (e.g., Cockram et al. 1998; Petersilia 1997; Santamour and West 1982a), although others have found no difference between the rates of these individuals in the corrections system and in the general population (Conley et al. 1992; MacEachron 1979; New York State Commission on Quality of Care for the Mentally Disabled 1991). Approximately 89% of individuals with mental retardation in the general population fall within the mild range (Ellis and Luckasson 1985); likewise, the majority of inmates with mental retardation fall in the mild range (Noble and Conley 1992). Therefore, the particular vulnerabilities and habilitation issues that present in individuals with mild mental retardation are most relevant to staff working with individuals with developmental disabilities within the correctional system. Offenders with moderate to profound mental retardation are unlikely to remain in the criminal justice system, because they are typically found not competent to stand trial and are sent to other, more appropriate institutions (Conley et al. 1992; Holland et al. 2002; Petrella 1992).

The distinction between *mental retardation* and *mental illness* is especially important in a discussion of appropriate interventions in corrections, although it is also relevant for pretrial concerns. An individual with a mental illness may be amenable to treatment, and the symptoms of the illness can be expected to ameliorate as a result of this treatment. In contrast, an individual with mental retardation or another developmental disability has, by definition, a condition that will continue indefinitely and is not necessarily responsive to treatment. Therefore, a discussion of interventions with such individuals must necessarily focus on habilitation rather than treatment. Additionally, identification of such inmates is of paramount importance, because many proceed through the criminal justice system undetected (Petrella 1992).

PREVALENCE

Prevalence rates of mental retardation in the general population vary depending on definitions, methods of study, and populations studied.

TABLE 18–1. Core aspects of developmental disability

The impairment manifests in childhood.

The impairment results in functional limitations.

The impairment is not expected to remediate, even with intervention.

The impairment can be any of a variety of disorders, although the most common is mental retardation.

According to DSM-IV-TR, the prevalence rate of individuals with mental retardation is estimated at about 1% of the population. The Arc of the United States (formerly the Association of Retarded Citizens of the United States) reviewed prevalence studies in the early 1980s and determined that 1.0%–3% of the general population had intellectual disabilities (The Arc of the United States 2004).

Unfortunately, the literature reporting the prevalence rates of incarcerated individuals with mental retardation contains many methodological problems. As previously noted, most studies indicate that individuals with mental retardation are overrepresented in correctional facilities; however, reported prevalence rates vary significantly. Jones (2009) noted that rates can vary from 2% to 40% depending on the method of assessment. As with the general population, differences in assessment, definition, and methodology, as well as regional differences, affect prevalence reports. Santamour and West (1982a) reported that the rate of adults with mental retardation in prison ranged from 8% to almost 30%. Specifically, the South Carolina Department of Corrections indicated a rate of 8%, Texas reported a rate of 10%, and Georgia reported a rate of 27%. Petersilia (1997) estimated that 6,400 adult and juvenile inmates have mental retardation in the California corrections system. An estimated 4%–10% of individuals in prison or jail in California have developmental disabilities (Petersilia 2000a). More recently, in a study conducted in the United Kingdom, 11% of younger male prisoners had at least borderline intellectual functioning (Herrington 2009). However, some reports suggest that the prevalence of individuals with mental retardation in correctional systems is comparable to the prevalence in the general population. For example, the New York State Commission on Quality of Care for the Mentally Disabled (1991) reported that 2% of approximately 53,400 inmates are developmentally disabled. Noble and Conley (1992) reported that approximately 14,000–20,000 inmates have developmental disabilities, constituting roughly 2% of all inmates in state and federal prisons. They also noted that rates of mental retardation ranged from 0.5% to almost 20% within state and federal prisons, asserting that the differences are secondary to methods of assessment. For example, group administrations of screening assessments are likely to overestimate the prevalence.

LEGAL ISSUES

Although Talent and Keldgord (1975) asserted that little effort has been expended on offenders with mental retardation, the management and treatment of individuals with developmental disabilities in the criminal justice system have received substantial legal attention in the past several decades. Case law and statutes have illuminated the scope of the problem and, in some instances, provided guidance as to reparative measures. One significant problem that has hampered the development of appropriate approaches with these individuals is the lack of distinction in the legal system between mental illness and mental retardation or developmental disabilities. As an example of this problem, the results of a survey of the attorneys general of the United States and four territories (McAfee and Gural 1988) suggest that the identification of individuals with developmental disabilities in the criminal justice system is unlikely to occur and that most protections for such individuals are contained in statutes pertaining to mental illness. In only one reporting state (South Carolina), the attorney general noted that judges routinely inquire about a defendant's IQ when a guilty plea is entered, presumably to ensure that the defendant has knowingly and intelligently entered the plea. Although many of the attorneys general described that special postconviction protections were in place for defendants with developmental disabilities, several reported that these protections were inconsistently employed. Eighty-six percent reported the use of a postconviction psychological evaluation, although no other named protection (e.g., reduced sentence, incarceration in a specialized unit, special training or education) was used in more than 50% of the respondent states.

Various courts in the United States have provided guidance to the correctional system regarding the management of offenders with developmental disabilities. For example, in *Estelle v. Gamble* (1976), the U.S. Supreme Court established the constitutional right of prisoners to medical treatment by holding that inmates could not be confined with "deliberate indifference" to their serious medical needs. Although individuals with developmental disabilities were not mentioned specifically, *Estelle* has been interpreted by lower courts to include psychiatric or psychological needs. One year later, in *Bowring v. Godwin* (1977), the Fourth Circuit Court of Appeals confirmed that psychiatric needs were included in the definition of severe medical needs: "We see no underlying distinction between the right to medical care for physical ills and its psychological or psychiatric counterpart." The U.S. District Court for the Southern District of Texas, in *Ruiz v. Estelle* (1980/1983), made specific references to "retarded inmates," noting repeatedly the injustices replete in the correctional system for these offenders, although the reparative measures suggested were generic to mental disorders. In *Kendrick v. Bland* (1981), the District Court for the Western District of Kentucky approved a consent decree requiring correction of conditions in Kentucky prisons, including the provision of education programs for "disadvantaged individuals under the age of 21 with learning problems and learning disabilities." This decision arose from the Education for all Handicapped Children Act of 1975 (EHA; P.L. 94-142), which has been interpreted to include incarcerated individuals age 21 or younger. This act requires that "free appropriate public education" be provided to all covered prisoners. The EHA was amended using "people-first" language and renamed the Individuals with Disabilities Education Act of 1990 (IDEA; P.L. 101-476).

Federal legislation has been interpreted to include the criminal justice system. In *Pennsylvania Department of Corrections v. Yeskey* (1998), the U.S. Supreme Court held in a unanimous decision that the Americans with Disabilities Act of 1990 (ADA; P.L. 101-336) applies to state prisoners: inmates with disabilities cannot be excluded from prison programs on the basis of a disability. In *Clark v. State of California* (1998), a class-action lawsuit was filed alleging that incarcerated individuals experienced discrimination as a result of their developmental disabilities, and injunctive relief was sought under the ADA. As a result of the *Yeskey* decision, California prison officials agreed to a settlement requiring the development and implementation of a plan to screen inmates for developmental disabilities and to provide these inmates with safe housing and supportive services.

These cases illustrate that the correctional system can no longer simply house inmates with developmental disabilities without appropriate screening and support. As a consequence, prisons increasingly are expected to develop specialized programs for these offenders.

DISPROPORTIONATE REPRESENTATION IN CORRECTIONAL SETTINGS

The literature is controversial regarding the disproportionate representation of offenders with mental retardation in correctional facilities. However, if such individuals are overrepresented, several factors may explain this disparity. The definitions of *mental retardation* and *developmental disability* require that the individual evidence impairments in adaptive functioning. These impairments can span numerous areas, often resulting in cognitive limitations that affect their decision-making skills, communication skills, social understanding, moral reasoning, and ability to learn from past mistakes (McGee and Menolascino 1992; Seay 2006). Deficits in these areas may lead to increased criminal behavior. Additionally, individuals with mental retardation are more likely to come from low-income minority groups residing in areas with increased police presence, a situation that places them at a higher risk of arrest (Petersilia 1997). Furthermore, individuals with developmental disabilities may often be manipulated into committing criminal acts by more functional friends and family members (Ebert and Long 2008; Jones 2007; Linhorst et al. 2002).

Once arrested, offenders with mental retardation may not understand their rights. For example, studies have shown that people with mental retardation often do not understand the Miranda warning against self-incrimination (Cloud et al. 2002; Ellis and Luckasson 1985; Everington and Fulero 1999; Fulero and Everington 1995; Petersilia 2000a). Given this lack of knowledge, an individual with mental retardation is more likely to waive his or her rights and provide incriminating information, increasing the likelihood of conviction and incarceration. Individuals with mental retardation are more vulnerable in interrogations because they are more susceptible to suggestion, acquiesce more often, and have a greater desire to please authority figures (Cloud et al. 2002; Everington and Fulero 1999; Jones 2007; Matikka and Vesala 1997; Pelka 1997; Petersilia 1997). These characteristics increase the likelihood of both false and legitimate confessions, which in turn increase the likelihood of conviction. Research has also indicated that offenders with mental retardation may not understand the differences between pleading guilty versus not guilty (S.A. Smith 1993).

Clinical Case 18–1

Mr. T, a 28-year-old man, was arrested and charged with petty theft. He was instructed by his older, more functional brother to steal a six-pack of beer from the local convenience store. Although Mr. T recognized that doing so was wrong, he wanted to please his brother and "fit in" with his brother's friends. A competence evaluation was requested by his attorney, who expressed concerns about Mr. T's judgment and intelligence. When the examiner began discussing pleas and possible defenses, Mr. T stated that he would have to plead guilty because "I did it."

Table 18–2 summarizes the cognitive and behavioral vulnerabilities of individuals with developmental disabilities that may contribute to the increased prevalence of arrest and incarceration.

TABLE 18–2.   Vulnerabilities of the offender with developmental
disabilities pretrial

Acquiescence	Offenders with developmental disabilities are eager to please and may be more vulnerable to interrogations.
Deference to authority	Offenders with developmental disabilities may interpret the actions of police officers as protective.
Masking their disability	Offenders with developmental disabilities may attempt to appear to possess a greater understanding than they do.
Concrete thinking	Offenders with developmental disabilities may have difficulty understanding the adversarial nature of the criminal justice system.
Language or educational deficits	Offenders with developmental disabilities may have difficulty understanding the Miranda warning and pleas or plea bargaining.

Santamour and West (1982a) proposed that probation is more likely given to individuals with higher intelligence, greater educational attainment, and an adequate work history. If this assertion is accurate, many people with mental retardation would not be granted probation, because they often are less educated and may not have a stable work history. Mason and Murphy (2002) studied a group of 90 probationers in southeast England and found no significant differences in two outcome measures of probation officer satisfaction for people with intellectual disability when compared with those functioning within the normal range of intelligence. Additionally, these two groups had no differences in number of probation violations. The authors noted that the lack of significant differences may be accounted for by the probation officers' ability to detect and counteract the difficulties of probationers with cognitive deficits. However, Mason and Murphy's study suggests that if Santamour and West's (1982a) supposition is accurate, the unwillingness to utilize probation is based on faulty beliefs about individuals with disabilities.

The number of individuals with mental retardation who are in prison is impacted by the individuals' impairments in decision making, communication, and moral reasoning; their susceptibility to suggestion and willingness to acquiesce; and a system that may not be inclined to release these offenders. These factors may explain the research that indicates that a disparity exists between the numbers of individuals with mental retardation in the general population versus the number of individuals with mental retardation in prisons. Clearly, the deficits described impair the ability of the offender with mental retardation to successfully navigate the criminal justice system prior to incarceration. These same vulnerabilities lead to predictable problems in the prison system.

PRETRIAL PROGRAMS FOR OFFENDERS WITH DEVELOPMENTAL DISABILITIES

Several programs have been developed to assist offenders with developmental disabilities in traversing the criminal justice system. For example, the Options for Justice program in St. Louis, Missouri, was developed to provide formal education to persons in the criminal justice system regarding the specific needs and vulnerabilities of these offenders (Linhorst et al. 2002). In Texas, an organization called Texas Appleseed has advocated for the rights of offenders with mental illness and mental retardation. The organization has published a number of handbooks, including "Opening the Door: Justice for Defendants With Mental Retardation," which is available to all attorneys (Texas Appleseed 2005). This handbook provides definitions of mental retardation and outlines specific vulnerabilities in such individuals. Recently, Georgia and Louisiana have adopted this handbook for attorneys working with individuals who have developmental disabilities.

The Options for Justice program, created in 1990, was funded by two county developmental disability boards in St. Louis, Missouri. The program was designed to provide a comprehensive range of services to employees of the criminal justice system and social service agencies, as well as offenders with developmental disabilities. The expressed goal of the program was to ensure that the treatment of offenders with developmental disabilities was equitable while they were held accountable for their behavior. In the following subsections, I describe several components of the program.

Education and Training

Education is provided to police officers, judges, attorneys, probation and parole officers, jail personnel, and social service workers regarding developmental disabilities; identifying offenders with such disabilities; and the manner in which disabilities might relate to the offense. The specific content of the training is tailored to the audience (e.g., police officers are provided with education regarding mental retardation and its possible effects on an individual's interrogation and understanding of Miranda warnings).

Direct Client Assistance

Case coordinators are provided to offenders with developmental disabilities to assist in both the pretrial and postdispositional phases. Pretrial assistance can include the provision of education to the court regarding the individual's specific disability, recommendations for alternative sentencing, and collaboration with community providers. Postdispositional activities include education of community agencies regarding the individual's disabilities, assistance in keeping scheduled appointments, and referrals to other community agencies.

Individual Justice Plan

The individual justice plan is developed based on the individual needs of the client and can include any of the following:

- Employment
- Counseling
- Housing
- Skills development
- Psychiatric treatment
- Substance abuse treatment
- Social activities
- Education
- Conditions of parole that affect the above

VULNERABILITY OF INDIVIDUALS WITH MENTAL RETARDATION IN CORRECTIONS

Prisoners with developmental disabilities are most often housed with the general population (Giamp and West 2003; New York State Commission on Quality of Care for the Mentally Disabled 1991; C. Smith et al. 1990). This housing situation places inmates with developmental disabilities at risk for victimization by other inmates. People with developmental disabilities are 4–10 times more likely to be victims of crime than those who do not have disabilities, and this trend holds true for persons with developmental disabilities in prison as well (Petersilia 2000b). Prisoners with mental retardation are more likely to be exploited, victimized, abused, and injured (Ellis and Luckasson 1985; Giamp and West 2003; Müller-Isberner and Hodgins 2000; Petersilia 1997; Santamour and West 1982a; C. Smith et al. 1990; Stavis 1991). Petersilia (1997) reported that offenders with mental retardation who are housed with the general population are more likely to have their property stolen, be raped, or be manipulated by other inmates to violate the rules. They have difficulty understanding the rules, which also increases the likelihood of disciplinary action. In *Ruiz v. Estelle* (1980/1983), the court opined,

> Mentally retarded persons meet with unremitting hardships in prison. They are slow to adjust to prison life and its requirements, principally because they have almost insurmountable difficulties in comprehending what is expected of them. Not understanding or remembering disciplinary rules, they tend to commit a large number of disciplinary infractions.

Clinical Case 18–2

Mr. J, age 39, was arrested on a federal fraud charge. He was evaluated for competence to stand trial because of significant concerns regarding his ability to understand the charges against him and to assist his attorneys in his defense. Mr. J was described as a "slow learner" and had dropped out of school in fifth grade. His mother described situations in which Mr. J was teased and taken advantage of or assaulted throughout his childhood. During the evaluation, Mr. J became tearful, stating that he was tired of people "messing" with him. He described an incident while incarcerated in which inmates who were more functional solicited him for oral sex. Although he was able to resist, he described continued harassment by these individuals. He reported the behavior to the correctional officers but received no assistance. Ultimately, Mr. J was "written up" for disruptive behavior when he became angry after continued solicitations.

In addition to the obvious consequences of maltreatment (e.g., physical injury, emotional turmoil), more subtle consequences ensue. Inmates with developmental disabilities are likely to resolve conflicts with others by using physical aggression due in part to limitations in communication skills (Petersilia 1997; C. Smith et al. 1990). People with mental retardation are more likely to have low frustration tolerance (Day 1990) and poor self-control (Benson 1994; Cullen 1993), increasing the likelihood of more disciplinary problems. C. Smith et al. (1990) found that youthful inmates with mental retardation received approximately three times as many disciplinary reports for noncompliant behavior and hygiene offenses (e.g., not showering) and assaulted other inmates or correctional staff over twice as often as other inmates. As a result of such disciplinary problems, inmates with mental retardation may serve longer prison sentences, be denied parole, or be transferred to a more secure prison (Ellis and Luckasson 1985; Giamp and West 2003; Petersilia 1997; Santamour and West 1982a; Stavis 1991). In *Ruiz v. Estelle* (1980/1983), the court noted,

It is common for mentally retarded inmates in TDC [Texas Department of Corrections] to serve longer sentences than inmates not fitting this category. Several reasons are evident. As previously noted, retarded inmates are more likely to have poor disciplinary records than their peers, which disqualify the former for early parole. They are frequently unable to succeed in institutional programs whose completion would increase their chances for parole, and they are also unlikely to be able to present well-defined employment and residential plans to the Parole Board.

Table 18–3 summarizes areas of vulnerabilities for offenders with developmental disabilities in a correctional environment.

RECEPTION AND ASSESSMENT PROCEDURES

Upon arrival at most correctional systems, inmates are subject to reception and assessment procedures used to identify any circumstance that would require specialized housing. During this classification process, some correctional systems attempt to identify offenders with developmental disabilities. A brief psychological and educational history may be obtained or certain testing may be performed to assess intelligence and adaptive functioning. For example, Giamp and West (2003) reported that a Colorado correctional facility uses the Culture Fair Intelligence Test (Cattell and Cattell 1973) and the Reading Level score from the Tests of Adult Basic Education (2005) to screen for mental retardation. If an inmate scores below a particular cutoff point, he or she is referred for further evaluation. This additional testing typically includes the Wechsler Adult Intelligence Scale—3rd Edition (WAIS-III; Wechsler 1997), which yields both Verbal and Performance IQ estimates, and an adaptive measure such as the Vineland Adaptive Behavior Scales (Sparrow et al. 2005) or the Adaptive Behavior Scale—Residential and Community, 2nd Edition (Nihira et al. 1993). In California, a screening tool was developed by the Department of Corrections to assess an inmate's cognitive abilities and functioning skills. The tool has several problems, however, most notably that compared with the assessment used by the Department of Developmental Services, the Department of Corrections tool overidentifies offenders with developmental disabilities.

Appropriate services are dependent on the use of valid and reliable instruments. As the AAIDD suggests, assessments must consider cultural and linguistic issues in addition to other sensory and communication factors (see http://www.aaidd.org/content_100.cfm?navID=21). MacEachron (1979) found that the prevalence of offenders with mental retardation dropped significantly when individual (rather than group) assessments of intelligence were administered. McGee and Menolascino

TABLE 18–3. Vulnerabilities of the offender with developmental disabilities in the correctional setting

Cognitive limitations
  Difficulty understanding and following rules
Adaptive skills deficits
  Difficulty following guidelines and routines
  More hygiene infractions
Impaired social understanding
  Vulnerability to manipulation and victimization
  Tendency to resolve conflicts with aggression
Lower educational and occupational functioning
  Less likely to be paroled

(1992) argued that even screening assessments should be administered individually, and only by professionals trained in such administration. They recommended using the Peabody Picture Vocabulary Test, now in its third edition (Dunn and Dunn 1997). Many jurisdictions, including North Carolina and South Carolina, use the Beta Examination, currently in its third revision (Beta-III; Kellogg and Morton 1999) and the Wide Range Achievement Test, now in its fourth edition (WRAT-4; Wilkinson and Robertson 2006), to screen for intellectual or academic deficits. Scores below a certain cutoff indicate the need for further assessment.

The assessments mentioned above are used primarily to identify inmates with deficits. Critical in formulating an individualized habilitation plan is use of a more comprehensive assessment that includes both strengths and deficit areas that may be most amenable to intervention. An individualized habilitation plan targets the areas most appropriate for each person. As noted previously, individuals with intellectual disabilities have varying levels of functioning and skills. As such, any treatment approach should be tailored for the specific person. Many jurisdictions (e.g., California, North Carolina) use their own assessments to identify functional deficits; however, rarely are these assessments normed or standardized. The AAIDD has published a comprehensive assessment called the Supports Intensity Scale (Tassé et al. 2005), which was designed to identify deficits in 57 specific life activities, 15 medical conditions, and 13 problem behaviors. This instrument was developed over a period of 5 years, and the developers performed an extensive literature review, a Q-sort, and three field tests. The Supports Intensity Scale is purported to have excellent psychometric properties. Research has indicated that the assessment possesses good interrater reliability, especially if the raters are trained (Thompson et al. 2008). The Service Need Assessment Profile (Gould 1998) also was designed to measure the support needs of individuals with developmental disabilities. Construct and criterion validity for this instrument are high (Guscia et al. 2006), indicating that it is a valid choice for attempting to delineate the needs of an individual with developmental disabilities. Table 18–4 provides a listing of the various instruments used in corrections for individuals with developmental delays and an estimate of the intensity of training required to use each one.

HABILITATION ISSUES

The management of inmates with developmental disabilities has presented correctional systems with significant problems. One controversy has been whether inmates with developmental disabilities should be housed in the general prison population. Those in favor of housing these inmates with the general prison population adhere to the principle of normalization, suggesting that individuals with mental retardation should be treated like others as much as possible (Santamour and West 1982a). However, as previously noted, much has been published on the disadvantages and risks to the prisoner with mental retardation when he or she is placed in the general prison population. Critics argue that normalization does not take these disadvantages into account. According to Petersilia (1997), "The emerging consensus within the profession seems to be that there are highly unique aspects to the correctional environment and that the normalization goals for the mentally retarded should not fully apply in this setting" (p. 6). Her statement suggests that specialized units may be more appropriate for such individuals.

Although court cases such as *Ruiz v. Estelle* (1980/1983) established that individuals with developmental disabilities have the right to treatment, Hall (1992) estimated that fewer than 10% of inmates with such deficits receive specialized services. In fact, many authors have indicated that specialized services for prisoners with mental retardation are inadequate (Giamp and West 2003; Müller-Isberner and Hodgins 2000). Although Hall (1992) noted that advocates for these offenders must be cautious in their expectations—"it is unreasonable to conceptualize prisons as care and treatment facilities" (p. 171)—services designed to aid the offender with mental retardation to adapt to incarceration and reintegrate into society are increasingly expected of correctional facilities.

Unlike programs for offenders with mental illness, specialized programs for offenders with developmental disabilities do not have remediation of disabilities as the goal. The goal of most programs is education,

TABLE 18–4. Common assessments used in the correctional setting for inmates with developmental disabilities

Test name	Training required
Intelligence assessments	
Beta-III (Kellogg and Morton 1999)	Minimal training
Culture Fair Intelligence Test (Cattell and Cattell 1973)	Requires training
Wechsler Adult Intelligence Scale, 3rd Edition (Wechsler 1997)	Extensive training
Educational assessments	
Peabody Picture Vocabulary Test, 3rd Edition (Dunn and Dunn 1997)	Minimal training
Tests of Adult Basic Education (2005)	Requires training
Wide Range Achievement Test, 4th Edition (Wilkinson and Robertson 2006)	Requires training
Adaptive skills	
Adaptive Behavior Scale—Residential and Community, 2nd Edition (Nihira et al. 1993)	Minimal training
Vineland Adaptive Behavior Scales (Sparrow et al. 2005)	Minimal training
Support assessments	
Service Need Assessment Profile (Gould 1998)	Minimal training
Supports Intensity Scale (Tassé et al. 2005)	Minimal training

training, and skills enhancement tailored to the inmate's specific needs. As with any other disorder, the diagnosis of mental retardation provides no information about the needs of the specific individual. Therefore, assessment is a critical component in any specialized program. For example, as a result of *Clark v. State of California* (1998), prison officials in California developed a "remedial plan" (known as the "Clark plan") for identifying prisoners with developmental disabilities and providing them with access to a variety of programs that would make early release more likely. This plan includes 1) screening for developmental disabilities; 2) housing inmates with developmental disabilities together based on level of functioning; 3) providing additional staff to these housing units; 4) training staff on interacting with inmates with developmental disabilities; 5) providing instructors with special education credentials for each developmental disability program responsible for developing individually tailored programs; and 6) providing parole agents to ensure that developmentally disabled inmates understand the terms of parole and are aware of services available in the community.

Programs for offenders with mental retardation generally focus on improving the functioning and adaptation of the inmate while incarcerated and upon release (Santamour 1987). The vulnerabilities outlined in the previous sections lead to logical interventions that include skills training, educational and vocational rehabilitation, and counseling and treatment specific to the needs of each offender.

Skills Training

Skills training for the offender with mental retardation can encompass a wide variety of areas. The assessment process is used to determine the areas most necessary for each individual, such as social skills training or training in areas of adaptive functioning. Day (1988) designed a program in the United Kingdom for offenders with intellectual deficits. An individualized treatment program was developed for each offender on the basis of a token economy system. The system consisted of a weekly grading scheme, which included both monetary and social incentives. A practical skills training package focused on skills such as maintaining a clean living area, laundering clothing, budgeting, and using community facilities. Leisure activities also were encouraged. Fifty-five percent of the participants evidenced a "good" response to treatment, and 30% were rated "fair." A reported 15% of enrollees did not benefit. Follow-up after approximately 3 years indicated that 70% of the participants who completed the program were evaluated as doing well in the community, especially those offenders who had committed crimes against persons rather than property.

Corrigan (1991) conducted a meta-analysis of social skills training programs and found that individuals with developmental disabilities evidenced the greatest improvement. However, generalization of skills learned was lowest for this group. Social skills training was least effective for the offender group. Interestingly, although the offenders acquired the requisite skills, these skills did not translate into behavior change. This study suggests that social skills training may improve institutional behavior, at least with those individuals with developmental disabilities, but may not generalize to other settings.

Cole et al. (1985) evaluated the efficacy of a self-management training program for adults with mental retardation and conduct problems in a vocational setting. The participants—six adults who exhibited significant behavior problems unresponsive to alternative treatments—were taught a variety of skills, including self-monitoring, self-evaluation, self-consequation, and self-instruction. An immediate decrease in disruptive behavior occurred and was maintained at 9-month follow-up.

An intensive behavior therapy unit in a Georgia maximum security prison for women has shown promising results (Daniel et al. 2003). This program, described as a weekly incentive program designed to improve skills and decrease inappropriate behaviors, was developed for inmates unable to adjust adequately in the general population.

Vocational Training

For several reasons, vocational training is an important part of a comprehensive program to treat inmates with developmental disabilities. Vocational training teaches inmates skills and information necessary to perform a job after release and allows the inmate to work in a sheltered environment before reentry into the community (Santamour and West 1982b). Vocational training also provides inmates with developmental disabilities the opportunity to engage in meaningful, productive work that decreases behavioral issues and increases feelings of self-worth (Shively 2004).

Harley (1996) advocated for a "multistage" vocational rehabilitation plan that deals with vocational training both before and after release from prison. Although this plan was not developed specifically for inmates with developmental disabilities, it involves the evaluation of individual strengths and needs, and conforms to the notion of an individualized habilitation plan. Harley recommended an initial vocational assessment during incarceration, including a comprehensive evaluation that would result in a diagnosis, a functional assessment, and prognosis for outcome. The second stage is to develop a specific habilitation plan that includes both pre- and postincarceration components. Harley recommended that transition goals and objectives be included in the plan, as well as "exit criteria" (i.e., the level of skill required for successful completion of the program).

Anger Management

Anger management is an important component in a treatment program for prisoners with mental retardation (Hall 1992). As previously noted, self-control and aggression can be problems for some inmates (Shively 2004). Lack of self-control in a prison environment can lead to negative consequences, such as increased disciplinary reports (C. Smith et al. 1990). The lack of communication and interpersonal skills can lead to frustration and an increased likelihood of acting out conflicts (C. Smith et al. 1990). However, administrators must necessarily be cautious regarding the methods of management. For example, in a study comparing the use of medication in controlling aggressive behavior, Elie et al. (1980) found that aggressive behavior was greater in patients who received thioridazine than in patients who received placebo.

Benson (1994) modified an anger management program for use with adults with mental retardation. Although this program was not developed specifically for offenders, it may be useful in an overall habilitation program that includes individualized treatment. According to Benson, self-control training may generalize from one situation to another and can reduce an inmate's incidents of aggression during incarceration and enable the inmate to control his or her anger in the community. The components of the program include 1) identification of feelings, 2) relaxation training, 3) self-instruction training, and 4) the development of problem-solving skills. Although additional research is necessary to establish the program's effectiveness, initial results indicate that it can have a therapeutic effect and may increase personal control.

Denkowski and Denkowski (1985) evaluated the effectiveness of a community-based treatment program for adolescent offenders with mental retardation. The program was based on a token economy system but was enhanced for one group by offering "social points." Additionally, this group was required to spend a fixed amount of time in a "timeout room" for any instance of aggression. The enhanced treatment group evidenced the greatest success in reducing physical and verbal aggression. Although this program was community based and was used with adolescents, a population likely more responsive to the use of timeouts, this study suggests that the appropriate use of social learning techniques can be effective in modifying problematic behavior in an offender population.

In the previous three paragraphs, I discuss various programs designed to modify aggressive behavior in individuals with mental retardation. Most research has indicated that behavior disorders are the most common co-occurring disturbance in offenders with mental retardation (Gardner et al. 1998). However, an offender with mental retardation may also be diagnosed with a major psychiatric disorder (e.g., schizophrenia, bipolar disorder). Treatment approaches for such offenders would necessarily address the psychiatric disturbance as well as the habilitative needs associated with the developmental disability. Chapter 13, "Creating Wellness Through Collaborative Mental Health Interventions," provides an excellent overview of treatment approaches for offenders with mental illness.

MODEL PROGRAMS FOR OFFENDERS WITH DEVELOPMENTAL DISABILITIES IN CORRECTIONS

South Carolina Habilitation Unit

The South Carolina Habilitation Unit (President's Committee on Mental Retardation 1992) was established in 1975 to provide residential services to male inmates with developmental disabilities and day treatment services to female inmates with developmental disabilities. The stated goal was to improve institutional adjustment and postrelease functioning. The unit houses a maximum of 40 male inmates and can provide services to 10 females. In general, eligibility includes individuals with intellectual or physical impairments that limit their ability to function in the general population and an expectation that they will benefit from the services. The South Carolina Department of Corrections adheres to the P.L. 106-402 definition of developmental disability (Developmental Disabilities Assistance and Bill of Rights Act of 2000). In addition, the department requires that the inmate agree to participate and demonstrate a potential for improvement. Prisoners in maximum security are not eligible. Referrals are generally made by regional classification coordinators or psychologists at reception and evaluation centers. Referred inmates suspected of having a developmental disability are administered the Beta-II, WAIS-III, and WRAT-3. They also are interviewed extensively. Inmates referred from other facilities are administered the Beta-II, the WRAT-3, and a Department of Corrections instrument designed to assess functional abilities. Entry requirements include a score of 60 or below on the Beta-II and a third-grade reading level or lower.

Each inmate has an Individual Habilitation Plan developed by a multidisciplinary team that consists of special education, work activity, a social work program (for life skills and counseling), and recreation. Inmates are involved in scheduled activities for a minimum of 38 hours per week.

Special Education

The South Carolina program includes ongoing educational assessment, curriculum and lesson plan development, and classroom instruction (both group and individual). This program is approved by the State Department of Education and receives funding for qualified inmates (age 21 or younger) under the IDEA.

Work Activity

One focus of the South Carolina program is on job acquisition and retention skills in a simulated work environment. The objectives are to develop positive work behavior, attitudes, and skills to maintain a job. A vocational assessment and on-the-job experience in various prison industries are provided to simulate a real-life work setting.

Social Work Program

The social work program focuses on the initial needs assessment and orientation as well as the development of the Individual Habilitation Plan. Each inmate is assigned a primary case manager who organizes all habilitative services, which might include individual counseling, group treatment, and community release planning. The life skills component emphasizes behaviors that will allow the inmate to function independently following release.

Recreation

The recreation program is designed to promote leisure skills and to develop effective interpersonal skills. Activities include team sports and arts and crafts.

Release Planning

Most inmates are released to the community rather than transferred to another facility. Release plans include organizing residential plans, vocational/occupational issues (job placement or training), follow-up treatment, and educational services. An attempt is made to involve family members, if appropriate. Social workers can be present at parole hearings to assist the inmate.

Utah Department of Corrections Adaptive Services for Environmental Needs Development

In 1999, the Utah Department of Corrections designated a segregated living space at the Utah State Prison to address the needs of offenders with IQs below 70. The Adaptive Services for Environmental Needs Development (ASEND) program provides programming for inmates with developmental disabilities who are unable to adequately adjust to the institutional environment. The goals of the ASEND program are to help inmates to adjust appropriately to incarceration, provide a safe environment for these individuals, and prepare them for their eventual release to the community.

Each inmate's written Individual Habilitation Plan can include services in any of the following areas:

- Education
- Life skills training

- Vocational training
- Specific areas indicated by the needs of the offender (e.g., psychiatric intervention, substance use treatment)
- Recreational activities
- Postrelease planning

In addition, staff assigned to the ASEND unit undergo training for working with this population. Inmates are screened using an assessment of grade level, which is followed by an in-depth IQ assessment (typically with the WAIS-III). The habilitative plan is developed within 30 days of arrival.

CONCLUSION

The habilitation of individuals with developmental disabilities in the correctional system cannot be ignored. Although Hall (1992) noted that correctional facilities should not be viewed as treatment facilities, such institutions cannot be deliberately indifferent to the needs of these offenders. Inmates with developmental delays may be more easily led, suggestible, and dependent. Lower levels of comprehension and poor adaptive skills can lead to more rule infractions and disciplinary action, leading to a decreased likelihood for parole. Research has indicated that these offenders serve more time for the same crime than do offenders without developmental disabilities (Petersilia 2000a).

Opinions are mixed as to whether appropriate services for such individuals should be provided on specialized units. Proponents of this approach cite the vulnerabilities of these offenders. However, all agree that specialized services must include appropriate assessment that takes into account culture and individualized approaches to habilitation. One cannot presume that services designed for the individual with mental illness will be appropriate for inmates with developmental disabilities.

Because little research has been conducted on the efficacy of specialized services for offenders with developmental disabilities, correctional facilities must draw on research based on nonoffending samples. An active collaboration between departments of corrections and agencies providing services for individuals with developmental disabilities can enhance service delivery and improve the integration of the offender into the community. As courts continue to protect the rights of offenders with developmental disabilities, correctional facilities must explore creative ways to deliver appropriate services.

SUMMARY POINTS

- Inmates with developmental disabilities have increased vulnerability secondary to cognitive and adaptive skills deficits.

- Early identification and detection are crucial in addressing the needs of these offenders.

- Pretrial programs can assist in diverting offenders with developmental disabilities from the criminal justice system to more appropriate treatment centers.

- Legislation requires that programs be developed to address these special needs in a correctional setting.

- Programs for offenders with developmental disabilities should include 1) skills development, 2) educational opportunities/vocational training, and 3) cognitive-behavioral interventions to address specific areas of concern.

REFERENCES

American Association on Intellectual and Developmental Disabilities: Definition of intellectual disability. 2009. Available at: http://www.aamr.org/content_100.cfm?navID=21. Accessed June 19, 2009.

American Psychiatric Association: Diagnostic and Statistical Manual of Mental Disorders, 4th Edition, Text Revision. Washington, DC, American Psychiatric Association, 2000

Americans with Disabilities Act of 1990, 42 U.S.C. § 12101 et seq

The Arc of the United States: Introduction to mental retardation. 2004. Available at: http://www.thearc.org/NetCommunity/Document.Doc?&id143. Accessed September 9, 2008.

Benson BA: Anger management training: a self-control programme for persons with mild mental retardation, in Mental Health in Mental Retardation: Recent Advances and Practices. Edited by Bouras N. New York, Cambridge University Press, 1994, pp 224–232

Bowring v Godwin, 551 F.2d 44 (4th Cir. 1977)

Cattell RB, Cattell AKS: Culture Fair Intelligence Test, 3rd Edition. Savoy, IL, Institute for Personality and Ability Testing, 1973

Centers for Disease Control and Prevention: State-specific rates of mental retardation—United States, 1993. MMWR Weekly 45:61–65, 1996. Available at: http://www.cdc.gov/mmwr/preview/mmwrhtml/00040023.htm. Accessed April 22, 2009.

Clark v State of California: 123 F.3d 1267 (9th Cir. 1997), cert. denied, 118 S.Ct 2340 (1998)

Cloud M, Shepherd GB, Barkoff A, et al: Words without meaning: the Constitution, confessions, and mentally retarded suspects. Univ Chic Law Rev 69:495–624, 2002

Cockram J, Jackson R, Underwood R: People with an intellectual disability and the criminal justice system: the family perspective. J Intellect Dev Disabil 23:41–56, 1998

Cole CL, Gardner WI, Karan OC: Self-management training of mentally retarded adults presenting severe conduct difficulties. Appl Res Ment Retard 6:337–347, 1985

Conley RW, Luckasson R, Bouthilet GN: The Criminal Justice System and Mental Retardation. Baltimore, MD, Paul H Brookes, 1992

Corrigan PW: Social skills training in adult psychiatric populations: a meta-analysis. J Behav Ther Exp Psychiatry 22:203–210, 1991

Cullen C: The treatment of people with learning disabilities who offend, in Clinical Approaches to the Mentally Disordered Offender. Edited by Howells K, Hollin CR. Chichester, UK, Wiley, 1993, pp 145–162

Daniel C, Jackson J, Watkins J: Utility of an intensive behavior therapy unit in a maximum security female prison. Behavior Therapist 26:211–212, 2003

Day K: A hospital based treatment programme for mentally handicapped offenders. Br J Psychiatry 153:635–644, 1988

Day K: Mental retardation: clinical aspects and management, in Principles and Practice of Forensic Psychiatry. Edited by Bluglass R, Bowden P. Edinburgh, UK, Churchill Livingstone, 1990, pp 399–418

Denkowski GC, Denkowski KM: Community based residential treatment of the mentally retarded adolescent offender, phase 1: reduction of aggressive behavior. J Community Psychol 13:299–305, 1985

Developmental Disabilities Assistance and Bill of Rights Act of 2000, 42 U.S.C. § 15001 et seq

Dunn LM, Dunn LM: Peabody Picture Vocabulary Test, 3rd Edition. Circle Pines, MN, AGS Publishing, 1997

Ebert RS, Long JS: Mental retardation and the criminal justice system: forensic issues, in Forensic Psychology and Neuropsychology for Criminal and Civil Cases. Edited by Hall HV. Boca Raton, FL, CRC Press, 2008, pp 375–392

Education for all Handicapped Children Act of 1975, 20 U.S.C. § 1400 et seq

Elie R, Langlois Y, Cooper SF, et al: Comparison of SCH-12679 and thioridazine in aggressive mental retardates. Can J Psychiatry 25:484–491, 1980

Ellis JW, Luckasson RA: Mentally retarded criminal defendants. George Washington Law Rev 53:414–493, 1985

Estelle v Gamble, 426 U.S. 97 (1976)

Everington C, Fulero SM: Competence to confess: measuring understanding and suggestibility of defendants with mental retardation. Ment Retard 37:212–220, 1999

Fulero SM, Everington C: Assessing competency to waive Miranda rights in defendants with mental retardation. Law Hum Behav 19:533–543, 1995

Gardner WI, Graeber JL, Machkovitz SJ: Treatment of offenders with mental retardation, in Treatment of Offenders With Mental Disorder. Edited by Wettstein RM. New York, Guilford, 1998, pp 329–364

Giamp JS, West ME: Delivering psychological services to incarcerated men with developmental disabilities, in Correctional Psychology: Practice, Programming, and Administration. Edited by Schwartz BK. Kingston, NJ, Civic Research Institute, 2003, pp 8.1–8.29

Gould A: The Service Need Assessment Profile. Sydney, New South Wales, ATG and Associates, 1998

Guscia R, Harries J, Kirby N, et al: Construct and criterion validities of the Service Need Assessment Profile (SNAP): a measure of support for people with disabilities. J Intellect Dev Disabil 31:145–155, 2006

Hall JN: Correctional services for inmates with mental retardation, in The Criminal Justice System and Mental Retardation: Defendants and Victims. Edited by Conley RW, Luckasson R, Bouthilet GN. Baltimore, MD, Paul H Brookes, 1992, pp 167–190

Harley DA: Vocational rehabilitation services for an offender population. J Rehabil 62:45–48, 1996

Herrington V: Assessing the prevalence of intellectual disability among young male prisoners. J Intellect Disabil Res 53:397–410, 2009

Holland AJ, Clare ICH, Mukhopadhyay T: Prevalence of "criminal offending" by men and women with intellectual disability and the characteristics of the "offenders": implications for research and service development. J Intellect Disabil Res 46:6–20, 2002

Individuals with Disabilities Education Act of 1990, 20 U.S.C. § 1400 et seq

Jones J: Persons with intellectual disabilities in the criminal justice system: review of issues. Int J Offender Ther Comp Criminol 51:723–733, 2007

Kellogg CE, Morton NW: Revised Beta Examination, 2nd Edition. San Antonio, TX, Psychological Corporation, 1974

Kellogg CE, Morton NW: Beta III Manual. San Antonio, TX, Pearson Education, 1999

Kendrick v Bland, 541 F.Supp. 21 (1981)

Lanterman Developmental Disabilities Services Act, California Welfare and Institutions Code, §§ 4500–4519, January 2009. Available at: http://www.dds.ca.gov/statutes/docs/LantermanAct_2009.pdf. Accessed September 9, 2008.

Linhorst DM, Bennett L, McCutchen T: Development and implementation of a program for offenders with developmental disabilities. Ment Retard 40:41–50, 2002

MacEachron AE: Mentally retarded offenders: prevalence and characteristics. Am J Ment Defic 84:165–176, 1979

Mason J, Murphy G: Intellectual disability amongst people on probation: prevalence and outcome. J Intellect Disabil Res 46:230–238, 2002

Matikka LM, Vesala HT: Acquiescence in quality-of-life interviews with adults who have mental retardation. Ment Retard 35:75–82, 1997

McAfee JK, Gural M: Individuals with mental retardation and the criminal justice system: the view from states' attorneys general. Ment Retard 26:5–12, 1988

McGee JJ, Menolascino FJ: The evaluation of defendants with mental retardation in the criminal justice system, in The Criminal Justice System and Mental Retardation: Defendants and Victims. Edited by Conley RW, Luckasson R, Bouthilet GN. Baltimore, MD, Paul H Brookes, 1992, pp 55–77

Müller-Isberner R, Hodgins S: Evidence-based treatment for mentally disordered offenders, in Violence, Crime and Mentally Disordered Offenders. Edited by Hodgins S, Müller-Isberner R. Chichester, UK, Wiley, 2000, pp 7–38

New York State Commission on Quality of Care for the Mentally Disabled: Inmates with developmental disabilities in NYS correctional facilities. March 1991. Available at: http://www.cqc.state.ny.us/publications/pubinmat.htm. Accessed April 22, 2009.

Nihira K, Leland H, Lambert N: Adaptive Behavior Scale—Residential and Community, 2nd Edition. Austin, TX, PRO-ED, 1993

Noble JH, Conley RW: Toward an epidemiology of relevant attributes, in The Criminal Justice System and Mental Retardation: Defendants and Victims. Edited by Conley RW, Luckasson R, Bouthilet GN. Baltimore, MD, Paul H Brookes, 1992, pp 17–53

Pelka F: Unequal justice: preserving the rights of the mentally retarded in the criminal justice system. Humanist 57:28–32, 1997

Pennsylvania Department of Corrections v Yeskey, 524 U.S. 206 (1998)

Petersilia J: Justice for all? Offenders with mental retardation and the California corrections system. Prison J 77:358–381, 1997

Petersilia J: Doing justice? Criminal offenders with developmental disabilities. California Policy Research Center Brief, Vol 12, No 4, University of California, August 2000a. Available at: http://www.ucop.edu/cprc/documents/dojustrpt.pdf. Accessed April 22, 2009.

Petersilia J: Invisible victims: violence against persons with developmental disabilities. Human Rights 27:9–13, 2000b

Petrella RC: Defendants with mental retardation in the forensic services system, in The Criminal Justice System and Mental Retardation: Defendants and Victims. Edited by Conley RW, Luckasson R, Bouthilet GN. Baltimore, MD, Paul H Brookes, 1992, pp 79–96

President's Committee on Mental Retardation: Correctional industries: background, planning and development guide for inmates with mental retardation. Hyattsville, MD, Sociometrics, March 27, 1992. Available at: http://www.nicic.org/pubs/1992/011245.pdf. Accessed April 22, 2009.

Ruiz v Estelle, 503 F.Supp. 1265 (S.D. Tex 1980), cert. denied, 103 S. Ct. 1438 (1983)

Santamour MB: The offender with mental retardation. Prison J 66:3–18, 1987

Santamour MB, West B: The mentally retarded offender: presentation of the facts and a discussion of issues, in The Retarded Offender. Edited by Santamour MB, Watson PS. New York, Praeger, 1982a, pp 7–36

Santamour MB, West B: Retarded offenders: habilitative program development, in The Retarded Offender. Edited by Santamour MB, Watson PS. New York, Praeger, 1982b, pp 272–296

Seay OJ: Evaluating mental retardation for forensic purposes. Applied Psychology in Criminal Justice 2:52–81, 2006

Shively R: Treating offenders with mental retardation and developmental disabilities. Corrections Today 66:84–87, 2004

Smith C, Algozzine B, Schmid R, et al: Prison adjustment of youthful inmates with mental retardation. Ment Retard 28:177–181, 1990

Smith SA: Confusing the terms "guilty" and "not guilty": implications for alleged offenders with mental retardation. Psychol Rep 73:675–678, 1993

Sparrow SA, Cicchetti DV, Balla DA: Vineland–II Survey Forms Manual. Minneapolis, MN, AGS Publishing, 2005

Stavis PF: Doing justice? The criminal justice system and persons with mental retardation. Quality of Care Newsletter, Issue 47, January–February 1991. Available at: http://www.cqc.state.ny.us/counsels_corner/cc47.htm. Accessed April 22, 2009.

Talent A, Keldgord R: The mentally retarded probationer. Fed Probat 2:39–46, 1975

Tassé MJ, Schalock R, Thompson JR, et al: Guidelines for Interviewing People With Disabilities: Supports Intensity Scale. Washington, DC, American Association on Intellectual and Developmental Disabilities, 2005. Available at: http://www.siswebsite.org/galleries/default-file/SISGuidelinesforinterviewing.pdf. Accessed April 22, 2009.

Tests of Adult Basic Education. Monterey, CA, CTB/McGraw-Hill, 2005

Texas Appleseed: Opening the door: justice for defendants with mental retardation. 2005. Available at: http://www.texasappleseed.net/pdf/hbook_MR_attorney_Opening.pdf. Accessed April 22, 2009.

Thompson JR, Tassé MJ, McLaughlin CA: Interrater reliability of the Supports Intensity Scale (SIS). Am J Ment Retard 113:231–237, 2008

Wechsler D: Wechsler Adult Intelligence Scale, 3rd Edition. San Antonio, TX, Pearson, 1997

Wilkinson GS, Robertson GJ: Wide Range Achievement Test, 4th Edition. Lutz, FL, Psychological Assessment Resources, 2006

CHAPTER 19

Juvenile Offenders

Stephen Wu, M.D.
Christopher Thompson, M.D.

The dramatic rise in the incarceration rate of juveniles (i.e., those under age 18) in the United States during the 1990s—a 43% increase over the course of the decade—has been followed by a modest decline in the rate since 2000. In 2006, just under 93,000 juveniles were in residential custody, a decrease of 14% from the peak population of over 107,000 in 1999 (Davis et al. 2008). Despite these declining figures, an estimated 88,000 more juveniles are incarcerated in the United States than in any western European country. The United States detains and holds approximately 1.4 per 100,000 youths. This rate is 2.5 times higher than that of the second-highest Western nation, the Netherlands (0.57), and more than five times that of England (0.25) and Germany (0.23) (Muncie 2008). In addition to being one of the world's "leaders" in juvenile incarceration, the United States is the only major country in the world that has refused to sign the 1989 United Nations Convention on the Rights of the Child (UNCRC), which declares that children have a right to protection, participation, personal development, and basic material provisions. With relation to juvenile justice, the UNCRC promotes the principle of the "best interests" of the child, custody as a last resort, separation from adults while in custody, and processes that respect the dignity of the child. By 2006, a total of 191 countries had ratified the UNCRC, making it one of the most widely agreed-upon set of principles in the annals of international human rights law (Krisberg 2006).

The "best interests" principle is the philosophical foundation upon which the United States' juvenile justice system was based at its outset in 1899. In contrast, developments in the late twentieth century suggest that more "punitive values" (e.g., retribution, incapacitation, individual responsibility, offender accountability) have eclipsed the more traditional principles of juvenile protection and support (Muncie 2008). Indeed, nearly all states have facilitated the transfer of juveniles to the adult criminal justice system, created mandatory minimum sentences for juveniles convicted of certain crimes, and undermined the principle of confidentiality by circulating the social histories of juvenile defendants among criminal justice, education, health, and social service agencies, as well as the media (Amnesty International 1998; Mears 2006; Snyder 2002). The profound changes in the core philosophy of the juvenile justice system have dramatically reshaped both the form and the function of youth detention in the United States and have had important and far-reaching implications for the provision of psychiatric care to youths in both the juvenile justice and adult criminal justice systems.

OVERVIEW OF JUVENILE ARREST AND VIOLENCE EPIDEMIOLOGY

The true extent of juvenile delinquency is difficult to ascertain. Many unlawful behaviors are never reported to law enforcement officials, and the majority of crimes that are reported remain unsolved. It is unclear how much of this "undocumented offending" is attributable to youths.

Current knowledge of juvenile crime in the United States is culled from two primary sources: official arrest records and self-report behavioral studies. Although official records reflect the actual number of youths entering the juvenile justice system, they may underestimate actual delinquent behavior because the records fail to account for crimes for which no arrests were made. At the same time, they may overestimate the extent of juvenile offending because they document the total numbers of youths taken into custody rather than those actually found delinquent by courts. Official records may also distort the understanding of the nature of delinquency by overrepresenting those specific behaviors that are targeted by law enforcement. On the other hand, self-report studies, which tend to report much higher offending rates than official records, capture information from youths who may have no contact with the justice system. However, these studies are limited by respondents' memories and willingness to disclose all delinquent behaviors (Krisberg and Wolf 2005). In an attempt to provide a more accurate and comprehensive picture of U.S. juvenile crime, reports from the Office of Juvenile Justice and Delinquency Prevention integrate both types of sources.

Data and Trends on Juvenile Crime

According to the Federal Bureau of Investigation (FBI; 2007), 1,268,950 juveniles were arrested in the United States in 2006. This accounted for 15.4% of the total arrests made that year. Juvenile arrests represented 15.9% of all violent crime arrests. For serious property crimes, including burglary, larceny-theft, motor vehicle theft, and arson, juveniles represented 26.5% of all arrests. Despite these high numbers, more than three-quarters of juvenile arrests are for less serious or trivial offenses. Unlike adults, juveniles may also be arrested for status offenses, or behaviors that are considered unlawful for youths because of their age (e.g., truancy, running away from home, underage drinking or smoking, incorrigibility, curfew violations). In 2006, status offenses accounted for over 10% of all juvenile arrests. Table 19–1 summarizes the 2006 arrest statistics in the United States.

Although arrest rates for juvenile violent crimes in the United States remained relatively stable from the early 1970s to the late 1980s, the 5-year period between 1989 and 1994 saw a dramatic, 60% increase in juvenile violent crime arrests; this trend, in conjunction with increasingly sensationalistic media coverage of particularly violent juvenile crimes and political pressure to "get tough on crime," led to an increase in public attention on juvenile delinquency and the eventual adoption of harsher, more punitive policies toward these young offenders (Krisberg 2005). Despite ongoing public concern that juvenile crime remains a large problem, juvenile violent crime rates appear to have steadily decreased over subsequent years. From 1997 to 2006, juvenile arrests for murder declined by 42%. Similar declines occurred in arrests for each category of violent crime, including 30.9% fewer arrests for rape, 15.9% fewer for robbery, and 20.9% fewer for aggravated assault (FBI 2007).

During the same 5-year period (1989–1994) that saw rising juvenile arrest rates for violent crimes, juvenile arrest rates for property crimes remained relatively stable. Over the past decade, however, the number of juveniles arrested for property crimes has decreased by 44%. By the late 1990s, arrest rates were as low as the rates in the 1960s. Over the past decade, a decline has also occurred in the arrest rate for juvenile drug abuse violations and for many status offenses, such as 30.9% fewer arrests for curfew violations and 45.3% fewer arrests for runaways (FBI 2007).

TABLE 19–1.   Arrests in the United States, 2006

Type of offense	All ages	Under age 18 years	Juvenile % of total
Total	8,241,244	1,268,950	15.4
Murder	7,515	710	9.5
Rape	14,127	2,104	14.9
Robbery	70,661	19,219	27.2
Aggravated assault	261,040	34,434	13.2
Violent crime	353,343	56,467	15.9
Property crime	896,146	237,458	26.5
Curfew violation	80,440	80,440	100.0
Runaway	68,127	68,127	100.0

Source. Adapted from Federal Bureau of Investigation: *Crime in the United States, 2006.* Washington, DC, U.S. Department of Justice, September 2007. Available at: http://www.fbi.gov/ucr/cius2006. Information derived from Table 32, "Ten-Year Arrest Trends."

Variability of Arrest Rates by Gender

Arrest rates for juvenile females have increased steadily since the 1980s. Nevertheless, over the past two decades, the number of juvenile females arrested has been consistently lower than that of juvenile males by a ratio of approximately 1:4. In 2006, females accounted for just over one-sixth of all juveniles arrested for violent crimes, including 4.9% of those arrested for murder, 9.3% of those arrested for robbery, and 23.2% of those arrested for aggravated assault. For serious property crimes, females accounted for just under one-third of juvenile arrests. The only arrest categories for which female adolescents outnumbered their male counterparts were running away from home (56.5%) and prostitution (74.5%) (Federal Bureau of Investigation 2007). Although these numbers generally confirm lower rates of offending behaviors among females, they may also be indicative of gender-biased law enforcement practices. For example, boys are arrested for substance abuse violations (e.g., possession of a controlled substance) five times more often than girls despite similar self-reported rates of substance use. Likewise, boys are arrested for vandalism six times more frequently than girls, although boys report engaging in this behavior only twice as much as girls. On the other hand, juvenile females are more likely than males to be arrested for certain status offenses (e.g., running away from home and incorrigibility), even when these behaviors may be a response to sexual or physical abuse at home rather than a disregard for parental authority (Chesney-Lind and Shelden 1992). The severity and gender specificity of female delinquent behavior are also potentially distorted by official records, which fail to distinguish among various types of offenses within particular categories. For example, one study cited by Krisberg (2005) revealed that juvenile females' assaultive behavior and subsequent arrests were almost entirely precipitated by family-centered arguments.

Variability of Arrest Rates by Race

Arrest data provided in the FBI's 2007 report indicate that black youths account for more than 27% of juvenile arrests, although they make up only 16% of the total juvenile population. This overrepresentation is even more dramatic for specific crime types; for example, black youths account for 37% of arrests for juvenile violent crimes and 50% of those for juvenile murder. Self-report studies have shown that the difference in arrest rates for black and white youths is not explained by corresponding rates of offending behaviors, but rather by the fact that black youths are more likely to be arrested than white youths for similar offenses (Huizinga and Elliott 1987). In fact, studies have repeatedly demonstrated that black youths face disparate treatment compared with white youths at every stage of the juvenile justice process. Blacks face higher rates of court referrals, of pretrial detention for both violent and property offenses, of transfer to adult criminal court, and of postadjudication incarceration, as well as longer periods in custody (Poe-Yamagata and Jones 2000). One systematic review of probation court cases revealed that delinquency in white youths was more likely to be attributed by probation officers to environmental factors, whereas delinquency in black youths was more likely to be considered a product of inherent psychopathic traits (e.g., "cold-blooded" and without remorse) (Bridges and Steen 1998).

Because the majority of Latino youths are classified as white by federal statistics, official arrest reports cannot be used to examine whether similar racial disparities exist when comparing Latinos and whites. Nevertheless, some studies demonstrate that Latino youths have higher arrests rates and face more severe penalties for similar offenses when compared with their white counterparts (Poe-Yamagata and Jones 2000; Villarruel et al. 2002). One study found that arrest rates for Latino youths were similar to those for black youths (Loeber and Farrington 1998).

Although national arrest rates for Asian and Pacific Islander youths appear to be lower than for other ethnic minorities, areas with concentrated populations of Asian and Pacific Islander youths have also shown disproportionate rates of arrest and confinement for these populations.

For example, according to arrest records from 1990 to 2003, Laotian and Vietnamese youths had the second and third highest arrest rates, respectively, for all ethnic groups in Richmond, California (Juneja 2006). Unfortunately, because self-report studies often fail to include these youths, accurately comparing them to other ethnic groups is difficult.

Reliable statistics are not available to indicate whether Native American youths experience many of the same disparities in treatment by the juvenile justice system as other minority youths. This lack of data is related to the fact that tribal territories are inconsistent in data collection and reporting. Additionally, poor coordination generally exists among the multiple tribal, local, state, and federal law enforcement agencies that share jurisdiction of a particular area. Suffice it to say that lack of local alternatives to detention commonly leads to higher confinement rates for Native American youths, either in nearby adult facilities or in juvenile facilities far from their home communities (Krisberg 2005).

As a whole, racial and ethnic minority youths arrested for violent crimes are 3.1 times more likely to be transferred to and convicted in adult criminal court than non-Hispanic white youths charged with similar crimes (Washburn et al. 2008). Minority youths are also more likely to be housed in secure facilities or in chronically overcrowded institutions. Reform efforts to deinstitutionalize youths in the 1970s resulted in larger reductions in incarceration rates for white youths than for minority youths, with racial disparities worsening during the 1980s and 1990s (Krisberg et al. 1987). Overrepresentation of minority youths increases at every stage of the juvenile justice process (Hamparian and Leiber 1997).

PERSISTENT OFFENDERS

Delinquency studies have found that offending behaviors are common during adolescence. According to data from the 2001 National Longitudinal Survey of Youth, a self-report study of 9,000 juveniles conducted annually since 1997, 33% of youths reported having been suspended from school at least once by age 17; by the same age, 37% admitted to vandalism, 43% to petty theft, and 16% to selling drugs (Snyder and Sickmund 2006). Such high rates of offending behavior during adolescence have led to speculation that participation in delinquency may be a transient consequence of the challenges of normal development. This suggestion is supported by statistics showing that arrest rates increase sharply during adolescence, peak around age 17, and then dramatically decline into early adulthood. Likewise, self-report studies indicate that two-thirds of juveniles who had admitted to offending behaviors at age 16 or 17 reported not repeating these behaviors during their early adult years. By age 28, almost 85% of former delinquents are no longer active offenders (Moffitt 1993). The transition away from delinquent behaviors may be delayed when negative consequences, such as injury, substance dependence, or a criminal record, are incurred (DeMatteo and Marczyk 2005; Moffitt et al. 2002). Risk factors that have been found to contribute to the development of more serious or persistent delinquency are noted in Table 19–2 (DeMatteo and Marczyk 2005).

For a smaller number of juvenile offenders, antisocial and illegal behaviors do not decline with the transition from adolescence to adulthood. These individuals are often referred to as "life-course-persistent" or "persistent" offenders. Compared with those who "outgrow" delinquency, persistent offenders generally begin offending at a younger age, commit more offenses, commit offenses at a greater frequency, and commit more severe offenses. Persistent offenders are also at a higher risk for substance abuse, school failure, employment difficulties, and mental health problems (DeMatteo and Marczyk 2005).

JUVENILE VERSUS ADULT LEGAL PROCESS

Because no uniform criminal justice system exists in the United States, details of the judicial process may vary from state to state. The following is a general summary of the differences between adult and juvenile proceedings.

Since its creation at the beginning of the twentieth century, the U.S. juvenile justice system has focused on the protection and rehabilitation of youthful offenders through supportive interventions, whereas the criminal (adult) justice system maintains the goal of deterrence through punishment. This difference is evident in crime prevention programs that focus on increasing community involvement to report on illicit activities committed by adults, but that employ schools and recreational programs to target and educate at-risk youths. At the same time, youthful offenders lack many of the rights and protections accorded to adults accused of crimes. Throughout its early history, the juvenile court was assumed to have benevolent motivations, and therefore few safeguards were extended to ensure the Fifth, Sixth, and Fourteenth Amendment rights of the accused (including notification of charges and the right to confront witnesses).

Many police agencies have special units that focus on juvenile offenders. Unlike adults, who primarily come to the attention of law enforcement through police discovery, victim or witness reports, or investigative work, juveniles may also be referred to police by their parents or schools,

TABLE 19–2.   Risk factors for increased juvenile delinquency rates

Individual risk factors

Childhood antisocial behaviors

Lower cognitive ability

Alcohol and illicit substance use

Poor school performance or truancy

Association with delinquent peers

Family factors

Parental divorce

Single-parent home

Large number of siblings

Erratic and harsh parental discipline

Lack of parental supervision, parental rejection

High levels of parent–child conflict

Physical abuse and neglect

Parents who model antisocial behaviors

Family or neighborhood poverty

Source.   DeMatteo and Marczyk 2005.

largely because, in addition to violent and property crimes, juveniles are targeted by law enforcement for status offenses. Law enforcement officers may decide whether to arrest an individual, release the individual with a warning, or divert the individual to a mental health program. In the case of juveniles, offenders may also be taken home to meet with their parents, especially in the case of minor offenses. Police typically divert into alternative programs or dismiss 25% of arrested youths and refer about two-thirds of cases to the juvenile court; 10% are transferred to the adult criminal court system or are referred to other community agencies (Krisberg 2005).

Once in custody, youths are taken either to a juvenile assessment center, where cases are evaluated by a multidisciplinary team and referred for appropriate community services, or to juvenile hall (the equivalent of a police station or local jail for adults) and booked. The booking process may include documenting personal information, fingerprinting, taking a mug shot, and conducting medical and mental health screenings. Many of those who are arrested are released within 1–2 days of booking. However, the average length of stay for detained youths is 15 days (Krisberg 2005). In contrast to adults, who are generally detained to maintain public safety, juveniles may also be held "for their own protection" (e.g., when there is inadequate supervision in the home environment).

In the criminal justice system, a prosecutor determines if charges are to be filed in court based on evidence provided by law enforcement agencies. In lieu of filing charges, the prosecutor may opt to revoke probation or parole for repeat offenders, recommend civil commitment to a mental health treatment facility, invoke civil sanctions such as revocation of the individual's driver's license, or reduce or dismiss the charges for assisting law enforcement in the prosecution of other crimes (Krisberg 2005). In the juvenile justice system, this process is handled by an intake unit consisting of probation staff that review the details of each case and make a recommendation whether to bring the case to court or refer it for a less restrictive intervention based on a combination of social service and legal factors.

When charges are filed against an adult, the defendant initially appears before a judge, who informs the accused of the charges and decides if there is probable cause for continued detention. For minor offenses, the judge may find the defendant guilty and assess a penalty (e.g., a fine); for more serious charges, defense counsel is retained by the individual or assigned by the court (i.e., a public defender). In contrast, juveniles are subject to a detention hearing, during which the district attorney files a petition asking the court to declare the youth a ward of the court. A juvenile court judge then decides if it is in the best interests of the youth or society to proceed with a formal hearing on the petition. Whereas adults are found guilty of committing specific criminal acts, the sustaining of a juvenile petition is based on a general pattern of behavior or family circumstances. Unlike adults, youths with cases under juvenile court jurisdiction have no automatic right to bail, and those who are not released home remain in detention during the course of their case proceedings.

Following their initial appearance in court, adult defendants undergo a series of court proceedings during their adjudicative process. These include a preliminary hearing to determine probable cause, a grand jury hearing for submission of the indictment, an arraignment hearing during which a plea is entered, a jury or bench trial to determine guilt, and a penalty phase to determine the sentence. In the case of juveniles, there may be a preplea hearing at which a probation officer submits a report containing social history and school information. This is followed soon after by an arraignment hearing, which takes place before a judge (juveniles do not have the right to a trial by jury). Adult criminal proceedings are considered matters of public record, whereas juvenile hearings are generally regarded as confidential, except those for the most serious offenses. For both juveniles and adults, the legal standard of proof for determination of guilt is "beyond a reasonable doubt" (i.e., 90%–95% certainty of guilt). The exception to this rule is status offenses, which only require proof by "a preponderance of the evidence" (i.e., at least 51% certainty of the offense). In both systems, defendants maintain the right to appeal the verdict.

Once they are found guilty, adult defendants are given a sentence that is based on, among other things, the gravity of their offense and their prior criminal record; sentencing length is usually rigidly determined by state statutes or U.S. sentencing guidelines. In general, offenders who are sentenced to less than 1 year are sent to county jails, and those with sentences of 1 year or longer are sent to state or federal prisons. For youths, the disposition determination includes consideration of multiple relevant social factors. Dispositions are often open-ended and may involve regular court supervision until the minor reaches the maximum age of the juvenile court's jurisdiction. Options for disposition include secure detention (at either state facilities or probation camps), "home on probation," suitable placement (with concomitant increased supervision or services than are available at home), house arrest with electronic monitoring, informal probation through a diversionary program, payment of monetary fines or restitution to the victim, and community service.

MENTAL DISORDERS IN THE JUVENILE JUSTICE SYSTEM

No reliable source of data exists on the prevalence of mental disorders among detained youths prior to the 1990s (Grisso 2004; Otto et al. 1992). Nevertheless, rising juvenile arrest rates in the United States during the early 1990s led many to presume that the number of detained youths with mental disorders was also increasing (Cocozza 1992). This notion was supported by epidemiological studies indicating that the rates of mental disorders among youths in general were higher than those measured during the first three-quarters of the twentieth century (Fombonne 1998; Grisso 2004).

In fact, research indicates that the prevalence of mental disorders is higher among youths in the juvenile justice system than in other public health or educational settings (Grisso 2004; Stiffman et al. 1997). However, the actual prevalence has been difficult to determine because prevalence studies have produced dramatically different numbers. Estimates of overall rates for mental disorders in the juvenile justice system have ranged from 50% to 100%. Studies assessing the prevalence of more specific disorders have shown the following rates: psychotic disorders, 1%–

45%; mood disorders, 10%–72%; anxiety disorders, 8%–52%; attention-deficit/hyperactivity disorder (ADHD), 2%–76%; and posttraumatic stress disorder, 3%–50% (Grisso 2004; Hennessey et al. 2004). Much of this variability has been attributed to study differences, including such factors as which disorders were included, how the disorders were defined, the duration of symptoms, the diagnostic methods and screening instruments used, the population sample size, and the types of facilities surveyed.

In his comparison of three large studies that employed similar methodologies for examining prevalence rates of mental disorders in youths in juvenile justice settings, Grisso (2004) noted general agreement that the number of youths meeting DSM-III or DSM-IV criteria for at least one disorder (including conduct disorder) varied between 60% and 70%. Many have argued that the inclusion of conduct disorder in the definition of *mental disorder* artificially and erroneously elevates the overall prevalence rates of mental disorders because the diagnosis of conduct disorder relies on the presence of persistent delinquent behaviors rather than emotional or cognitive symptoms. Excluding individuals with conduct disorder alone from the analysis, however, did not lower the rates significantly (Teplin et al. 2002). Table 19–3 summarizes prevalence rates of mental disorders in juveniles noted in several studies (Atkins et al. 1999; Teplin et al. 2002; Wasserman et al. 2002).

Prevalence rates for nearly all mental disorders were as high or somewhat higher for girls than for boys. One study reported higher prevalence rates in white youths (82%) when compared with black (65%) or Latino (70%) youths (Teplin et al. 2002).

Washburn et al. (2008) examined the rates of psychiatric disorders among 1,715 youths held in juvenile detention facilities in Cook County, Illinois. The researchers found that 68% of these youths had a mental disorder as defined by DSM-IV. As in Teplin et al.'s (2002) study, excluding conduct disorder alone from the definition of *mental disorder* reduced this figure by only 6%, indicating that the vast majority of youths diagnosed with conduct disorder also met criteria for at least one other major Axis I disorder. In Washburn et al.'s (2008) study, 20% of these youths had an affective disorder, 22% had an anxiety disorder, 1% had a psychotic disorder, 12% had posttraumatic stress disorder, 44% had a disruptive behavior disorder (e.g., conduct disorder, oppositional defiant disorder, or ADHD), and 51% had a substance use disorder (i.e., substance abuse or dependence). Of these youths, 43% had at least two mental disorders, 19% had at least three mental disorders, and 7% met DSM-IV criteria for four mental disorders. The highest rates of comorbidity were seen with disruptive behavior disorders and substance use disor-

TABLE 19–3.   Prevalence rates of mental disorder in juvenile detainees

Disorder	Prevalence rate
Attention-deficit/hyperactivity disorder	2%–16%
Oppositional defiant disorder	3%–14%
Conduct disorder	23%–28%
Major depressive disorder	7%–13%
Posttraumatic stress disorder	3%–50%

Source.   Atkins et al. 1999; Hennessey et al. 2004; Teplin et al. 2002; Wasserman et al. 2002.

ders. The prevalence rates for specific and comorbid disorders were as high or higher for youths who had their cases transferred to adult court for adjudication (Washburn et al. 2008). Among detained youths, the three most frequently diagnosed disorders are conduct disorder, ADHD, and substance abuse or dependence; these youths also commonly have higher rates of learning disorders and mental retardation, as well as overall lower intelligence levels (Sevin Goldstein et al. 2005).

These findings have numerous implications, most of which have been recognized in the adult correctional population. First, public agencies that detain and incarcerate individuals are legally and ethically responsible for attending to these individuals' mental health needs because detainees or prisoners are not free to seek out mental health services on their own. Second, because mental illness may impair an individual's adjudicative competence, recognition of certain mental disorders and their potential effects on competence is vital to ensure due process and fairness of the legal process. Finally, to the extent that mental illness may contribute to offending behavior, treatment is a necessary part of the rehabilitative process to reduce recidivism and protect the public.

SCREENING AND ASSESSMENT

Many juveniles exhibit symptoms that could indicate different diagnoses or combinations of diagnoses. Substance use disorders (i.e., abuse or dependence) or problem use frequently complicates the diagnostic process and compromises the accuracy of diagnoses. Additionally, collateral information is frequently limited and youths typically are not the most reliable historians, for a variety of reasons such as poorer memory retention and recall, higher susceptibility to suggestion, and tendencies toward elaboration. Despite these problems, a comprehensive assessment of all aspects of a juvenile's history and presentation is crucial to improve diagnostic accuracy and the ability to implement effective treatment modalities.

Clinical Case 19–1

A 17-year-old female being held in juvenile hall on a charge of attempted murder against her brother is noted by probation staff to appear extremely depressed. On mental health screening with the Massachusetts Youth Screening Instrument—2nd Version (MAYSI-2), she is found to have elevated scores on a number of symptom scales. When interviewed, she complains of frequent mood swings, daily anxiety, low self-esteem, nightmares, restlessness, poor concentration, and impaired memory, although she is unable to characterize the time of onset of any of these symptoms. At home, she frequently stays up all night and constantly checks to make sure that all doors are locked. Her social history is significant for being bitten in the face and disfigured by a dog as a toddler, experiencing years of physical abuse by her mother, being frequently threatened with violence by her brother, and having been sexually assaulted multiple times by various men, including a neighbor, a foster parent, and an employee at a recent placement. She relates that both of her parents have a history of either depression or substance abuse, but neither parent can be reached for further information.

For many youths, the juvenile justice system offers their first contact with mental health professionals. Initial mental health assessments help determine which individuals are referred for ongoing care. Because resources are limited, reliable assessment is crucial so that appropriate mental health treatment can be offered to individuals most likely to benefit from such treatment. Standardized, validated assessment instruments can aid in this process. The following are descriptions of well-researched, validated assessment tools that are commonly used within the juvenile justice system. The first two assessments discussed were developed for use in the juvenile justice system. The remaining instruments were not developed specifically for use with the juvenile justice population, but they have utility in identifying certain disorders or other issues of concern in that population.

Massachusetts Youth Screening Instrument—2nd Version

The MAYSI-2 (Grisso et al. 2001), which is currently employed in 39 states, is the most widely used mental health screening tool in the U.S. juvenile justice system. Unlike other assessments, the MAYSI-2 was designed specifically for youths in juvenile justice facilities and normed by age, gender, and ethnic background. Therefore, it may provide the most clinically relevant information for this population. The instrument is designed for youths ages 12–17 with at least a fifth-grade reading ability. It consists of 52 self-report, yes-no questions; takes 10–15 minutes to administer; and requires 3 minutes to score. The MAYSI-2 is available in both English and Spanish and can be administered either in paper-and-pencil fashion or on a computer.

The inventory focuses on the presence of specific symptoms rather than diagnoses and consists of the following seven scales: alcohol and drug use, anger and irritability, depression and anxiety, somatic complaints, suicidal ideation, thought disturbance, and traumatic experience. Although most of the scales assess for the presence of symptoms over the "past few months," the traumatic experience items assess events or feelings that have occurred during the youth's entire lifetime. There are separate traumatic experience scales for boys and girls, and the thought disturbance scale is valid only for males.

Los Angeles Risk and Resiliency Check-up

The Los Angeles Risk and Resiliency Check-up (LARRC; Turner et al. 2005) is a 60-item assessment tool that focuses on six domains of a youth's life that may affect his or her criminal recidivism. These domains include delinquency, education, family, peer relations, substance use, and individual factors. Half of the items inquire about risk factors that increase the likelihood of initiating or continuing criminal activity, and the other half identify protective factors that reduce the likelihood of further criminal behavior. A total resiliency score is obtained by subtracting risk factor scores from protective factor scores. This instrument helps match individuals with programs and services that are likely to be effective in reducing their unique recidivism risk factors. The LARRC may be administered by nonclinical staff in juvenile intake, diversion, probation, detention, group home placement, and aftercare settings. It is completed after a 45-minute interview with the juvenile and the collection and examination of collateral data. LARRC scores have been correlated with information on the general recidivism in males and females from all ethnic groups who are wards of the Los Angeles and San Diego County probation systems.

Diagnostic Interview Schedule for Children, Version IV

The National Institute of Mental Health's Diagnostic Interview Schedule for Children, Version IV (DISC-IV; Shaffer et al. 2000) is a highly structured instrument that was designed to assess more than 30 psychiatric disorders that commonly occur in children and adolescents. It consists of a series of carefully worded and specifically ordered questions, although the interviewer may focus on current, recent, or past diagnoses or limit the interview to questions about specific disorders. It also assesses the youth's level of functioning. The DISC-IV can be administered by lay interviewers who have received some training with the instrument. It usually requires 1–2 hours to administer and is available in both English and Spanish versions.

Swanson, Nolan, and Pelham Parent and Teacher Questionnaire

The Swanson, Nolan, and Pelham Parent and Teacher Questionnaire (SNAP-IV; Swanson 1995) was designed for use with children and adolescents ages 6–18 to detect and ascertain the severity of symptoms of ADHD, oppositional defiant disorder, and aggression. It contains 90 items and takes about 10 minutes to administer (Collett et al. 2003).

Children's Depression Inventory

The Children's Depression Inventory (CDI; Kovacs 1995) was derived from the Beck Depression Inventory (Beck et al. 1961) and can be used with children and adolescents ages 7–17. Parents and teachers provide perspectives on various academic, social, and emotional behaviors and functional problems observed in a child or adolescent over the previous 2-week period in the home and school environments. The child or adolescent also reports on a number of symptoms, such as negative mood, interpersonal problems, ineffectiveness, depressed facial affect, and negative self-esteem. The CDI requires a first-grade reading level and takes 10–15 minutes to complete. The parent version includes 17 items, the teacher version contains 12 items, and the youth self-report component includes 27 items.

Hamilton Rating Scale for Depression

The Hamilton Rating Scale for Depression (HAM-D; Hamilton 1960) is the most widely studied rating instrument for depression. This scale quantifies the degree of depression and, based on the score, categorizes an individual as not depressed, mildly depressed, moderately depressed, or severely depressed. The HAM-D is often used to measure treatment response or achievement of remission. The scale should be administered by a mental health clinician and requires approximately 20 minutes to complete. Several versions exist, differing only in the number of items (between 6 and 31) included.

CRAFFT

The CRAFFT is a brief, six-question screening tool for assessing adolescent drug and alcohol abuse (Knight et al. 2002). It is based on adult screening tools but includes situations that are more relevant for adolescents. The questions relate to the letters in the tool's acronym and refer to the use of drugs or alcohol while in a **C**ar, for **R**elaxation or fitting in, and while **A**lone, and that causes **F**orgetfulness, that is criticized by **F**amily or friends, or that results in the youth's getting into **T**rouble.

Teen Addiction Severity Index

The Teen Addiction Severity Index (T-ASI; Kaminer et al. 1991) is a 154-item semistructured interview that was modified from the adult Addiction Severity Index (McLellan et al. 1980) for use with adolescents. It provides severity ratings in seven domains, including substance use, school, employment status, family functioning, peer and social relationships, involvement with the juvenile justice system, and psychiatric status. It can be used to determine substance use severity upon initial assessment and can be repeated periodically to monitor and quantify response or lack of response to treatment. The interview takes 30–45 minutes to administer and 5 minutes to score.

Wide Range Achievement Test

The Wide Range Achievement Test (WRAT-4; Wilkinson et al. 2006) is designed to determine basic academic functioning and skills deficits and can be used with individuals ages 5–94. The instrument takes 15–30 minutes to complete and consists of subtests for reading, spelling, and arithmetic. However, it contains no items designed to assess reading comprehension or understanding of math word problems.

Kaufman Brief Intelligence Test

The Kaufman Brief Intelligence Test (K-BIT; Kaufman 1990) provides a quick, noncomprehensive estimate of intelligence and is particularly useful when evaluation time is limited or when individuals have difficulty completing a more time-intensive intelligence measure. The test can be administered by trained nonclinicians to individuals ages 4–90 and requires 15–30 minutes to complete. The K-BIT assesses both vocabulary and nonverbal intellectual reasoning and permits the examiner to teach during the test to obtain a more accurate picture of the individual's potential intelligence.

TREATMENT AND MANAGEMENT

Safety should always be a primary concern in treating and managing juvenile offenders, especially when they have a history of self-injurious behavior, suicide attempts, or violence. Parental support for both the minor and the treatment regimen is crucial in increasing the probability of treatment success. Also, addressing an individual's concerns about the type of treatment pursued increases the likelihood of adherence and subsequent positive outcomes. Clinical Case 19–2 touches on a number of overarching issues that arise in the treatment of juveniles.

Clinical Case 19–2

A 15-year-old male who was arrested for making terrorist threats against his stepfather is referred to mental health services because of his history of depression and two prior suicide attempts (by cutting his wrists and overdose). He has been treated in the past with antidepressant medication, with unclear benefit. In addition to having multiple arrests for running away from home, he reports being physically abused by his father, constantly criticized by his stepmother, and ignored and neglected by his mother and stepfather. The boy has intermittently been placed in foster care. He reports that his depressive symptoms occur only when he is living at home, and that his mood and behavior seem consistently better when in foster placements or while housed in juvenile detention facilities. He is hesitant to restart antidepressant medication and, following a discussion of treatment alternatives, requests psychotherapy to address his depressive symptoms. He is willing to remain on increased observation status by probation staff during his adjustment period to juvenile hall.

Suicide

Suicide is the third leading cause of death among adolescents. Although more adults commit suicide before trial than after trial, the suicide rate among youths housed in pretrial detention centers is lower (just under 1 in 100,000) than that of youths housed in postadjudication facilities (approximately 5 in 100,000). In part, this difference may be related to the ages of juveniles housed in these types of facilities (i.e., overall suicide rates are higher in adolescence, particularly late adolescence, than in childhood). The rate of suicide attempts, suicidal gestures, and self-mutilations is about 2,500 in 100,000 (Grisso 2004). Conditions associated with extended detention (e.g., separation from loved ones, crowding, solitary confinement) may serve as significant stressors that increase the risk of suicide. Hanging is the most common method of suicide within juvenile detention facilities. One study of juvenile detainees found that among detainees who hung themselves, 21% used door hinges or doorknobs, 20% used air grates, 20% used bunk frames or holes, and 15% used window frames (Hayes 2005a). The primary means of deterring suicide attempts in detention facilities is through identification and increased observation of those thought to be at risk. National correctional facility standards recommend 30-minute checks for "special management detainees" (those who demonstrate significant behavior problems), 15-minute checks for those demonstrating concerning behaviors or expressing suicidal ideation, and constant observation for those reporting or engaging in suicidal behavior (Hayes 2005b).

Informed Consent

Informed consent is a legal and ethical requirement for appropriate mental health treatment for youths, as for adults. Youths should receive a fair and reasonable explanation of the risks and potential benefits of any proposed intervention; however, they have limited authority to make mental health treatment decisions and are generally considered incompetent to consent for medical treatment, although there are exceptions (e.g., abortion in many states). In most cases, before treatment with psychotropic medications can be initiated, informed consent must first be obtained from a minor's legal guardian, along with "informed assent" by the youth. Exceptions to this doctrine include medical emergencies, treatment of emancipated minors or minors meeting "mature minor" provision requirements, and instances in which necessary treatment might not be pursued if parental consent or notification is required (e.g., substance abuse treatment). Although informed consent should generally be obtained from a youth's legal guardian before initiating psychotherapy, the age of consent for this treatment modality is often lower than that for psychotropic medications or other medical procedures. For example, in California, youths age 12 and older can consent for their own psychotherapy or substance abuse treatment (not involving medications) as long as certain other criteria are met.

Psychotropic Medications: Issues Related to Adherence

Significantly fewer medications have U.S. Food and Drug Administration approval for use in children and adolescents than in adults; therefore, adherence to well-accepted practice guidelines and treatment algorithms should be followed when treating youths. Because of the stigma associated with having a psychiatric diagnosis, many youths are reluctant to assent to treatment with psychotropic medications, especially in detention facilities, where spacing and staffing limitations can lead to discovery by probation staff and peers that a youth takes psychotropic medication.

This stigma may also result in the refusing or "cheeking" of medications and should be taken into account when addressing concerns about adherence. Conversely, minors sometimes make mental health complaints with the goal of obtaining medications for misuse, such as recreational use, abuse, or diversion. The extent to which this problem exists within a facility is important in considering if and when to start medication treatment.

Expected length of stay is another factor to consider when deciding whether to have a youth start taking psychotropic medications. Many minors are released within 2 days of being taken into custody; for most, the average stay is no more than 2 weeks (Krisberg 2005). This brief amount of custodial time may limit the types of treatments that should be started during a youth's detention. For example, during pretrial detention, when periods of incarceration are indeterminate and likely relatively brief, most group therapies would be a waste of both time and resources (Grisso 2004). Starting treatment with medications may also be inappropriate because of insufficient time to gather sufficient collateral data, to complete an adequate medical workup, or to follow up on the response to treatment. However, continuing medications that a youth has been taking in the community and that have proven helpful is usually appropriate.

Parents and Custody Staff

Although minors in detention are generally seen alone (i.e., without their parents present), parental support is generally crucial to the success of any treatment plan. Minors are often influenced by their parents' opinions about receiving mental health treatment and may refuse medications if their parents have significant concerns, whether based on realistic fears or significant misconceptions. Parents may also be responsible for a minor's remaining in treatment after release from custody. In many cases, parents are the primary cause of termination of treatment; reasons may include parental disagreement with the diagnosis and proposed treatment, lack of transportation to clinics or pharmacies, and differing family priorities. The stress of having one's child in custody may also produce an adversarial relationship between parents and individuals associated with the juvenile justice system or detention facility. Therefore, the mental health care provider may be perceived as authoritarian rather than supportive. Frequently, the clinician can rectify this misunderstanding by speaking with parents and addressing their concerns.

Within juvenile correctional facilities, probation officers serve as de facto parents and are the adults with whom juveniles have the most contact. Although probation officers may be a source of stress and conflict for detainees, just as often they are a source of support and counsel. Therefore, probation staff should receive training about how mental disorders or symptoms are likely to affect incarcerated youths. In addition to learning about common diagnoses and treatment effects, probation staff should become familiar with behavioral interventions that address physical safety and de-escalate anxiety, anger, and other emotions associated with problematic behaviors.

Managing Juveniles in Adult Correctional Facilities

During the 1990s, many states changed their statutes to facilitate the transfer of juvenile cases to the adult criminal justice system for adjudication. One consequence of this change has been an increase in the number of adolescents who are incarcerated in adult correctional facilities. From 1983 to 1998, the number of juveniles housed in adult correctional facilities increased by approximately 366%, and by 1998 approximately 5,400 convicted youths were being held in adult prison facilities (Austin et al. 2000).

Additionally, prior to incarceration, transferred youths are held in custody for longer periods of time than their juvenile court counterparts and therefore may be at greater risk for developing psychiatric problems because of their extended periods of confinement. Compared with juveniles housed in juvenile detention facilities, juveniles housed in adult correctional facilities are 30% more likely to be assaulted with a weapon and twice as likely to be beaten by staff. The suicide rate for juveniles in adult correctional facilities is five times greater than that of the adult correctional facility general population and eight times greater than that of the juvenile detention facility population (Austin et al. 2000).

Although little has been written about the treatment of juveniles in adult correctional settings, the few known facts are alarming. Transferred youths who are sentenced to adult prisons have a significantly greater prevalence of disruptive behavior disorders, substance use disorders, and comorbid affective and anxiety disorders than do youths who remain in the juvenile justice system. The majority of youths who are incarcerated with adults have at least one of these psychiatric disorders, and up to 15% have all four of these disorders (Washburn et al. 2008). One study found that the 6-month rate of major depressive disorder for transferred youths was three times greater than the lifetime rate for adult male prisoners (Teplin 1994). This finding suggests that transferred youths may have a greater need for mental health services than their adult counterparts, although adult facilities may not be equipped to perform age-appropriate assessments or provide age-appropriate treatment for youths. Specific interventions, such as adolescent group therapies, may not be available in adult facilities (Woolard et al. 2005), and treatment within adult facilities is less likely to focus on offender rehabilitation.

Evidence-Based Therapies

The trend has been toward the use of evidence-based treatments for youths in general, and for youths in detention settings in particular. To some extent, this trend has been tempered by the limited amount of information available on effective treatments for youths. However, the knowledge in this area is growing rapidly. A number of well-researched and validated interventions that have been developed are discussed below.

Cognitive-Behavioral Therapy

Cognitive-behavioral therapy is an empirically based practice that is useful in the treatment of a wide range of mental disorders. Individuals are first educated about the complex relationship that exists among one's thoughts, emotions, and behaviors. They then are introduced to and practice a variety of techniques, with the goal of reshaping distorted thoughts, negative feelings, and problematic behaviors. Specific techniques are chosen according to the diagnosis and characteristics of the individual in treatment (Landenberger and Lipsey 2005).

Cognitive-Behavioral Intervention for Trauma in Schools

Cognitive-behavioral intervention for trauma in schools is an evidence-based program that was developed specifically for youths ages 11–15 who have been exposed to trauma and who demonstrate moderate symptoms of posttraumatic stress disorder, depression, and anxiety. The program consists of symptom-focused group therapy and skill-building techniques and has been demonstrated to reduce symptom severity and improve psychosocial functioning. The program was designed and tested for use within the school system and has been used in the treatment of individuals with single or multiple trauma exposures. The program is currently being piloted for use in juvenile detention settings (mainly postadjudication camps), and adaptations are being considered that will improve the efficacy of this intervention in juvenile justice populations (Stein et al. 2003).

Anger Management Training

Anger management training is a specific form of cognitive-behavioral therapy that has shown some efficacy in reducing anger and aggression in adolescents. Numerous manuals have been developed on this topic, and this training can be offered to juvenile offenders in both individual and group therapy settings. Areas of focus may include managing negative feelings, identifying triggers, practicing conflict resolution, and developing communication skills (Feindler and Scalley 1998).

Motivational Interviewing

Motivational interviewing is a form of supportive counseling that has demonstrated effectiveness in achieving behavioral change. In motivational interviewing, the clinician avoids persuasion and confrontation by employing an interpersonal style that demonstrates an individual's ambivalence about change and then helps the individual explore and eventually resolve this ambivalence. The technique was developed by William Miller, Ph.D., based on clinical experience he gained in the treatment of alcohol dependence. In one recent study, the technique was shown to reduce negative engagement in incarcerated adolescents in substance abuse treatment (Stein et al. 2006). Motivational interviewing is also useful in addressing other problematic behaviors not related to substance use (Miller and Rollnick 2002).

Girls...Moving On

Girls...Moving On is a program that was developed for females ages 12–21 who have a history of antisocial behavior and risk for continued involvement in the juvenile or adult criminal justice systems. The program is open-ended with regard to length, and either an individual or a group format can be used. It employs relational theory, which proposes that social connections are central to growth and maturation, to increase the participants' capacity for developing healthy and supportive relationships. This program combines the evidence-based components of motivational interviewing and cognitive-behavioral therapy that have demonstrated efficacy in decreasing the risk of recidivism, increasing life satisfaction, and improving skills related to coping with trauma, abuse, and neglect (Van Dieten 2004).

COMMUNITY PROGRAMS AND ALTERNATIVE PLACEMENTS

During the 1960s, several states introduced alternatives to juvenile detention facilities to improve rehabilitation efforts. Reformers argued that community-based programs that provide intensive probation supervision in combination with individual therapy would be more cost-effective than conventional detention facilities. This idea was based on the theory that juvenile offenders were more likely to succeed when given increased support within their communities than when removed from the community and its attendant support networks. Group homes, partial release programs, and halfway houses were established to decrease commitment rates to juvenile institutions and to reduce tension and violence within overcrowded juvenile detention settings.

More recent programs have engaged school districts to provide dropout services; positive school engagement opportunities; goal-oriented educational programs; and workforce development programs that include skills assessment and training, community service, work training opportunities, and paid work experience internships. The goals of victim restitution programs are to monitor and enforce these obligations and offer workshops for teaching employment preparation skills, stipends for competency development, connection to workforce skills training, and job opportunities to assist youths in meeting their legal financial obligations. Awareness programs are used in an attempt to instill an understanding of the impact of crime on individuals and the community (DeMatteo and Marczyk 2005).

Diversion Programs

Juvenile diversion programs, which evolved in the 1970s, attempt to steer youthful offenders away from the justice system by deferring adjudication and requiring participation in treatment; in most cases, the charges are dropped if the youth successfully completes treatment. Treatment may include individual and family therapies, as well as educational, employment, and recreational interventions. Diversion programs, which tend to involve referrals for lesser crimes, may actually increase the number of juveniles incorporated into the justice system by including many of those for whom charges would have been dropped (Chapin and Griffin 2005). Although recidivism rates appear to be as high for youths in diversion programs as for those in the juvenile justice system, the former treatment appears to be no worse than traditional entry into the juvenile justice system (DePrato and Hammer 2002).

Two specific types of diversion programs are the juvenile drug court and the juvenile mental health court. These programs oversee first-time offenders facing drug-related charges or youths with mental health and developmental disabilities who are referred from delinquency court. A courtroom-based team approach allows collaboration among judge, district attorney, public defender, probation staff, mental health staff, social workers, and school liaisons to provide intensive case management with a focus on individual reform and social reintegration. Drug-related offenders are often involved in outpatient substance abuse treatment, which might include detoxification, counseling, and educational or vocational assessment and training. Youths in mental health court may receive medication management and therapy as part of treatment. Cases are often monitored simultaneously through delinquency court and through regular judicial review within the specific diversion program. Unfortunately, the frequent number of required court appearances often results in increased failure-to-appear rates (DePrato and Hammer 2002).

Community-Based Programs

Community-based interventions are intended to provide services within the normal environment of the adolescent in lieu of detention, with the goal of strengthening the minor's support systems while avoiding the ensuing difficulties associated with transition back to the community. Services are targeted at areas of concern within the family, neighborhood, or school, and frequently take place across multiple settings.

Multisystemic Therapy

Multisystemic therapy is the community-based intervention with the highest rate of treatment efficacy for juvenile delinquency. Treatment services are tailored to each case and may combine individual, family, or marital therapy; peer group counseling; and case management. These services are administered across a variety of settings, including home, school, and neighborhood clinics. Various studies have demonstrated the effectiveness of multisystemic therapy in reducing adolescent drug use, increasing school attendance, reducing future violent offending, improving family and peer relations, and decreasing psychiatric symptoms (Sheidow and Henggler 2005).

Multidimensional Treatment Foster Care

Multidimensional treatment foster care is an intensive behavioral treatment program in which juvenile offenders are placed with trained foster parents who work with biological parents, case managers, individual and family therapists, and other resource staff to provide a viable and effective alternative to incarceration or residential placement. Youths are provided with social and problem-solving skills training and are rewarded with privileges for normative behaviors. Families are trained to provide consistent and noncoercive behavioral management, and treatment may be extended to the school environment. Two empirical studies indicate that compared with standard care, multidimensional treatment foster care results in higher rates of treatment completion, lower rates of running away from treatment settings, fewer days spent in detention facilities, more days spent with biological families, and fewer posttreatment offenses (Chamberlain 1990; Chamberlain and Reid 1998).

Functional Family Therapy

Functional family therapy involves three sequential phases of treatment: engagement and motivation, behavior change, and generalization. In the first phase, the therapist establishes an alliance with the family and reduces negative emotions and behaviors that may interfere with desired changes. In the second phase, parent training and communication skills training are used to enhance interpersonal and problem-solving skills. The final phase resembles case management and focuses on connecting the family with supportive community services. Several studies have supported the efficacy of this treatment in reducing recidivism rates compared with no treatment or "usual community services" (Sheidow and Henggler 2005).

Alternative Programs

Other juvenile intervention programs include boot camps, which are military-style programs focusing on rule adherence and moral development through intensive work and exercise regimens; wilderness programs that place youths in remote locations and emphasize teamwork, peer support, and goal setting; and Scared Straight programs, which expose youthful offenders to prison settings through lectures, tours, and "scare tactics." Research studies indicate that these interventions may not be effective at reducing recidivism and may, in fact, produce harmful results (DePrato and Hammer 2002).

ETHICAL ISSUES

As in all fields of medicine, the psychiatrist who works within the correctional system is obligated to act in the best medical interest of the patient. Sometimes, however, this obligation becomes complicated by the conditions imposed by the correctional system. Although the duty to maintain confidentiality must be respected, a certain degree of communication with probation staff about issues that are revealed during mental health care may be necessary to ensure a minor's safety. On the other hand, data collected during the course of assessment and treatment may increase a juvenile's risk for delinquency adjudication and the imposition of a more restrictive sentence by the courts. Despite some existing protections to reduce this risk, it is impossible to eliminate given the general loss of privacy and autonomy that youths face while in state custody as defendants in legal proceedings. For this reason, the data collected during screening, assessment, and treatment should be limited to those data considered necessary for adequate and appropriate care, thereby limiting the risk of harm without adequate justification (Grisso 2004).

Even when mental health concerns are identified, the clinician should give careful consideration to the appropriateness of initiating treatment. Clinical care is potentially harmful in many instances. For example, when group therapy is not carefully implemented, it may result in the exposure of minors to negative peer influences that actually promote further delinquency (Grisso 2004). Poor response to inappropriate treatment may cause parents and minors to regard mental health care as ineffective and judges to regard a minor as incorrigible. In addition, many medications are associated with unpleasant or dangerous side effects (e.g., the development of diabetes mellitus from atypical antipsychotic medications), and medical care that is not closely monitored may produce unanticipated risks (e.g., falls resulting from the effects of sedating medications).

CONCLUSION

The juvenile justice system has a mandate to address the serious mental health care needs of its wards. This is a daunting task given the unique conditions of incarceration, the large number of detained youths, and the high rates of mental illness that exist within this population. The provision of adequate psychiatric care in juvenile detention facilities requires the development of specialized knowledge and specific techniques, as well as familiarity with the obstacles and stressors that minors within the system face on a daily basis. The growing number of youths transferred to the adult criminal justice system further compounds the already difficult task of providing good care to incarcerated minors. Successful treatment depends on adequate assessment of the particular needs and situations of incarcerated youths and the availability of effective interventions.

SUMMARY POINTS

- The United States has the world's highest juvenile incarceration rates.
- Minority youths are disproportionately represented in the U.S. correctional system.
- Most juveniles who engage in delinquency do not continue to offend as adults.
- The prevalence of DSM-IV-TR mental disorders among incarcerated youths is between 60% and 70% and may be somewhat higher for juveniles transferred to the adult criminal justice system.

- The most common mental health diagnoses among incarcerated youths are conduct disorder, attention-deficit/hyperactivity disorder, and substance use disorders.

- Evidence-based treatments exist for delinquent youths but should be carefully tailored to meet each individual's needs.

- The juvenile justice system has historically prioritized rehabilitation over retribution.

REFERENCES

Amnesty International: Betraying the young: human rights violations against children in the U.S. justice system. November 1998. Available at: http:// www.amnesty.org/en/library/info/AMR51/057/1998. Accessed April 27, 2009.

Atkins D, Pumariega W, Rogers K: Mental health and incarcerated youth, I: prevalence and nature of psychopathology. J Child Fam Stud 8:193–204, 1999

Austin J, Johnson KD, Gregoriou M: Juveniles in adult prisons and jails: a national assessment (ED450323). Washington, DC, Bureau of Justice Assistance, 2000

Beck AT, Ward CH, Mendelson M, et al: Beck Depression Inventory (BDI): an inventory for measuring depression. Arch Gen Psychiatry 4:561–571, 1961

Bridges GS, Steen S: Racial disparities in official assessments of juvenile offenders: attributional stereotypes as mediating mechanisms. Am Sociol Rev 63:554–570, 1998

Chamberlain P: Comparative evaluation of specialized foster care for seriously delinquent youths: a first step. Community Alternatives: International Journal of Family Care 2:21–36, 1990

Chamberlain P, Reid JB: Comparison of two community alternatives to incarceration for chronic juvenile offenders. J Consult Clin Psychol 66:624–633, 1998

Chapin DA, Grffin PA: Juvenile diversion, in Juvenile Delinquency: Prevention, Assessment, and Intervention. Edited by Heilbrun K, Sevin Goldstein NE, Redding RE. New York, Oxford University Press, 2005, pp 161–178

Chesney-Lind M, Shelden RG: Girls: Delinquency and Juvenile Justice. Belmont, CA, Wadsworth, 1992

Cocozza JJ: Responding to the Mental Health Needs of Youth in the Juvenile Justice System. Seattle, WA, National Coalition for the Mentally Ill in the Criminal Justice System, 1992

Collett BR, Ohan JL, Myers KM: Ten-year review of rating scales, V: scales assessing attention deficit/hyperactivity disorder. J Am Acad Child Adolesc Psychiatry 42:1015–1037, 2003

Davis A, Tsukida C, Marchionna S, et al: The declining number of youth in custody in the juvenile justice system. Focus: Research From the National Council on Crime and Delinquency, August 2008. Available at: http://www.nccd-crc.org/nccd/pubs/2008_focus_JJS_custody_decline.pdf. Accessed April 27, 2009.

DeMatteo D, Marczyk G: Risk factors, protective factors, and the prevention of antisocial behavior among juveniles, in Juvenile Delinquency: Prevention, Assessment, and Intervention. Edited by Heilbrun K, Sevin Goldstein NE, Redding RE. New York, Oxford University Press, 2005, pp 19–44

DePrato DK, Hammer JH: Assessment and treatment of juvenile offenders, in Principles and Practice of Child and Adolescent Forensic Psychiatry. Edited by Schetky DH, Benedek EP. Washington, DC, American Psychiatric Publishing, 2002, pp 267–278

Federal Bureau of Investigation: Crime in the United States, 2006. Washington, DC, U.S. Department of Justice, September 2007. Available at: http://www.fbi.gov/ucr/cius2006. Accessed April 27, 2009.

Feindler EL, Scalley M: Adolescent anger management groups for violence reduction, in Group Interventions in School and Community. Edited by Ollendick T, Storber K. Needham Heights, UK, Allyn & Bacon, 1998, pp 100–118

Fombonne E: Increased rates of psychosocial disorders in youth. Eur Arch Psychiatry Clin Neurosci 248:14–21, 1998

Grisso T: Double Jeopardy: Adolescent Offenders With Mental Disorders. Chicago, University of Chicago, 2004

Grisso T, Barnum R, Fletcher KE, et al: Massachusetts Youth Screening Instrument for mental health needs of juvenile justice youths. J Am Acad Child Adolesc Psychiatry 40:541–548, 2001

Hamilton M: A rating scale for depression. J Neurol Neurosurg Psychiatry 23:56–62, 1960

Hamparian D, Leiber M: Disproportionate Confinement of Minority Juveniles in Secure Facilities: 1996 National Report. Champaign, IL, Community Research Associates, 1997

Hayes LM: Juvenile suicide in confinement in the United States results from a national survey. Crisis 26:146–148, 2005a

Hayes LM: Suicide prevention in correctional facilities, in Correctional Mental Health. Edited by Scott CL, Gerbasi JB. Washington, DC, American Psychiatric Publishing, 2005b, pp 69–88

Hennessey M, Ford JD, Mahoney K, et al: Trauma among girls in the juvenile justice system. Los Angeles, National Traumatic Stress Network, 2004

Huizinga D, Elliott DS: Juvenile offenders: prevalence, offender incidence, and arrest rates by race. Crime Delinq 33:206–223, 1987

Juneja P: Juvenile justice and education issues affecting Asian and Pacific Islander (API) youth in Richmond, California. National Council on Crime and Delinquency. October 5, 2006. Available at: http://www.ncjrs.gov/App/Publications/abstract.aspx?ID=237419. Accessed April 27, 2009.

Kaminer Y, Bukstein OG, Tarter RE: The Teen Addiction Severity Index: rationale and reliability. Int J Addict 26:219–226, 1991

Kaufman AS: Assessing Adolescent and Adult Intelligence. Boston, Allyn & Bacon, 1990

Knight JR, Sherritt L, Shrier LA, et al: Validity of the CRAFFT substance abuse screening test among adolescent clinic patients. Arch Pediatr Adolesc Med 156:607–614, 2002

Kovacs M: The Children's Depression Inventory. Psychopharmacol Bull 21:995–998, 1985

Krisberg B: Juvenile Justice: Redeeming Our Children. Thousand Oaks, CA, Sage, 2005

Krisberg B: Rediscovering the juvenile justice ideal in the United States, in Comparative Youth Justice. Edited by Muncie J, Goldsan B. London, Sage, 2006, pp 6–18

Krisberg B, Wolf AM: Juvenile offending, in Juvenile Delinquency: Prevention, Assessment, and Intervention. Edited by Heilbrun K, Sevin Goldstein NE, Redding RE. New York, Oxford University Press, 2005, pp 67–84

Krisberg B, Schwartz I, Fishman G, et al: The incarceration of minority youth. Crime Delinq 33:173–205, 1987

Landenberger NA, Lipsey MW: The positive effects of cognitive-behavioral programs for offenders: a meta-analysis of factors associated with effective treatment. Journal of Experimental Criminology 1:451–476, 2005

Loeber R, Farrington DP (eds): Serious and Violent Juvenile Offenders: Risk Factors and Successful Interventions. Thousand Oaks, CA, Sage, 1998, pp 30–46

McLellan AT, Luborsky L, Woody GE, et al: An improved diagnostic evaluation index for substance abuse patients: the Addiction Severity Index. J Nerv Ment Dis 168:1–2, 1980

Mears D: Exploring state-level variation in juvenile incarceration rates. Prison J 86:470–490, 2006

Miller WR, Rollnick S: Motivational Interviewing: Preparing People for Change, 2nd Edition. New York, Guilford, 2002

Moffitt TE: Adolescence-limited and life-course-persistent antisocial behavior: a developmental taxonomy. Psychol Rev 100:674–701, 1993

Moffitt TE, Caspi A, Harrington H, et al: Males on the life-course-persistent and adolescence-limited antisocial pathways: follow-up at age 26. Dev Psychopathol 14:179–207, 2002

Muncie J: The punitive turn in juvenile justice: culture of control and rights compliance in western Europe and the USA. Youth Justice 8:107–121, 2008

Otto RK, Greenstein JJ, Johnson MK, et al: Prevalence of mental disorders in the juvenile justice system, in Responding to the Mental Health Needs of Youth in the Juvenile Justice System. Edited by Cocozza JJ. Seattle, WA, National Coalition for the Mentally Ill in the Criminal Justice System, 1992

Poe-Yamagata E, Jones M: And Justice for Some. New York, National Council on Crime and Delinquency, 2000

Sevin Goldstein NE, Olubadewo O, Redding RE, et al: Mental health disorders: the neglected risk factor in juvenile delinquency, in Juvenile Delinquency: Prevention, Assessment, and Intervention. Edited by Heilbrun K, Sevin Goldstein NE, Redding RE. New York, Oxford University Press, 2005, pp 85–110

Shaffer D, Fisher P, Lucas CP, et al: NIMH Diagnostic Interview Schedule for Children Version IV (NIMH DISC-IV): description, differences from previous versions, and reliability of some common diagnoses. J Am Acad Child Adolesc Psychiatry 39:28–38, 2000

Sheidow AJ, Henggeler SW: Community-based treatments, in Juvenile Delinquency: Prevention, Assessment, and Intervention. Edited by Heilbrun K, Sevin Goldstein NE, Redding RE. New York, Oxford University Press, 2005, pp 257–281

Snyder HN: Juvenile crime and justice in the United States of America, in Juvenile Justice Systems: An International Comparison of Problems and Solutions. Edited by Bala N, Nornick J, Snyder H, et al. Toronto, ON, Thompson, 2002

Snyder HN, Sickmund M: Juvenile offenders and victims: 2006 national reports (NCJ 212906). 2006. Available at: http://www.ojjdp.ncjrs.org/Publications. Accessed April 27, 2009.

Stein BD, Jaycox LH, Kataoka SH, et al: A mental health intervention for schoolchildren exposed to violence: a randomized control trial. JAMA 290:603–611, 2003

Stein LA, Colby SM, Barnett NP, et al: Enhancing substance abuse treatment engagement in incarcerated adolescents. Psychological Services 3:25–34, 2006

Stiffman A, Chen Y, Elze D, et al: Adolescents' and providers' perspectives on the need for and use of mental health services. J Adolesc Health 21:335–342, 1997

Swanson JM: SNAP-IV Scale. Irvine, University of California Child Development Center, 1995

Teplin LA: Psychiatric and substance abuse disorders among male urban jail detainees. Am J Public Health 84:290–293, 1994

Teplin LA, Abram KM, McClelland GM, et al: Psychiatric disorders in youth in juvenile detention. Arch Gen Psychiatry 59:1133–1143, 2002

Turner S, Fain T, Sehgal A: Validation of the risk and resiliency assessment tool for juveniles in the Los Angeles County probation system. Santa Monica, CA, RAND, 2005. Available at: http://www.rand.org/pubs/technical_reports/2005/RAND_TR291.sum.pdf. Accessed April 27, 2009.

Van Dieten M: Girls...Moving On. Toronto, ON, Orbis Partners, 2004

Villarruel FA, Walker NE, Minifree P, et al: Donde está la justicia? A call to action on behalf of Latino and Latina youth in the U.S. justice system. Lansing, MI, Michigan State University Institute for Children, Youth and Families, 2002

Washburn JJ, Teplin LA, Voss LS, et al: Psychiatric disorders among detained youths: a comparison of youths processed in juvenile court and adult criminal court. Psychiatr Serv 59:965–973, 2008

Wasserman G, McReynolds L, Lucas C, et al: The voice DISC-IV with incarcerated male youths: prevalence of disorder. J Am Acad Child Adolesc Psychiatry 41:314–321, 2002

Wilkinson GS, Robertson GJ: Wide Range Achievement Test, 4th Edition. Lutz, FL, Psychological Assessment Resources, 2006

Woolard JL, Odgers C, Lanza-Kaduce L, et al: Juveniles within adult correctional settings: legal pathways and developmental considerations. International Journal of Forensic Mental Health 4:1–18, 2005

CHAPTER 20

Geriatric Offenders

Jason G. Roof, M.D.

Americans are getting older. In 1900, people over age 65 represented only 4% of the total population of the United States. By 2050, approximately 78.9 million people, or 20% of the population, will be age 65 and older (Malmgren 2000). As the overall age of the general U.S. population increases, the age of the population of incarcerated individuals also continues to rise. Geriatric inmate populations, however, are increasing at a disproportionately higher rate than younger inmate populations, and this increase is a result of more than population growth alone. Additional factors that play a part in this disproportionate increase include an increase in the average age of inmates at the time of incarceration and legislative changes that have limited judicial discretion, lengthened sentences, and toughened parole requirements (Glaser et al. 1990; Raimer and Stobo 2004). Table 20–1 illustrates the projected growth of the geriatric population in the United States from 1900 to 2050.

In 2003, over 2 million inmates were incarcerated in the United States. This number represents a 500% increase from the 325,400 inmates in prisons and jails in 1970. Inmates who were age 50 years or older represented 5.7% of all inmates in 1992 and 8.6% of all inmates in 2002 (Mitka 2004). The Texas Department of Criminal Justice reported that the state's population of inmates age 55 years or older increased by 148% between 1994 and 2002, compared with a 32% overall increase in the inmate population (Texas Department of Corrections 2003). California has

TABLE 20–1.　Population age 65 or older—United States, 1990–2050

Population	1900	1950	1955	2010	2030	2050
Age 65 and older						
Population, in millions	3.1	12.3	33.5	39.4	69.4	78.9
Percentage of total population	4.1	8.1	12.8	13.2	20.0	20.0
Age 85 and older						
Population, in millions	0.1	0.6	3.6	5.7	8.5	18.2
Percentage of 65+ population	4.0	4.7	10.8	14.4	12.2	23.1

Source.　Malmgren 2000.

reported at least a 350% increase in geriatric female offenders in the past 12 years (Williams et al. 2006). The average age of inmates at the time of admission is increasing (Raimer and Stobo 2004). In 1990, the average age of an inmate was 29.9 years; in 1998, the average age was 31.5 years (Linder and Meyers 2007). This evidence indicates that not only are the populations of U.S. jails and prisons increasing, but they are also getting older.

UNIQUE CHARACTERISTICS OF GERIATRIC OFFENDERS

Because incarcerated individuals as a whole are more likely to experience physical stressors at a higher rate than the general population, an individual as young as age 50 may be considered a "geriatric" patient (Lewis et al. 2006; Loeb et al. 2007). On average, incarcerated individuals come from lower socioeconomic status, have lifestyle practices that can cause accelerated aging, have decreased access to medical and mental health treatment and maintenance, and experience the ongoing deleterious effects of incarceration (Loeb et al. 2007). For many inmates, health care during incarceration may be the first consistent access to health care that they have had in their lives (Linder and Meyers 2007).

Studies have demonstrated that individuals older than age 65 are less likely to be arrested for all types of crimes (Covey and Menard 1987; Lewis et al. 2006). Like younger populations, older offenders are more likely to be abusing or dependent on alcohol than any other substance; however, they differ from younger populations in that they are more likely to have only one substance of abuse and are more likely to be arrested for a drug-related crime (Arndt et al. 2002; Lewis et al. 2006). In a study by Arndt et al. (2002), 71% of inmates age 55 and older reported substance abuse problems upon entering prison; of these individuals, 85% reported alcohol as their primary problem substance, and 7% reported cocaine/crack, which was the second most common substance reported. The Virginia Department of Corrections' special needs correctional center contains geriatric offenders, 75% of whom are incarcerated for violent offenses, most often rape or sexual assault (Virginia Department of Corrections 2007). Geriatric individuals referred for evaluation for criminal responsibility or competency to stand trial, as a population, were found to be poorly educated, divorced or separated instead of widowed, and recidivists with a high prevalence of violent and substance-related crimes (Lewis et al. 2006).

In addition to understanding unique characteristics of geriatric offenders compared with their younger peers, the clinician should also be familiar with the most frequent concerns of older inmates. Table 20–2 summarizes the most common concerns in this population.

Kracoski and Babb (1990) interviewed staff members and administrators of various correctional facilities. The authors reported a general consensus that geriatric offenders, when compared with younger offenders, tended to isolate from the inmate subculture, were less likely to receive assistance from friends and family members, and were more fearful of the consequences of release.

COMMON HEALTH PROBLEMS OF GERIATRIC INMATES

A remarkable series of events over the past 20 years have improved the health and quality of life of many persons over age 50. Better financial security, medical advances, greater awareness of medical conditions, and the pursuit of healthier lifestyles have extended and improved the quality of life for people as they age (AARP 2002).

Unfortunately, the geriatric offender population has not benefited as greatly from these developments. Nearly 85% of older inmates live with multiple medical conditions and on average will experience three chronic health conditions (Fazel et al. 2001; Loeb et al. 2007). Management of these conditions has been estimated to increase housing costs for older patients by as much as five times when compared with costs for younger inmates (Loeb et al. 2007; Virginia Department of Corrections 2007). Individuals who are incarcerated for long periods of time are at

TABLE 20–2.   Most common concerns of inmates age 50 and older

Fear of victimization by younger inmates

Inconsiderate younger inmates

Decreased privacy

Ongoing noise in their environment

Lack of friendships within their facility

Desire to be housed with same-age peers

Inadequate space and poor ventilation in housing environment

Housed too far away from bathroom and dining facilities

Source. Vito and Wilson 1985.

increased risk for having HIV infection, tuberculosis, and liver disease (Linder and Meyers 2007). Whether their infections were acquired inside correctional facilities or outside in the general population, inmates, who typically engage in more high-risk sexual and drug-related behaviors than the general population, become burdened with a disproportionately high rate of serious infectious disease (Hammett 2006). The Department of Justice reported that 1.8% of state prison inmates and 0.9% of federal prison inmates were infected with HIV as of 2006. Of those known to be HIV positive, inmates with AIDS accounted for 0.5% of the state prison population and 0.4% of federal inmates (Maruschak 2008). Despite the increased rate of infectious disease, improved treatments for HIV have resulted in significantly longer life expectancies for patients with HIV. This trend has been demonstrated at the California Medical Facility, Vacaville, where AIDS deaths as a percentage of all deaths decreased from 48.1% in 1993 to 19.7% in 2000 (Linder et al. 2002). A similar burden exists with hepatitis C. Although U.S. prisoners are not universally tested for hepatitis C, the U.S. Department of Justice reported that 31% of prisoners who were tested for hepatitis C between July 1, 1999, and June 30, 2000, tested positive for hepatitis C (Beck and Maruschak 2004). Liver dysfunction and physiological changes of aging can significantly complicate an older inmate's course of treatment.

Also, individuals who have been incarcerated for more than 6 years have an increased probability of medical problems (Voelker 2004). The most commonly reported health conditions are cardiovascular diseases, arthritis/back problems, respiratory diseases, endocrine disorders, and sensory deficits (Loeb et al. 2007). Loeb et al. (2007) asked inmates to comment on their health and the effects of incarceration on their health. Inmates frequently expressed concerns about perceived health deterioration, such as the development or worsening of diabetes, bone or joint disorders, cardiovascular problems, weight problems, or decreasing fitness.

The U.S. Department of Health and Human Services noted that the most prevalent chronic medical conditions from 2005 to 2006 for men and women of all races over age 65 were hypertension (53.3%), arthritis (49.6%), chronic joint symptoms (43.4%), and all types of heart disease (31%) (National Center for Health Statistics 2008). A more specific focus on older inmates by the U.S. Department of Justice found several significant medical issues: muscle weakness, decreased muscular flexibility and renal mass, decreased immune function, decreased function of the senses, requirement of different diets due to changes in the gastrointestinal system, incontinence, and falls (Morton 1992).

In 2004, the leading causes of death in all adults were, in decreasing order, diseases of the heart; malignant neoplasms; cerebrovascular diseases; chronic lower respiratory diseases; accidents (unintentional injuries); diabetes mellitus; Alzheimer's disease; influenza and pneumonia; nephritis, nephrotic syndrome, and nephrosis; and septicemia. Alzheimer's disease ranked as the tenth leading cause of death for men and the fifth for women. For individuals ages 45–74, cancer and then heart disease were the leading causes of death. For those over age 74, heart disease and cancer were still the top two causes, but heart disease was a more likely cause of death (Heron 2007).

Significant changes in the aging human body include decreased drug absorption through the gastrointestinal tract, increased total body fat resulting in increased lipophilic drug absorption, changes in plasma protein binding, decreased hepatic metabolism and clearance, and decreased renal clearance (Chutka et al. 2004; Zubenko and Sunderland 2000). These changes, coupled with the significant risk of chronic disease, contribute to a significantly complicated treatment course for this population.

COMMON MENTAL HEALTH PROBLEMS OF GERIATRIC INMATES

Studies have shown that at least half of geriatric inmates and forensic evaluees have a psychiatric disorder and up to 80% of geriatric offenders have had a previous psychiatric hospitalization (Lewis et al. 2006). Table 20–3 summarizes the most common mental health diagnoses in the older populations referred for forensic evaluation.

TABLE 20–3. Prevalence of psychiatric disorders in inmates 60 and older referred for forensic evaluation

Diagnosis	Percentage of population
Alcohol abuse/dependence	67
Dementia	44
Antisocial personality disorder	32
Drug abuse/dependence	17
Schizophrenia	14
Borderline intellectual functioning	11
Delusional disorder	6
Major depressive disorder	6
Schizoaffective disorder	4
Organic personality disorder	4
Adjustment disorder or bereavement	4

Source. Lewis et al. 2006.

Changes in Cognition

Changes in Memory Related to Normal Aging

Nonpathological changes in memory related to normal aging are often identified using terms such as "benign senescence" or "age-associated memory decline" or can be included in the age-related cognitive decline diagnosis from the *Diagnostic and Statistical Manual of Mental Disorders,* 4th Edition, Text Revision (DMS-IV-TR; American Psychiatric Association 2000). Recently, the Aging, Demographics, and Memory Study found that 22.2% of Americans over age 71 had cognitive impairment without dementia (Plassman et al. 2008). Researchers with the Baltimore Longitudinal Study of Aging, the longest-running scientific study of human aging, have reported several significant findings in age-related alterations in cognition. Abilities to problem-solve and to learn rapidly are not significantly impaired for most individuals until late in life; visuospatial abilities, fluency of language, and general intelligence may also decline. Tests have indicated the preservation of verbal abilities into the 80s (Price 2000). Typically, older individuals have a shortened attention span, slower incorporation of new ideas, increased sleep fragmentation, and a decrease of brain weight. Additionally, frontal lobe functioning may be increasingly impaired during aging (Ratcliff and Saxton 2000).

Based on a study of 50 randomly selected male patients being held in a maximum security state hospital for offenders with mental disorders, Martell (1992) reported that 64% of those examined had multiple indicators of potential brain dysfunction and 84% had at least one indicator. These indicators included a history of head injury with loss of consciousness; cognitive impairment; seizure disorder; neurological abnormalities; and a diagnosed organic brain syndrome. Because of the significant prevalence of cognitive dysfunction, the ability of many geriatric inmates to follow the numerous rules and regulations of a correctional environment may be substantially impaired.

Dementia

Although cognitive impairment without dementia is quite common, of those individuals who have cognitive impairment without dementia, 10%–15% progress to dementia annually (Plassman et al. 2008). Dementia is characterized by cognitive deficits caused by medical conditions, substances, or a combination of several conditions. DSM-IV-TR lists several diagnoses, which include dementia of the Alzheimer's type, dementia due to various general medical conditions, substance-induced persisting dementia, dementia due to multiple etiologies, and dementia not otherwise specified if the etiology is indeterminate (American Psychiatric Association 2000).

Medications or medical problems may induce what appears to be dementia or delirium. The most common offending drug classes are anticholinergics, antihypertensives, psychotropics, sedative-hypnotics, and narcotic analgesics (Chutka et al. 2004). Medications may cause such an effect when, for example, a geriatric patient's dosage of medication is too high, the geriatric patient does not appropriately follow dosing directions, the patient has an increased sensitivity to or impaired metabolism for a certain medication, and/or drug-drug interactions occur. Also, several medical conditions, including heart disease, renal disease, congestive heart failure, thyroid dysfunction, and vitamin deficiencies, may present as manageable sources of dementia-type symptoms.

Alzheimer's disease is the most frequent cause of dementia. An estimated 60%–70% of dementia cases are of the Alzheimer's type (Alzheimer's Association 2005). Studies have shown that Alzheimer's disease has a cumulative incidence as high as 4.7% by age 70, 18.2% by age 80, and 49.6% by age 90 (Santacruz and Swagerty 2001). The Alzheimer's Association (2005) estimates that 4.5 million Americans have Alzheimer's disease.

In a setting of incarceration, such as a jail or prison, the early stages of Alzheimer's disease may be seen as a subtle loss of short-term memory.

Inmates may become easily lost within the facility or demonstrate problems with word finding and the naming of standard objects. Individuals in this early stage of Alzheimer's disease may demonstrate apraxia (an inability to perform complex movements) or may have difficulty dressing or eating. During the late stages of Alzheimer's disease, an individual's judgment often becomes impaired and personality changes may become apparent. Such personality changes may present as increased apathy or hostility toward, or withdrawal from, peers or custody staff (Santacruz and Swagerty 2001). Also, patients with late-stage Alzheimer's disease often experience a significant disturbance in the sleep cycle and may experience depression, anxiety, delusions, or hallucinations. DSM-IV-TR lists the diagnostic criteria for dementia of the Alzheimer's type (see Table 20–4).

Delirium

Although abnormal changes in memory, judgment, and cognition may occur in both dementia and delirium, one of the best methods to differentiate the two is the presence or absence of a clouding of consciousness that fluctuates over the course of a short time (e.g., in a single day). This fluctuation is characteristic of delirium. Additionally, an acute or subacute onset of symptoms more often indicates delirium as opposed to dementia (Sadock and Sadock 2003). DSM-IV-TR defines delirium due to a general medical condition (see Table 20–5).

Clinical Case 20–1

Mr. J is a 75-year-old man who has been incarcerated for 3 years. Custody staff asked the facility's psychiatric service to evaluate Mr. J due to observations that he has been isolating, refusing meals, inadequately caring for himself, and appearing disoriented at times. He has been unable to follow directions given to him by custody staff and appears to have great difficulty returning to the appropriate cell or reporting to officers when asked. On evaluation, he appears to have significant cognitive impairment and appears to be poorly oriented. Notably, he appears very poorly motivated to respond to the interviewer's questions and answers "I don't know" or "No" to most questions. Although he is resistant to providing family history, he consents to allowing the clinician to speak with his family. Family interviews indicate that the family has a positive history of depression and that Mr. J had a recent family visit during which he appeared generally well-oriented and was able to converse without difficulty.

Clinical Case 20–1 demonstrates the difficulty of determining whether an individual has dementia or depression, because the clinical pictures may look similar. Depression that may look like dementia has been

TABLE 20–4. DSM-IV-TR diagnostic criteria for dementia of the Alzheimer's type

A. The development of multiple cognitive deficits manifested by both

    (1) memory impairment (impaired ability to learn new information or to recall previously learned information)

    (2) one (or more) of the following cognitive disturbances:

        (a) aphasia (language disturbance)

        (b) apraxia (impaired ability to carry out motor activities despite intact motor function)

        (c) agnosia (failure to recognize or identify objects despite intact sensory function)

        (d) disturbance in executive functioning (i.e., planning, organizing, sequencing, abstracting)

B. The cognitive deficits in Criteria A1 and A2 each cause significant impairment in social or occupational functioning and represent a significant decline from a previous level of functioning.

C. The course is characterized by gradual onset and continuing cognitive decline.

D. The cognitive deficits in Criteria A1 and A2 are not due to any of the following:

    (1) other central nervous system conditions that cause progressive deficits in memory and cognition (e.g., cerebrovascular disease, Parkinson's disease, Huntington's disease, subdural hematoma, normal-pressure hydrocephalus, brain tumor)

    (2) systemic conditions that are known to cause dementia (e.g., hypothyroidism, vitamin B_{12} or folic acid deficiency, niacin deficiency, hypercalcemia, neurosyphilis, HIV infection)

    (3) substance-induced conditions

E. The deficits do not occur exclusively during the course of a delirium.

F. The disturbance is not better accounted for by another Axis I disorder (e.g., major depressive disorder, schizophrenia).

Code based on presence or absence of a clinically significant behavioral disturbance:

    294.10 Without Behavioral Disturbance: if the cognitive disturbance is not accompanied by any clinically significant behavioral disturbance.

    294.11 With Behavioral Disturbance: if the cognitive disturbance is accompanied by a clinically significant behavioral disturbance (e.g., wandering, agitation).

TABLE 20–4.   DSM-IV-TR diagnostic criteria for dementia of the Alzheimer's type *(continued)*

Specify subtype:
  With Early Onset: if onset is at age 65 years or below
  With Late Onset: if onset is after age 65 years

Coding note: Also code 331.0 Alzheimer's disease on Axis III. Indicate other prominent clinical features related to the Alzheimer's disease on Axis I (e.g., 293.83 Mood disorder due to Alzheimer's disease, with depressive features, and 310.1 Personality change due to Alzheimer's disease, aggressive type).

Source.   Reprinted from American Psychiatric Association: *Diagnostic and Statistical Manual of Mental Disorders*, 4th Edition, Text Revision. Washington, DC, American Psychiatric Association, 2000, pp. 157–158. Copyright 2000, American Psychiatric Publishing. Used with permission.

TABLE 20–5.   DSM-IV-TR diagnostic criteria for delirium due to...[indicate the general medical condition]

A.   Disturbance of consciousness (i.e., reduced clarity of awareness of the environment) with reduced ability to focus, sustain, or shift attention.

B.   A change in cognition (such as memory deficit, disorientation, language disturbance) or the development of a perceptual disturbance that is not better accounted for by a preexisting, established, or evolving dementia.

C.   The disturbance develops over a short period of time (usually hours to days) and tends to fluctuate during the course of the day.

D.   There is evidence from the history, physical examination, or laboratory findings that the disturbance is caused by the direct physiological consequences of a general medical condition.

Coding note: If delirium is superimposed on a preexisting vascular dementia, indicate the delirium by coding 290.41 Vascular dementia, with delirium.

Coding note: Include the name of the general medical condition on Axis I, e.g., 293.0 Delirium due to hepatic encephalopathy; also code the general medical condition on Axis III.

Source.   Reprinted from American Psychiatric Association: *Diagnostic and Statistical Manual of Mental Disorders*, 4th Edition, Text Revision. Washington, DC, American Psychiatric Association, 2000, p. 143. Copyright 2000, American Psychiatric Publishing. Used with permission.

termed *pseudodementia* or *depression-related cognitive dysfunction* (Sadock and Sadock 2003). Certain unique features may indicate the presence of depression over dementia. Features indicating pseudodementia include better premorbid functioning, a rapid onset of symptoms, a patient's detailed complaints of cognitive dysfunction, poor motivation to perform even simple tasks, negativistic answers to questions, and a personal or familial history of depression (Sadock and Sadock 2003).

Suicide

As a population, geriatric offenders may face multiple stressors. Older offenders face an increased likelihood of medical illness, an increased probability of needing to cope with chronic and terminal illnesses, and the loss of family and friends while incarcerated (Revier 2004). American white men over age 85 have been found to have the highest rate of suicide when variables such as race, sex, and age are examined (AARP 2002). Suicide is the eighth leading cause of death for men and the sixteenth leading cause of death for women (Heron 2007).

The risk of incarcerated individuals committing suicide while in custody is higher in jails than in prisons (Kuhlmann and Ruddell 2005). Increased surveillance of high-risk inmates during periods of increased stress, such as during the first hours of arrest and after important judicial decisions, may result in reductions of suicide in custody settings. The California Department of Corrections and Rehabilitation performed a review of all completed suicides occurring between 1999 and 2004 and found several significant characteristics related to inmate suicide (Patterson and Hughes 2008). These characteristics are summarized in Table 20–6.

ASSESSMENT OF THE GERIATRIC OFFENDER

Intake Into the Correctional Facility

Many jail and prison systems use preliminary screening to determine if an inmate has any significant medical issues, such as disability, illness, current medication use, or allergies. Additional questions may then be used to assess the individual's psychiatric history or attempt to obtain information related to suicidality. Correctional institutions in some states, such as Ohio, then assign inmates a certain numerical medical classification rating to indicate the level of medical management (e.g., from 1 for *stable* to 4 for *requiring constant medical care*). If the individual is entering prison, he or she will be assigned to the particular facility that may best satisfy the individual's medical requirements (Anno et al. 2004). Should

TABLE 20–6.   Characteristics of inmates that suggest an increased need for monitoring for suicidality

History of serious mental illness

History of suicide attempts

Prisoners housed in a single cell (particularly in administrative segregation or a secure housing unit)

Prisoners with safety concerns, particularly if associated with anxiety and agitation

Prisoners with serious medical concerns

Coexisting severe personality disorders and coexisting mental illness

Significant change in legal status

Caucasian

Source.   Patterson and Hughes 2008.

initial screening indicate a need, further psychiatric evaluation will be performed.

Rating Scales

A clinician's ability to assess a geriatric patient may be improved through the use of specialized rating scales. Burns et al. (1999) identified 162 scales for use with older patients. Scales typically address one or more general domains and may help the clinician better understand an individual's mood, ability to perform activities of daily living, overall functionality, ability to think and remember, or quality of life (Burns et al. 2002). Before choosing a scale, the clinician must consider multiple elements, including the following: the population for which the scale was first designed, the specific illness for which the scale was designed, the patient's ability to understand written and/or verbal instructions, time limitations, and training required to administer the scale. For example, a clinician may find that the Hamilton Rating Scale for Depression is less sensitive in detecting clinically significant depression in a geriatric patient because of unique symptoms of depression present in elderly individuals (Burns et al. 2002).

A commonly used scale to screen for depression in elderly individuals is the Geriatric Depression Scale (Yesavage et al. 1982). The patient answers yes-no questions. Although the original scale has 30 questions, a shortened 15-item version by Shiekh and Yesavage (1986) is available and more frequently used (Burns et al. 2002). Easily administered, brief scales such as this may be quite effective in screening for symptoms of mental illness in various correctional settings.

A frequently used examination, for both clinical and research purposes, is the Geriatric Mental State (GMS) schedule (Geriatric Mental State Resource Centre 2007). The GMS was designed to detect a wide range of mental illnesses as well as organic brain syndrome. This schedule, presented as a semistructured interview, has been translated into at least 17 languages. A complementary schedule, the History and Aetiology Schedule (HAS; Geriatric Mental State Resource Centre 2007), was created to be given to the interviewee's most relevant significant other. Designating a significant other in a correctional population may be problematic, and the utility of the HAS in a correctional setting may be complicated. The Automated Geriatric Examination for Computer Assisted Taxonomy (Geriatric Mental State Resource Centre 2007) is a computerized combination of the GMS and HAS. Administration of this series of instruments is complicated by the requirements that the test administrator be trained, that a computer and software be present, and that approximately 45 minutes of time be available to administer the testing (Burns et al. 2002; Geriatric Mental State Resource Centre 2007).

A clinician may wish to screen an inmate for the presence of cognitive deficits. Two useful instruments are the Mini-Mental State Examination, which requires 5–10 minutes and examines components such as the individual's orientation, memory, attention, and language abilities (Folstein et al. 1975), and the Clock Drawing Test, which is highly portable and requires only a few minutes to administer and interpret (Brodaty and Moore 1997).

To assess an individual's ability to care for himself or herself, particularly in the presence of dementia, the clinician can choose from several scales. Such evaluations may be useful when a geriatric offender's release plan is being considered. One such scale, the Bristol Activities of Daily Living Scale, was designed specifically for use with individuals who have dementia. This scale examines 20 separate abilities that are important in an individual's life (Bucks et al. 1996), including the ability to attend to personal hygiene, the ability to understand speech, and orientation. If Alzheimer's dementia is suspected or diagnosed, the clinician might determine a patient's ability to attend to activities of daily living using the Alzheimer's Disease Functional Assessment and Change Scale (Galasko et al. 1997), the Disability Assessment for Dementia (Gelinas et al. 1999), or the Interview for Deterioration in Daily Living Activities in Dementia (Teunisse et al. 1991).

TREATMENT OF THE GERIATRIC OFFENDER: COMMON ADVERSE EFFECTS OF DRUGS

Geriatric patients can be particularly sensitive to various drugs and may demonstrate a constellation of side effects that might exacerbate or cause additional health problems. Institutionalized elderly individuals have been found to be taking an average of seven different daily medications (Chutka et al. 2004). The use of so many medications, although frequently necessary, can increase the likelihood of adverse reactions. Studies have shown that elderly individuals over age 70 are seven times more likely to experience adverse reactions to medications than are individuals in their 20s. Additional studies have demonstrated that 17%–30% of all hospital admissions of elderly individuals may be the result of medication-related adverse reactions (Chutka et al. 2004; Fick et al. 2003).

A clinician may interpret a patient's adverse reactions as treatable symptoms and be tempted to treat the adverse reaction with additional medications. Such treatments, however, can cause an even greater likelihood of other adverse reactions and side effects (see Table 20–7).

TABLE 20–7.   Common adverse effects of psychotropic drugs in elderly individuals

Central nervous system	Sedation, confusion, disorientation, memory impairment, delirium
Peripheral (anticholinergic)	Constipation, dry mouth, blurred vision, urinary retention
Motor	Extrapyramidal symptoms, tremor, impaired gait, increased body sway, falling
Cardiovascular	Hypotension, cardiac conduction delay
Other	Agitation, mood and perceptual disturbances, headache, sweating, sexual dysfunction, gastrointestinal disturbances (nausea, anorexia, changes in weight or bowel habits, hyponatremia)

Source.   Zubenko and Sunderland 2000.

Beers et al. (1991, 1992) described medications that were not appropriate for use in a nursing home population. These guidelines were updated in 1997, and specific drugs listed by Beers were reviewed in 2004 (Chutka et al. 2004). The results of this review are listed in Table 20–8.

TABLE 20–8. Recommendations regarding inappropriate drugs for elderly persons

Drug	Reasons drug is inappropriate	Comment
Anticholinergics	Cardiac arrhythmia, dry mouth and eyes, urinary retention	Avoid if possible
Barbiturates	Respiratory depression, habituation, falls/hip fractures, better/safer alternatives available	Appropriate for patients with seizure disorders
First- and second-generation antipsychotics	Anticholinergic effects extrapyramidal effects, tardive dyskinesia, better alternatives available with newer medications	Patients require intramuscular or intravenous medication
First-generation antihistamines	Sedation, falls, impaired driving, safer alternatives available	Avoid if possible
Long-acting benzodiazepines	Falls/hip fractures, safer alternatives available with shorter duration	Avoid if possible
Meprobamate	Respiratory depression, falls/hip fractures, tolerance, safer alternatives available	Avoid if possible
Pentazocine	Hallucinations, central nervous system impairment	Avoid high doses or prolonged use
Tricyclic antidepressants	Anticholinergic effects, cardiac toxicity, orthostatic hypotension	Low dose for neuropathic pain is appropriate

Source. Chutka et al. 2004.

Clinical Case 20–2

Mr. H is a 75-year-old man currently serving a life sentence for murder. He has a long history of depression that has been well controlled with antidepressant medication. Despite years of stabilization on a standard medication, he reports having experienced significant stress for the past 6 months. Approximately 7 months ago, Mr. H was transferred from a facility that separated geriatric inmates from younger inmates and had programs designed specifically for geriatric inmates. He describes significant fear related to being unable to respond quickly enough to the demands of officers, the threat of victimization by younger inmates, and his inability to participate in recreational activities due to the presence of younger and more aggressive inmates. Despite continued compliance with his antidepressant medications, he reports increasing anxiety related to the conditions of his incarceration and is requesting additional medication from the facility's psychiatric service.

CORRECTIONS PROGRAMS AND HOUSING FOR GERIATRIC OFFENDERS

Geriatric populations require conditions that may differ significantly from those of younger inmate populations. Federal and state correctional systems that segregate older offenders often place them in specialized segregated housing units, segregate them in a separate portion of the facility, or use a combination of these two methods (Thivierge-Rikard and Thompson 2007). States that have created housing units or separate facilities for geriatric populations include Alabama, Arkansas, Colorado, the District of Columbia, Georgia, Idaho, Illinois, Kentucky, Louisiana, Michigan, Minnesota, Mississippi, New Mexico, North Carolina, Ohio, Pennsylvania, South Carolina, Texas, Virginia, and Washington (Kempker 2003). Physical accessibility issues, such as providing alternatives to stairways, must be considered when housing geriatric inmates. Additionally, the medical and mental health service needs of geriatric offenders may vary significantly and need to be considered (Kracoski and Babb 1990). The U.S. Department of Justice (1997) surveyed various corrections departments and listed several frequently used methods of geriatric care, which include increased physical examinations, the use of chronic care clinics, preventive care, special diets, compassionate release, and specialized housing.

Recognizing that geriatric inmates have a unique set of challenges associated with their care, Virginia's Department of Corrections has designated a specialized Continuing Care Community to better address such issues (Virginia Department of Corrections 2007). For example, geriatric inmates are not placed in bunk beds or made to perform difficult physical work. Virginia has also enacted specialized programs for the geriatric inmate, including horticulture, large-print library books, assisted living services, and "reality orientation to check for dementia, Alzheimer's disease and cognitive abilities" (Virginia Department of Corrections 2007). Due to a demonstrated reluctance by geriatric inmates to participate in typical recreational activities with younger populations, some facilities offer activities that require less physical exertion, such as age-limited sports activities or less strenuous activities such as playing checkers or card games (Kracoski and Babb 1990). Less physically demanding work assignments, such as assembling mailing packets or operating self-service elevators, have been made available to older inmates in some institutions to address the issue of reduced strength and the presence of physical disabilities (Kracoski and Babb 1990).

McCain Correctional Hospital in North Carolina is a converted tuberculosis sanatorium, which was deeded over to the North Carolina Division of Prisons in 1983. This facility has nursing care beds, X-ray equipment, and respiratory therapy and pharmacy capabilities. North Carolina also created a separate 222-bed area within this facility for inmates who are disabled and elderly and who would best be served in a nursing home–type environment. Activities geared toward older inmates include recreational programs such as horseshoes, morning exercise, ceramics, and horticulture, as well as group sessions referred to as "reminiscent therapy." Additional efforts have been made by this facility to offer activities that integrate geriatric offenders with community senior citizen clubs. Finally, social workers within the facility help to provide geriatric offenders with release planning, nursing home placement, and aftercare for their mental and medical illnesses (North Carolina Department of Correction 2009).

SPECIAL RELEASE PROGRAMS

Due to the costs associated with housing an inmate with special needs, or because an inmate may be chronically ill and in severe declining health, many states have enacted conditional early-release programs. In 2001, U.S. jurisdictions were asked to respond to a survey assessing the presence of medical parole or "compassionate release." Of the 49 jurisdictions that responded, 43 reported that they had some form of medical parole or compassionate release program. Of the few inmates who were granted such a release, most were near death (Linder and Meyers 2007). Virginia has a conditional release program, called a "geriatric release" clause, for 60-year-old inmates not convicted of a Class 1 felony who have served at least 10 years and for 65-year-old inmates who have served at least 5 years. From 1999 to 2006, of the 400 inmates eligible for geriatric release, 35 applied but only four releases were granted (Virginia Department of Corrections 2007).

HOSPICE FOR GERIATRIC OFFENDERS

As the inmate population ages, the percentage of inmate deaths due to natural causes also increases (Linder and Meyers 2007). To address end-of-life issues, hospice services in prison began in the early 1980s. In 2001, Linder and Meyers (2007) surveyed 49 jurisdictions for the presence of palliative care services. This survey showed that 25 of the 49 respondents had hospice programs, and five of these programs were freestanding units. Despite the presence of such programs, the authors noted several challenges with inmate palliative care services (see Table 20–9).

PLACEMENT PROBLEMS

Nursing homes and group homes may be resistant to accepting elderly clients with significant legal histories, and families may resist helping or be unable to assist elderly family members. Geriatric offenders may have a significantly reduced ability to become gainfully employed or to interface effectively with aftercare organizations. Aftercare organizations may include difficult-to-follow plans, extensive travel, and long periods of waiting to obtain care and services. For example, a constellation of problems is involved in trying to place a geriatric inmate with dementia who has a violent criminal history.

Project for Older Prisoners (POPS), a program created by Jonathan Turley at Tulane Law School, attempts to bring about awareness of the needs of aging prisoners and present alternatives to traditional incarceration models. In 2003, POPS proposed a risk-based approach to addressing the rising number of geriatric inmates and the costs associated with their care. Turley (2006) suggested the creation of other POPS programs through other law schools; the creation of a system for supervised release of low-risk, high-cost prisoners; the creation of alternative incarceration for mid-risk older prisoners; and, to address the need to protect society from high-risk older prisoners, the establishment of geriatric housing units while incarceration continues.

Once a geriatric offender is released, his or her reentry into society presents several significant areas of concern. Stojkovic (2007) listed five major areas of problems: personal adjustment issues, family issues, em-

TABLE 20–9. Challenges with inmate palliative care services

Restrictions on inmate and staff movements

Limited access to urgent care facilities

Restricted pharmacy formularies

Impediments to dispensing medications on an "as needed" basis

Limited patient autonomy, because corrections department policies sometimes restrict the use of do-not-resuscitate orders and advance medical directives

Finding, training, and employing hospice volunteers

Defining patients' "families" and determining when and how to work with them

Source. Linder and Meyers 2007.

ployment, housing, and health issues. Personal adjustment issues include difficulty adapting to the outside world. An individual who has lived for many years within the walls of a facility that dictates a daily schedule and provides food and shelter may find adapting to a less structured environment difficult. Family issues include the loss of the geriatric offender's family network due to long-term incarceration. Family members may have died or may be unwilling or unable to address the needs of the recently released geriatric offender, who may require substantial supervision. Reduced employability can complicate the ability of the newly released geriatric offender to obtain adequate housing, as well as mental health and general health care (Stojkovic 2007).

CONCLUSION

The requirement to address the needs of geriatric offenders increases as the U.S. population and incarcerated individuals become older. Geriatric offenders as patients are uniquely complicated on many fronts. To address these complications, many states have initiated specialized training and programs related to geriatric inmate populations; however, an increasingly important goal is for all states to address the needs of this significant large and growing population.

Geriatric offenders create the need for increased training and dialogue about capacity. According to Lewis et al. (2006), the ability of an aging individual to understand the complexities of his or her legal situation, medical and psychiatric illnesses, and placement options after release may be compromised. An increased sensitivity to facilitating the release and aftercare of geriatric inmates must be fostered in the correctional system. Administration of systematic screening and monitoring instruments to assess the geriatric offender's understanding of his or her medicolegal situation and to detect any undiagnosed condition(s) is necessary to reduce inappropriate and inhumane situations for the inmate. Although many states have initiated specialized housing and treatment programs for specific geriatric inmates, a critical need exists for the nation to address the needs of this population and to further the national dialogue about aging and incarceration.

SUMMARY POINTS

- The geriatric inmate population is increasing at a significantly higher rate than the younger inmate population.
- Incarcerated individuals as young as age 50 may be considered "geriatric."
- Significant changes that occur in the aging human body may complicate treatment.
- The most common health conditions of older inmates are cardiovascular diseases, arthritis/back problems, respiratory diseases, endocrine disorders, and sensory deficits.
- The most common psychiatric diagnoses in this population are dementia, substance abuse and/or dependence, depression, and personality disorders.
- An estimated 60%–70% of cases of dementia are due to Alzheimer's disease.
- Dementia, delirium, and depression must be carefully differentiated.
- Many medications must be cautiously used or avoided in geriatric populations.

REFERENCES

AARP: Beyond 50: a report to the nation on economic security. 2002. Available at: http://assets.aarp.org/rgcenter/econ/beyond_50_econ.pdf. Accessed April 29, 2009.

Alzheimer's Association: Basics of Alzheimer's disease: what it is and what you can do. 2005. Available at: http://www.alz.org/national/documents/brochure_basicsofalz_low.pdf. Accessed April 30, 2009.

American Psychiatric Association: Diagnostic and Statistical Manual of Mental Disorders, 4th Edition, Text Revision. Washington, DC, American Psychiatric Association, 2000

Anno BJ, Graham C, Lawrence JE, et al: Correctional health care: addressing the needs of elderly, chronically ill, and terminally ill inmates. Middletown, CT, U.S. Department of Justice, National Institute of Corrections, 2004

Arndt S, Turvey CL, Flaum M: Older offenders, substance abuse, and treatment. Am J Geriatr Psychiatry 10:733–739, 2002

Beck AJ, Maruschak LM: Hepatitis testing and treatment in state prisons (NCJ 199173C). U.S. Department of Justice, Office of Justice Programs, April 2004. Available at: http://www.ojp.usdoj.gov/bjs/pub/pdf/httsp.pdf. Accessed April 30, 2009.

Beers MH, Ouslander JG, Rollingher I, et al: Explicit criteria for determining inappropriate medication use in nursing home residents. UCLA Division of Geriatric Medicine. Arch Intern Med 151:1825–1832, 1991

Beers MH, Ouslander JG, Fingold SF, et al: Inappropriate medication prescribing in skilled-nursing facilities, Ann Intern Med 117:684–689, 1992

Brodaty H, Moore CM: The Clock Drawing Test for dementia of the Alzheimer's type: a comparison of three scoring methods in a memory disorders clinic. Int J Geriatr Psychiatry 12:619–627, 1997

Bucks RS, Ashworth DL, Wilcock GK, et al: Assessment of activities of daily living in dementia: development of the Bristol Activities of Daily Living Scale. Age Ageing 25:113–120, 1996

Burns A, Beevor A, Lelliott P, et al: Health of the Nation Outcome Scales for elderly people (HoNOS 65+): glossary for HoNOS 65+ score sheet. Br J Psychiatry 174:435–438, 1999

Burns A, Lawlor B, Craig S: Rating scales in old age psychiatry. Br J Psychiatry 180:161–167, 2002

Chutka DS, Takahashi PY, Hoel RW: Inappropriate medications for elderly patients. Mayo Clin Proc 79:122–139, 2004

Covey HC, Menard S: Trends in arrests among the elderly. Gerontologist 27:666–672, 1987

Fazel S, Hope T, O'Donnell I, et al: Health of elderly male prisoners: worse than the general population, worse than younger prisoners. Age Ageing 30:403–407, 2001

Fick DM, Cooper JW, Wade WE, et al: Updating the Beers criteria for potentially inappropriate medication use in older adults: results of a U.S. consensus panel of experts. Arch Intern Med 163:2716–2724, 2003

Folstein MF, Folstein SE, McHugh PR: "Mini-mental state": a practical method for grading the cognitive state of patients for the clinician. J Psychiatr Res 12:189–198, 1975

Galasko D, Bennett D, Sano M, et al: An inventory to assess activities of daily living for clinical trials in Alzheimer's disease: the Alzheimer's Disease Cooperative Study. Alzheimer Dis Assoc Disord 11 (suppl 2):S33–S39, 1997

Gelinas I, Gauthier L, McIntyre M, et al: Development of a functional measure for persons with Alzheimer's disease: the Disability Assessment for Dementia. Am J Occup Ther 53:471–481, 1999

Geriatric Mental State Resource Centre: GMS Resource Centre. February 19, 2007. Available at: http://www.liv.ac.uk/gms/index.htm. Accessed April 30, 2009.

Glaser JB, Warchol A, D'Angelo D, et al: Infectious diseases of geriatric inmates. Rev Infect Dis 12:683–692, 1990

Hammett TM: HIV/AIDS and other infectious diseases among correctional inmates: transmission, burden, and an appropriate response. Am J Public Health 96:974–978, 2006

Heron M: Deaths: leading causes for 2004. Natl Vital Stat Rep 56:1–95, 2007

Kempker E: The graying of American prisons: addressing the continued increase in geriatric inmates. Corrections Compendium 28:1–2, 4, 22–26, 2003

Kracoski PC, Babb S: Adjustment of older inmates: an analysis by institutional structure and gender. J Contemp Crim Justice 6:264–281, 1990

Kuhlmann R, Ruddell R: Elderly jail inmates: problems, prevalence and public health. Californian J Health Promot 3:49–60, 2005

Lewis CF, Fields C, Rainey E: A study of geriatric forensic evaluees: who are the violent elderly? J Am Acad Psychiatry Law 34:324–332, 2006

Linder JF, Meyers FJ: Palliative care for prison inmates: "Don't let me die in prison." JAMA 298:894–901, 2007

Linder JF, Knauf K, Enders SR, et al: Prison hospice and pastoral care services in California. J Palliat Med 5:903–908, 2002

Loeb SJ, Steffensmeier D, Myco PM: In their own words: older male prisoners' health beliefs and concerns for the future. Geriatr Nurs 28:319–329, 2007

Malmgren R: Epidemiology of aging, in Textbook of Geriatric Neuropsychiatry. Edited by Cummings JL, Coffey CE. Washington, DC, American Psychiatric Press, 2000, pp 17–31

Martell DA: Estimating the prevalence of organic brain dysfunction in maximum-security forensic psychiatric patients. J Forensic Sci 37:878–893, 1992

Maruschak LM: HIV in prisons, 2006 (NCJ 222179). Washington, DC, U.S. Department of Justice, Bureau of Justice Statistics, 2008

Mitka M: Aging prisoners stressing health care system. JAMA 292:423–424, 2004

Morton J: An administrative overview of the older inmate. U.S. Department of Justice, National Institute of Corrections, August 1992. Available at: http://www.nicic.org/pubs/1992/010937.pdf. Accessed April 30, 2009.

National Center for Health Statistics: Prevalence of selected chronic conditions by age, sex, and race/ethnicity: United States, 1997–2006. Hyattsville, MD, National Center for Health Statistics, 2008

North Carolina Department of Correction: McCain Correctional Hospital. 2009. Available at: http://www.doc.state.nc.us/dop/prisons/mccain.htm. Accessed April 30, 2009.

Patterson RF, Hughes K: Review of completed suicides in the California Department of Corrections and Rehabilitation, 1999 to 2004. Psychiatr Serv 59:676–682, 2008

Plassman BL, Langa KM, Fisher GG, et al: Prevalence of cognitive impairment without dementia in the United States. Ann Intern Med 148:427–434, 2008

Price DL: Aging of the brain and dementia of the Alzheimer type, in Principles of Neural Science, 4th Edition. Edited by Kandel ER, Schwartz JH, Jessell TM. New York, McGraw-Hill, 2000, pp 1149–1161

Raimer BG, Stobo JD: Health care delivery in the Texas prison system: the role of academic medicine. JAMA 292:485–489, 2004

Ratcliff G, Saxton J: Age-associated memory impairment, in Textbook of Geriatric Neuropsychiatry. Edited by Cummings JL, Coffey CE. Washington, DC, American Psychiatric Press, 2000, pp 165–179

Revier R: Aging behind bars: health care for older female inmates. J Women Aging 16:55–69, 2004

Sadock BJ, Sadock VA: Delirium, dementia, and amnestic and other cognitive disorders and mental disorders due to a general medical condition, in Kaplan and Sadock's Synopsis of Psychiatry: Behavioral Sciences/Clinical Psychiatry, 9th Edition. Edited by Sadock BJ, Sadock VA. Philadelphia, Lippincott Williams & Wilkins, 2003, pp 319–370

Santacruz KS, Swagerty D: Early diagnosis of dementia. Am Fam Physician 63:703–713, 717–718, 2001

Shiekh J, Yesavage J: Geriatric Depression Scale: recent findings in development of a shorter version, in Clinical Gerontology: A Guide to Assessment and Intervention. Edited by Brink J. New York, Haworth, 1986, pp 165–173

Stojkovic S: Elderly prisoners: a growing and forgotten group within correctional systems vulnerable to elder abuse. J Elder Abuse Negl 19:97–117, 2007

Teunisse S, Derix MM, van Crevel H: Assessing the severity of dementia: patient and caregiver. Arch Neurol 48:274–277, 1991

Texas Department of Corrections: Texas Department of Criminal Justice Fiscal Year 2002 Statistical Report. Texas Department of Corrections, 2003

Thivierge-Rikard RV, Thompson MS: The association between aging inmate housing management models and non-geriatric health services in state correctional institutions. J Aging Soc Policy 19:39–56, 2007

Turley J: An "old" prison solution. Los Angeles Times, October 7, 2006, B17

U.S. Department of Justice: Prison medical care: special needs populations and cost control. Longmont, CO, National Institute of Corrections Information Center, September 1997. Available at: http://www.nicic.org/pubs/1997/013964.pdf. Accessed April 30, 2009.

Virginia Department of Corrections: Report on the response of the Department of Corrections to the impact of the aging of Virginia's population. November 15, 2007. Available at: http://www.vda.virginia.gov/pdfdocs/2624-DeptofCorrections.pdf. Accessed April 30, 2009.

Vito G, Wilson D: Forgotten people: elderly inmates. Fed Probat 49:18–24, 1985

Voelker R: New initiatives target inmates' health. JAMA 291:1549–1551, 2004

Williams BA, Lindquist K, Sudore RL, et al: Being old and doing time: functional impairment and adverse experiences of geriatric female prisoners. J Am Geriatr Soc 54:702–707, 2006

Yesavage JA, Brink TL, Rose TL, et al: Development and validation of a geriatric depression screening scale: a preliminary report. J Psychiatr Res 17:37–49, 1982

Zubenko GS, Sunderland T: Geriatric neuropsychopharmacology, in Textbook of Geriatric Neuropsychiatry. Edited by Cummings JL, Coffey CE. Washington, DC, American Psychiatric Press, 2000, pp 749–778

Index

*Page numbers printed in **boldface** type refer to tables or figures.*